Kai-Ming G. Fu • Michael Y. Wang
Michael S. Virk • John R. Dimar II
Praveen V. Mummaneni
Editors

Treatment of Spine Disease in the Elderly

Cutting Edge Techniques and Technologies

Springer

Editors
Kai-Ming G. Fu
Weill Cornell Medical College
New York, NY, USA

Michael S. Virk
Department of Neurological Surgery
Weill Cornell Medical Center
New York, NY, USA

Praveen V. Mummaneni
UCSF Neurosurgery
San Francisco, CA, USA

Michael Y. Wang
Departments of Neurosurgery & Rehab Medicine
University of Miami School of Medicine
Miami, FL, USA

John R. Dimar II
Dept. of Orthopedic Surgery
Leatherman Spine Center, University of Louisville
Louisville, KY, USA

ISBN 978-3-031-12614-7 ISBN 978-3-031-12612-3 (eBook)
https://doi.org/10.1007/978-3-031-12612-3

This Springer imprint is published by the registered company Springer Nature Switzerland AG
The registered company address is: Gewerbestrasse 11, 6330 Cham, Switzerland

Treatment of Spine Disease in the Elderly

Foreword

Advances in spine care in both technology and technique have created significant improvements in the lives of many. As the population throughout the world ages, spinal pathology affecting the elderly will become an increasingly important public health concern. Previous literature has focused on different populations, such as spinal trauma in young patients and degenerative disease in the middle aged. Older patients suffer from high rates of spinal trauma, spinal deformity, oncology, and of course progressive degenerative disease. These patients often present differently than those in younger groups. Different fracture patterns, oncological etiologies, and deformity issues are some common examples. Comorbidities increase in number and severity with age, with elderly patients requiring treatment that considers frailty and osteoporosis among other severe pathology. Elderly patients require a tailored approach to their spine care. Previous textbooks have presented the advances and current concepts of modern surgical spinal care. However, this textbook is unique in its sole focus on advances in spinal care for the elderly. The editors sought to present a comprehensive text on all aspects of spinal care in the elderly. From evaluation of the medical comorbidities and bone health to advanced techniques in pain management, physiatry, and less invasive surgical means, this text provides a reference for all of those that treat elderly patients.

Christopher I. Shaffrey MD
Professor of Neurosurgery
Professor of Orthopedic Surgery
Chief: Duke Spine Center
Duke University
Durham NC, USA

Elderly Specific Considerations in Spine Disease

The human spine is unique because of its upright posture and, as a result, is subject to predictable, progressive degenerative changes that may lead to a wide variety of pathological conditions with aging. Many of these changes are due to repetitive environmental trauma that accelerates the genetically programmed temporal aging processes of the intervertebral discs, ligaments, and facet joints. This frequently leads to loss of sagittal or coronal alignment and balance. As a consequence of the increasing elderly population, the medical community is experiencing a dramatic increase in patients with spinal disease in this age demographic (>65 years old). Aging pathology can be *intrinsic to the spine*, such as degenerative disc disease, spondylolisthesis, spinal stenosis, and adult spinal deformity, which individually or collectively frequently cause back pain, spinal cord compression, and nerve root compression. Additionally, the spine is subjected to *extrinsic causes of spinal disease* with aging including trauma and metabolic bone diseases such as osteoporosis, metastatic tumors, and infections. The purpose of this textbook is to familiarize spine surgeons with a wide variety of pathologic spinal conditions that *affect the elderly population*. These conditions often require a combination of operative and conservative treatment making it essential that spine surgeons understand the state-of-the-art techniques required to treat these conditions.

Trauma

As a consequence of aging of the spine there is a gradual loss of muscle strength, disc integrity with collapse and spondylosis/ankylosis, and misalignment. As a consequence of these changes there is a loss of flexibility and resilience of the cervical and thoracolumbar spine in the elderly when subjected to traumatic events. For example, with an aging cervical spine type 2 odontoid fractures are common and carry a high nonunion rate with bracing and may require surgery. Minor injuries of the thoracolumbar spine such as falls result in spinal compression fractures while high energy injuries result in severe fracture/dislocations, burst injuries, Chance injuries and in the case of elderly kyphotic ankylosed spines that suffer a hyperextension injury, a complete 3 column disruption. Perhaps the most important intrinsic clinical modifier as to the type of fracture in the elderly population is the quality of the bone while there are extrinsic factors, such as metastatic tumor that has destroyed the integrity of the vertebra resulting in a pathological fracture.

Elderly patients have a broad spectrum of preexisting comorbidities that need assessment and treatment prior to surgical treatment, if feasible, since the risk of perioperative complications is higher in this challenging population [1]. For example, the treatment of odontoid fractures is controversial with more recent studies recommending open reduction and fusion [2]. Low energy compression fractures of the thoracolumbar spine account for the most osteoporotic common fractures suffered in elderly adults costing 1 billion dollars annually to treat [3]. Most require simple brace treatment or minimally invasive vertebroplasty or kyphoplasty [4, 5]. Many low-energy burst fractures can be treated with bracing but thoracolumbar ones can be quite problematic because they tend to kyphos due to lack of anterior support requiring surgical stabilization and deformity correction and potentially with anterior column support. Most demand a metastatic and metabolic work up for osteoporosis, and heal uneventfully except for a few that either have neurologic compression or develop avascular necrosis, with both conditions requiring difficult surgical reconstructions. In the case of fracture dislocations that exhibit instability or displacement, especially with neurologic injury, expedient surgical stabilization of the traumatic deformity (anterolisthesis, lateral translation, slice injury) combined with fusion and decompression should be done immediately since studies have shown improved outcomes. Hyperextension injuries in a kyphotic ankylosed spine are notoriously problematic and underappreciated. They can be very unstable, similar to ankylosing spondylitis, requiring an MRI to appreciate the 3-column nature of the injury and most likely surgical stabilization. Elderly patients often require unique surgical correction techniques to enhance fixation and address poor bone quality including concurrent vertebroplasties, hydroxyapatite-coated pedicle screws, and construct matching with less rigid titanium rods.

Tumor

Spine tumors are more common in elderly populations and can be very challenging to treat due to the patients' comorbidities, intractable back pain, possible spinal column instability, and a progressive neurologic deficit. Primary bone tumors of the spine account for less than 10% of all bone tumors with the most common type being benign vertebral hemangiomas. Far more common are metastatic spine tumors that have been reported to spread to the spine at some point during the disease process anywhere from 30% to 70% of the time. The bony spinal column is the most common site for bone metastasis with the most common cancers being breast, lung, thyroid, kidney, prostate, melanoma, and gastrointestinal (due to the larger number of GI cancers). Once diagnosed a percutaneous open biopsy is required followed by the optional use of one of the available scoring systems which have limited value as far as prognosis [6]. Following diagnosis, an experienced multidisciplinary team is recommended to develop a meticulous treatment plan that includes various combinations of chemotherapy, radiation therapy (conventional, focused, and proton beam), and surgery. Surgery is indicated if there is sufficient vertebral column destruction to render the spine unstable and the tumor is not sensitive to chemotherapy or radiation such as a myeloma or other hematogenous tumors [7]. Another strong indication is an epidural extension of the tumor causing progressive neurologic compromise, where a prospective study has clearly shown that patients treated with direct decompressive surgery plus postoperative radiation therapy retain the ability to walk for longer duration and regain the ability to ambulate more often (ambulatory rate surgery 84% vs. radiation 57%) [8]. Surgical decompression with stabilization when required allows most elderly patients to remain ambulatory. Still, the 2-year survival rates following spinal metastasis have been reported to be 10% to 20% following diagnosis with certain cancers such as breast and prostate having a longer survival up to a 44% survival rate [9].

Adult Deformity

Degeneration of the spine is inevitable due to gradual deterioration of the discs, ligaments, and facet joints. A recent review of a Medicare database showed the overall prevalence of diagnosed spinal degenerative disease was 27.3% and increased with age [10]. These changes are subdivided into five general categories: herniated nucleus pulposus (HNP), degenerative disc disease (DDD), spinal stenosis (SS), spondylolisthesis, and adult spinal deformity (ASD). The vast majority of patients with these conditions can be treated nonoperatively with medications, bracing, physical therapy, and pain management techniques. Conditions that cannot be treated by traditional conservative treatment modalities and require surgical intervention will be discussed in the following chapters, including disc excision or artificial disc replacement for degenerative disc disease, a decompression for bony stenosis, and spinal fusion in instances of instability or deformity, and adult deformity correction.

Adult spinal deformity (ASD) is perhaps one of the most challenging degenerative spinal diseases since it involves disruption of the sagittal and/or coronal balance with pathological changes in the normal spinopelvic parameters, specifically pelvic tilt and sacral slope leading to positive sagittal balance [11, 12]. The incidence of degenerative scoliosis in the elderly ranges from 6% to 68% and is frequently associated with spondylosis, degenerative disc disease, spondylolisthesis, and spinal stenosis [13].

Surgery for ASD consists of decompression alone, posterior fusion alone, decompression with limited fusion, fusion with deformity correction, and decompression with fusion and deformity correction [13]. Anterior surgery has had a renaissance over the past decade following decades of the prevalence of posterior spinal osteotomies which have waned in popularity and are used primarily for rigidly fused flatback deformities. The evolution back to anterior surgery has been supported by improved fusion rates and the findings that the majority of lordosis is located at L4-S1 (average 62%) which lends itself nicely to the use of hyperlordotic cages to restore lumbar lordosis in a relatively controlled manner [14]. All of these techniques will be discussed and can be used selectively or collectively to correct adult spinal deformity in concert within suggested age-adjusted goals [15].

Osteoporosis

Osteoporosis is a skeletal disease that affects over 40 million people and is defined by poor bone quality. The condition typically will exhibit low bone mineral density and has resulted in an increasing incidence of fragility fractures prevalent in the aging population. The spine is the most common site of osteoporotic fracture and unfortunately there is only a 20% chance that further assessment of the patient's bone health will be done resulting in serious morbidity and potential mortality [16]. The combined incidence of these osteoporotic fragility fractures in all locations is estimated to be 2.3 million yearly and fractures of the spine are estimated to be 700,000 annually [17, 18]. The mortality at 2 and 3 years has been found to be 32.7% and 46.1% while 20% of patients with one fracture will experience another fracture within 1 year [16–18]. Spinal osteoporosis additionally creates significant economic and medical burdens on the health care system, being estimated to be $27,500 per hospitalization and the combined cost of treatment being estimated at 17 billion dollars yearly and climbing [16–18]. Unfortunately, the condition is often underdiagnosed in elderly patients undergoing spinal reconstruction surgery and consequently it results in increased complications, increased risk of pseudarthrosis, adjacent fractures, and worse outcomes. This steadily led to a greater appreciation of bone physiology and to the absolute need to ensure optimal bone health prior to elective spine surgery by spine surgeons over the past decade [19]. As a consequence of the severe morbidity, mortality, and the cost of not treating metabolic bone disease prior to an osteoporotic fragility fracture, there has been significant emphasis on medical treatment education and a quantum leap in basic science research directed at developing effective treatment regimens to address osteoporosis. A significant need has been identified and is being addressed for the education of both primary care providers and orthopedic surgeons in the critical importance of the treatment of osteoporosis with various treatment regimens and medications. Additionally, there has been increasing implementation of diagnostic testing to identify the disease utilizing DEXA scans and the growing use of the "Surrogate" Hounsfield Units (HU) measured on CT scanning [20].

Intensive basic science research over the past two decades has resulted in the discovery of the critical cellular pathways that are responsible for normal bone physiology by utilizing both genetic analysis of normal bone metabolism and genetic abnormalities that cause bone disease to guide the development of targeted drugs to treat osteoporosis. Finally, there have been many excellent studies that have identified the influence of Vitamin D_3 deficiency on poor bone quality on the success of fusion, instrumentation failure, and complications in adult spine surgery [21–26]. Beyond ensuring surgical patients have adequate bone density along with adequate Vitamin D_3 and calcium intake [21, 22, 26], perhaps one of the most important offshoots of osteoporotic research has been the development of targeted drug therapy to effectively treat the disease. There are currently five major classes of osteoporotic drug therapies available. The first were three catabolic compounds that slow bone resorption including the bisphosphonates in the 1990s, followed by the Selective Estrogen Receptor Modifiers (SERMs), and then Denosumab the first biologic monoclonal antibody therapy. The next were the anabolic teriparatides which are parathyroid hormone peptides and recently a second monoclonal antibody has been approved, romosozumab. This fifth osteoporotic medication blocks sclerostin activating osteoblastic proliferation promoting bone formation, while slowing resorption and does not carry a risk of promoting cancer [27–30]. These osteoporotic medications are often used with vitamin D_3, calcium supplements, and are administered sequentially to maintain efficacy. Multiple authors have also shown that vitamin D_3 combined with certain of these medications to treat osteoporosis increases fusion rates, decreases instrumentation failure, and decreases complications demonstrating their significant clinical efficacy [21, 22, 31, 32]. Understanding bone metabolism, the diagnosis of osteoporosis, and how osteoporosis influences surgical complications and outcomes is critical to promote high-quality surgical outcomes and prevent complications. Additionally, they review the current metabolic bone disease treatments available to improve bone quality, how they are incorporated into preoperative treatment regimens to improve bone quality prior to surgical intervention [33], and current surgical techniques available to improve outcomes in elderly patients with osteoporosis. In conclusion, the following chapters review the importance of understanding the treatment of tumors, trauma, adult spinal deformity, osteoporosis, and other elderly specific considerations to ensure proper treatment.

John R. Dimar II

References

1. Dimar JR, Fisher C, Vaccaro AR, Carreon LY, et al. Predictors of complications after spinal stabilization of thoracolumbar spine injuries. J Trauma Inj Infect Crit Care. 2010;69(6):1497–503.
2. Carvalho AD, Figueiredo J, Schroeder GD, Vaccaro AR, Rodrigues-Pinto R. Odontoid fractures: a critical review of current management and future directions. Clin Spine Surg. 2019;32(8):313–23.
3. Goldstein CL, Chutkan NB, Choma TJ, Orr RD. Management of the elderly with vertebral compression fractures. Neurosurgery. 2015;77(Suppl 4):S33–45.
4. Buchbinder R, et al. A randomized trial of vertebroplasty for painful osteoporotic vertebral fractures. NEJM. 2009;361:557.
5. Kallmes DF, et al. A randomized trial of vertebroplasty for osteoporotic spinal fractures. N Engl J Med. 2012;366(10):970.
6. Ahmed AK, Goodwin CR, Sciubba DM, et al. Predicting survival for metastatic spine disease: a comparison of nine scoring systems. Spine J. 2018;18:1804–14.

7. Dimar JR, Voor MJ, Zhang YM, Glassman SD. A Human cadaver model for determination of pathologic fracture threshold resulting from tumorous destruction of the vertebral body. Spine. 1998;23(11):1209–14.
8. Patchell RA, Tibbs PA, Regine WF, Payne R, Saris S, Kryscio RJ, Mohiuddin M, Young B. Direct decompressive surgical resection in the treatment of spinal cord compression caused by metastatic cancer: a randomized trial. Lancet. 2005;366:643.
9. Delank K-S, Wendtner C, Eich HT, Eysel P. The treatment of spinal metastases. Dtsch Arztebl Int. 2011;108(5):71–80.
10. Parenteau CS, Lau EC, Campbell IC, Courtney A. Prevalence of spine degeneration diagnosis by type, age, gender, and obesity using Medicare data. Sci Rep. 2021;11:5389.
11. Lagaye J, Duval-Beupère G, et al. Pelvic incidence: a fundamental pelvic parameter for three –dimensional regulation of spinal sagittal curves. Eur Spine J. 1998;7:99–103.
12. Glassman SD, Bridwell K, Dimar JR, et al. The impact of positive sagittal balance in adult spinal deformity. Spine. 2006;30(18):2024–9.
13. Guey-Chi P, Daubs MD, Berven S, et al. Surgery for degenerative scoliosis, the development of appropriate use criteria. Spine. 2016;41(10):910–8.
14. Pesenti S, Lafage R, Stein D, Lafage V, et al. The amount of proximal lumbar lordosis is related to pelvic incidence. Clin Orthop Relat Res. 2018;476:1603–11.
15. Lafage R, Schwab FJ, Glassman S, Bess S, Lafage V, et al. Age adjusted alignment goals have the potential to reduce PJK. Spine. 2017;42(17):1275–82.
16. Anderson P, Jeray K, Lane J, Binkley N. AOA critical issues: bone health optimization: beyond own the bone. J Bone Joint Surg Am. 2019;101:1413–9.
17. Carlson BC, Anderson PA, et al. A review and clinical perspective of the impact of osteoporosis on the spine. Geriatr Orthop Surg Rehabil. 2019;10:1–8.
18. Weisenthal BW, et al. Healthcare burden of osteoporosis. Semin Spine Surg. 2018;30:2–7.
19. Dimar J, Anderson P. The basics of bone physiology, healing, and osteoporosis. Instr Course Lect. 2021;Chapter 33:527–35.
20. Schreiber JJ, Hughes AP, Taher F, Girardi FP. An association can be found between Hounsfield units and success of lumbar spine fusion. HSS J. 2014;10(1):25–9.
21. Ravindra VM. Prevalence of vitamin D deficiency in patients undergoing elective spine surgery: a cross-sectional analysis. World Neurosurg. 2015;83(6):1114–9.
22. Ravindra VM, Godzik J, Dailey AT, et al. Vitamin D levels and 1 year fusion outcomes in elective spine surgery. Spine. 2015;40(19):1536–41.
23. Yagi M, King AB, Boachie-Adjei O. Characterization of osteopenia/osteoporosis in adult scoliosis. Spine. 2011;36(20):1652–7.
24. Yagi M, Fujita N, Tsuji O, et al. Low bone-mineral density is a significant risk for proximal junctional failure after surgical correction of adult spinal deformity. Spine. 2018;43(7):485–91.
25. Bjerke BT, et al. Incidence of osteoporosis related complications following posterior lumbar fusion. Glob Spine J. 2018;8(6):563–9. Epub 2017 Dec 10.
26. Stoker GE, et al. Preoperative vitamin D status of adults undergoing surgical spine fusion. Spine. 2013;38(6):507.
27. McClung MR, et al. Denosumab in postmenopausal women with low bone mineral density. N Engl J Med. 2006;354(8):821–31.
28. Lehman R. Management of osteoporosis in spine surgery. J Am Acad Orthop Surg. 2015;23:4.
29. Robling AG, Drake MT. Sclerostin: from bedside to bench, and back to the bedside. Bone. 2017;96:1–2.
30. Prather C, Adams E. Romosozumab: a first in class sclerostin inhibitor for osteoporosis. Am J Health Syst Pharm. 2020;77(23):1949–56.
31. Ohtori S, Inoue G, Orita S, et al. Teriparatide accelerates lumbar posterolateral fusion in women with postmenopausal osteoporosis. Spine. 2012;37(23):E1464–8.
32. Ohtori S, Inoue G, Orita S, et al. Comparison of teriparatide and bisphosphonate treatment to reduce pedicle screw loosening after lumbar spinal fusion in postmenopausal women with osteoporosis from a bone quality standpoint. Spine. 2013;38(8):E487–92.
33. Anderson P, Dimar J. Rationale for bone health optimization in patients undergoing spine surgery. Instr Course Lect. 2021;Chapter 21:355–66.

Contents

Part I
Special Perioperative Considerations in the Elderly

Chapter 1
Bone Health, Advances in Assessment and Treatment

Panagiota Andreopoulou

Introduction

Invasive spinal procedures that require instrumentation are performed in more than 400,000 patients annually in the United States for degenerative disc disease, spinal stenosis, spondylolisthesis, spondylosis, spinal fractures, scoliosis, and kyphosis [1–3] Cases have been increasing among patients over age 65 with otherwise long life expectancy [3] who are seeking relief from chronic pain and neurologic symptoms.

However, complications are frequent in up to 45% of cases [4–6] and are associated with substantial morbidity and healthcare costs [7, 8]. Those include pseudoarthrosis, hardware loosening and failure, proximal junctional kyphosis (PJK), graft or interbody cage subsidence, adjacent-level disc degeneration, and vertebral compression fractures [9]. A successful approach aiming to minimize risk of complications should include preoperative identification and treatment of modifiable risk factors, especially skeletal deficits that may compromise early stability of instrumentation. The precise quantification of bone strength and the treatment of compromised bone quality have been challenging for clinicians attempting to predict and optimize surgical outcomes.

P. Andreopoulou (✉)
Weill Cornell Medical School, New York, NY, USA
e-mail: Paa2655@med.cornell.edu

K.-M. G. Fu et al. (eds.), *Treatment of Spine Disease in the Elderly*,
https://doi.org/10.1007/978-3-031-12612-3_1

Identification of Patients at Risk for Postoperative Complications

Assessment of factors and medical conditions that may be compromising bone health is imperative in elderly patients who are planning spine surgery especially invasive procedures such as spinal fusion and instrumentation. The aging population has higher prevalence of osteoporosis due to increased bone resorption and decreased bone formation leading to decreased bone strength and high risk of fractures. In addition, the elderly are particularly susceptible to medical issues related to aging and directly affecting bone health, such as vitamin D deficiency and osteomalacia, decreased calcium absorption and other nutrient malabsorption, diabetes mellitus, primary hyperparathyroidism, paraprotein production (monoclonal gammopathy of undetermined significance (MGUS), multiple myeloma), malignancies treated with agents adversely affecting bone mass (e.g., aromatase inhibitors for breast cancer and androgen deprivation therapy for prostate cancer), rheumatologic disorders, medications including psychotropic medications, proton pump inhibitors, anticoagulants [10], and often a long history of multiple epidural steroid injections that tend to precede spinal surgery. Therefore, a meticulous history, physical examination, and pertinent laboratory and imaging testing could unveil potentially significant concurrent medical issues that are treatable and can be corrected in time for surgery.

Osteoporosis is a skeletal condition characterized by compromised bone strength usually due to a combination of low bone mineral density (BMD) and poor bone quality, predisposing to increased risk of fracture [11]. It is a highly prevalent condition especially in women. The World Health Organization (WHO) has defined osteoporosis using a BMD score derived from DXA, that is, 2.5 standard deviations below the mean for healthy young adults at the spine, femoral neck, or total hip (T-score) [12]. T-scores between −1.0 and −2.5 are consistent with low bone mass, and those above −1.0 are considered normal.

Osteoporosis is strongly associated with increasing age and negatively affects surgical outcomes, need for revision surgery, and risk of complications. In a study of 144 spine surgery candidates over the age of 50, 27% had osteoporosis, 37.5% had evidence of prior fracture (mostly radiographic vertebral fractures), and 75% had vitamin D deficiency [13]. In a larger study of 759 patients older than age 50 undergoing spinal instrumentation at a single center, 51.3% of females and 14.5% of males had osteoporosis. Another 41.4% and 46.1% had T-scores consistent with low bone mass [14].

Another important consideration is that quite commonly skeletal quality in the spine of candidates for surgery is compromised by prior multiple epidural steroid injections (ESIs) that provide relief of symptoms of spinal radiculopathy. There is some systemic glucocorticoid absorption associated with use of ESIs [15] that is enough to cause suppression of the hypothalamic-pituitary-adrenal axis [16, 17] and hyperglycemia in patients with diabetes [18]. It has been shown that volumetric

BMD by central QCT is lower in patients receiving ESIs compared to age- and sex-matched controls [19].

Currently poor bone quality is often noted intraoperatively; therefore, risk of complications may not be optimally addressed. Standard modes of fracture risk assessment may not detect osteoporosis in spine surgery candidates, and newer methodologies are being investigated.

Dual-Energy X-ray Absorptiometry (DXA)

Measurement of areal bone mineral density (aBMD) is an assessment of the mineral content in key skeletal regions by dual-energy X-ray absorptiometry (DXA) and is the standard of care for the diagnosis of osteoporosis and fracture risk assessment. DXA is widely available at low cost with immediately interpretable results and very low radiation exposure [20]. DXA-measured BMD strongly correlated with bone strength based on biomechanical studies [21] and with fracture risk based on epidemiological studies. The risk of fracture exponentially increases as BMD decreases at the spine, hip, and forearm [22, 23]. Additionally, DXA may include an assessment of lower thoracic and lumbar (T4–L4) vertebral compression deformities via a concurrent lateral view of the spine [24].

Based on several studies, low BMD is a risk factor for PJK [25–28], adjacent fractures [28, 29], screw loosening [28, 30, 31], and hardware subsidence [32]. The stability of spinal instrumentation relies on good bone quality, and the pullout strength of pedicle screws is highly correlated with spinal BMD [33].

However, patients that are candidates for spinal fusion by definition have baseline degenerative disease (significant deformity, osteosclerosis, osteophytes, scoliosis, spondylolisthesis, degenerative disc disease, vertebral fractures, prior spine surgery) that render the spine BMD values falsely elevated and unreliable due to artifact [22, 34, 35]. Areal BMD measurements are also affected by bone size and shape, soft tissue composition, and concurrent obesity and do not allow discrimination between undermineralized bone (osteomalacia) and osteoporosis.

Assessment of bone quality by DXA in patients with lumbar scoliosis is limited [36, 37]. Younger patients with scoliosis have been shown to have low BMD [38, 39]; however, in adult patients that require surgery, many spinal segments are degenerated and sclerotic resulting in falsely normal to high BMD readings on DXA [36].

Peripheral DXA measurements of the forearm, heel, or hand BMD correlate less well with central DXA measurements and are not used in clinical practice to assess bone mass [40].

Lastly, DXA does not measure volumetric bone mineral density (vBMD) or assess bone microarchitecture that are important parameters of bone strength. Therefore, assessment of trabecular structure, cortical thickness, and focal defects must be considered for a complete risk assessment.

Computed Tomography (CT)-Based Techniques

Computed tomography (CT)-based techniques, such as use of Hounsfield units (HUs) and central quantitative computed tomography (cQCT), are emerging methods alternative to DXA for assessment of bone strength. These assessments can be performed in pre-existing CT images, thus avoiding extra radiation exposure or time commitment [41].

cQCT provides a three-dimensional measurement of vBMD in trabecular or cortical bone at the spine and hip, which is less affected by sclerotic changes, vascular calcifications [42], obesity [43], and other artifacts that compromise DXA results [44, 45]. Low BMD measurements by CT are common in patients presenting for fusion [25, 26, 28, 46, 47].

In a retrospective study of patients who underwent lumbar interbody fusion, those with pseudoarthrosis tended to have lower vBMD on postoperative CT, compared to patients with successful fusion [48]. Seventy-eight percent of patients with low BMD by CT had hardware instability, adjacent fractures, and other complications [29]. Patients with low preoperative spine vBMD not only had higher rates of postoperative skeletal complications but also earlier occurrence of complications than those with higher vBMD [47].

Another method of estimating trabecular bone BMD is measurement of Hounsfield units (HUs) of lumbar spine vertebrae in an already available CT of the spine. HUs are measured based on preoperative CT (within 6 months before surgery) from L1 to L5, in a circular region within the vertebral body, excluding cortical bone, lateral walls, endplates, or osteophytes, at the midsagittal plane, midbody axial plane, axial plane just below the superior endplate, and axial plane just above the inferior endplate [49].

A correlation between HU values and presence of osteoporosis [50–53] and success of lumbar fusion has been shown [53]. An HU value of 110 has previously been reported as a cutoff for osteoporosis [54, 55]; however, there are differences in values depending on the CT model.

Trabecular Bone Score (TBS)

Trabecular bone score (TBS) is a fairly recent advance in DXA methodology that has greatly expanded its functionality. Application of this software on the DXA spine image (TBSiNsight, Medimaps Group, Switzerland) estimates trabecular bone texture, which correlates with bone microarchitecture [56]. A relationship between 3D bone characteristics, mechanical parameters, and TBS has been established [56, 57]. TBS predicts fragility fracture risk in osteoporosis independently of BMD and of clinical risk factors and has value in monitoring response to treatment [58, 59]. TBS may elucidate the etiology of increased fractures in the setting of secondary osteoporosis with abnormal trabecular microarchitecture at a higher

BMD (e.g., diabetes, rheumatoid arthritis, glucocorticoid-induced osteoporosis). Recommended TBS reference ranges for postmenopausal women are >1.35 normal microarchitecture, 1.2–1.35 partially degraded bone, and <1.2 completely degraded bone [60].

TBS may also be falsely elevated due to spine artifact although to a lesser degree than BMD by DXA [58].

High-Resolution Peripheral QCT (HR-pQCT)

High-resolution peripheral QCT (HR-pQCT) measurement [61] involves peripheral skeletal sites that are composed predominantly by cortical bone (the distal radius and distal tibia); however, abnormal cortical bone values are associated with higher risk of vertebral fractures [62, 63]. The cortical bone rim of vertebral bodies, although thin, contributes to their bone strength [64, 65]. In a recent prospective study, abnormalities of both trabecular and cortical microarchitecture as measured by HR-pQCT were associated with the development of early complications within the first 6 months following spine fusion surgery [66].

At this time HR-pQCT is not widely available for clinical use and is mainly utilized in the research setting.

Studies suggest that higher bone mass and intact microarchitecture is critical for enabling new bone formation, increasing early hardware stability, promoting successful healing, and minimizing complications. Identification of high-risk patients prior to surgery could lead to early treatment intervention and might ultimately minimize these types of complications.

Optimization of Bone Strength Perioperatively

Deficiencies in calcium and vitamin D intake can accelerate the rate of bone loss and lead to osteomalacia.

During bone remodeling, which is a constant process throughout an individual's lifetime, calcium diffuses into and out of the skeleton. As much as 10,000 mg of calcium is filtered by the kidneys daily, and more than 98% of that is reabsorbed. Inadequate calcium intake in the setting of calcium loss by the kidneys, gastrointestinal tract, and skin can eventually lead to bone demineralization. Therefore, calcium supplementation may be indicated if dietary calcium is limited. The recommended total daily calcium intake is 1200 mg for postmenopausal women and men over age 70 and 1000 mg for men over age 50 in order to replenish the daily calcium losses (National Osteoporosis Foundation).

Vitamin D levels (25OHD) positively correlate with BMD and muscle function (e.g., walking speed). Supplementation with at least 800 IU of vitamin D daily is associated with improved balance and lower extremity function and reduced falls

[67, 68]. 25OHD levels less than 30 ng/mL are associated with secondary hyperparathyroidism, and intestinal calcium transport increases at 25OHD levels greater than 32 ng/mL.

Following a fusion surgery, endochondral and intramembranous ossification forms a solid stabilizing bony bridge across decompressed segments [69–73]; however, this process may be hindered by biological and biomechanical challenges [74].

Antiresorptive and anabolic therapies that are standard treatment for osteoporosis appear effective at improving spinal surgery outcomes and reducing complications [75]. Bisphosphonates and teriparatide have been tested in patients undergoing spinal fusion for their effects on arthrodesis, vertebral bone density, adjacent vertebral fractures, instrumentation failure, fusion mass catabolism, and graft or cage subsidence [9].

Overall, prior treatment of underlying osteoporosis is associated with lower risk of osteoporosis-related complications after spinal fusion. In a large retrospective study that included 849 patients (predominantly white (86%) females (83%) age 60–79 (80%)), treated patients and not-treated patients had 1-year complication incidence of 9.1% and 15.0%, respectively. Treated patients comprised only 14.3% of the cohort of which 88% were treated with bisphosphonates and 12.4% with teriparatide. Eighteen percent of the untreated patients with complications had to undergo a revision surgery [76].

Bisphosphonates

Bisphosphonates are the most widely prescribed treatment for osteoporosis. They are antiresorptive therapies that inhibit osteoclastogenesis in the bone marrow, decrease osteoclast activity at the bone surface, and decrease the osteoclast life span by increasing apoptotic cell death [77].

In humans bisphosphonates may be beneficial in bridging bone formation and decreasing vertebral fracture risk in patients undergoing interbody lumbar fusion but without difference in clinical outcomes. In a small prospective study, 36 patients with osteopenia undergoing single-level posterior lumbar interbody fusion were randomized to either alendronate 35 mg or vitamin D for 1 year. Fusion was assessed via radiographs and CT reconstruction. Patients treated with alendronate had a significantly higher fusion rate when compared with controls (95% vs. 65%) and decreased risk of vertebral compression fracture (VCF) (0% vs. 24%) at 1 year after surgery. Despite that, the incidence of cage subsidence, defined as more than 2 mm vertical migration from baseline on CT scan, was not significantly different between the two groups, and there was no significant difference in clinical outcome [78]. However, in another study of 44 patients, there was no difference in fusion rate between alendronate and no treatment in patients with and without endplate degeneration after posterior lumbar fusion (PLF) [79].

Two small retrospective studies looked into the effects of zoledronate intravenous infusion. The first evaluated 44 patients at 6-month follow-up after one- or two-level PLF but found no significant difference between fusion rate, volume of fusion mass, clinical outcomes, and complications rates between zoledronate and control groups [80]. The other study evaluated 64 patients at a longer follow-up of 24 months and showed higher fusion rate (75% vs. 56%), lower risk of VCF (19% vs. 51%), cage subsidence (28% vs. 54%), and pedicle screw loosening (PSL) (18% vs. 45%) as well as significant improvement in clinical outcomes [81].

In a randomized, placebo-controlled study of 79 patients treated with zoledronic acid vs. placebo, investigators noted earlier fusion (significant difference at 3, 6, and 9 months, but nonsignificant difference at 12 months), reduced risk of VCF (0% vs. 17%), and improved clinical outcomes at 9 and 12 months post-op; however, there was no difference in overall fusion rate (82% vs. 83%). Three patients (9%) in the zoledronic acid group and five patients (14%) in the placebo group had fusion failure [82]. Similar observations were made among 30 patients receiving zoledronic acid and 34 untreated patients. No significant difference was observed between overall fusion rates at 12 months (92% vs. 92.86%), and improved clinical outcomes were observed at 12 and 24 months in the zoledronic acid group on multiple score scales. Rates of VCF (0 vs. 5 cases) and PSL (0 vs. 6 cases) were reduced in the treatment group [83].

In summary, data on effect of bisphosphonates on rate of fusion and clinical outcome measures are inconsistent; however, it appears that bisphosphonates induce earlier fusion, and reduce the risk of cage subsidence, VCF, and PSL.

Anabolic Agents: Teriparatide

Teriparatide is part of the PTH (parathyroid hormone) peptide (hPTH 1–34) [84]. Intermittent administration has an anabolic effect via the activation of osteoblast cell surface receptors that further induce the production of several growth factors, including insulin-like growth factor 1 (IGF1), and lead to primarily increase of trabecular bone mass [85].

Several small and mostly retrospective studies have demonstrated a beneficial effect of teriparatide treatment on fusion outcomes [86–92].

Higher fusion rate was noted 6 months after PLF or transforaminal lumbar interbody fusion (TLIF) in 29 patients treated with teriparatide monotherapy compared to 37 untreated patients (69% vs. 35%). However, there was no significant difference in Japanese Orthopedic Association Pain Evaluation Questionnaires (JOA-BPEQ) or ODI scores between the two groups [92].

Sequential/cyclical treatment was studied in 47 patients after PLIF for spinal stenosis who were treated with 3 months of teriparatide alternating with 3 months alendronate for a total of 12 months compared to risedronate alone for at least 12 months. The first group had earlier fusion (6.0 ± 4.8 months vs. 10.4 ± 7.2 months) and improved BMD recovery range (T-score) at 24-month follow-up compared to alendronate alone (0.7 ± 1.4 vs. 0.1 ± 0.5). However, again no significant difference in ODI, VAS, or Prolo scale scores was observed at 24 months, and no significant difference in overall fusion rate (92.6% vs. 96.4%) [93].

Anabolic therapy is likely superior to antiresorptives in the setting of spinal fusion surgery. In a study of 57 patients treated either with teriparatide starting at 2 months preoperatively and continuing for 8 months postoperatively or with risedronate, earlier fusion and higher fusion rate was noted at 12 months after one or two-level PLF (82% vs. 68%). However, there was no significant difference in low back pain or lower extremity pain [86].

Teriparatide was shown to be superior to bisphosphonate in reducing the incidence of PSL in 62 postmenopausal women treated with teriparatide for 2 months preoperatively and 10 months postoperatively after one- or two-level PLF compared to risedronate and to untreated patients, based on radiographic and CT analysis (7–13% vs. 13–26% and 15–25%). Unlike other bisphosphonates, risedronate did not significantly reduce the rate of PSL [88]. It appears however that any benefit of teriparatide in reducing PSL is significant after the first 6 months post-op as observed in 84 patients treated with teriparatide for 6 months post-op followed by risedronate compared to patients treated with risedronate monotherapy. In that group the number of loosened screws detected between 6 and 12 months was significantly different (2.3% vs. 9.2%) despite the opposite effect early on after surgery [89].

A retrospective clinical review of 159 patients from 27 different centers in Japan undergoing instrumented fusion for osteoporotic vertebral fracture showed a lower rate of mechanical complications (BP vs. TP: 73.1% vs. 58.2%) in those receiving postoperative teriparatide therapy for 2 years vs. those receiving oral bisphosphonate therapy [94]. However, a placebo-controlled trial in patients with PMO undergoing non-instrumented PLF showed no radiographic or clinical improvements with teriparatide initiated immediately postoperatively [95].

In summary teriparatide use is associated with earlier fusion, higher overall fusion rates in some but not all studies, and reduced PSL compared to bisphosphonates. Data regarding potential higher benefit with treatment starting preoperatively are lacking, and this is problematic given the frequent dilemma regarding timing of surgery and need for potential delay in order to treat underlying osteoporosis.

Anabolic Agents: Abaloparatide

Abaloparatide is a peptide analog of PTH-related protein (PTH-rP) and thus a PTH receptor agonist with stronger affinity compared to teriparatide. It increases bone formation in women with postmenopausal osteoporosis, leading to greater increases in spine BMD compared to teriparatide during the first year of therapy and an overall 86% reduction in vertebral fracture risk compared to placebo [96].

In a rat posterior lumbar fusion model, treatment with abaloparatide was associated with improved fusion mass architecture by micro-computed tomography (micro-CT), and a onefold higher fusion rate compared with vehicle, although the latter was not clinically significant [97].

A recent case report of a 66-year-old woman with cervical fusion nonunion and two failed revision surgeries showed successful fusion after 12 weeks of abaloparatide therapy, starting 2 weeks prior to corpectomy and fusion [98].

Combination Therapy

A novel approach in the treatment of osteoporosis is the combination of anabolic agent with a potent antiresorptive. The later addition of denosumab to teriparatide treatment has been shown to be highly effective in reducing risk of fractures [99]. Denosumab is a RANKL inhibitor and the most potent antiresorptive available. The same approach may be useful in the setting of spinal surgery. In a small clinical trial, 16 patients with osteoporosis and lumbar spinal stenosis were randomized to treatment with teriparatide alone (starting a month before the surgery and continued for 12 months after surgery) vs. teriparatide and denosumab (administered at 2 months and 8 months postoperatively). All patients underwent posterior lumbar interbody fusion with local bone grafts. Femoral neck BMD and bone turnover markers were measured at 3, 6.9, and 12 months following surgery and fusion rates assessed via CT at baseline, 6, and 12 months postoperatively. The combination group had a higher fusion rate at month 6 compared with patients receiving teriparatide alone [100].

Overall, there is insignificant difference in short-term clinical results despite radiographic union [101]. However, in the long term solid union is associated with better functional outcomes [28].

Conclusion

Whereas the great majority of candidates for spinal surgery have underlying poor bone quality, several advances in preoperative fragility assessment via imaging as well as treatment modalities to improve bone strength are available and allow us to optimize surgical outcomes.

References

1. Hall MJ, DeFrances CJ, Williams SN, Golosinskiy A, Schwartzman S. National Hospital discharge survey: 2007 summary. Natl Health Stat Rep. 2010;29:1–20, 24.
2. Rajaee SS, Bae HW, Kanim LE, Delamarter RB. Spinal fusion in the United States: analysis of trends from 1998 to 2008. Spine. 2012;37(1):67–76.
3. Martin BI, Mirza SK, Spina N, Spiker WR, Lawrence B, Brodke DS. Trends in lumbar fusion procedure rates and associated hospital costs for degenerative spinal diseases in the United States, 2004 to 2015. Spine. 2019;44(5):369–76.

4. Uribe JS, Deukmedjian AR, Mummaneni PV, Fu KM, Mundis GM Jr, Okonkwo DO, Kanter AS, Eastlack R, Wang MY, Anand N, Fessler RG, La Marca F, Park P, Lafage V, Deviren V, Bess S, Shaffrey CI, G. International Spine Study. Complications in adult spinal deformity surgery: an analysis of minimally invasive, hybrid, and open surgical techniques. Neurosurg Focus. 2014;36(5):E15.
5. Dede O, Thuillier D, Pekmezci M, Ames CP, Hu SS, Berven SH, Deviren V. Revision surgery for lumbar pseudarthrosis. Spine. 2015;15(5):977–82.
6. Yoon ST, Boden SD. Spine fusion by gene therapy. Gene Ther. 2004;11(4):360–7.
7. Bess S, BoachieAdjei O, Burton D, Cunningham M, Shaffrey C, Shelokov A, Hostin R, Schwab F, Wood K, Akbarnia B, G. International Spine Study. Pain and disability determine treatment modality for older patients with adult scoliosis, while deformity guides treatment for younger patients. Spine. 2009;34(20):2186–90.
8. Pichelmann MA, Lenke LG, Bridwell KH, Good CR, O'Leary PT, Sides BA. Revision rates following primary adult spinal deformity surgery: six hundred forty-three consecutive patients followed-up to twenty-two years postoperative. Spine. 2010;35(2):219–26.
9. McCoy S, Tundo F, Chidambaram S, Baaj AA. Clinical considerations for spinal surgery in the osteoporotic patient: a comprehensive review. Clin Neurol Neurosurg. 2019;180:40–7.
10. Mirza F, Canalis E. Secondary osteoporosis: pathophysiology and management. Eur J Endocrinol. 2015;173:R131–51.
11. Eur. Found. Osteoporos. Bone Dis. Osteoporosis prevention, diagnosis, and therapy. Development Panel on Osteoporosis Prevention, Diagnosis, and Therapy. NIH consensus. JAMA. 2001;285:78S.
12. Lewiecki EM, Gordon CM, Baim S, et al. International Society for Clinical Densitometry 2007 adult and pediatric official positions. Bone. 2008;43:1115–21.
13. Schmidt T, Ebert K, Rolvien T. A retrospective analysis of bone mineral status in patients requiring spinal surgery. BMC Musculoskelet Disord. 2018;19(1):53.
14. Chin DK, Park JY, Yoon YS, et al. Prevalence of osteoporosis in patients requiring spine surgery: incidence and significance of osteoporosis in spine disease. Osteoporos Int. 2007;18:1219–24.
15. Moon HJ, Choi KH, Lee SI, Lee OJ, Shin JW, Kim TW. Changes in blood glucose and cortisol levels after epidural or shoulder intra-articular glucocorticoid injections in diabetic or nondiabetic patients. Am J Phys Med Rehabil. 2014;93(5):372–8.
16. Chon JY, Moon HS. Salivary cortisol concentration changes after epidural steroid injection. Pain Physician. 2012;15(6):461–6.
17. Kay J, Findling JW, Raff H. Epidural triamcinolone suppresses the pituitary-adrenal axis in human subjects. Anesth Analg. 1994;79(3):501–5.
18. Kim WH, Sim WS, Shin BS, Lee CJ, Jin HS, Lee JY, Roe HJ, Kim CS, Lee SM. Effects of two different doses of epidural steroid on blood glucose levels and pain control in patients with diabetes mellitus. Pain Physician. 2013;16(6):557–68.
19. Liu Y, Carrino JA, Dash AS, Chukir T, Do H, Bockman RS, Hughes AP, Press JM, Stein EM. Lower spine volumetric bone density in patients with a history of epidural steroid injections. J Clin Endocrinol Metab. 2018;103(9):3405–10. https://doi.org/10.1210/jc.2018-00558. PMID: 29982535.
20. Njeh CF, Fuerst T, Hans D, et al. Radiation exposure in bone mineral density assessment. Appl Radiat Isot. 1999;50(1):215–36.
21. Lotz JC, Cheal EJ, Hayes WC. Fracture prediction for the proximal femur using finite element models: Part I — Linear analysis. J Biomech Eng. 1991;113:353–60.
22. Stone KL, Seeley DG, Lui LY, Cauley JA, Ensrud K, Browner WS, Nevitt MC, Cummings SR, G. Osteoporotic Fractures Research. BMD at multiple sites and risk of fracture of multiple types: long-term results from the study of osteoporotic fractures. J Bone Miner Res. 2003;18(11):1947–54.
23. Johnell O, Kanis JA, Oden A, et al. Predictive value of BMD for hip and other fractures. J Bone Miner Res. 2005;20:1185–94.

24. Schousboe JT, Vokes T, Broy SB, et al. Vertebral fracture assessment: the 2007 ISCD official positions. J Clin Densitom. 2008;11:92–108.
25. Balci A, Kalemci O, Kaya FG, Akyoldas G, Yucesoy K, Ozaksoy D. Early and long-term changes in adjacent vertebral body bone mineral density determined by quantitative computed tomography after posterolateral fusion with transpedicular screw fixation. Clin Neurol Neurosurg. 2016;145:84–8.
26. Wang H, Ma L, Yang D, Wang T, Yang S, Wang Y, Wang Q, Zhang F, Ding W. Incidence and risk factors for the progression of proximal junctional kyphosis in degenerative lumbar scoliosis following long instrumented posterior spinal fusion. Medicine. 2016;95(32):e4443.
27. Liu FY, Wang T, Yang SD, Wang H, Yang DL, Ding WY. Incidence and risk factors for proximal junctional kyphosis: a meta-analysis. Eur Spine J. 2016;25(8):2376–83.
28. Bjerke BT, Zarrabian M, Aleem IS, Fogelson JL, Currier BL, Freedman BA, Bydon M, Nassr A. Incidence of osteoporosis-related complications following posterior lumbar fusion. Glob Spine J. 2018;8(6):563–9.
29. Formby PM, Kang DG, Helgeson MD, Wagner SC. Clinical and radiographic outcomes of transforaminal lumbar interbody fusion in patients with osteoporosis. Glob Spine J. 2016;6(7):660–4.
30. Bredow J, Boese CK, Werner CM, Siewe J, Lohrer L, Zarghooni K, Eysel P, Scheyerer MJ. Predictive validity of preoperative CT scans and the risk of pedicle screw loosening in spinal surgery. Arch Orthop Trauma Surg. 2016;136(8):1063–7.
31. Schwaiger BJ, Gersing AS, Baum T, Noel PB, Zimmer C, Bauer JS. Bone mineral density values derived from routine lumbar spine multidetector row CT predict osteoporotic vertebral fractures and screw loosening. AJNR Am J Neuroradiol. 2014;35(8):1628–33.
32. Tempel ZJ, Gandhoke GS, Okonkwo DO, Kanter AS. Impaired bone mineral density as a predictor of graft subsidence following minimally invasive transpsoas lateral lumbar interbody fusion. Eur Spine J. 2015;24(Suppl. 3):414–9.
33. Halvorson TL, Kelley LA, Thomas KA, Whitecloud TS III, Cook SD. Effects of bone mineral density on pedicle screw fixation. Spine. 1994;19(21):2415–20. Epub 1994/11/01. PMID:7846594.
34. Schuit SC, van der Klift M, Weel AE, de Laet CE, Burger H, Seeman E, Hofman A, Uitterlinden AG, van Leeuwen JP, Pols HA. Fracture incidence and association with bone mineral density in elderly men and women: the Rotterdam study. Bone. 2004;34(1):195–202.
35. Blake GM, Fogelman I. The role of DXA bone density scans in the diagnosis and treatment of osteoporosis. Postgrad Med J. 2007;83(982):509–17.
36. Pappou IP, Girardi FP, Sandhu HS, Parvataneni HK, Cammisa FP Jr, Schneider R, Frelinghuysen P, Lane JM. Discordantly high spinal bone mineral density values in patients with adult lumbar scoliosis. Spine. 2006;31(14):1614–20.
37. Sarioglu O, Gezer S, Sarioglu FC, Koremezli N, Kara T, Akcali O, Ozaksoy D, Balci A. Evaluation of vertebral bone mineral density in scoliosis by using quantitative computed tomography. Pol J Radiol. 2019;84:e131–5.
38. Cheng JC, Guo X, Sher AH. Persistent osteopenia in adolescent idiopathic scoliosis. A longitudinal follow up study. Spine. 1999;24(12):1218–22.
39. Cheng JC, Hung VW, Lee WT, Yeung HY, Lam TP, Ng BK, Guo X, Qin L. Persistent osteopenia in adolescent idiopathic scoliosis—longitudinal monitoring of bone mineral density until skeletal maturity. Stud Health Technol Inform. 2006;123:47–51.
40. Blake GM, Chinn DJ, Steel SA, et al. A list of device-specific thresholds for the clinical interpretation of peripheral x-ray absorptiometry examinations. Osteoporos Int. 2005;16:2149–56.
41. Pickhardt PJ, Lee LJ, del Rio AM, Lauder T, Bruce RJ, Summers RM, Pooler BD, Binkley N. Simultaneous screening for osteoporosis at CT colonography: bone mineral density assessment using MDCT attenuation techniques compared with the DXA reference standard. J Bone Miner Res. 2011;26(9):2194–203.
42. Smith JA, Vento JA, Spencer RP, Tendler BE. Aortic calcification contributing to bone densitometry measurement. J Clin Densitom. 1999;2:181–3.

43. Yu EW, Thomas BJ, Brown JK, Finkelstein JS. Simulated increases in body fat and errors in bone mineral density measurements by DXA and QCT. J Bone Miner Res. 2012;27:119–24.
44. Farhat GN, Cauley JA, Matthews KA, Newman AB, Johnston J, Mackey R, Edmundowicz D, Sutton-Tyrrell K. Volumetric BMD and vascular calcification in middle-aged women: the study of women's health across the nation. J Bone Miner Res. 2006;21(12):1839–46.
45. Rehman Q, Lang T, Modin G, Lane NE. Quantitative computed tomography of the lumbar spine, not dual x-ray absorptiometry, is an independent predictor of prevalent vertebral fractures in postmenopausal women with osteopenia receiving long-term glucocorticoid and hormone-replacement therapy. Arthritis Rheum. 2002;46(5):1292–7.
46. Burch S, Feldstein M, Hoffmann PF, Keaveny TM. Prevalence of poor bone quality in women undergoing spinal fusion using biomechanical-CT analysis. Spine. 2016;41(3):246–52.
47. Liu Y, Dash A, Krez A, Kim HJ, Cunningham M, Schwab F, Hughes A, Carlson B, Samuel A, Marty E, Moore H, McMahon DJ, Carrino JA, Bockman RS, Stein EM. Low volumetric bone density is a risk factor for early complications after spine fusion surgery. Osteoporos Int. 2020;31:647–54. https://doi.org/10.1007/s00198-019-05245-7.
48. Schreiber JJ, Hughes AP, Taher F, Girardi FP. An association can be found between hounsfield units and success of lumbar spine fusion. HSS J. 2014;10(1):25–9.
49. Hendrickson NR, Pickhardt PJ, Del Rio AM. Bone mineral density T-scores derived from CT attenuation numbers (Hounsfield units): clinical utility and correlation with dual-energy X-ray absorptiometry. Iowa Orthop J. 2018;38:25–31.
50. Kim KJ, Kim DH, Lee JI. Hounsfield units on lumbar computed tomography for predicting regional bone mineral density. Open Med. 2019;14:545–51.
51. Schreiber JJ, Anderson PA, Hsu WK. Use of computed tomography for assessing bone mineral density. Neurosurg Focus. 2014;37(1):E4.
52. Anderson PA, Polly DW, Binkley NC, Pickhardt PJ. Clinical use of opportunistic computed tomography screening for osteoporosis. J Bone Joint Surg Am. 2018;100(23):2073–81.
53. Zaidi Q, Danisa OA, Cheng W. Measurement techniques and utility of Hounsfield unit values for assessment of bone quality prior to spinal instrumentation: a review of current literature. Spine. 2019;44(4):E239–44.
54. Pickhardt PJ, Pooler BD, Lauder T. Opportunistic screening for osteoporosis using abdominal computed tomography scans obtained for other indications. Ann Intern Med. 2013;158(8):588–95.
55. Jang S, Graffy PM, Ziemlewicz TJ. Opportunistic osteoporosis screening at routine abdominal and thoracic CT: normative L1 trabecular attenuation values in more than 20 000 adults. Radiology. 2019;291(2):360–7.
56. Hans D, Barthe N, Boutroy S, et al. Correlations between trabecular bone score, measured using anteroposterior dual-energy X-ray absorptiometry acquisition, and 3-dimensional parameters of bone microarchitecture: an experimental study on human cadaver vertebrae. J Clin Densitom. 2011;14:302–12.
57. Silva BC, Walker MD, Abraham A, et al. Trabecular bone score is associated with volumetric bone density and microarchitecture as assessed by central QCT and HRpQCT in Chinese American and white women. J Clin Densitom. 2013;16:554–61.
58. Silva BC, Leslie WD, Resch H, Lamy O, Lesnyak O, Binkley N, McCloskey EV, Kanis JA, Bilezikian JP. Trabecular bone score: a noninvasive analytical method based upon the DXA image. J Bone Miner Res. 2014;29(3):518–30.
59. Hans D, Goertzen AL, Krieg MA, Leslie WD. Bone microarchitecture assessed by TBS predicts osteoporotic fractures independent of bone density: the Manitoba study. J Bone Miner Res. 2011;26:2762–9.
60. Cormier C, Lamy O, Poriau S. TBS in routine medical practice: proposals of use. Plan-les-Ouates.: Medimaps Group; 2012. http://www.medimapsgroup.com/upload/MEDIMAPS-UK-WEB.pdf.

61. Boutroy S, Bouxsein ML, Munoz F, Delmas PD. In vivo assessment of trabecular bone microarchitecture by high-resolution peripheral quantitative computed tomography. J Clin Endocrinol Metab. 2005;90:6508–15.
62. Sornay-Rendu E, Cabrera-Bravo JL, Boutroy S, Munoz F, Delmas PD. Severity of vertebral fractures is associated with alterations of cortical architecture in postmenopausal women. J Bone Miner Res. 2009;24(4):737–43.
63. Stein EM, Liu XS, Nickolas TL, Cohen A, McMahon DJ, Zhou B, Zhang C, Kamanda-Kosseh M, Cosman F, Nieves J, Guo XE, Shane E. Microarchitectural abnormalities are more severe in postmenopausal women with vertebral compared to nonvertebral fractures. J Clin Endocrinol Metab. 2012;97(10):E1918–26.
64. Roux JP, Wegrzyn J, Arlot ME, Guyen O, Delmas PD, Chapurlat R, Bouxsein ML. Contribution of trabecular and cortical components to biomechanical behavior of human vertebrae: an ex vivo study. J Bone Miner Res. 2010;25(2):356–61.
65. Seeman E, Delmas PD. Bone quality—the material and structural basis of bone strength and fragility. N Engl J Med. 2006;354(21):2250–61.
66. Kim HJ, Dash A, Cunningham M, Schwab F, Dowdell J, Harrison J, Zaworski C, Krez A, Lafage V, Agarwal S, Carlson B, McMahon DJ, Stein EM. Patients with abnormal microarchitecture have an increased risk of early complications after spinal fusion surgery. Bone. 2021;143:115731. https://doi.org/10.1016/j.bone.2020.115731. Epub 2020 Nov 4. PMID: 33157283.
67. Bischoff-Ferrari HA, Willett WC, Wong JB, Giovannucci E, Dietrich T, Dawson-Hughes B. Fracture prevention with vitamin D supplementation: a meta-analysis of randomized controlled trials. JAMA. 2005;293(18):2257–64. https://doi.org/10.1001/jama.293.18.2257. PMID: 15886381.
68. Chapuy MC, Arlot ME, Duboeuf F, Brun J, Crouzet B, Arnaud S, Delmas PD, Meunier PJ. Vitamin D3 and calcium to prevent hip fractures in elderly women. N Engl J Med. 1992;327(23):1637–42. https://doi.org/10.1056/NEJM199212033272305. PMID: 1331788.
69. Boden SD, Schimandle JH, Hutton WC. An experimental lumbar intertransverse process spinal fusion model. Radiographic, histologic, and biomechanical healing characteristics. Spine. 1995;20:412–20.
70. Lawrence JP, Ennis F, White AP, et al. Effect of daily parathyroid hormone (1-34) on lumbar fusion in a rat model. Spine J. 2006;6:385–90.
71. O'Loughlin PF, Cunningham ME, Bukata SV, et al. Parathyroid hormone (1-34) augments spinal fusion, fusion mass volume, and fusion mass quality in a rabbit spinal fusion model. Spine. 2009;34:121–30.
72. Kaiser MG, Groff MW, Watters WC III, et al. Guideline update for the performance of fusion procedures for degenerative disease of the lumbar spine. Part 16: bone graft extenders and substitutes as an adjunct for lumbar fusion. J Neurosurg Spine. 2014;21:106–32.
73. Okamoto S, Ikeda T, Sawamura K, et al. Positive effect on bone fusion by the combination of platelet-rich plasma and a gelatin beta-tricalcium phosphate sponge: a study using a posterolateral fusion model of lumbar vertebrae in rats. Tissue Eng Part A. 2012;18:157–66.
74. Reid JJ, Johnson JS, Wang JC. Challenges to bone formation in spinal fusion. J Biomech. 2011;44:213–20.
75. Hirsch BP, Unnanuntana A, Cunningham ME, Lane JM. The effect of therapies for osteoporosis on spine fusion: a systematic review. Spine J. 2013;13:190–9.
76. Jain N, Labaran L, Phillips FM, Khan SN, Jain A, Kebaish KM, Hassanzadeh H. Prevalence of osteoporosis treatment and its effect on post-operative complications, revision surgery and costs after multi-level spinal fusion. Glob Spine J. 2022;12:1119. https://doi.org/10.1177/2192568220976560. PMID: 33334188.
77. Rodan GA, Fleisch HA. Bisphosphonates: mechanisms of action. J Clin Invest. 1996;97:2692–6.

78. Nagahama K, Kanayama M, Togawa D, Hashimoto T, Minami A. Does alendronate disturb the healing process of posterior lumbar interbody fusion? A prospective randomized trial. J Neurosurg Spine. 2011;14:500–7.
79. Kim SM, Rhee W, Ha S, Lim JH, Jang IT. Influence of alendronate and endplate degeneration to single level posterior lumbar spinal interbody fusion. Korean J Spine. 2014;11:221–6.
80. Park YS, Kim HS, Baek SW, Kong DY, Ryu JA. The effect of zoledronic acid on the volume of the fusion-mass in lumbar spinal fusion. Clin Orthop Surg. 2013;5:292–7.
81. Tu CW, Huang KF, Hsu HT, Li HY, Yang SSD, Chen YC. Zoledronic acid infusion for lumbar interbody fusion in osteoporosis. J Surg Res. 2014;192:112–6.
82. Chen F, Dai Z, Kang Y, Lv G, Keller ET, Jiang Y. Effects of zoledronic acid on bone fusion in osteoporotic patients after lumbar fusion. Osteoporos Int. 2016;27:1469–76.
83. Ding Q, Chen J, Fan J, Li Q, Yin G, Yu L. Effect of zoledronic acid on lumbar spinal fusion in osteoporotic patients. Eur Spine J. 2017;26:2969–77.
84. Neer RM, Arnaud CD, Zanchetta JR, Prince R, Gaich GA, Reginster JY, et al. Effect of parathyroid hormone (1–34) on fractures and bone mineral density in postmenopausal women with osteoporosis. N Engl J Med. 2001;344(19):1434–41. Epub 2001/05/11. PMID:11346808.
85. Rosen CJ, Bilezikian JP. Clinical review 123: anabolic therapy for osteoporosis. J Clin Endocrinol Metab. 2001;86:957–64.
86. Ohtori S, Inoue G, Orita S, Yamauchi K, Eguchi Y, Ochiai N, Kishida S, Kuniyoshi K, Aoki Y, Nakamura J, Ishikawa T, Miyagi M, Kamoda H, Suzuki M, Kubota G, Sakuma Y, Oikawa Y, Inage K, Sainoh T, Takaso M, Ozawa T, Takahashi K, Toyone T. Teriparatide accelerates lumbar posterolateral fusion in women with postmenopausal osteoporosis: prospective study. Spine. 2012;37(23):E1464–8.
87. Inoue G, Ueno M, Nakazawa T, Imura T, Saito W, Uchida K, Ohtori S, Toyone T, Takahira N, Takaso M. Teriparatide increases the insertional torque of pedicle screws during fusion surgery in patients with postmenopausal osteoporosis. J Neurosurg Spine. 2014;21(3):425–31.
88. Ohtori S, Inoue G, Orita S, Yamauchi K, Eguchi Y, Ochiai N, Kishida S, Kuniyoshi K, Aoki Y, Nakamura J, Ishikawa T, Miyagi M, Kamoda H, Suzuki M, Kubota G, Sakuma Y, Oikawa Y, Inage K, Sainoh T, Takaso M, Toyone T, Takahashi K. Comparison of teriparatide and bisphosphonate treatment to reduce pedicle screw loosening after lumbar spinal fusion surgery in postmenopausal women with osteoporosis from a bone quality perspective. Spine. 2013;38(8):E487–92.
89. Kim JW, Park SW, Kim YB, Ko MJ. The effect of postoperative use of Teriparatide reducing screw loosening in osteoporotic patients. J Korean Neurosurg Soc. 2018;61(4):494–502.
90. Ohtori S, Orita S, Yamauchi K, Eguchi Y, Ochiai N, Kuniyoshi K, Aoki Y, Nakamura J, Miyagi M, Suzuki M, Kubota G, Inage K, Sainoh T, Sato J, Shiga Y, Abe K, Fujimoto K, Kanamoto H, Inoue G, Takahashi K. More than 6 months of teriparatide treatment was more effective for bone union than shorter treatment following lumbar posterolateral fusion surgery. Asian Spine J. 2015;9(4):573–80.
91. Yagi M, Ohne H, Konomi T, Fujiyoshi K, Kaneko S, Komiyama T, Takemitsu M, Yato Y, Machida M, Asazuma T. Teriparatide improves volumetric bone mineral density and fine bone structure in the UIV+1 vertebra, and reduces bone failure type PJK after surgery for adult spinal deformity. Osteoporos Int. 2016;27(12):3495–502.
92. Ebata S, Takahashi J, Hasegawa T, Mukaiyama K, Isogai Y, Ohba T, Shibata Y, Ojima T, Yamagata Z, Matsuyama Y, Haro H. Role of weekly teriparatide administration in osseous union enhancement within six months after posterior or transforaminal lumbar interbody fusion for osteoporosis-associated lumbar degenerative disorders: a multicenter, prospective randomized study. J Bone Joint Surg Am. 2017;99(5):365–72.
93. Cho PG, Ji GY, Shin DA, Ha Y, Yoon DH, Kim KN. An effect comparison of teriparatide and bisphosphonate on posterior lumbar interbody fusion in patients with osteoporosis: a prospective cohort study and preliminary data. Eur Spine J. 2017;26:691–7.

94. Kawabata A, Yoshii T, Hirai T, et al. Effect of bisphosphonates or teriparatide on mechanical complications after posterior instrumented fusion for osteoporotic vertebral fracture: a multi-center retrospective study. BMC Musculoskelet Disord. 2020;21:420.
95. Jespersen AB, Andresen ADK, Jacobsen MK, Andersen MO, Carreon LY. Does systemic administration of parathyroid hormone after noninstrumented spinal fusion surgery improve fusion rates and fusion mass in elderly patients compared to placebo in patients with degenerative lumbar spondylolisthesis? Spine. 2019;44(3):157–62.
96. Miller PD, Hattersley G, Riis BJ, et al. Effect of abaloparatide vs placebo on new vertebral fractures in postmenopausal women with osteoporosis: a randomized clinical trial. JAMA. 2016;316:722–33.
97. Arlt H, Besschetnova T, Ominsky MS, Fredericks DC, Lanske B. Effects of systemically administered abaloparatide, an osteoanabolic PTHrP analog, as an adjuvant therapy for spinal fusion in rats. JOR Spine. 2020;4(1):e1132. https://doi.org/10.1002/jsp2.1132. eCollection 2021 Mar. PMID: 33778406.
98. Parikh S, Lubitz SE, Sharma A. Novel use of abaloparatide to augment spinal fusion in patient undergoing cervicothoracic revision surgery. J Endocrine Soc. 2020;4(Suppl 1):MON-365.
99. Leder BZ, Tsai JN, Uihlein AV, Burnett-Bowie SA, Zhu Y, Foley K, et al. Two years of Denosumab and teriparatide administration in postmenopausal women with osteoporosis (The DATA Extension Study): a randomized controlled trial. J Clin Endocrinol Metab. 2014;99(5):1694–700. Epub 2014/02/13. PMID:24517156; PubMed Central PMCID: PMC4010689.
100. Ide M, Yamada K, Kaneko K, et al. Combined teriparatide and denosumab therapy accelerates spinal fusion following posterior lumbar interbody fusion. Orthop Traumatol Surg Res. 2018;104:1043–8.
101. Tsutsumimoto T, Shimogata M, Yoshimura Y, Misawa H. Union versus nonunion after posterolateral lumbar fusion: a comparison of long-term surgical outcomes in patients with degenerative lumbar spondylolisthesis. Eur Spine J. 2008;17(8):1107–12. Epub 2008/06/10. PMID:18536941; PubMed Central PMCID: PMC2518764.

Chapter 2
Antithrombotic Management in Spine Surgery in the Elderly

Nallammai Muthiah, Nitin Agarwal, and David Kojo Hamilton

Introduction

Spine surgery, as with any surgery, is a risk factor for thromboembolic events [1–9]. The estimated incidence of perioperative deep venous thrombosis or pulmonary thromboembolism for spine surgery varies widely, with rates reported between 0.03%and 31% [10–15]. This large range likely reflects the variability in power of studies, thromboembolism prophylaxis protocols, extent of surgery, changes in chemoprophylaxis medications, changes in techniques over time, and patient population. Still, patient safety is among the foremost considerations for spine surgeons, and spine surgery carries a significant risk for venous thrombosis or thromboembolism regardless of protocols, medications, techniques, or patient population. Several sets of guidelines exist for antithrombotic management before and after spine surgery, though many of these guidelines are loosely based on retrospective and prospective trials. There is no single standardized protocol for VTE prophylaxis, especially for

N. Muthiah
Department of Neurological Surgery, University of Pittsburgh Medical Center, Pittsburgh, PA, USA
e-mail: muthiahn@upmc.edu

N. Agarwal
Department of Neurological Surgery, University of Pittsburgh Medical Center, Pittsburgh, PA, USA

Neurotrauma, Department of Neurosurgery, Washington University in St. Louis, St. Louis, MO, USA
e-mail: nitin.agarwal@wustl.edu

D. K. Hamilton (✉)
Spine Fellowship Program, Residency Site Program, Department of Neurological Surgery, UPMC Mercy, University of Pittsburgh Medical Center, Pittsburgh, PA, USA
e-mail: hamiltondk@upmc.edu

K.-M. G. Fu et al. (eds.), *Treatment of Spine Disease in the Elderly*,
https://doi.org/10.1007/978-3-031-12612-3_2

patients with multiple comorbidities. This chapter draws from this existing literature and will provide suggested guidelines for VTE prophylaxis. Ultimately, however, antithrombotic medications should be managed in complete clinical context.

Age is among the most important risk factors for cardiovascular disease, though the exact mechanism of aging on cardiovascular health has yet to be fully understood [16–18]. Aging is thought to decrease platelet aggregation and fibrinolysis secondary to endothelial cell senescence [19, 20], exhaustion of endothelial cell repair mechanisms [20], the increased likelihood of comorbidities (i.e., hypertension, hepatic disease, renal disease, etc.) [18], and lifestyle changes which may increase sedentary time [21]. The incidence of thromboembolism among adults at age 80 is about three time that at age 60 [22]. For this reason, many older adults are started on venous thromboembolism prophylaxis.

To that end, one of the greatest challenges in perioperative management for elderly spine surgery patients is anticoagulation. Both vessel thrombosis and uncontrolled bleeding—entities on opposite ends of the spectrum—are major complications associated with spine surgery [2, 4, 5, 8, 9]. Several medication classes are currently approved for anticoagulation in older adults. The rest of this chapter will offer an algorithmic approach to managing antithrombotic agents, delineated by medication class, for the elderly spine surgery patient. The first section of this chapter will outline antithrombotic agent management for elective neurosurgical procedures, the next section will discuss management in urgent or emergent procedures, and the final section will review special considerations for managing antithrombotic agents in older adults.

Preoperative Antithrombotic Therapy

When considering preoperative anticoagulation management in the elderly, first spine surgeons must estimate perioperative thrombotic risk. To do so, three risk factors must always be considered: mechanical heart valves, prior thromboembolism, and atrial fibrillation [23].

Atrial fibrillation is the most common arrythmias diagnosed in clinical practice [24]. Age is the most important risk factor for atrial fibrillation [25], and the prevalence of this arrythmia is 12% among US adults older than 65 [26]. Atrial fibrillation is also a major risk factor for thromboembolism among adults in this age group [27]. The risk of stroke among patients with atrial fibrillation is fivefold greater than in the general population [28]. Appropriate anticoagulation can decrease the risk of stroke for patients with atrial fibrillation by 66% [29, 30]. The CHA_2DS_2-VASc score has been used to stratify patients with atrial fibrillation into low-, moderate-, and high-risk groups for perioperative thrombosis [3], though this risk classification is based on indirect evidence and should always be supplemented with patient-specific clinical reasoning. The presence of mechanical heart valves and/or prior thromboembolism generally increases the risk of perioperative thrombosis [3], further allowing spine surgeons to risk-stratify older adult patients.

Antithrombotic Agent Classes

Medication-specific considerations are also vital to preoperative antithrombotic management. These considerations are discussed in the following sections.

Antiplatelets

Aspirin (Acetylsalicylic Acid, ASA)

Aspirin is among the most commonly prescribed medications in the United States today [31]. It is relatively inexpensive, is available over the counter, is easy to take, and has multiple dose-based physiologic effects. At low doses, aspirin is primarily an antiplatelet; at high doses, it has anti-inflammatory properties [32]. In other words, aspirin is a versatile and easily accessible medication.

ASA is an irreversible cyclooxygenase-1 and cyclooxygenase-2 inhibitor, which prevents the formation of thromboxane-A_2 and ultimately inhibits platelet aggregation. As an irreversible agent, aspirin's effects last the life of the platelet (7–10 days). Peak serum levels are achieved at 30 min following administration, with a half-life of 20 min. Aspirin has been used for primary prevention of cardiovascular disease in the past, though recent studies suggest that the benefits of taking ASA as a primary preventative agent do not necessarily outweigh the risks. As per the 2019 American Heart Association (AHA) guidelines, aspirin should not be used in patients older than 70 years at risk for bleeding [33–36]. For this reason, aspirin is used mainly for the secondary prevention of cardiovascular disease in at-risk patients aged 40–70 [33–37].

An estimated 44.6% of adults aged 70–79 and 46.2% of adults older than 80—a total of approximately 9.5 million adults—use daily aspirin [34]. Interestingly, the prevalence of cardiovascular disease in adults aged 60–79 is approximately 75%, and in adults ≥80, the prevalence is approximately 80% [38]. This discrepancy in prevalence of cardiovascular disease and rates of aspirin use among older adults is not surprising. Not all adults with cardiovascular disease require antithrombotic therapy. Those who do require antithrombotic therapy may also require nonaspirin medications. At the same time, older adults can easily use aspirin for reasons other than for the secondary prevention of thromboembolism. There is evidence to suggest that a substantial portion of patients may be taking aspirin without the explicit advice or possibly knowledge of their physicians [34]. All this to say, it is vital to ascertain all nonprescription medications, especially those like aspirin, which can increase intraoperative bleeding risk. Plans for management of these medications should be created by medical and surgical teams several weeks before surgery.

It is recommended that ASA be held 5–10 days before spine surgery for patients taking the medication for cardiac risk [5, 39]. Some patients take aspirin along with another antiplatelet agent for the purpose of bare-metal or drug-eluting stent thrombosis prevention. For those on such dual antiplatelet therapy, current recommendations are to delay spine surgery by 6 months if feasible and continue both medications

[23, 40, 41]. If it is not feasible to wait 6 months for surgery, the risks and benefits of bleeding must be considered carefully with medicine and anesthesiology colleagues as well as the patient. If the risk of bleeding is expected to be minimal, discontinuing the P2Y12 receptor antagonist while continuing aspirin is recommended [23, 40, 41]. However, for major procedures where intraoperative or postoperative bleeding could be catastrophic, both agents may need to be held [23, 40, 41].

Clopidogrel and Other P2Y12 Receptor Antagonists

P2Y12 receptor inhibitors are thienopyridines which function as antiplatelet medications by inhibiting ADP-mediated platelet aggregation, thereby preventing clotting [42, 43]. Among the thienopyridines, clopidogrel (second generation), prasugrel (third generation), ticagrelor, and cangrelor (fourth generation) are used most commonly in clinical practice [42].

Clopidogrel is a prodrug which is metabolized into active compounds by the cytochrome P450 (CYP450) system in the liver. While prasugrel and ticagrelor are often used in the setting of STEMI to reduce ischemic outcomes [43], for the older spine surgery patient, P2Y12 receptor inhibitors (especially clopidogrel [42]) are more likely to be seen in combination with aspirin for thromboembolism prophylaxis in patients with intracardiac stents. For patients with cardiac stents, stopping such dual antiplatelet therapy significantly increases the risk of thromboembolism. Therefore, as previously mentioned, it is recommended to stop only the P2Y12 receptor antagonist when some increased intraoperative bleeding can be tolerated [41, 43].

Dipyridamole is another medication which falls into the class of P2Y12 receptor antagonists. It acts as both a vasodilator and antiplatelet agent. To date, there is no rigorous data to guide preoperative management of dipyridamole for spine surgery patients. Consultation with medical and anesthesia colleagues will be important to determine the risk/benefit profile of drug cessation. If the decision is made to hold dipyridamole, it is suggested to be stopped for 2 days prior to surgery [44]. Importantly, formulations of dipyridamole and aspirin (i.e., Aggrenox) exist. Such formulations should be stopped 7–10 days before surgery.

Figure 2.1 depicts a suggested algorithm for preoperative antiplatelet agent management among elderly spine surgery patients.

Oral Anticoagulants

Warfarin

Warfarin is among the most common anticoagulants used for treatment of non-valvular heart diseases [31]. Warfarin's therapeutic effect is secondary to its properties as a vitamin K epoxide reductase antagonist, an enzyme which activates vitamin K. Vitamin K is necessary for the gamma carboxylation of factors II, VII, IX, and X of the coagulation cascade. Warfarin has a half-life of 36–42 h, necessitating it be stopped earlier than

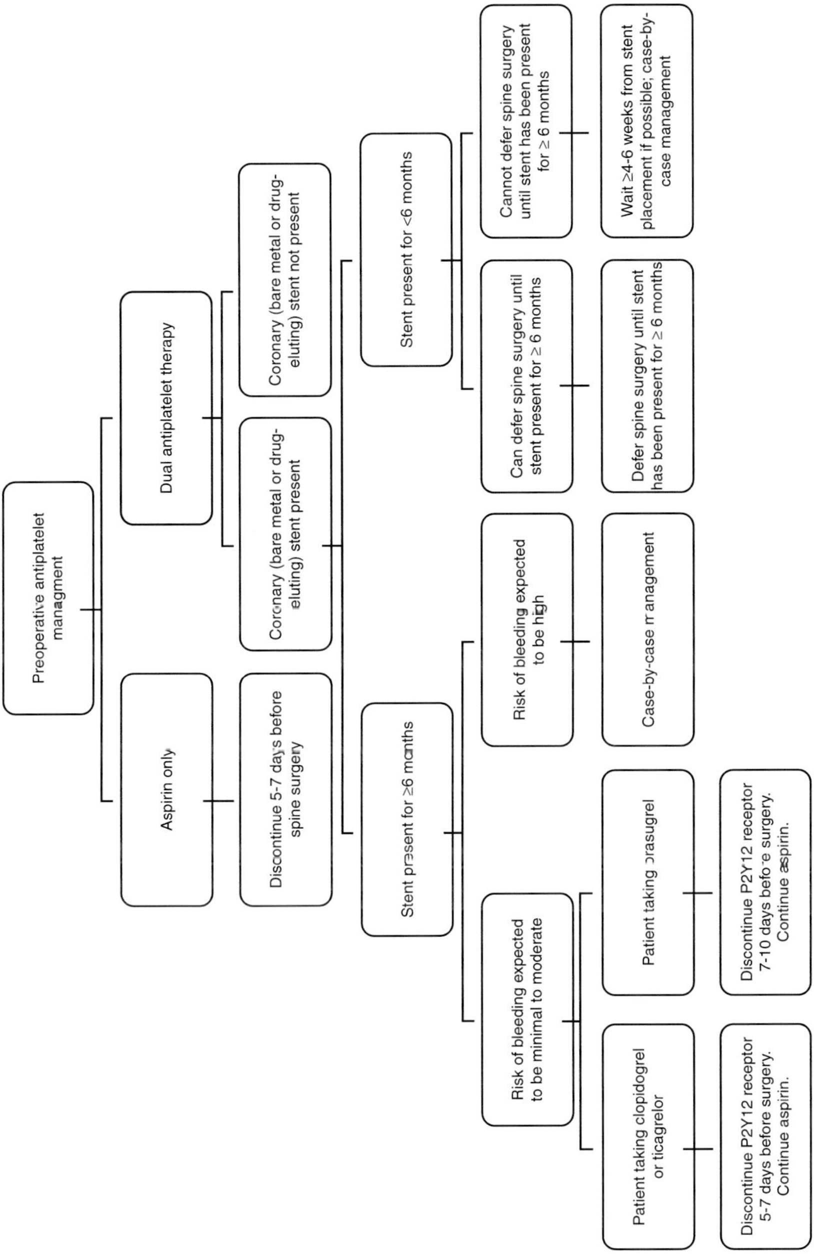

Fig. 2.1 Algorithm for preoperative antiplatelet management

other anticoagulants prior to surgery. Warfarin's therapeutic effect is traditionally measured by the international normalized ratio (INR). Current guidelines suggest that warfarin be stopped 5 days before surgery or until a goal INR of ≤1.5 is achieved.

Within the first 12–16 h of warfarin intake, factor VII levels are approximately 40%, which is enough for the coagulation cascade to remain relatively clinically functional. For that reason, warfarin is unique among anticoagulants in that it is safe to perform neuraxial anesthesia or remove an epidural catheter within 24 h of first warfarin intake. There is no clear consensus as to how long following warfarin intake it becomes unsafe to perform neuraxial anesthesia or epidural catheter manipulation, though it is recommended that such procedures be preceded by an INR of ≤1.4.

Figure 2.2 depicts a suggested algorithm for preoperative warfarin management among elderly spine surgery patients.

Direct Oral Anticoagulants (DOACs)

DOACs have become more popular anticoagulation agents since their introduction. Today, the AHA recommends use of DOACs over warfarin in patients with atrial fibrillation requiring anticoagulation [45]. Agents in this class include drugs with the suffix *-xaban* (i.e., apixaban, rivaroxaban) and *-gatran* (dabigatran). Dabigatran is a prodrug whose active product functions as reversible direct thrombin (factor II) inhibitor. It binds the active site of thrombin, attenuating formation of fibrin and inhibiting the coagulation cascade. Apixaban and rivaroxaban are irreversible factor Xa inhibitors, which also impair the common pathway in the coagulation cascade, thereby attenuating the formation of fibrin. DOACs have a rapid onset and offset, need not be monitored via serial blood levels, are easy to take, and have been shown to have fewer bleeding complications than warfarin in older adults [46, 47]. DOACs are becoming increasingly common among traditional spine surgery patients.

There is no reliable method of laboratory monitoring of DOAC levels, so perioperative management for elderly patients can be challenging [48, 49]. Furthermore, DOACs are cleared renally. Among adults aged 65–79 years, the prevalence of chronic kidney disease is approximately 22%, and among those older than 80 years, that prevalence jumps to 51% [50]. As many spine surgery patients are older adults, renal function (often approximated by creatinine clearance) must be considered well in advance of surgery. In general, patients with poorer renal function require earlier DOAC cessation than those with good renal function [48, 49]. Each DOAC also has its own half-life, which also should be accounted for when determining preoperative DOAC cessation timing [48, 49]. Because DOACs have such a rapid offset, bridging with heparin compounds is often performed [48, 49].

For patients with creatinine clearance ≥30 mL/min who are taking apixaban twice daily or rivaroxaban once daily, the last dose should be given 3 days before spine surgery [48, 49]. Patients taking dabigatran twice daily with creatinine clearance ≥50 mL/min should take their last dose 3 days before surgery, while those with a creatinine clearance of 30–49 should take their last dose 5 days before surgery [48, 49]. If creatinine clearance is ≤30, usually DOACs are not started in the first place, so preoperative management is unclear.

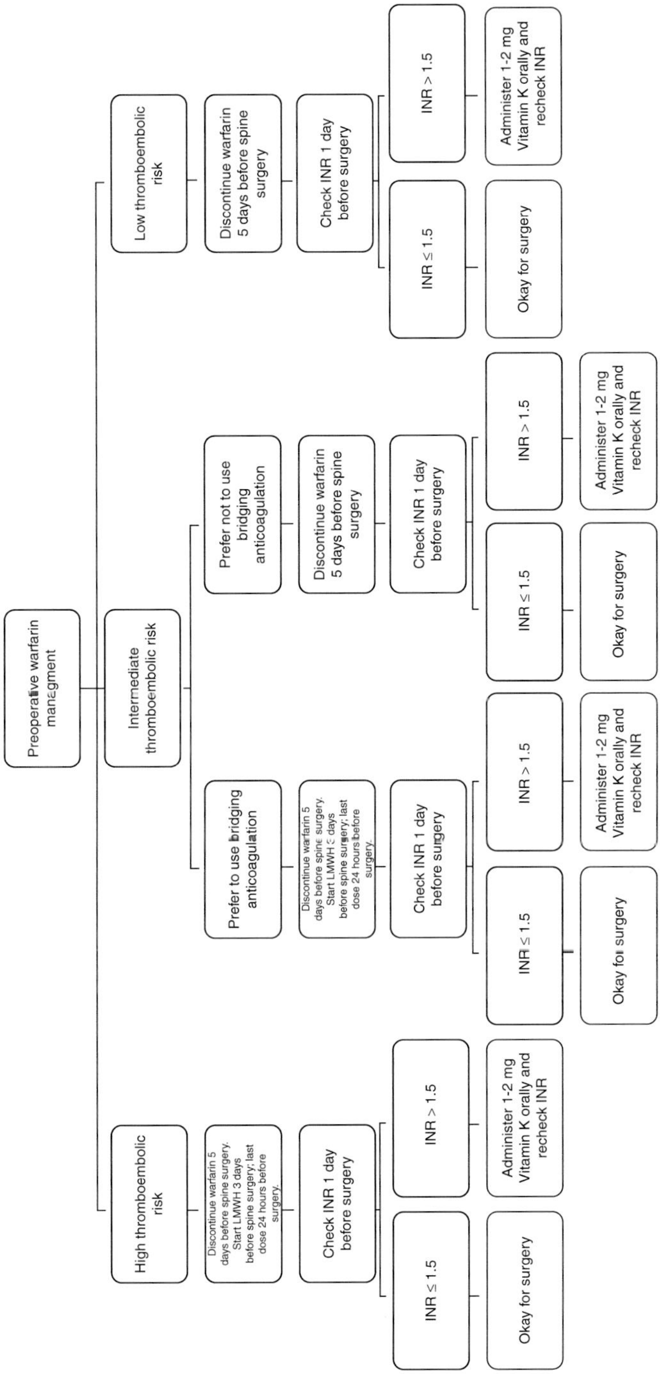

Fig. 2.2 Algorithm for preoperative warfarin management

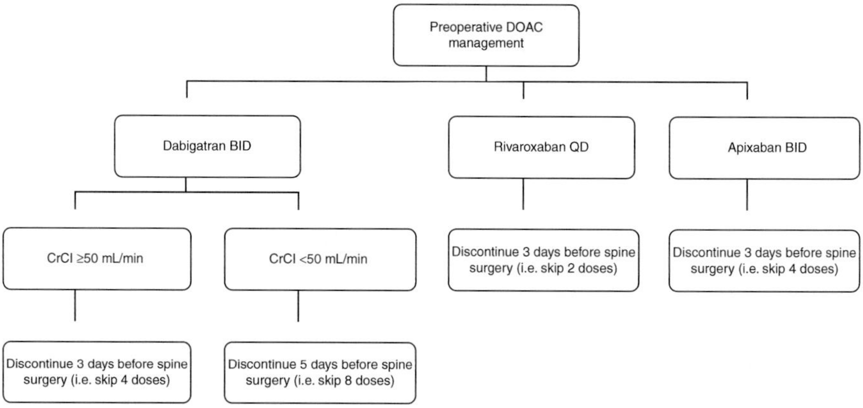

Fig. 2.3 Algorithm for preoperative DOAC management

Figure 2.3 depicts a suggested algorithm for preoperative DOAC management among elderly spine surgery patients.

Heparin Compounds

Unfractionated Heparin (UFH)

Unfractionated heparin is a compound which binds to antithrombin III to serve as a factor Xa and, to a lesser extent, direct thrombin inhibitor. In vivo, antithrombin III inhibits factor Xa of the coagulation cascade, preventing formation of activated thrombin from prothrombin. UFH binds to antithrombin III and inhibits factors Xa and thrombin. UFH is a compound used typically in hospital settings due to its route of administration and necessity to closely monitor its therapeutic effect. UFH has a short half-life of only 1–2 h and is easily reversed with protamine, making this medication a good choice for patients who are at high risk of VTE before surgery. The American Society of Regional Anesthesia (ASRA) recommends stopping UFH 4–6 h before surgery or until the aPTT is <35.7 s (regardless of whether the patient is on a therapeutic dose or a prophylactic dose) [51]. For prophylactic dose UFH (5000 units every 8 h), it is also okay to continue the medication throughout surgery if the procedure is expected to have minimal bleeding [51].

Low Molecular Weight Heparin (LMWH)

LMWHs have a similar mechanism of action as UFH. However, as the compounds are fractionated into various-sized smaller molecules, fewer molecules within the LMWH mixture are large enough to directly inhibit thrombin when compared to UFH. LMWHs are gaining popularity as they have a lower incidence of heparin-induced thrombocytopenia than UFH and do not require constant monitoring. These benefits, however, come at the cost of inability to easily reverse supra-therapeutic effects. Prior to surgery, the ARSA recommends stopping therapeutic doses of enoxaparin (>40 mg four times per day) 1 day before surgery and stopping prophylactic doses (30 mg twice per day to 40 mg four times per day) 12–24 h before spine surgery with the caveat that it may be okay to continue prophylactic enoxaparin depending on the risk for thromboembolism [52].

Fondaparinux

Fondaparinux is another heparin compound. There are currently no rigorous studies to date evaluating the safety and efficacy of fondaparinux in the population of older spine surgery patients, so surgeons must rely on their clinical judgment when deciding when to start this medication postoperatively. The ASRA recommends stopping prophylactic dose fondaparinux 2–3 days before spine surgery with the caveat that there is no strong evidence against simply continuing the medication [52, 53]. For therapeutic dose fondaparinux, the last dose should be 4–5 days before spine surgery [52, 53].

Bridging Anticoagulation

When oral anticoagulants are stopped preoperatively, it is possible to "bridge" the period between anticoagulant cessation and surgery with a short-acting agent. Heparin compounds are traditionally used for bridging. It is important to note that no clinical trial evidence exists to guide the use of bridging, though bridging has been retrospectively shown to increase bleeding intra- and postoperatively while not substantially decreasing thromboembolism risk preoperatively [49]. Ultimately the decision to bridge requires weighing the risk of VTE in clinical context against the risk of bleeding during and after spine surgery [49].

If it is decided that bridging anticoagulation will be net beneficial to the patient, low molecular weight heparins (LMWHs) are often the first choice [49] because they do not need to be monitored, have lower incidence of heparin-induced thrombocytopenia, and have similar clinical outcomes as unfractionated heparin (UFH). Importantly, bridging does not seem to decrease the incidence of VTE but does increase bleeding risk [49]. Thus, it is recommended to avoid bridging when possible, even in most patients with recent VTE [54, 55] or those with atrial fibrillation [49, 56]. UFH allows for easy reversal with protamine if necessary, which can become useful in the case of excessive intraoperative bleeding. Figure 2.4 is an adaptation of a useful algorithm advocated by Tafur and Douketis for anticoagulation bridging in the preoperative period [49].

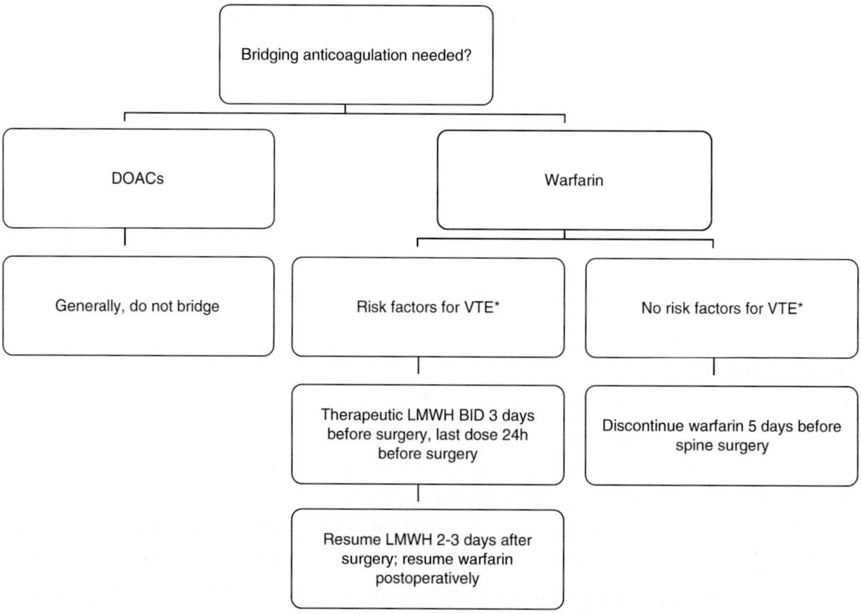

Fig. 2.4 Algorithm for deciding whether to bridge warfarin with low molecular weight heparin (LMWH). Risk factors for venous thromboembolism from highest to lowest odds ratios of developing venous thromboembolism include expected major surgery (OR ≥ 10), spinal cord injury (OR ≥ 10) or major trauma (OR ≥ 10), previous deep venous thrombosis (2 ≥ OR ≥ 9), malignancy (2 ≥ OR ≥ 9), chemotherapy (2 ≥ OR ≥ 9), paralytic stroke (2 ≥ OR ≥ 9), congestive heart failure (2 ≥ OR ≥ 9), hormone replacement therapy (2 ≥ OR ≥ 9), bed rest >3 days (OR ≤ 2), increasing age (OR ≤ 2), obesity (OR ≤ 2), and varicose veins (OR ≤ 2). *VTE* venous thromboembolism, *LMWH* low molecular weight heparin [57]

Intraoperative Anticoagulation

Intraoperative anticoagulation is an option for patients undergoing specific spinal procedures [58, 59]. The main risk in giving anticoagulants intraoperatively is bleeding. However, sometimes the risk of bleeding is predicted to be less than the risk of thrombosis. For example, anterior approaches to the lumbar spine are associated with iliac artery thrombosis secondary to the necessary retraction of arteries for exposure [58]. The incidence of iliac artery thrombosis is estimated to be as high as 0.9% [60]. Though limited, existing data suggest that intraoperative heparin for anterior surgical approaches to the lumbar spine are not associated with increased bleeding and can be safely used to prevent iliac artery thrombosis [59]. Some studies have assessed the safety and efficacy of intraoperative heparin in preventing microvascular thrombosis during free flap procedures [61]. These data suggests that neither the incidence of microvascular thrombosis nor that of hematoma formation are significantly increased with the use of a single dose of unfractionated heparin intraoperatively [61]. While these data are based on analyses of patients undergoing free flap reconstructions and may not necessarily be applicable to typical spine surgery patients, they do suggest that intraoperative heparinization with UFH can be safe for appropriately chosen patients. There is unfortunately no clear guidance to date on indications, appropriate timing, and optimal dosing of intraoperative anticoagulation for older adults during spine surgery when the risk of thrombosis is perceived to be higher than the risk of bleeding.

Postoperative Antithrombotic Therapy

Older patients who have just undergone spine surgery, especially those with malignancies or movement-limiting neurologic deficits, are at moderate to high risk for venous thromboembolism [57]. Conservative measures are usually used as first-line treatment to prevent venous stasis and thrombosis [62–64]. The value of early ambulation and sequential compression devices (SCDs) in the early postoperative period cannot be overstated [62–64]. The North American Spine Society (NASS) guidelines for mechanical thromboembolism prophylaxis state that despite the lack of evidence for specific timings and durations, "... initiation of mechanical compression just prior to or at the beginning of surgery and continuation until the patient is fully ambulatory is a reasonable practice" [65]. When these conservative measures are not sufficient to reasonably prevent thrombosis, antithrombotic therapy can be used. Recent studies have suggested that multimodal therapy with both SCDs, early ambulation, and aggressive anticoagulation in the early postoperative period was associated with decreased incidence of VTE without increased risk of bleeding [10]. It should be noted that the NASS does recommend cautious use of postoperative anticoagulation since many elective spine surgeries inherently have a relatively low risk for VTE. Indeed, some older adults may be healthy enough to not require postoperative antithrombotic therapy, but this decision should be made on a case-by-case basis. When required, the most common medications of choice for VTE prophylaxis in the immediate postoperative period are unfractionated heparin and enoxaparin [10, 54, 66].

It is also important to remain cognizant of common practices following spine surgery which may, in and of themselves, increase the risk for postoperative VTE. For example, steroids, often given to decrease swelling in the acute postoperative period, have been associated with a 1.47 times increased risk of pulmonary embolism and 1.55 times increased risk of deep vein thrombosis in a sample of over 94,000 neurosurgical patients [67]. The risk for VTE is even greater when spine surgery patients have underlying malignancies [57], have ambulation-limiting neurologic deficits [10, 57, 68], or spend longer in the hospital [57]. Longer postoperative stays are associated with worse outcomes, especially for older patients who tend to be less physiologically resilient and at high risk for delirium [69, 70].

The following sections will outline suggested algorithms for *restarting* antiplatelet and anticoagulant medications following spine surgery. In other words, the rest of this section is dedicated to management of patients who had preoperatively used (or had preoperative indications to chronically use) a given anticoagulant or antiplatelet. The best way to utilize this section, therefore, is to note which medications a patient was taking preoperatively and identify the suggested algorithm for restarting that specific medication. In that way, all the following sections will not apply to every patient.

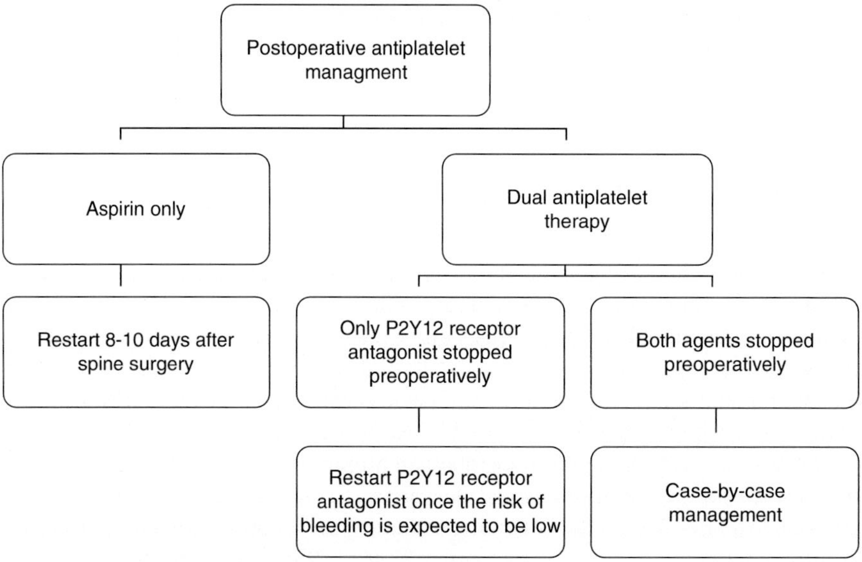

Fig. 2.5 Algorithm for postoperative antiplatelet management

Antiplatelets

Figure 2.5 depicts a suggested algorithm for restarting antiplatelet medications in the postoperative period for the older spine surgery patient.

Aspirin (Acetylsalicylic Acid, ASA)

For spinal surgery, aspirin is recommended to be held for 8–10 days following the procedure [71], once the risk of significant bleeding has passed. For patients with bare-metal or drug-eluting stents, aspirin is usually continued throughout the perioperative period due to the significant risk for thromboembolism [71]. In the case that aspirin needs to be stopped for major spinal surgeries, decisions should be made on a case-by-case basis with medical and anesthesia colleagues, taking into account patient age, comorbidities, medications, extent of surgery, expected recovery time, duration of hospital stay, and socioeconomic factors which may influence compliance with treatment or follow-up [71, 72].

Clopidogrel and Other P2Y12 Receptor Antagonists

Clopidogrel and ticagrelor should be started as soon as the risk of postoperative bleeding is reasonably low [73]. Patients usually are taking these medications because they have a bare-metal or drug-eluting stent, and therefore have high risk of thromboembolism.

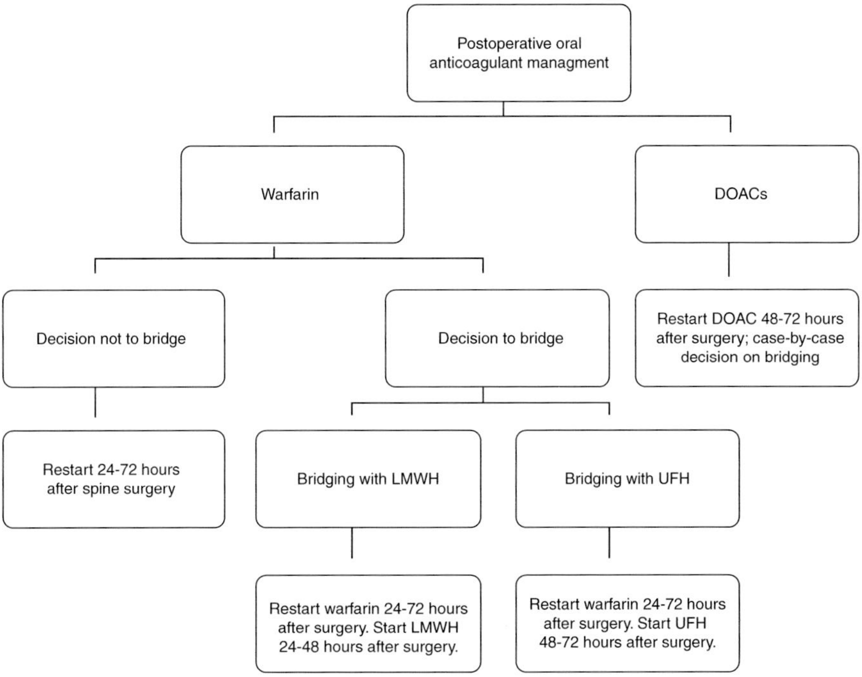

Fig. 2.6 Algorithm for postoperative anticoagulant management

Oral Anticoagulants

Figure 2.6 depicts a suggested algorithm for starting oral anticoagulant agents in the postoperative period for the older spine surgery patient.

Warfarin

Warfarin is recommended to be restarted 1–3 days after surgery [56]. While waiting to restart warfarin, patients can be bridged with prophylactic or therapeutic dose heparin compounds ≥24 h after surgery. Evidence has shown that foregoing bridging is non-inferior to bridging with low molecular weight heparin [56]. Still, the decision to postoperatively bridge back to warfarin with LMWH or UFH is often made on a case-by-case basis. If postoperative bridging is desired, surgeons can choose to start either therapeutic dose LMWH/unfractionated heparin 2–3 days after surgery or prophylactic dose LMWH/unfractionated heparin 1–2 days after surgery. The alternative is to also simply start warfarin 1–3 days after surgery without heparin bridging [56].

Direct Oral Anticoagulants (DOACs)

DOACs can usually be restarted 2–3 days after surgery [74], during which time prophylactic anticoagulants can be used in the interim if patients are unable to ambulate or have other risk factors for thrombosis (i.e., active malignancy). Low-dose enoxaparin (40 mg) is commonly used for prophylaxis.

Studies suggest that DOACs have a lower bleeding risk than warfarin in the postoperative period [48]. Moreover, compared to oral anticoagulants (DOACs and warfarin), antiplatelet agents (heparin compounds) have been shown to carry an increased risk of intracerebral hemorrhage. DOACs have been associated with fewer deaths, cardiovascular events, hemorrhagic strokes, and hospitalizations with bleeding complications than warfarin [46].

Heparin Compounds

Figure 2.7 depicts a suggested algorithm for starting heparin compounds in the postoperative period for the older spine surgery patient. It is important to note that the NASS guidelines currently recommend mechanical prophylaxis and early ambulation as first-line treatment for surgeries with low VTE risk, such as most elective

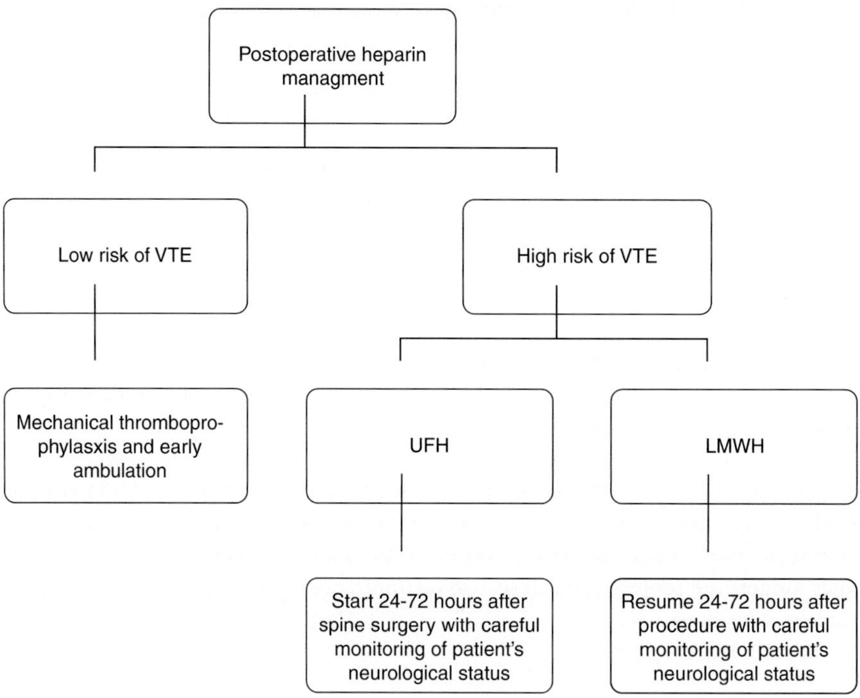

Fig. 2.7 Algorithm for postoperative heparin compound management

procedures performed through a posterior approach [65]. For procedures with high risk of VTE, heparin compounds can be started to decrease risk of thrombosis. Some evidence exists to suggest that starting heparin immediately after spine surgery was not associated with increased incidence of symptomatic epidural hematomas [10]. At the same time, the NASS guidelines issue caution about use of heparin and enoxaparin following spine surgery due to the known reports of symptomatic epidural hematomas [65]. That said, UFH and LMWH are frequently used following spine procedures in clinical practice. Ultimately, current evidence is conflicting regarding the use of postoperative heparin, but regardless, the decision to start antithrombotic agents postoperatively should take into account patient age, comorbidities, extent of procedure, neurologic deficits, and any other risk factors for VTE or bleeding [57]. If heparin is started, the neurological exam must be carefully monitored for the duration of the hospital stay [65].

Unfractionated Heparin and LMWH

When the decision is made to use heparin compounds postoperatively, UFH and LMWH are typically started 24 h after surgery, or at the next scheduled dose [51, 75]. They have short half-lives and fast onset. In the appropriate clinical context, as outlined above, UFH or LMWH can be used to bridge back to warfarin or DOACs in the postoperative period.

Antithrombotic Management in the Emergent Setting

Elective spine procedures afford the surgical team time for gradual, controlled antithrombotic management. Spinal emergencies due to myriad etiologies such as trauma and infection do not offer the luxury of time. As mentioned earlier in this chapter, many adults over age 65 take antiplatelet or oral anticoagulant agents chronically. For spine emergencies in the elderly, it is vital to identify any medications that have the potential to increase perioperative bleeding and develop efficient plans for management. This section will review management of antiplatelets and anticoagulants for older adults in need of urgent or emergent spinal procedures.

Antiplatelets

Aspirin

As aforementioned, many older adults take aspirin, at times, even without a prescription by a physician. In the emergency setting, it is important to gather patients' medication history and the last time at which they took their medications. If not from the patient, this information should be sought from family members. In the case that no information is available about patient medication history, it is possible to perform platelet function assays, which easily assesses the extent of platelet function [76]. However, these studies may not be time-effective, especially in the acute neurosurgical setting.

Aspirin's effects can typically be reversed with an infusion of platelets preoperatively [76].

Clopidogrel

Similar to aspirin, it is important to identify whether the acute spine surgery patient is taking clopidogrel and, if so, the timing of the last dose. When this information is not available, clopidogrel's effects can be measured using platelet aggregation tests. Again, such tests are not particularly time-efficient when patients require acute neurosurgical intervention. Clopidogrel tends to lead to more platelet dysfunction than aspirin [76]. When clopidogrel reversal is needed, additional units of platelets may be required in the acute neurosurgical setting [76].

Oral Anticoagulants

Warfarin

Since warfarin works by inhibiting activation of vitamin K by vitamin K epoxide reductase, it prevents synthesis of coagulation cascade factors II, VI, IX, and X. Warfarin has a half-life of 36–42 h [77]. For this reason, simply stopping warfarin immediately before a surgical procedure is often not sufficient to normalize INR in the urgent or emergent setting [78]. Likewise, administration of vitamin K itself is usually not enough to normalize INR before surgery since vitamin K takes 12–24 h to take full effect [78]. Consequently, transfusion of activated coagulation cascade factors is frequently necessary. The volume of fresh frozen plasma (FFP) required to normalize INR in the setting of therapeutic anticoagulation with warfarin may be prohibitively large [78, 79]. Therefore, for urgent or emergent spine surgeries, warfarin is typically reversed with prothrombin complex concentrates (PCC) [78, 79]. PCC can either contain four factors (four-factor PCC, factors II, VII, IX, and X) or three factors (three-factor PCC: factors II, IX, and X with small amounts of VII).

If surgery can be safely delayed for 6–12 h, intravenous infusion of vitamin K may be sufficient to normalize INR (INR < 1.5) [79]. If surgery cannot be delayed, current guidelines recommend using 20–50 IU/kg of four-factor PCC with concomitant intravenous vitamin K (5–10 mg) for warfarin reversal [79, 80]. Notably, there is a small risk of thrombotic complications following warfarin reversal [79, 81]. That said, the risk/benefit profile for PCC should be weighed carefully based on each patient's comorbidities, the extent of the planned surgical procedure, and the preoperative INR.

DOACs

As previously mentioned, the DOACs predominantly work via inhibition of either factor II or factor Xa. The DOACs are not easily monitored or reversed, so quick planning for urgent/emergent DOAC management is challenging. Nevertheless, spine surgeons can still optimize the risk of perioperative bleeding and thrombosis.

DOACs have a faster onset and offset than warfarin, so it is important to confirm when patients took their last dose. DOACs achieve peak effects at 1–3 h, and they are cleared rapidly enough such that if surgery can be delayed by 8–12 h, no reversal agent may be necessary for major surgical procedures [77, 79]. Prior to urgent or emergent spine surgery, renal function should also be checked in patients taking DOACs. DOACs are all, to some extent, renally cleared. Especially in the setting of bleeding secondary to trauma, acute kidney injury can develop, thereby leading to accumulation of DOACs in the blood [77, 79]. Thus, estimating creatinine clearance is important to determine the extent to which DOAC clearance may be delayed.

Idarucizumab is, as its name suggests, a monoclonal antibody. It binds dabigatran with high affinity. While expensive, it is the only non-vitamin K oral anticoagulant reversal agent approved by the US Food and Drug Administration in the setting of urgent surgical procedures [77]. Idarucizumab is typically given as two boluses or infusions of 2.0–2.5 g doses at intervals less than 15 min apart [77]. In the United States, its efficacy is measured using the activated partial thromboplastin time (aPTT) or diluted thrombin time, though emergent procedures should not necessarily need to be delayed to check these levels [77]. The major clinical trial assessing the efficacy of idarucizumab showed that the median time to maximum dabigatran reversal was within 4 h and that the median time from antibody infusion to surgery was 1.6 h [82]. Moreover, 93% of surgeons reported that hemostasis was normal during surgery [82]. About 67% of patients requiring urgent surgery restarted antithrombotic therapy within 72 h of surgery [79, 82].

Chronic kidney disease (CKD) is associated with increased bleeding risk secondary to both uremic platelet dysfunction and accumulation of renally cleared DOACs, like dabigatran, in the blood [83, 84]. A subsequent reanalysis of data from the idarucizumab clinical trial further found that regardless of baseline renal function, idarucizumab completely reverses dabigatran [85]. After reversal with idarucizumab, 94.4% of patients with severe renal impairment (CrCl <30 mL/min, $n = 91$) achieved normal surgeon-perceived hemostasis and 0% experienced any bleeding 24 h postoperatively [85]. Comparatively, 93.6% of patients with normal baseline renal function (CrCl ≥80 mL/min, $n = 108$) achieved normal surgeon-perceived hemostasis, and 2.1% experienced bleeding 24 h postoperatively [85]. Patients with severe renal impairment were found to experience re-elevation of dabigatran levels 12–24 h after reversal [85]. Thus, in the setting of urgent or emergent spine surgery, idarucizumab can reverse dabigatran in patients with renal impairment. That said, signs of bleeding should be carefully monitored in the postoperative period.

Andexanet is a recombinant factor Xa variant used to reverse the factor Xa antagonists, like rivaroxaban, apixaban, and edoxaban. Andexanet has been shown to effectively reduce factor Xa activity and allow for excellent or good hemostatic efficacy (defined for intracranial hemorrhage as excellent: ≤20% increase in hemorrhage volume at 12 h compared to 1 h, and good, ≤35% increase in hemorrhage volume at 12 h compared to 1 h) 12 h after administration [86]. With that said, andexanet is currently approved only for the purpose of reversing major bleeding associated with factor Xa inhibitors.

Ciraparantag is a small, synthetic cation which purportedly binds to all non-vitamin K antagonists as well as heparins and calcium channel chelators [77]. To date, clinical trials are still assessing its safety and efficacy in reversing edoxaban, LMWH, and UFH.

Since no direct reversal agents are currently approved for factor Xa inhibitor reversal in the setting of urgent or emergent surgical procedures, alternative methods of reversing anticoagulation have been considered. Current guidelines state that four-factor PCC is a viable option [77, 79, 87, 88], though the safety and efficacy of PCC for factor Xa antagonists have yet to be rigorously studied in the general population, let alone among older adults [89]. Ultimately, while it may be feasible to reverse factor Xa inhibitors with PCC, the decision to do so requires consideration of both clinical context and the prospect of bleeding during surgery.

Heparin Compounds

Unfractionated Heparin

Generally, patients will only be taking UFH while in the hospital. Since UFH has a plasma half-life of 45–90 min, reversal of its anticoagulant effects can often be achieved by simply stopping UFH administration, even in the setting of emergent surgery [80].

Andexanet, the recombinant factor Xa variant from the previous section, has also been purported to reverse UFH. In the case that it is not possible surgery cannot be delayed while UFH is stopped, protamine sulfate has been approved for the reversal of UFH. Protamine is typically administered gradually at a dose of 1 mg protamine sulfate for every 80–100 units of UFH given in within 30 min, 0.5 mg protamine sulfate for every 80–100 units of UFH given in the last 30–60 min, and 0.25–0.35 mg protamine sulfate for every 80–100 units of UFH given more than 2 h ago [76]. By itself, protamine is an anticoagulant, so excess protamine can lead to increased bleeding [76]. It is therefore suggested to err on the side of less protamine when reversing UFH.

LMWH

LMWH has a longer half-life than UFH (4 h vs. 45–90 min), so its effects can sometimes be reversed by simple cessation of the agent. When surgery cannot be delayed, protamine sulfate can still be administered. Notably, protamine sulfate is less effective at reversing the effects of LMWH than UFH, and its safety and efficacy has only been demonstrated in small retrospective studies. When reversing LMWH, protamine sulfate is dosed at 1 mg for every 1000 units of LMWH given within 4–8 h [76, 80]. Lower doses can be used if the last dose of LMWH was given longer than 8 h ago [80].

Fondaparinux

To date, there is no FDA-approved reversal agent for fondaparinux. Importantly, protamine sulfate has no activity against fondaparinux. While recombinant factor VIIa has been given in the setting of major bleeding to attenuate the effects of fondaparinux [80], no studies to date have assessed safe and effective methods for agent reversal in the setting of urgent/emergent surgery, let alone among the older adult population specifically.

Special Considerations

Changes in Body Composition

Natural aging leads to changes in body composition, which must be considered when managing medications for the elderly prior to spine surgery. Notably, older adults tend to have a lower proportion of lean muscle and total body water, which ultimately leads to a relative increased proportion of total body fat [90, 91]. These changes alter the pharmacokinetics and pharmacodynamics of antithrombotic agents.

Pharmacokinetics

Pharmacokinetics refers to the absorption, distribution, metabolism, and elimination of compounds which enter the body. As adults age, pharmacokinetics change based on alterations in body composition and physiologic function. The rest of this section will focus on age-related changes in the pharmacokinetics for antithrombotic agents important for spine surgery patients.

Absorption

To date, there is no consensus on the effects of aging on the absorption of most drugs [91], let alone antithrombotic agents. While studies have shown that older adults have decreased gastric enzyme secretion [92] and decreased intestinal absorption [93], the clinical implications of these changes are not yet clear. To date, there exists no standardized method of measuring drug absorption for older adults. Likely for that reason, studies assessing the clinical significance of drug absorption in humans have provided mixed results. Regardless, changes in absorption are unlikely to significantly impact clinical outcomes for older spine surgery patients [94].

Volume of Distribution

The major pharmacokinetic change that occurs with aging is a decreased volume of distribution (V_D) for water-soluble drugs [91] due to an increased relative proportion of total body fat. Among anticoagulants, warfarin and heparin are both relatively water-soluble and therefore have a low V_D. For older adults, the V_D of these medications becomes even lower, resulting in higher serum concentrations and increased risk for drug toxicity.

Protein Binding

Warfarin is a polar, acidic compound which remains bound to albumin in vivo. As adults age, the production of albumin decreases. Theoretically, this could lead to higher serum levels of free warfarin and increased drug-drug interactions [91]. However, decreased protein binding has been shown to have minimal clinical significance [95].

Clearance

Reduced clearance is a major change associated with age. Clearance of most medications occurs through the liver or kidneys [94]. Reduced physiologic functioning of these organs contributes to increased toxicity associated with these medications [94]. Anticoagulants differ in the organ by which they are cleared. For example, warfarin is primarily cleared by the liver, while all DOACs are at least partially cleared by the kidneys [90]. The rest of this section will discuss the effects of impaired hepatic and renal function on the clearance of relevant anticoagulants.

Hepatic Impairment

The liver produces several molecules vital for clotting and fibrinogenesis, including antithrombin III and the factors of the coagulation cascade. Patients with hepatic impairment have a decreased ability to produce these compounds. However, contrary to popular belief, patients with liver disease are not protected from thrombotic events. Patients with hepatic impairment are, in fact, at risk for both bleeding and thrombosis simultaneously [96]. Today, nonalcoholic fatty liver disease (NAFLD) is the most common cause of liver disease in the United States, with an estimated prevalence of 30–40% among US adults [97]. Patients with liver impairment secondary to NAFLD are likely to also have cardiovascular compromise associated with obesity and are at greater risk for hepatocellular carcinoma [97]—both risk factors for VTE [57] As most clinical trials studying the effects of oral anticoagulants excluded patients with liver disease, management of oral anticoagulants for patients with liver disease is unclear.

Renal Impairment

Among adults 60 years and older, 39.4% have chronic kidney disease (CKD) [98]. CKD, akin to liver disease, puts patients at increased risk for both VTE and bleeding [99]. The risk of VTE increases secondary to increased levels of procoagulant factors, potential treatment with erythropoietin analogs, and decreased levels of endogenous anticoagulant and fibrinolytic factors [99]. The risk of bleeding, on the other hand, is at least partially due to dysfunctional platelets secondary to uremic toxin accumulation [99]. The risk of bleeding increases when patients with renal impairment take oral anticoagulants. In fact, patients with CKD are four times more likely to have an INR > 4.0 than patients without CKD [100], which significantly increases the risk of bleeding intra- and postoperatively. Risk scores have been used to predict the risk of bleeding following initiation of warfarin, including the HEMORR$_2$HAGES and HAS-BLED scores (Table 2.1) [101, 102].

Among the DOACs, dabigatran has the largest extent of renal clearance [103]. Therefore, especially for spine surgery patients on dabigatran with CKD, glomerular filtration rate must be closely monitored throughout their hospital stay. Management of DOACs should consider the patient's other comorbidities, other medications, need for dialysis, and extent of surgery.

Warfarin, though primarily cleared by the liver, exhibits decreased clearance among patients with CKD when compared to healthy controls [100]. The pharmacokinetics and pharmacodynamics of renally cleared anticoagulants are not well-established in patients with CKD receiving hemodialysis [104]. Moreover, consultation with anticoagulation services is important to assure individualized weight of risks and benefits for patients with CKD who are taking anticoagulants in the perioperative period [99].

Table 2.1 Two alternative score-based guidelines: (a) HEMORR$_2$HAGES and (b) HAS-BLED utilized to estimate the risk of bleeding following initiation of warfarin

HEMORR$_2$HAGES score		
H	Hepatic or renal disease	1
E	Ethanol abuse	1
M	Malignancy	1
O	Older age	1
R	Reduced platelet count or function	1
R$_2$	Rebleeding risk	2
H	Hypertension	1
A	Anemia	1
G	Genetic factors	1
E	Excessive fall risk	1
S	Stroke	1
Maximum score		12
HAS-BLED score		
H	Hypertension	1
A	Abnormal liver or renal function	1 or 2
S	Stroke	1
B	Bleeding	1
L	Labile INR	1
E	Elderly (age >65)	2
D	Drugs or alcohol	1 or 2
Maximum score		9

Among antiplatelets, unfractionated heparin is preferred over LMWH compounds when required for perioperative anticoagulation or bridging therapy in patients with CKD since UFH levels are easily monitored with the aPTT and the effects are easily reversible [99].

Fall Risk

Falls are the most common unintentional cause of hospitalization for patients older than 65 years of age [105]. In fact, one fall doubles the risk of a subsequent fall [106]. For older spine surgery patients, the risk of falls is significant and must be considered when managing antithrombotic therapy. Patients taking antithrombotic agents are at risk of bleeding from even minor trauma. Pre-fall anticoagulation with warfarin has been associated with a sixfold increased fall-related mortality than no anticoagulation [107]. Furthermore, in a patient population in which osteoporosis/osteopenia is a significant medical comorbidity, ground-level falls have the potential to cause extensive damage.

Depending on presenting neurologic deficits, patients undergoing spine surgery could be at greater risk for falls than non-spine surgical procedures. However, there is no evidence to date to suggest that spine surgery itself is associated with increased falls.

Diet

With age, dietary habits sometimes change. Older adults may alter their lifestyle to adjust to the social changes of retirement, their physical ability, and socioeconomic factors. The prevalence of depression peaks among older adults, which can further alter dietary habits. Older adults may also be on medications which have gastrointestinal side effects such that some foods are poorly tolerated, contributing more to changes in diet.

Among anticoagulants, warfarin pharmacokinetics are most likely to be associated with dietary intake. As mentioned earlier in this chapter, warfarin effectively decreases vitamin K activity. Increased vitamin K intake (perhaps via supplements or consumption of leafy green vegetables) can decrease the clinical efficacy of warfarin [108]. Therefore, it is important for spine surgeons to discuss dietary habits with their older patients prior to surgery.

Polypharmacy

Among the medications discussed in this chapter, oral anticoagulants have been most extensively studied with respect to polypharmacy. Warfarin is metabolized through the CYP450 system in the liver [109]. This makes it vulnerable to many drug-drug interactions [109, 110]. Specifically, the risk of bleeding is significantly greater for patients taking warfarin and any other medication with anticoagulant properties, including aspirin [111], nonsteroidal anti-inflammatory drugs (NSAIDs) [111], and selective serotonin reuptake inhibitors (SSRIs) [112]. Among adults aged 65 years and older, the prevalence of major depressive disorder is approximately 1–5% [113], though clinically significant symptoms of depression manifest in 15% of older adults [114]. Furthermore, the prevalence of depression is estimated to be 10–12% among hospitalized older adult patients [114]. It is vital for spine surgeons to thoroughly review medications with their patient prior to spine surgery. The risk of bleeding when taking warfarin and one or more of these medications increases even in the absence of an increase in INR [110].

Several antimicrobials classically affect the function of warfarin through two mechanisms: (1) elimination of vitamin K-producing gut bacteria (minor) and (2) altering metabolism through the CYP450 system (major) [108]. Inhibitors of the CYP450 system like metronidazole, trimethoprim-sulfamethoxazole, and ciprofloxacin tend to potentiate the anticoagulant effects of warfarin [109]. Inducers of the CYP450 system, like rifampin, attenuate warfarin's anticoagulant properties [109]. Spine surgery patients, especially when they have indwelling Foley catheters in the postoperative period, may develop urinary tract infections (UTIs) and require treatment with one of the aforementioned medications. UTIs in the setting of recent spine surgery necessitate a discussion about warfarin management.

Changes in thyroid function also alter INR. In patients with hyperthyroidism, for example, INR increases [110]. Therefore, patients with thyroid disorders on thyroid replacement medication (i.e., levothyroxine) or those on thyroid suppressant medications (i.e., methimazole) should be counseled to take those medications as directed by their endocrinologist. Furthermore, medications that alter thyroid function (i.e., amiodarone) must also be carefully managed during the perioperative period, usually with input from the physician prescribing the given medication [110].

Dyslipidemia is a chronic condition which predisposes cardiovascular disease. The prevalence of dyslipidemia, not surprisingly, increases with age [115]. Some older adults may be started on fibrates to lower triglycerides and increase HDL [115]. Spine surgeons should be cautious when managing perioperative warfarin for patients concomitantly taking fibrates, for fibrates have been shown to potentiate the effects of warfarin [110].

Future Directions

This chapter provided approximate guidelines for antithrombotic therapy management by medication. There has been immense progress in the understanding of the risks and benefits of antithrombotic therapy for older spine surgery patients. However, no standardized guidelines have garnered acceptance among spine surgeons to date, let alone management for older adults with multiple medical comorbidities. The American population is aging, and more adults are living with chronic medical conditions. Therefore, while it is challenging to perform randomized control trials to assess the effects of antithrombotic therapy on patient outcomes, developing standardized guidelines for spine surgery patients will be important for the future of spine surgery. Some potential directions for future work include randomized control trials (1) assessing the risks of bleeding versus thrombosis for intraoperative anticoagulation in patients undergoing lumbar spine surgery via anterior approaches, (2) comparing LMWH to UFH in perioperative anticoagulant bridging, and (3) identifying ideal antiplatelet management for older adults on dual antiplatelet therapy for intracardiac stents.

References

1. Bracey AW. Perioperative management of antithrombotic and antiplatelet therapy. Tex Heart Inst J. 2015;42(3):239–42. https://doi.org/10.14503/THIJ-15-5066.

2. Cheng JS, Arnold PM, Anderson PA, Fischer D, Dettori JR. Anticoagulation risk in spine surgery. Spine. 2010;35(9 Suppl):S117–24. https://doi.org/10.1097/BRS.0b013e3181d833d4.
3. Douketis JD, Bakhsh E. Perioperative management of antithrombotic therapy. Pol Arch Med Wewn. 2008;118(4):201–8.
4. Kepler CK, McKenzie J, Kreitz T, Vaccaro A. Venous thromboembolism prophylaxis in spine surgery. J Am Acad Orthop Surg. 2018;26(14):489–500. https://doi.org/10.5435/JAAOS-D-17-00561.
5. Porto GBF, Jeffrey Wessell DO, Alvarado A, Arnold PM, Buchholz AL. Anticoagulation and Spine Surgery. Glob Spine J. 2020;10(1 Suppl):53S–64S. https://doi.org/10.1177/2192568219852051.
6. Rockson HB, DiPaola CP, Connolly PJ, Stauff MP. Venous thromboembolism prophylaxis for patients having elective spine surgery: when, why, and how much. J Bone Joint Surg Am. 2019;101(13):1220–9. https://doi.org/10.2106/JBJS.18.00849.
7. Solaru S, Alluri RK, Wang JC, Hah RJ. Venous thromboembolism prophylaxis in elective spine surgery. Glob Spine J. 2021;11:1148. https://doi.org/10.1177/2192568220962439.
8. Takahashi H, Yokoyama Y, Iida Y, Terashima F, Hasegawa K, Saito T, et al. Incidence of venous thromboembolism after spine surgery. J Orthop Sci. 2012;17(2):114–7. https://doi.org/10.1007/s00776-011-0188-2.
9. Wang T, Yang SD, Huang WZ, Liu FY, Wang H, Ding WY. Factors predicting venous thromboembolism after spine surgery. Medicine. 2016;95(52):e5776. https://doi.org/10.1097/MD.0000000000005776.
10. Cox JB, Weaver KJ, Neal DW, Jacob RP, Hoh DJ. Decreased incidence of venous thromboembolism after spine surgery with early multimodal prophylaxis: clinical article. J Neurosurg Spine. 2014;21(4):677–84. https://doi.org/10.3171/2014.6.SPINE13447.
11. Catre MG. Anticoagulation in spinal surgery. A critical review of the literature. Can J Surg. 1997;40(6):413–9.
12. Ferree BA. Deep venous thrombosis following lumbar laminotomy and laminectomy Orthopedics. 1994;17(1):35–8.
13. Ferree BA, Stern PJ, Jolson RS, Roberts JM, Kahn A III. Deep venous thrombosis after spinal surgery. Spine. 1993;18(3):315–9. https://doi.org/10.1097/00007632-199303000-00001.
14. Oda T, Fuji T, Kato Y, Fujita S, Kanemitsu N. Deep venous thrombosis after posterior spinal surgery. Spine. 2000;25(22):2962–7. https://doi.org/10.1097/00007632-200011150-00019.
15. Rokito SE, Schwartz MC, Neuwirth MG. Deep vein thrombosis after major reconstructive spinal surgery. Spine. 1996;21(7):853–8. https://doi.org/10.1097/00007632-199604010-00016; discussion 9.
16. Paneni F, Diaz Canestro C, Libby P, Luscher TF, Camici GG. The aging cardiovascular system: understanding it at the cellular and clinical levels. J Am Coll Cardiol. 2017;69(15):1952–67. https://doi.org/10.1016/j.jacc.2017.01.064.
17. North BJ, Sinclair DA. The intersection between aging and cardiovascular disease. Circ Res. 2012;110(8):1097–108. https://doi.org/10.1161/CIRCRESAHA.111.246876.
18. Rosendaal FR. Venous thrombosis: prevalence and interaction of risk factors. Haemostasis. 1999;29(Suppl S1):1–9. https://doi.org/10.1159/000054106.
19. Kovacic JC, Moreno P, Nabel EG, Hachinski V, Fuster V. Cellular senescence, vascular disease, and aging: part 2 of a 2-part review: clinical vascular disease in the elderly. Circulation. 2011;123(17):1900–10. https://doi.org/10.1161/CIRCULATIONAHA.110.009118.
20. Bochenek ML, Schutz E, Schafer K. Endothelial cell senescence and thrombosis: ageing clots. Thromb Res. 2016;147:36–45. https://doi.org/10.1016/j.thromres.2016.09.019.
21. Dominguez LJ, Galioto A, Ferlisi A, Pineo A, Putignano E, Belvedere M, et al. Ageing, lifestyle modifications, and cardiovascular disease in developing countries. J Nutr Health Aging. 2006;10(2):143–9.
22. Engbers MJ, van Hylckama VA, Rosendaal FR. Venous thrombosis in the elderly: incidence, risk factors and risk groups. J Thromb Haemost. 2010;8(10):2105–12. https://doi.org/10.1111/j.1538-7836.2010.03986.x.

23. Douketis JD, Spyropoulos AC, Spencer FA, Mayr M, Jaffer AK, Eckman MH, et al. Perioperative management of antithrombotic therapy: antithrombotic therapy and prevention of thrombosis, 9th ed: American College of Chest Physicians Evidence-Based Clinical Practice Guidelines. Chest. 2012;141(2 Suppl):e326S–e50S. https://doi.org/10.1378/chest.11-2298.
24. Chugh SS, Havmoeller R, Narayanan K, Singh D, Rienstra M, Benjamin EJ, et al. Worldwide epidemiology of atrial fibrillation: a global burden of disease 2010 study. Circulation. 2014;129(8):837–47. https://doi.org/10.1161/CIRCULATIONAHA.113.005119.
25. Kornej J, Borschel CS, Benjamin EJ, Schnabel RB. Epidemiology of atrial fibrillation in the 21st century: novel methods and new insights. Circ Res. 2020;127(1):4–20. https://doi.org/10.1161/CIRCRESAHA.120.316340.
26. Heidenreich PA, Trogdon JG, Khavjou OA, Butler J, Dracup K, Ezekowitz MD, et al. Forecasting the future of cardiovascular disease in the United States: a policy statement from the American Heart Association. Circulation. 2011;123(8):933–44. https://doi.org/10.1161/CIR.0b013e31820a55f5.
27. Lutsey PL, Norby FL, Alonso A, Cushman M, Chen LY, Michos ED, et al. Atrial fibrillation and venous thromboembolism: evidence of bidirectionality in the Atherosclerosis Risk in Communities Study. J Thromb Haemost. 2018;16(4):670–9. https://doi.org/10.1111/jth.13974.
28. Wolf PA, Abbott RD, Kannel WB. Atrial fibrillation as an independent risk factor for stroke: the Framingham Study. Stroke. 1991;22(8):983–8. https://doi.org/10.1161/01.str.22.8.983.
29. Hart RG, Pearce LA, Aguilar MI. Meta-analysis: antithrombotic therapy to prevent stroke in patients who have nonvalvular atrial fibrillation. Ann Intern Med. 2007;146(12):857–67. https://doi.org/10.7326/0003-4819-146-12-200706190-00007.
30. Ruff CT, Giugliano RP, Braunwald E, Hoffman EB, Deenadayalu N, Ezekowitz MD, et al. Comparison of the efficacy and safety of new oral anticoagulants with warfarin in patients with atrial fibrillation: a meta-analysis of randomised trials. Lancet. 2014;383(9921):955–62. https://doi.org/10.1016/S0140-6736(13)62343-0.
31. Fuentes AV, Pineda MD, Venkata KCN. Comprehension of top 200 prescribed drugs in the US as a resource for pharmacy teaching, training and practice. Pharmacy. 2018;6(2):43. https://doi.org/10.3390/pharmacy6020043.
32. Oprea AD, Popescu WM. Perioperative management of antiplatelet therapy. Br J Anaesth. 2013;111(Suppl 1):i3–17. https://doi.org/10.1093/bja/aet402.
33. Peters AT, Mutharasan RK. Aspirin for prevention of cardiovascular disease. JAMA. 2020;323(7):676. https://doi.org/10.1001/jama.2019.18425.
34. O'Brien CW, Juraschek SP, Wee CC. Prevalence of aspirin use for primary prevention of cardiovascular disease in the united states: results from the 2017 national health interview survey. Ann Intern Med. 2019;171(8):596–8. https://doi.org/10.7326/M19-0953.
35. McNeil JJ, Woods RL, Nelson MR, Reid CM, Kirpach B, Wolfe R, et al. Effect of aspirin on disability-free survival in the healthy elderly. N Engl J Med. 2018;379(16):1499–508. https://doi.org/10.1056/NEJMoa1800722.
36. McNeil JJ, Wolfe R, Woods RL, Tonkin AM, Donnan GA, Nelson MR, et al. Effect of aspirin on cardiovascular events and bleeding in the healthy elderly. N Engl J Med. 2018;379(16):1509–18. https://doi.org/10.1056/NEJMoa1805819.
37. Shufelt CL, Manson JE. Aspirin for primary prevention of cardiovascular disease in women. Menopause. 2020;27(5):605–6. https://doi.org/10.1097/GME.0000000000001547.
38. Yazdanyar A, Newman AB. The burden of cardiovascular disease in the elderly: morbidity, mortality, and costs. Clin Geriatr Med. 2009;25(4):563–77, vii. https://doi.org/10.1016/j.cger.2009.07.007.
39. Epstein NE. When to stop anticoagulation, anti-platelet aggregates, and non-steroidal anti-inflammatories (NSAIDs) prior to spine surgery. Surg Neurol Int. 2019;10:45. https://doi.org/10.25259/SNI-54-2019.

40. Douketis JD, Darvish-Kazem S, Spencer N, Tafur A. Perioperative management of patients who are receiving antiplatelet therapy: a case-based, evidence-informed approach. Pol Arch Intern Med. 2018;128(12):771–8. https://doi.org/10.20452/pamw.4403.
41. Levine GN, Bates ER, Bittl JA, Brindis RG, Fihn SD, Fleisher LA et al. 2016 ACC/AHA guideline focused update on duration of dual antiplatelet therapy in patients with coronary artery disease: a report of the American College of Cardiology/American Heart Association Task Force on Clinical Practice Guidelines: An Update of the 2011 ACCF/AHA/SCAI Guideline for Percutaneous Coronary Intervention, 2011 ACCF/AHA Guideline for Coronary Artery Bypass Graft Surgery, 2012 ACC/AHA/ACP/AATS/PCNA/SCAI/STS Guideline for the Diagnosis and Management of Patients With Stable Ischemic Heart Disease, 2013 ACCF/AHA Guideline for the Management of ST-Elevation Myocardial Infarction, 2014 AHA/ACC Guideline for the Management of Patients With Non-ST-Elevation Acute Coronary Syndromes, and 2014 ACC/AHA Guideline on perioperative cardiovascular evaluation and management of patients undergoing noncardiac surgery. Circulation 2016;134(10):e123–55. https://doi.org/10.1161/CIR.0000000000000404.
42. Secco GG, Parisi R, Mirabella F, Fattori R, Genoni G, Agostoni P, et al. P2Y12 inhibitors: pharmacologic mechanism and clinical relevance. Cardiovasc Hematol Agents Med Chem. 2013;11(2):101–5. https://doi.org/10.2174/1871525711311020005.
43. Damman P, Woudstra P, Kuijt WJ, de Winter RJ, James SK. P2Y12 platelet inhibition in clinical practice. J Thromb Thrombolysis. 2012;33(2):143–53. https://doi.org/10.1007/s11239-011-0667-5.
44. Diener HC, Cunha L, Forbes C, Sivenius J, Smets P, Lowenthal A. European Stroke Prevention Study. 2. Dipyridamole and acetylsalicylic acid in the secondary prevention of stroke. J Neurol Sci. 1996;143(1–2):1–13. https://doi.org/10.1016/s0022-510x(96)00308-5.
45. January CT, Wann LS, Calkins H, Chen LY, Cigarroa JE, Cleveland JC, Jr. et al. 2019 AHA/ACC/HRS Focused Update of the 2014 AHA/ACC/HRS Guideline for the Management of Patients With Atrial Fibrillation: a report of the American College of Cardiology/American Heart Association Task Force on Clinical Practice Guidelines and the Heart Rhythm Society. J Am Coll Cardiol 2019;74(1):104–32. https://doi.org/10.1016/j.jacc.2019.01.011.
46. Scotti P, Seguin C, Lo BWY, de Guise E, Troquet JM, Marcoux J. Antithrombotic agents and traumatic brain injury in the elderly population: hemorrhage patterns and outcomes. J Neurosurg. 2019;133:486–95. https://doi.org/10.3171/2019.4.JNS19252.
47. Xian Y, Xu H, O'Brien EC, Shah S, Thomas L, Pencina MJ, et al. Clinical effectiveness of direct oral anticoagulants vs warfarin in older patients with atrial fibrillation and ischemic stroke: findings from the patient-centered research into outcomes stroke patients prefer and effectiveness research (PROSPER) study. JAMA Neurol. 2019;76:1192. https://doi.org/10.1001/jamaneurol.2019.2099.
48. Shaw JR, Woodfine JD, Douketis J, Schulman S, Carrier M. Perioperative interruption of direct oral anticoagulants in patients with atrial fibrillation: a systematic review and meta-analysis. Res Pract Thromb Haemost. 2018;2(2):282–90. https://doi.org/10.1002/rth2.12076.
49. Tafur A, Douketis J. Perioperative management of anticoagulant and antiplatelet therapy. Heart. 2018;104(17):1461–7. https://doi.org/10.1136/heartjnl-2016-310581.
50. Murphy D, McCulloch CE, Lin F, Banerjee T, Bragg-Gresham JL, Eberhardt MS, et al. Trends in prevalence of chronic kidney disease in the United States. Ann Intern Med. 2016;165(7):473–81. https://doi.org/10.7326/M16-0273.
51. Horlocker TT, Vandermeuelen E, Kopp SL, Gogarten W, Leffert LR, Benzon HT. Regional anesthesia in the patient receiving antithrombotic or thrombolytic therapy: American Society of Regional Anesthesia and Pain Medicine evidence-based guidelines (Fourth Edition). Reg Anesth Pain Med. 2018;43(3):263–309. https://doi.org/10.1097/AAP.0000000000000763.
52. Narouze S, Benzon HT, Provenzano D, Buvanendran A, De Andres J, Deer T et al. Interventional Spine and Pain Procedures in Patients on Antiplatelet and Anticoagulant Medications (Second Edition): Guidelines From the American Society of Regional Anesthesia

and Pain Medicine, the European Society of Regional Anaesthesia and Pain Therapy, the American Academy of Pain Medicine, the International Neuromodulation Society, the North American Neuromodulation Society, and the World Institute of Pain. Reg Anesth Pain Med 2018;43(3):225–62. https://doi.org/10.1097/AAP.0000000000000700.
53. Bauer KA. Fondaparinux: basic properties and efficacy and safety in venous thromboembolism prophylaxis. Am J Orthop. 2002;31(11 Suppl):4–10.
54. Baumgartner C, de Kouchkovsky I, Whitaker E, Fang MC. Periprocedural bridging in patients with venous thromboembolism: a systematic review. Am J Med. 2019;132(6):722–32.e7. https://doi.org/10.1016/j.amjmed.2019.01.004.
55. Siegal D, Yudin J, Kaatz S, Douketis JD, Lim W, Spyropoulos AC. Periprocedural heparin bridging in patients receiving vitamin K antagonists: systematic review and meta-analysis of bleeding and thromboembolic rates. Circulation. 2012;126(13):1630–9. https://doi.org/10.1161/CIRCULATIONAHA.112.105221.
56. Douketis JD, Spyropoulos AC, Kaatz S, Becker RC, Caprini JA, Dunn AS, et al. Perioperative bridging anticoagulation in patients with atrial fibrillation. N Engl J Med. 2015;373(9):823–33. https://doi.org/10.1056/NEJMoa1501035.
57. Anderson FA Jr, Spencer FA. Risk factors for venous thromboembolism. Circulation. 2003;107(23 Suppl 1):I9–16. https://doi.org/10.1161/01.CIR.0000078469.07362.E6.
58. Kulkarni SS, Lowery GL, Ross RE, Ravi Sankar K, Lykomitros V. Arterial complications following anterior lumbar interbody fusion: report of eight cases. Eur Spine J. 2003;12(1):48–54. https://doi.org/10.1007/s00586-002-0460-4.
59. Sim EM, Claydon MH, Parker RM, Malham GM. Brief intraoperative heparinization and blood loss in anterior lumbar spine surgery. J Neurosurg Spine. 2015;23(3):309–13. https://doi.org/10.3171/2014.12.SPINE14888.
60. Inamasu J, Guiot BH. Vascular injury and complication in neurosurgical spine surgery. Acta Neurochir. 2006;148(4):375–87. https://doi.org/10.1007/s00701-005-0669-1.
61. Chen CM, Ashjian P, Disa JJ, Cordeiro PG, Pusic AL, Mehrara BJ. Is the use of intraoperative heparin safe? Plast Reconstr Surg. 2008;121(3):49e–53e. https://doi.org/10.1097/01.prs.0000299267.84139.2a.
62. Geerts WH, Bergqvist D, Pineo GF, Heit JA, Samama CM, Lassen MR, et al. Prevention of venous thromboembolism: American College of Chest Physicians Evidence-Based Clinical Practice Guidelines (8th Edition). Chest. 2008;133(6 Suppl):381S–453S. https://doi.org/10.1378/chest.08-0656.
63. Gould MK, Garcia DA, Wren SM, Karanicolas PJ, Arcelus JI, Heit JA, et al. Prevention of VTE in nonorthopedic surgical patients: antithrombotic therapy and prevention of thrombosis, 9th ed: American College of Chest Physicians Evidence-Based Clinical Practice Guidelines. Chest. 2012;141(2 Suppl):e227S–e77S. https://doi.org/10.1378/chest.11-2297.
64. Kearon C, Akl EA, Comerota AJ, Prandoni P, Bounameaux H, Goldhaber SZ, et al. Antithrombotic therapy for VTE disease: antithrombotic therapy and prevention of thrombosis, 9th ed: American College of Chest Physicians Evidence-Based Clinical Practice Guidelines. Chest. 2012;141(2 Suppl):e419S–e96S. https://doi.org/10.1378/chest.11-2301.
65. Bono CM, Watters WC III, Heggeness MH, Resnick DK, Shaffer WO, Baisden J, et al. An evidence-based clinical guideline for the use of antithrombotic therapies in spine surgery. Spine J. 2009;9(12):1046–51. https://doi.org/10.1016/j.spinee.2009.09.005.
66. Agarwal N, Zenonos GA, Agarwal P, Walch FJ, Roach E, Stokes SJ, et al. Risk-to-benefit ratio of venous thromboembolism prophylaxis for neurosurgical procedures at a quaternary referral center. Neurosurgery. 2019;84(2):355–61. https://doi.org/10.1093/neuros/nyy035.
67. Lieber BA, Han J, Appelboom G, Taylor BE, Han B, Agarwal N, et al. Association of steroid use with deep venous thrombosis and pulmonary embolism in neurosurgical patients: a national database analysis. World Neurosurg. 2016;89:126–32. https://doi.org/10.1016/j.wneu.2016.01.033.
68. Gibbs NM. Venous thrombosis of the lower limbs with particular reference to bed-rest. Br J Surg. 1957;45(191):209–36. https://doi.org/10.1002/bjs.18004519102.

69. Fineberg SJ, Nandyala SV, Marquez-Lara A, Oglesby M, Patel AA, Singh K. Incidence and risk factors for postoperative delirium after lumbar spine surgery. Spine. 2013;38(20):1790–6. https://doi.org/10.1097/BRS.0b013e3182a0d507.
70. Kobayashi K, Ando K, Kato F, Kanemura T, Sato K, Hachiya Y, et al. Predictors of prolonged length of stay after lumbar interbody fusion: a multicenter study. Glob Spine J. 2019;9(5):466–72. https://doi.org/10.1177/2192568218800054.
71. Devereaux PJ, Mrkobrada M, Sessler DI, Leslie K, Alonso-Coello P, Kurz A, et al. Aspirin in patients undergoing noncardiac surgery. N Engl J Med. 2014;370(16):1494–503. https://doi.org/10.1056/NEJMoa1401105.
72. Graham MM, Sessler DI, Parlow JL, Biccard BM, Guyatt G, Leslie K, et al. Aspirin in patients with previous percutaneous coronary intervention undergoing noncardiac surgery. Ann Intern Med. 2018;168(4):237–44. https://doi.org/10.7326/M17-2341.
73. Mehta SR, Bainey KR, Cantor WJ, Lordkipanidze M, Marquis-Gravel G, Robinson SD, et al. 2018 Canadian Cardiovascular Society/Canadian Association of Interventional Cardiology focused update of the guidelines for the use of antiplatelet therapy. Can J Cardiol. 2018;34(3):214–33. https://doi.org/10.1016/j.cjca.2017.12.012.
74. Douketis JD, Spyropoulos AC, Duncan J, Carrier M, Le Gal G, Tafur AJ, et al. Perioperative management of patients with atrial fibrillation receiving a direct oral anticoagulant. JAMA Intern Med. 2019;179:1469. https://doi.org/10.1001/jamainternmed.2019.2431.
75. Strom RG, Frempong-Boadu AK. Low-molecular-weight heparin prophylaxis 24 to 36 hours after degenerative spine surgery: risk of hemorrhage and venous thromboembolism. Spine. 2013;38(23):E1498–502. https://doi.org/10.1097/BRS.0b013e3182a4408d.
76. Campbell PG, Sen A, Yadla S, Jabbour P, Jallo J. Emergency reversal of antiplatelet agents in patients presenting with an intracranial hemorrhage: a clinical review. World Neurosurg. 2010;74(2–3):279–85. https://doi.org/10.1016/j.wneu.2010.05.030.
77. Levy JH, Douketis J, Weitz JI. Reversal agents for non-vitamin K antagonist oral anticoagulants. Nat Rev Cardiol. 2018;15(5):273–81. https://doi.org/10.1038/nrcardio.2017.223.
78. Angelo M, Gutmann B, Adami M, Zagler B, Zelger A, Pechlaner C, et al. Emergency correction of coagulation before major surgery in two elderly patients on oral anticoagulation. Thromb J. 2007;5:1. https://doi.org/10.1186/1477-9560-5-1.
79. Levy JH, Douketis J, Steiner T, Goldstein JN, Milling TJ. Prothrombin complex concentrates for perioperative vitamin K antagonist and non-vitamin K anticoagulant reversal. Anesthesiology. 2018;129(6):1171–84. https://doi.org/10.1097/ALN.0000000000002399.
80. Thomas S, Makris M. The reversal of anticoagulation in clinical practice. Clin Med. 2018;18(4):314–9. https://doi.org/10.7861/clinmedicine.18-4-314.
81. Agarwal P, Abdullah KG, Ramayya AG, Nayak NR, Lucas TH. A Retrospective propensity score-matched early thromboembolic event analysis of prothrombin complex concentrate vs fresh frozen plasma for warfarin reversal prior to emergency neurosurgical procedures. Neurosurgery. 2018;82(6):877–86. https://doi.org/10.1093/neuros/nyx327.
82. Pollack CV Jr, Reilly PA, Eikelboom J, Glund S, Verhamme P, Bernstein RA, et al. Idarucizumab for dabigatran reversal. N Engl J Med. 2015;373(6):511–20. https://doi.org/10.1056/NEJMoa1502000.
83. Ocak G, Rookmaaker MB, Algra A, de Borst GJ, Doevendans PA, Kappelle LJ, et al. Chronic kidney disease and bleeding risk in patients at high cardiovascular risk: a cohort study. J Thromb Haemost. 2018;16(1):65–73. https://doi.org/10.1111/jth.13904.
84. Molnar AO, Bota SE, Garg AX, Harel Z, Lam N, McArthur E, et al. The risk of major hemorrhage with CKD. J Am Soc Nephrol. 2016;27(9):2825–32. https://doi.org/10.1681/ASN.2015050535.
85. Eikelboom JW, van Ryn J, Reilly P, Hylek EM, Elsaesser A, Glund S, et al. Dabigatran reversal with idarucizumab in patients with renal impairment. J Am Coll Cardiol. 2019;74(14):1760–8. https://doi.org/10.1016/j.jacc.2019.07.070.
86. Connolly SJ, Crowther M, Eikelboom JW, Gibson CM, Curnutte JT, Lawrence JH, et al. Full study report of andexanet alfa for bleeding associated with factor Xa inhibitors. N Engl J Med. 2019;380(14):1326–35. https://doi.org/10.1056/NEJMoa1814051.

87. Eerenberg ES, Kamphuisen PW, Sijpkens MK, Meijers JC, Buller HR, Levi M. Reversal of rivaroxaban and dabigatran by prothrombin complex concentrate: a randomized, placebo-controlled, crossover study in healthy subjects. Circulation. 2011;124(14):1573–9. https://doi.org/10.1161/CIRCULATIONAHA.111.029017.
88. Raval AN, Cigarroa JE, Chung MK, Diaz-Sandoval LJ, Diercks D, Piccini JP, et al. Management of patients on non-vitamin k antagonist oral anticoagulants in the acute care and periprocedural setting: a scientific statement from the American Heart Association. Circulation. 2017;135(10):e604–e33. https://doi.org/10.1161/CIR.0000000000000477.
89. Beynon C, Potzy A, Unterberg AW, Sakowitz OW. Emergency neurosurgical care in patients treated with apixaban: report of 2 cases. Am J Emerg Med. 2015;33(6):858.e5–7. https://doi.org/10.1016/j.ajem.2014.12.017.
90. Bauersachs RM, Herold J. Oral anticoagulation in the elderly and frail. Hamostaseologie. 2020;40(1):74–83. https://doi.org/10.1055/s-0040-1701476.
91. Mangoni AA, Jackson SH. Age-related changes in pharmacokinetics and pharmacodynamics: basic principles and practical applications. Br J Clin Pharmacol. 2004;57(1):6–14. https://doi.org/10.1046/j.1365-2125.2003.02007.x.
92. Kekki M, Samloff IM, Ihamaki T, Varis K, Siurala M. Age- and sex-related behaviour of gastric acid secretion at the population level. Scand J Gastroenterol. 1982;17(6):737–43. https://doi.org/10.3109/00365528209181087.
93. Corazza GR, Frazzoni M, Gatto MR, Gasbarrini G. Ageing and small-bowel mucosa: a morphometric study. Gerontology. 1986;32(1):60–5. https://doi.org/10.1159/000212766.
94. Crooks J, O'Malley K, Stevenson IH. Pharmacokinetics in the elderly. Clin Pharmacokinet. 1976;1(4):280–96. https://doi.org/10.2165/00003088-197601040-00003.
95. Benet LZ, Hoener BA. Changes in plasma protein binding have little clinical relevance. Clin Pharmacol Ther. 2002;71(3):115–21. https://doi.org/10.1067/mcp.2002.121829.
96. Qamar A, Vaduganathan M, Greenberger NJ, Giugliano RP. Oral anticoagulation in patients with liver disease. J Am Coll Cardiol. 2018;71(19):2162–75. https://doi.org/10.1016/j.jacc.2018.03.023.
97. Mitra S, De A, Chowdhury A. Epidemiology of non-alcoholic and alcoholic fatty liver diseases. Transl Gastroenterol Hepatol. 2020;5:16. https://doi.org/10.21037/tgh.2019.09.08.
98. Mallappallil M, Friedman EA, Delano BG, McFarlane SI, Salifu MO. Chronic kidney disease in the elderly: evaluation and management. Clin Pract. 2014;11(5):525–35. https://doi.org/10.2217/cpr.14.46.
99. Dager WE, Kiser TH. Systemic anticoagulation considerations in chronic kidney disease. Adv Chronic Kidney Dis. 2010;17(5):420–7. https://doi.org/10.1053/j.ackd.2010.06.002.
100. Limdi NA, Beasley TM, Baird MF, Goldstein JA, McGwin G, Arnett DK, et al. Kidney function influences warfarin responsiveness and hemorrhagic complications. J Am Soc Nephrol. 2009;20(4):912–21. https://doi.org/10.1681/ASN.2008070802.
101. Pisters R, Lane DA, Nieuwlaat R, de Vos CB, Crijns HJ, Lip GY. A novel user-friendly score (HAS-BLED) to assess 1-year risk of major bleeding in patients with atrial fibrillation: the Euro Heart Survey. Chest. 2010;138(5):1093–100. https://doi.org/10.1378/chest.10-0134.
102. Gage BF, Yan Y, Milligan PE, Waterman AD, Culverhouse R, Rich MW, et al. Clinical classification schemes for predicting hemorrhage: results from the National Registry of Atrial Fibrillation (NRAF). Am Heart J. 2006;151(3):713–9. https://doi.org/10.1016/j.ahj.2005.04.017.
103. Padrini R. Clinical pharmacokinetics and pharmacodynamics of direct oral anticoagulants in patients with renal failure. Eur J Drug Metab Pharmacokinet. 2019;44(1):1–12. https://doi.org/10.1007/s13318-018-0501-y.
104. Jain N, Reilly RF. Clinical pharmacology of oral anticoagulants in patients with kidney disease. Clin J Am Soc Nephrol. 2019;14(2):278–87. https://doi.org/10.2215/CJN.02170218.
105. Bergen G, Stevens MR, Burns ER. Falls and fall injuries among adults aged >/=65 years - United States, 2014. MMWR Morb Mortal Wkly Rep. 2016;65(37):993–8. https://doi.org/10.15585/mmwr.mm6537a2.

106. O'Loughlin JL, Robitaille Y, Boivin JF, Suissa S. Incidence of and risk factors for falls and injurious falls among the community-dwelling elderly. Am J Epidemiol. 1993;137(3):342–54. https://doi.org/10.1093/oxfordjournals.aje.a116681.
107. Franko J, Kish KJ, O'Connell BG, Subramanian S, Yuschak JV. Advanced age and preinjury warfarin anticoagulation increase the risk of mortality after head trauma. J Trauma. 2006;61(1):107–10. https://doi.org/10.1097/01.ta.0000224220.89528.fc.
108. Shearer MJ, Fu X, Booth SL. Vitamin K nutrition, metabolism, and requirements: current concepts and future research. Adv Nutr. 2012;3(2):182–95. https://doi.org/10.3945/an.111.001800.
109. Holbrook AM, Pereira JA, Labiris R, McDonald H, Douketis JD, Crowther M, et al. Systematic overview of warfarin and its drug and food interactions. Arch Intern Med. 2005;165(10):1095–106. https://doi.org/10.1001/archinte.165.10.1095.
110. Crader MF, Johns T, Arnold JK. Warfarin drug interactions. Treasure Island, FL: StatPearls; 2020.
111. Shireman TI, Howard PA, Kresowik TF, Ellerbeck EF. Combined anticoagulant-antiplatelet use and major bleeding events in elderly atrial fibrillation patients. Stroke. 2004;35(10):2362–7. https://doi.org/10.1161/01.STR.0000141933.75462.c2.
112. Cochran KA, Cavallari LH, Shapiro NL, Bishop JR. Bleeding incidence with concomitant use of antidepressants and warfarin. Ther Drug Monit. 2011;33(4):433–8. https://doi.org/10.1097/FTD.0b013e318224996e.
113. Fiske A, Wetherell JL, Gatz M. Depression in older adults. Annu Rev Clin Psychol. 2009;5:363–89. https://doi.org/10.1146/annurev.clinpsy.032408.153621.
114. Blazer DG. Depression in late life: review and commentary. J Gerontol A Biol Sci Med Sci. 2003;58(3):249–65. https://doi.org/10.1093/gerona/58.3.m249.
115. Shao H, Chen LQ, Xu J. Treatment of dyslipidemia in the elderly. J Geriatr Cardiol. 2011;8(1):55–64. https://doi.org/10.3724/SP.J.1263.2011.00055.

Chapter 3
Managing Multiple Medical Comorbidities

Sujatha Sankaran

Pre-operative Risk Stratification and Communication of Risk

Pre-operative risk stratification in older adults helps to quantify the patient's risk of perioperative complications. There are a variety of risk stratification tools that are used to quantify perioperative risk, but none are geriatric-specific. The American College of Surgeons National Quality Improvement Program (ACP-NSQIP) has created and validated a risk assessment tool that takes into consideration the surgery-specific risk of the procedure, and incorporates a number of patient-specific variables, including geriatric variables such as age, functional status, and nutritional status. The other variables also include risk factors that are more common in older adults, such as respiratory disease, heart failure, and disseminated cancer. The ACS NSQIP tool quantifies risk of any complication, serious complication, post-op infections, thromboembolism, return to OR, readmission, and overall mortality. Other risk stratification tools, such as the Revised Cardiac Risk Index (RCRI) and the Gupta risk assessment, focus more on risk of major perioperative cardiovascular adverse events such as myocardial infarction.

After risk is assessed, surgical teams should assess whether the patient has capacity to make medical decisions about his or her care. Subsequently, surgical teams should discuss with patients and families their overall goals for treatment in the context of the patient's life expectancy. Many spine procedures are performed to reduce pain, and a realistic discussion of the recovery trajectory is important to elucidate the rate at which pain control can be achieved and whether this is consistent with the patient's overall goals of care. Open communication and shared decision-making are essential components of this process.

S. Sankaran (✉)
University of California at San Francisco, San Francisco, CA, USA
e-mail: Sujatha.sankaran@ucsf.edu

K.-M. G. Fu et al. (eds.), *Treatment of Spine Disease in the Elderly*,
https://doi.org/10.1007/978-3-031-12612-3_3

Geriatric-Specific Risk Factors

There are a number of medical conditions that older adults are predisposed to and that increase risk of complications perioperatively. Older adults are more likely to have renal, cardiac, and pulmonary disease than their younger counterparts. There are four specific areas that should be assessed in older adults before spine surgery—cognitive status, functional status, nutrition, and overall frailty.

Patients with cognitive deficits are more likely to experience delirium in the hospital, which can in turn increase length of stay and lead to other post-operative complications. Cognitive function should be assessed prior to surgery, and patients with cognitive deficits should be referred to a geriatrician. Patients should be assessed for other conditions that predispose to cognitive deficits, such as hearing and vision loss, alcohol and other substance use, and side effects from medications.

Functional status is another important predictor of post-operative complications. Patients should be assessed for their ability to perform activities of daily living (ADLs), and a timed "up and go" test can be administered. This test measures the patient's ability to get up from a seated position, walk 10 ft, turn around, and sit back in the chair. An up and go test that takes longer than 15 s is associated with increased risk of post-op complications, and these patients should receive pre-operative physical and occupational therapy, and early PT should be initiated post-operatively.

Nutrition is another important predictor of post-operative complications. Malnutrition risk increases as people age, and poor nutrition is associated with increased risk of post-operative complications. Nutritional status can be assessed by checking pre-albumin and albumin levels, taking a history on unintentional weight loss from patients, and measuring body mass indices. In some cases, pre-operative nutritional support can improve post-operative outcomes.

These individual predictors can be combined to estimate overall frailty. Studies have shown that four of the following risk factors increase 6-month mortality: cognitive score of less than 3, albumin less than or equal to 3.3 g/dL, more than one fall in the last 6 months, hematocrit less than 35%, dependence with at least one ADL, and presence of at least three comorbidities.

Age as a Risk Factor

Mortality risk increases linearly with increasing age, but the risk of a major adverse cardiovascular event only increases slightly with increasing age, and age is not a predictor of cardiac complications in patients receiving spine surgery. There is, however, a significant risk of increased pulmonary complications as patients age.

Though age does increase risk of some post-operative complications, there is no evidence that increased age correlates with increases in mortality. When there is an increased mortality risk with increased age, this correlates with increasing numbers of comorbidities, such as cognitive and functional decline, malnutrition, and frailty.

Obesity

Obesity in itself does not increase risk of post-operative mortality and most post-operative complications. Obesity does increase risk of perioperative deep venous thrombosis, pulmonary embolism, wound infections, mechanical ventilation, and overall hospital length of stay.

Management of Diabetes

Release of neuroendocrine hormones perioperatively can cause hyperglycemia in patients with diabetes mellitus, and blood glucose levels should be monitored closely during the perioperative period in elderly patients receiving spine surgery. In addition, patients with diabetes have higher rates of coronary artery disease when compared to those without diabetes, so detailed cardiovascular pre-operative examination is important. The American Diabetes Association recommends post-operative blood glucose goals ranging from 80 to 180 mg/dL, though the data varies as to what an optimal target is for the perioperative period. Hypoglycemia below 70 mg/dL should be avoided. For patients already on oral diabetes medication, SGLT inhibitors should be held 3–4 days prior to surgery, as these medications can increase risk of UTI, volume depletion, acute kidney injury, and diabetic ketoacidosis in the post op setting. Other oral medications can be taken until surgery but should be held on the morning of surgery. For patients on insulin, daily or twice daily basal insulin should generally be given at normal doses, but prandial insulin should be held. For premixed fixed-ratio insulin, approximately 20% of the normal insulin dose should be given the night before surgery, and 50% of the normal insulin dose should be given on the day of surgery. For complicated regimens, pre-operative evaluation with the patient's endocrinologist may be warranted. Post-operatively, most oral hypoglycemic and insulin regimens can be resumed once the patient is eating normally again. Metformin should be held if the patient has acute kidney injury or congestive heart failure, and SGLT-2 inhibitors should not be restarted in the hospital due to the risks of volume depletion and urinary tract infections. Patients who are receiving steroids are prone to hyperglycemia and may require higher doses of insulin.

Cardiac and Pulmonary Disease

Patients with advanced age who are receiving spine surgery have an increased chance of cardiac and pulmonary comorbidities, and should be evaluated thoroughly prior to surgery and risk stratified according to scoring systems such as the RCRI. Once risk stratification has taken place, discussions should take place with the patient and family members to discuss the relative risks and benefits of surgery. If the decision is made to proceed with surgery, on the day of surgery, ACE inhibitors, angiotensin receptor blockers, mineralocorticoid antagonists, and digoxin can generally be held, while beta-blockers are generally continued pre-operatively and in the post-op period.

Studies have consistently shown that age increases risk of pulmonary complications from spine surgery, including post-op atelectasis, pulmonary infection, COPD exacerbations, and respiratory failure. Obstructive sleep apnea (OSA) increases risk of post-operative complications including hypoxemia, respiratory failure, need for mechanical ventilation, and transfer to the ICU, and all patients should be screened pre-operatively for OSA. COPD and pulmonary hypertension also increase risk for pulmonary complications from spine surgery, but there is no clear established increase in risk for pulmonary complications in patients with asthma.

Venous Thromboembolism

Risk of post-operative deep venous thrombosis or pulmonary embolism is between 0% and 15% in spine surgeries. Patients with coexisting malignancies have increased risk of perioperative thromboembolism. All patients over the age of 75 are considered at moderate or high risk for post-operative venous thromboembolism. All of these patients with low bleeding risk should receive pharmacological prophylaxis. Studies have shown superiority of low molecular weight heparin or unfractionated heparin for the prevention of venous thromboembolism, so unfractionated heparin should only be used for prophylaxis in patients who have a contraindication to low molecular weight heparin such as renal insufficiency. In patients who are at high risk for a bleeding complication for whom anticoagulant prophylaxis may be contraindicated, mechanical prophylaxis using intermittent pneumatic compression is a reasonable approach.

Anemia

Older patients receiving major spinal surgery are prone to large amounts of blood loss. Patients should be transfused in the perioperative setting for hemoglobin levels greater than 7 or 8 g/dL.

Delirium

Post-operative delirium is an acute intermittent confusional state that is characterized by fluctuations in attention with or without cognitive changes that did not exist prior to surgery. Advanced age increases susceptibility to delirium, and in some studies, up to 62% of older patients receiving major surgery experienced delirium. Reversible causes of delirium include infection, electrolyte disturbances, uncontrolled pain, pre-existing dementia, medication side effects, and withdrawal from substances such as alcohol. Strategies to prevent post-operative delirium include non-pharmacological measures such as supplying aids to maintain sensory input such as glasses and hearing aids, reorientation and cognitive stimulation, and early mobilization. Medications that increase risk of delirium and should be avoided include benzodiazepines, anticholinergics, and opioids, though uncontrolled pain can also cause delirium, so opioid treatment may be necessary. If a patient is severely agitated due to delirium, reversible causes have been addressed, and non-pharmacological interventions such as redirection have failed, it is appropriate to treat with small doses of antipsychotic medications such as haloperidol. Benzodiazepines are not recommended in the setting for elderly patients, as they can worsen confusion and are sedating.

Pain Management Before and After Surgery

Pain management for patients receiving spine surgery may be challenging, as many of these patients are opioid-tolerant and have chronic pain. In addition, opioids have the potential to incite delirium and confusion in elderly patients, but poor pain control can also cause delirium, so thorough patient evaluation is essential. Multimodal analgesia, combining non-opioid medications with opioid medications for pain control, is an integrated approach that can improve overall pain management. Ketamine can be an effective adjuvant pain medication in patients who are opioid-tolerant. Gabapentinoids such as gabapentin and pregabalin are also an appropriate medication class that can decrease opioid requirements for post-op spine patients, but can also cause sedation and respiratory depression, so caution should be exercised when using these agents in elderly patients. Acetaminophen has a small but statistically significant benefit in pain control for patients who have undergone spine surgery, and has a favorable side effect profile. Nonsteroidal anti-inflammatory drugs (NSAIDs) are relatively contraindicated in many spinal procedures due to risk of nonunion, so discussion between anesthesiologist, internal medicine consultant, and spine surgeon in the pre-operative setting is important to establish whether these agents can be safely used for individual patients. In the post-operative setting, it is important to taper down opioid pain medications and to provide patients with a continuing tapering schedule on discharge from the hospital. Patients should be advised about the risk of opioid overdose and side effects, and if a patient is discharged on greater than 90 oral morphine equivalents, he or she should receive intranasal naloxone and teaching of patient and family members on how to administer it in the case of opioid overdose.

Smoking, Alcohol, and Substance Use

Smoking increases risk of post-operative complications, including overall morbidity, wound infections, general complications, and pulmonary complications. Tobacco cessation interventions should be offered to all smokers, and there is evidence that the longer an individual is not smoking for, the greater the benefit. Alcohol misuse also is associated with increased risk of post-operative complications, including surgical site and general infections, cardiopulmonary complications, prolonged length of stay, increased ICU days, and higher rates of unexpected returns to OR. While there is little evidence that alcohol cessation pre-operatively decreases risk, there is little harm, so is a reasonable approach. It is also important to obtain a thorough substance use history, as this may reveal opioid use disorder, stimulant use disorder, or other substance use disorders that could affect the post-op course in areas such as pain management and risk of withdrawal from substance use.

Post-operative Disposition

Older patients who receive spine surgery often require prolonged inpatient stays and, in some cases, ICU-level care. Up to 10% of patients who have received lumbar spinal fusion have been shown to require care in an ICU, and patients who are older, are male, and have other comorbidities and more prone to post-operative complications require hospitalization. Procedures that take longer than 5 h and that require an anterior thoracic approach are associated with higher lengths of stay in the hospital. In addition, older patients who receive spine surgery have an increased risk of discharge to a healthcare facility other than home for recovery. This recovery period at a facility helps to provide consistent physical therapy, mobilization, and fall prevention to facilitate eventual discharge home.

Conclusions

Older adults undergoing spinal procedures often have multiple comorbidities that predispose them to longer hospital lengths of stay and post-operative complications. The effects of many of these complications can be mitigated by thorough pre-operative evaluation and communication between primary care physicians, the surgeon, and other consultants. It is paramount that the risks and benefits of surgery are explained in a thorough manner with patients and families to ensure that they are making informed decisions about pursuing surgery and have a realistic sense of what the surgical and post-operative course will entail. Understanding patient priorities, providing comprehensive information with all options presented in a clear fashion, and consistent communication are essential to ensuring that older patients achieve success when receiving spine surgery.

Bibliography

1. Oresanya LB, Lyons WL, Finlayson E. Preoperative assessment of the older patient: a narrative review. JAMA. 2014;311(20):2110–20. https://doi.org/10.1001/jama.2014.4573. PMID: 24867014.
2. Lee TH, Marcantonio ER, Mangione CM, Thomas EJ, Polanczyk CA, Cook EF, Sugarbaker DJ, Donaldson MC, Poss R, Ho KK, Ludwig LE, Pedan A, Goldman L. Derivation and prospective validation of a simple index for prediction of cardiac risk of major noncardiac surgery. Circulation. 1999;100(10):1043–9. https://doi.org/10.1161/01.cir.100.10.1043. PMID: 10477528.
3. Polanczyk CA, Marcantonio E, Goldman L, Rohde LE, Orav J, Mangione CM, Lee TH. Impact of age on perioperative complications and length of stay in patients undergoing noncardiac surgery. Ann Intern Med. 2001;134(8):637–43. https://doi.org/10.7326/0003-4819-134-8-200104170-00008. PMID: 11304103.
4. Mullen JT, Moorman DW, Davenport DL. The obesity paradox: body mass index and outcomes in patients undergoing nonbariatric general surgery. Ann Surg. 2009;250(1):166–72. https://doi.org/10.1097/SLA.0b013e3181ad8935. PMID: 19561456.
5. Kaw R, Pasupuleti V, Walker E, Ramaswamy A, Foldvary-Schafer N. Postoperative complications in patients with obstructive sleep apnea. Chest. 2012;141(2):436–41. https://doi.org/10.1378/chest.11-0283. Epub 2011 Aug 25. PMID: 21868464.
6. Tønnesen H, Nielsen PR, Lauritzen JB, Møller AM. Smoking and alcohol intervention before surgery: evidence for best practice. Br J Anaesth. 2009;102(3):297–306. https://doi.org/10.1093/bja/aen401. PMID: 19218371.
7. Lenoir B, Merckx P, Paugam-Burtz C, Dauzac C, Agostini MM, Guigui P, Mantz J. Individual probability of allogeneic erythrocyte transfusion in elective spine surgery: the predictive model of transfusion in spine surgery. Anesthesiology. 2009;110(5):1050–60. https://doi.org/10.1097/ALN.0b013e31819df9e0. PMID: 19352170.
8. Bell RF, Dahl JB, Moore RA, Kalso E. Perioperative ketamine for acute postoperative pain. Cochrane Database Syst Rev. 2006;(1):CD004603. https://doi.org/10.1002/14651858.CD004603.pub2. Update in: Cochrane Database Syst Rev. 2015;7: CD004603. PMID: 16437490.
9. Pandey CK, Navkar DV, Giri PJ, Raza M, Behari S, Singh RB, Singh U, Singh PK. Evaluation of the optimal preemptive dose of gabapentin for postoperative pain relief after lumbar diskectomy: a randomized, double-blind, placebo-controlled study. J Neurosurg Anesthesiol. 2005;17(2):65–8. https://doi.org/10.1097/01.ana.0000151407.62650.51. PMID: 15840990.
10. Fu KM, Smith JS, Polly DW Jr, Ames CP, Berven SH, Perra JH, McCarthy RE, Knapp DR Jr, Shaffrey CI, Scoliosis Research Society Morbidity and Mortality Committee. Correlation of higher preoperative American Society of Anesthesiology grade and increased morbidity and mortality rates in patients undergoing spine surgery. J Neurosurg Spine. 2011;14(4):470–4. https://doi.org/10.3171/2010.12.SPINE10486. Epub 2011 Feb 4. PMID: 21294615.

Chapter 4
Anesthetic Concerns for Spinal Surgery in the Elderly

Priscilla Nelson and Philip C. Kuo

Introduction

Geriatric patients can benefit significantly from spinal surgery, particularly for degenerative diseases. Surgical management of spinal pathology can lead to improved quality of life with a similar complication profile compared to younger patients [1–3]. Furthermore, studies have demonstrated that the improved cost-effectiveness of operative management was similar for both primary and revision surgery [1–3]. However, there are additional studies, some of which are based on nationwide representative samples, presenting conflicting information, which suggests that complications, reoperations, and readmissions may be significantly higher in elderly patients [4–7]. Given the potential for increased complications, perioperative optimization is warranted in the geriatric population. This requires a focused approach to each phase of surgical patient care.

Age-Related Physiologic Changes

Aging involves multiple biologic pathways impacting the molecular, biologic, and organ-level mechanisms (Table 4.1) [8]. The initial workup of the geriatric patient is performed, keeping these differences in mind.

P. Nelson (✉) · P. C. Kuo
Division of Neuroanesthesiology, Department of Anesthesiology, Weill Cornell Medical College, New York, NY, USA
e-mail: Prn9012@med.cornell.edu; phk9011@med.cornell.edu

K.-M. G. Fu et al. (eds.), *Treatment of Spine Disease in the Elderly*,
https://doi.org/10.1007/978-3-031-12612-3_4

Table 4.1 Age-related physiologic changes and perioperative considerations by organ system

System	Physiologic changes	Perioperative considerations
Central nervous	Decreased brain weight and volume	Preoperative cognitive assessment
	Decreased cerebral blood flow and cerebral oxygen consumption	Prehabilitation
	Blunted autonomic neural response	Postoperative delirium prevention and screening
	Lowered threshold to neurodegeneration	
Cardiovascular	Loss of myocytes with increase in myocyte volume	Preoperative cardiac clearance when indicated
	Myocardial and large vessel stiffening	Maintenance of intraoperative normotension to assure appropriate perfusion
	Decreased sympathetic tone	
	Myocardial conduction abnormalities	
Respiratory	Weakening of respiratory musculature	Critical airway protection and management
	Increased chest wall rigidity	Judicious titration of opioid analgesics
	Blunted central responses to physiologic changes	
	Decreased cough and airway protection	
	Increased closing capacity	
Renal	Cortical tissue loss	Close attention to volume management needed as physiologic volume adjustment impaired
	Decreased glomerular filtration rate	
Hepatobiliary/ gastrointestinal	Decreased liver size	Hepatically cleared drugs will have longer half-life
	Decreased blood flow	Decreased overall nausea and vomiting
Cutaneous/ muscular	Loss of muscle mass	Environmental temperature regulation
	Impaired temperature regulation	Positioning changes to prevent pressure points
		Prehabilitation

Central Nervous System

Aging in the central nervous system can lead to numerous challenges, including cognitive decline, memory loss, dementia, movement disorders, depression, sleep challenges, and increased risk of delirium [9]. Aging does not change the number of neurons; however, it does lead to decreased synapses and fewer dendrites, which leads to decreased brain volume [9]. Age-related changes in neuronal transmission and firing, calcium metabolism, and gene expression alter connectivity and cognitive plasticity [9]. Such alterations can contribute to postoperative delirium and postoperative cognitive dysfunction, which can impact upwards of 10% of geriatric patients in the postoperative period.

Cardiovascular

Aging of the circulatory system leads to arterial stiffening, changes in sympathetic tone, alterations of baroreceptor function, loss of elasticity in the myocardium, and conduction system abnormalities. These changes also put the geriatric patient at a higher risk of venous thromboembolism. The loss of elasticity in the vasculature leads to a dependence on preload, and small decreases in circulating blood volume can lead to a significant drop in cardiac output. In spinal cases where moderate to large volumes of blood loss are expected, one may see significant cardiovascular decompensation. Cardiac arrhythmias like atrial fibrillation can also lead to a drop in cardiac output because of the lack of atrial kick. The ability of the heart to deal with autonomic changes also decreases with age.

Respiratory

The geriatric respiratory system is less compliant, with weaker musculature, and a higher incidence of pulmonary pathology. There is a blunted central response to hypercapnia and hypoxia, which leads to an increased risk of anesthetic-induced respiratory depression. A decrease in pharyngeal tone, ability to clear secretions, mucociliary transport, and cough reflex can lead to a higher risk of aspiration and pneumonia postoperatively. Additionally, closing capacity, the critical lung volume during expiration at which airway closure can be detected, increases with age leading to higher risk for atelectasis and age-related decrease in oxygenation due to shunt.

Renal

After age 40, the kidney begins to decrease in size and weight, mainly due to glomerulosclerosis [8]. This results in a decrease in the glomerular filtration rate. Many common chronic diseases hasten this reduction. While most elderly patients have a normal creatinine level, their muscle mass and overall creatinine are less. As a result, a normal creatinine should be viewed with caution in the context of the individual older patient. The older patient may also have a decreased ability to adjust volume status, which may result in acid-base alterations. This is coupled with a decrease in serum renin, renin activity, and aldosterone and alterations in sodium excretion. Due to the inappropriate sodium excretion, hypovolemia can result in hypotension and acute kidney injury [10].

Gastrointestinal

Aging leads to a decrease in hepatic blood flow and hepatocytes, yet despite this, the liver retains normal synthetic function. Drugs that are dependent on hepatic blood flow for clearance like ketamine, fentanyl, morphine, and lidocaine may, however, have a longer-acting effect. The incidence of postoperative nausea and vomiting decreases with age.

Musculoskeletal and Cutaneous

Lean muscle mass decreases while total body fat increases with age. Even short periods of bedrest result in significant loss of muscle mass. One study showed that older individuals placed on bedrest for 10 days had greater muscle loss than their younger counterparts who were placed on bedrest for 28 days [11]. It is critical to engage physical therapy to prevent muscle loss in the perioperative period. Temperature dysregulation in cold operating rooms can occur quickly from a decrease in the amount of subcutaneous or insulating fat. There is also dysregulation of the cutaneous microcirculation, which can lead to poor wound healing. Finally, positioning the patient from supine to prone or extending the neck for good surgical access and exposure can be challenging as older adults have limited joint mobility because of the high prevalence of osteoarthritis. It is important to document preoperatively the patient's range of motion to not worsen preexisting joint conditions.

Preanesthetic Consultation

For the geriatric patient, the preoperative assessment follows the same standards of care with additional attention to frailty, functional status, polypharmacy, cognitive ability, and risk of delirium postoperatively [7, 12]. The American College of Surgeons has established a best practice guideline to aid in preoperative management of the geriatric patient [13, 14].

Frailty

Frailty is a relatively new concept that tries to capture an individual's reserve to physiologic stress. Physiologic reserve can be conceptualized as a decline in organ systems that leads to a physiologically vulnerable state. In spinal surgery, frailty index independently correlates with multiple adverse surgical events [15–17]. Further, frailty has been correlated with increased risk of delirium in surgical patients [18, 19].

Prehabilitation

Prehabilitation has been demonstrated to improve surgical and patient-reported outcomes and can decrease length of stay in spine patients with results based on randomized controlled trials [20, 21]. Such prehabilitation involves participation in an intensive exercise program and optimization of analgesic treatment [21, 22]. Of note, elderly patients were included in the study groups, and as a result, the findings can be applied to this cohort. A detailed understanding of prehabilitation in elderly patients, though, is lacking and requires further examination with an increased sample size.

Cognition and Dementia

It is important to obtain baseline cognitive status as this helps to stratify patients who are at risk for delirium after surgery. Upwards of 20% of patients over the age of 65 have some form of cognitive impairment [23]. Although many clinicians are hesitant to discuss cognition with patients, patients are generally accepting of the screening [23]. Some of the tests that can be administered quickly with good sensitivity are the MiniCog [24], Montreal Cognitive Assessment (MoCA) [25], Mini-Mental State Exam (MMSE) [26], Clock-drawing Test and [27], Cognitive Disorder Examination (CODEX) [9, 28]. Studies have shown that patients with impaired cognition preoperatively are at higher risk for delirium postoperatively, so it is important to establish a baseline of their cognitive function [29]. Such patients with preoperative impairment are also less likely to return home after surgery, requiring a significantly higher level of care [30]. Screening can help risk-stratify elderly patients to aid with decision-making.

Medication Management

Identification of medications taken by the geriatric patient is considered best practice and can avoid polypharmacy and identify potential drug interactions. It is important to avoid medications listed on the American Geriatrics Society's Beers Criteria for Potentially Inappropriate Medication Use in Older Adults [31]. Some of the medications we routinely use as part of a standard anesthetic may be inappropriate in the elderly patient [9]. They include anticholinergics like diphenhydramine, scopolamine, and hydroxyzine, which increase the risk of confusion. The older patient can be more sensitive to benzodiazepines as the metabolism of these drugs may be slower. Benzodiazepines, which are commonly used as premedication for anxiety, can put the elderly patient at increased risk of delirium, cognitive impairment, and falls in the postoperative period.

Intraoperative Management

Once a preoperative assessment has been done, the task of the anesthesiologist is to design an intraoperative plan that is unique to the needs of the older individual. The main goals of any intraoperative anesthetic are the same: analgesia, amnesia, akinesia, and hemodynamic stability. Temperature regulation in the geriatric patient is also critical. Given the heterogeneity found in the geriatric population, it is difficult to make broad statements regarding intraoperative management, and as such individualized care must be provided.

Anesthetic Techniques: General and Regional Anesthesia and Monitored Anesthesia Care

Most spine cases require general anesthesia with an endotracheal tube and prone positioning. However, given the increase in minimally invasive surgery, non-general anesthesia alternatives such as neuraxial (regional) anesthesia and monitored anesthesia care with local anesthesia are at times utilized in certain institutions. No specific anesthetic technique has been shown to decrease the incidence of delirium, postoperative neurologic disorders, or cognitive dysfunction [9].

The standards for monitored anesthesia care (MAC) are the same as those undergoing general anesthesia. However, because of the lack of reserve, older patients are extremely susceptible to airway obstruction, hypoxia, hypercarbia, and aspiration. Progression from a light plane to a deep plane of anesthesia may occur suddenly and quickly. Deep sedation during procedures where older adults were given neuraxial anesthesia as the primary anesthetic was associated with higher mortality [32].

Depth of Sedation

The American Society of Anesthesiology new Brain Heath Initiate suggests using age-adjusted concentrations of inhaled anesthetics and using processed EEG to titrate and maintain anesthetic depth [33]. The goal of depth of anesthesia monitors is to avoid excessively deep planes of anesthetics that can result in low blood pressure and hemodynamic instability.

Hemodynamic Perfusion Monitoring

In spinal surgery patients, hemodynamic monitoring can be monitored through invasive or noninvasive techniques. Typically, at our institution, an arterial line is utilized to monitor minute-by-minute variations in blood pressure, with an external blood pressure cuff utilized to also allow for correlation. Pulse and tissue oxygenation monitoring can be performed with a variety of pulse oximeters, some of which can also guide fluid management.

Perfusion monitoring is critical for several reasons in the geriatric patient. Primarily, maintaining appropriate cerebral perfusion is critical, as the geriatric patient can have decreased cerebrovascular reactivity [34]. Given this decreased reserve, transient periods of hypotension can result in downstream defects, which may not be seen in younger individuals who have a more appropriate cerebral dilatory response to hypotension. Secondarily, maintaining appropriate peripheral perfusion as well as cord perfusion is critical to surgical outcomes. Hypotension should be treated in standard fashion, with prudent use of fluid administration and use of vasopressor agents, keeping in close communication with the surgeon to determine if the perfusion is related to blood loss or due to the vascular impact of anesthetic agents. Blood pressure goals should be set based on the geriatric patient's preoperative state.

Intraoperative Neurophysiological Monitoring

Intraoperative neurophysiological monitoring is standard of care in spine surgery and does not change for geriatric patients [35, 36]. Cerebral monitoring can be performed with numerous monitors, but at our institution, we use the bispectral index monitor (BIS monitor) or the SedLine index (Masimo monitor) [37–40]. These monitors allow for the assessment of depth of anesthesia. Neuronal transmission monitoring is performed by examining the integrity of the nervous system with a combination of EMG, MEPS, SSEPs, and EEG, depending on the procedure. A multimodal approach has been shown to be more effective and accurate when possible [41], although there is significant heterogeneity of available studies examining the utilization of intraoperative neurophysiological monitoring in spine surgery [42].

Postoperative Management

The goals of postoperative anesthetic care include adequate pain control and prevention of common geriatric-associated adverse events. The American College of Surgeons has established a best practice guideline for the care of the geriatric surgery patient, which includes a checklist to enhance the prevention of delirium, pulmonary complications, falls, postoperative urinary complications, and pressure ulcers and improve care transitions [14]. These are not specific to only spine surgery cases; the overarching principles and concepts can be broadly applied. There are no specific recommendations for the geriatric patient in the postanesthesia care unit; however, additional attention should be placed on the increased risk for desaturation and aspiration [9]. Pain control must be carefully administered to adequately control pain while minimizing the possibility for oversedation, ideally employing a multimodal approach. Long-acting opioids and gabapentin should be avoided.

Screening for Delirium

Delirium prevention is a critical aspect of postoperative geriatric care, as delirium can impact upwards of 40% of older patients undergoing spine surgery [43]. This is most successful when utilizing a multidisciplinary approach that focuses on behavior restoration and not pharmacologic management of delirium. One such program, the Hospital Elder Life Program (HELP), has components that focus on reorientation, mobilization, and restoration of normal sleep cycles and has been shown to improve related outcomes and be cost-effective in non-spine surgery [44, 45]. Preventing delirium is of particular interest given the association of delirium with numerous downstream adverse outcomes, including worse cognitive outcomes and increased risk of dementia [46, 47]. Postoperative delirium has been associated with a longer and more costly hospital course, increased risk of institutionalization, functional decline, and higher likelihood of death at 6 months postoperatively [48]. However, other studies suggest that delirium may be related to early cognitive dysfunction, but not a later impact [49, 50]. At least one recent study has suggested that longer-term postoperative cognitive dysfunction (POCD) may be a different process related to neurocognitive deficits [50].

Postoperative Cognitive Dysfunction

Postoperative cognitive dysfunction (POCD) is a memory or thinking impairment that has been corroborated by neurophysiologic testing [51, 52]. Postoperative delirium is an independent risk factor for cognitive dysfunction [47], which can have a major impact on postoperative quality of life. It is a broad area of current research given the continued aging of the population and the impact that surgical events can have on cognition. Numerous recent studies have begun to dive deeper into this topic in spine surgery, both from the risk standpoint and the treatment. A recent systematic review suggests that in noncardiac surgery, a significant proportion of patients demonstrate POCD in the early weeks postoperatively, but that minimal evidence exists linking the continuation to long-term dysfunction [53].

Management Strategies

A recent randomized controlled trial examining general anesthesia compared to a combined anesthetic with general and epidural anesthesia in lumbar decompression and fusion patients demonstrated that the treatment cohort had less pain and less cognitive dysfunction in the first 48 h compared to general anesthesia alone [54]. Systematic reviews that have compared general anesthesia to regional anesthesia, however, have not found conclusive differences [55, 56]. Other randomized studies have suggested intravenous lidocaine infusions may improve postoperative cognition at 3 days based on the mini-mental status exam [57] and that anesthesia with inhalational agents compared to intravenous agents may also contribute to higher rates of postoperative cognitive challenges [58]. Generally speaking, this is an area of active research currently lacking a detailed understanding.

Conclusions

Geriatric spine surgery patients have a unique perioperative physiologic profile and require additional preoperative workup and focused management postoperatively. Such patients are at particularly high risk for postoperative delirium, which is best managed through a multidisciplinary, non-pharmacologic approach. Further research on the impact of frailty on perioperative outcomes and prehabilitation impact in geriatric patients is warranted given the importance of these two concepts.

Conflicts of Interest None.

References

1. Devin CJ, Chotai S, Parker SL, Tetreault L, Fehlings MG, McGirt MJ. A Cost-utility analysis of lumbar decompression with and without fusion for degenerative spine disease in the elderly. Neurosurgery. 2015;77(Suppl 4):S116–24.
2. Adogwa O, Carr RK, Kudyba K, Karikari I, Bagley CA, Gokaslan ZL, et al. Revision lumbar surgery in elderly patients with symptomatic pseudarthrosis, adjacent-segment disease, or same-level recurrent stenosis. Part 1. Two-year outcomes and clinical efficacy: clinical article. J Neurosurg Spine. 2013;18(2):139–46.
3. Adogwa O, Owens R, Karikari I, Agarwal V, Gottfried ON, Bagley CA, et al. Revision lumbar surgery in elderly patients with symptomatic pseudarthrosis, adjacent-segment disease, or same-level recurrent stenosis. Part 2. A cost-effectiveness analysis: clinical article. J Neurosurg Spine. 2013;18(2):147–53.
4. Drazin D, Al-Khouja L, Lagman C, Ugiliweneza B, Shweikeh F, Johnson JP, et al. Scoliosis surgery in the elderly: complications, readmissions, reoperations and mortality. J Clin Neurosci. 2016;34:158–61.
5. Worley N, Marascalchi B, Jalai CM, Yang S, Diebo B, Vira S, et al. Predictors of inpatient morbidity and mortality in adult spinal deformity surgery. Eur Spine J. 2016;25(3):819–27.
6. Daubs MD, Lenke LG, Cheh G, Stobbs G, Bridwell KH. Adult spinal deformity surgery: complications and outcomes in patients over age 60. Spine. 2007;32(20):2238–44.
7. Thomas K, Wong KH, Steelman SC, Rodriguez A. Surgical risk assessment and prevention in elderly spinal deformity patients. Geriatr Orthop Surg Rehabil. 2019;10:2151459319851681.
8. Aalami OO, Fang TD, Song HM, Nacamuli RP. Physiological features of aging persons. Arch Surg. 2003;138(10):1068–76.
9. Gropper DM, Hemmings M, Pamnani P, Wu H, Hugh C, Malhotra V, Pamnani A, Pryor KO, Wu CL. Miller's anesthesia. 9th ed. Philadelphia, PA: Elsevier; 2020.
10. Schlanger LE, Bailey JL, Sands JM. Electrolytes in the aging. Adv Chronic Kidney Dis. 2010;17(4):308–19.
11. Kortebein P, Ferrando A, Lombeida J, Wolfe R, Evans WJ. Effect of 10 days of bed rest on skeletal muscle in healthy older adults. JAMA. 2007;297(16):1772–4.
12. Kurrek MM, Barnett S, Minville V. Considerations for the perioperative care of elderly and frail patients. J Frail Aging. 2014;3(4):230–3.
13. Chow WB, Rosenthal RA, Merkow RP, Ko CY, Esnaola NF. Optimal preoperative assessment of the geriatric surgical patient: a best practices guideline from the American College of Surgeons National Surgical Quality Improvement Program and the American Geriatrics Society. J Am Coll Surg. 2012;215(4):453–66.
14. Mohanty S, Rosenthal RA, Russell MM, Neuman MD, Ko CY, Esnaola NF. Optimal perioperative management of the geriatric patient: a best practices guideline from the American College of Surgeons NSQIP and the American Geriatrics Society. J Am Coll Surg. 2016;222(5):930–47.
15. Yagi M, Michikawa T, Hosogane N, Fujita N, Okada E, Suzuki S, et al. The 5-item modified frailty index is predictive of severe adverse events in patients undergoing surgery for adult spinal deformity. Spine. 2019;44(18):E1083–e91.
16. Leven DM, Lee NJ, Kothari P, Steinberger J, Guzman J, Skovrlj B, et al. Frailty index is a significant predictor of complications and mortality after surgery for adult spinal deformity. Spine. 2016;41(23):E1394–e401.
17. Flexman AM, Charest-Morin R, Stobart L, Street J, Ryerson CJ. Frailty and postoperative outcomes in patients undergoing surgery for degenerative spine disease. Spine J. 2016;16(11):1315–23.
18. Nomura Y, Nakano M, Bush B, Tian J, Yamaguchi A, Walston J, et al. Observational study examining the association of baseline frailty and postcardiac surgery delirium and cognitive change. Anesth Analg. 2019;129(2):507–14.

19. Goudzwaard JA, de Ronde-Tillmans M, El Faquir N, Acar F, Van Mieghem NM, Lenzen MJ, et al. The Erasmus Frailty Score is associated with delirium and 1-year mortality after Transcatheter Aortic Valve Implantation in older patients. The TAVI Care & Cure program. Int J Cardiol. 2019;276:48–52.
20. Lindbäck Y, Tropp H, Enthoven P, Abbott A, Öberg B. PREPARE: presurgery physiotherapy for patients with degenerative lumbar spine disorder: a randomized controlled trial. Spine J. 2018;18(8):1347–55.
21. Nielsen PR, Jørgensen LD, Dahl B, Pedersen T, Tønnesen H. Prehabilitation and early rehabilitation after spinal surgery: randomized clinical trial. Clin Rehabil. 2010;24(2):137–48.
22. Nielsen PR, Andreasen J, Asmussen M, Tønnesen H. Costs and quality of life for prehabilitation and early rehabilitation after surgery of the lumbar spine. BMC Health Serv Res. 2008;8:209.
23. Culley DJ, Flaherty D, Reddy S, Fahey MC, Rudolph J, Huang CC, et al. Preoperative cognitive stratification of older elective surgical patients: a cross-sectional study. Anesth Analg. 2016;123(1):186–92.
24. Lin JS, O'Connor E, Rossom RC, Perdue LA, Eckstrom E. Screening for cognitive impairment in older adults: a systematic review for the U.S. Preventive Services Task Force. Ann Intern Med. 2013;159(9):601–12.
25. Nasreddine ZS, Phillips NA, Bédirian V, Charbonneau S, Whitehead V, Collin I, et al. The Montreal Cognitive Assessment, MoCA: a brief screening tool for mild cognitive impairment. J Am Geriatr Soc. 2005;53(4):695–9.
26. Veliz-Reissmüller G, Agüero Torres H, van der Linden J, Lindblom D, Eriksdotter JM. Pre-operative mild cognitive dysfunction predicts risk for post-operative delirium after elective cardiac surgery. Aging Clin Exp Res. 2007;19(3):172–7.
27. Puustinen J, Luostarinen L, Luostarinen M, Pulliainen V, Huhtala H, Soini M, et al. The use of MoCA and other cognitive tests in evaluation of cognitive impairment in elderly patients undergoing arthroplasty. Geriatr Orthop Surg Rehabil. 2016;7(4):183–7.
28. Belmin J, Pariel-Madjlessi S, Surun P, Bentot C, Feteanu D, Lefebvre des Noettes V, et al. The cognitive disorders examination (Codex) is a reliable 3-minute test for detection of dementia in the elderly (validation study on 323 subjects). Presse Med. 2007;36(9 Pt 1):1183–90.
29. Racine AM, Fong TG, Gou Y, Travison TG, Tommet D, Erickson K, et al. Clinical outcomes in older surgical patients with mild cognitive impairment. Alzheimers Dement. 2018;14(5):590–600.
30. Adogwa O, Elsamadicy AA, Sergesketter A, Vuong VD, Moreno J, Cheng J, et al. Independent association between preoperative cognitive status and discharge location after surgery: a strategy to reduce resource use after surgery for deformity. World Neurosurg. 2018;110:e67–72.
31. American Geriatrics Society. 2015 Updated beers criteria for potentially inappropriate medication use in older adults. J Am Geriatr Soc. 2015;63(11):2227–46.
32. Brown CHT, Azman AS, Gottschalk A, Mears SC, Sieber FE. Sedation depth during spinal anesthesia and survival in elderly patients undergoing hip fracture repair. Anesth Analg. 2014;118(5):977–80.
33. Mahanna-Gabrielli E, Schenning KJ, Eriksson LI, Browndyke JN, Wright CB, Culley DJ, et al. State of the clinical science of perioperative brain health: report from the American Society of Anesthesiologists Brain Health Initiative Summit 2018. Br J Anaesth. 2019;123(4):464–78.
34. McKetton L, Sobczyk O, Duffin J, Poublanc J, Sam K, Crawley AP, et al. The aging brain and cerebrovascular reactivity. NeuroImage. 2018;181:132–41.
35. Gonzalez AA, Jeyanandarajan D, Hansen C, Zada G, Hsieh PC. Intraoperative neurophysiological monitoring during spine surgery: a review. Neurosurg Focus. 2009;27(4):E6.
36. Malhotra NR, Shaffrey CI. Intraoperative electrophysiological monitoring in spine surgery. Spine. 2010;35(25):2167–79.
37. Oliveira CR, Bernardo WM, Nunes VM. Benefit of general anesthesia monitored by bispectral index compared with monitoring guided only by clinical parameters. Systematic review and meta-analysis. Braz J Anesthesiol. 2017;67(1):72–84.

38. Sudhakaran R, Makkar JK, Jain D, Wig J, Chabra R. Comparison of bispectral index and end-tidal anaesthetic concentration monitoring on recovery profile of desflurane in patients undergoing lumbar spine surgery. Ind J Anaesth. 2018;62(7):516–23.
39. Karwacki Z, Niewiadomski S, Rzaska M, Witkowska M. The effect of bispectral index monitoring on anaesthetic requirements in target-controlled infusion for lumbar microdiscectomy. Anaesthesiol Intens Ther. 2014;46(4):284–8.
40. Purdon PL, Sampson A, Pavone KJ, Brown EN. Clinical electroencephalography for anesthesiologists: Part I: Background and basic signatures. Anesthesiology. 2015;123(4):937–60.
41. Sutter M, Eggspuehler A, Jeszenszky D, Kleinstueck F, Fekete TF, Haschtmann D, et al. The impact and value of uni- and multimodal intraoperative neurophysiological monitoring (IONM) on neurological complications during spine surgery: a prospective study of 2728 patients. Eur Spine J. 2019;28(3):599–610.
42. Daniel JW, Botelho RV, Milano JB, Dantas FR, Onishi FJ, Neto ER, et al. Intraoperative neurophysiological monitoring in spine surgery: a systematic review and meta-analysis. Spine. 2018;43(16):1154–60.
43. Brown CHT, LaFlam A, Max L, Wyrobek J, Neufeld KJ, Kebaish KM, et al. Delirium after spine surgery in older adults: incidence, risk factors, and outcomes. J Am Geriatr Soc. 2016;64(10):2101–8.
44. Rubin FH, Neal K, Fenlon K, Hassan S, Inouye SK. Sustainability and scalability of the hospital elder life program at a community hospital. J Am Geriatr Soc. 2011;59(2):359–65.
45. Chen CC, Li HC, Liang JT, Lai IR, Purnomo JDT, Yang YT, et al. Effect of a modified hospital elder life program on delirium and length of hospital stay in patients undergoing abdominal surgery: a cluster randomized clinical trial. JAMA Surg. 2017;152(9):827–34.
46. Wacker P, Nunes PV, Cabrita H, Forlenza OV. Post-operative delirium is associated with poor cognitive outcome and dementia. Dement Geriatr Cogn Disord. 2006;21(4):221–7.
47. Bickel H, Gradinger R, Kochs E, Förstl H. High risk of cognitive and functional decline after postoperative delirium. A three-year prospective study. Dement Geriatr Cogn Disord. 2008;26(1):26–31.
48. Adogwa O, Elsamadicy AA, Vuong VD, Fialkoff J, Cheng J, Karikari IO, et al. Association between baseline cognitive impairment and postoperative delirium in elderly patients undergoing surgery for adult spinal deformity. J Neurosurg Spine. 2018;28(1):103–8.
49. Rudolph JL, Marcantonio ER, Culley DJ, Silverstein JH, Rasmussen LS, Crosby GJ, et al. Delirium is associated with early postoperative cognitive dysfunction. Anaesthesia. 2008;63(9):941–7.
50. Daiello LA, Racine AM, Yun Gou R, Marcantonio ER, Xie Z, Kunze LJ, et al. Postoperative delirium and postoperative cognitive dysfunction: overlap and divergence. Anesthesiology. 2019;131(3):477–91.
51. Ramaiah R, Lam AM. Postoperative cognitive dysfunction in the elderly. Anesthesiol Clin. 2009;27(3):485–96, table of contents.
52. Fong HK, Sands LP, Leung JM. The role of postoperative analgesia in delirium and cognitive decline in elderly patients: a systematic review. Anesth Analg. 2006;102(4):1255–66.
53. Newman S, Stygall J, Hirani S, Shaefi S, Maze M. Postoperative cognitive dysfunction after noncardiac surgery: a systematic review. Anesthesiology. 2007;106(3):572–90.
54. Ezhevskaya AA, Ovechkin AM, Prusakova ZB, Zagrekov VI, Mlyavykh SG, Anderson DG. Relationship among anesthesia technique, surgical stress, and cognitive dysfunction following spinal surgery: a randomized trial. Journal of neurosurgery. Spine. 2019;31:1–8.
55. Wu CL, Hsu W, Richman JM, Raja SN. Postoperative cognitive function as an outcome of regional anesthesia and analgesia. Reg Anesth Pain Med. 2004;29(3):257–68.
56. Davis N, Lee M, Lin AY, Lynch L, Monteleone M, Falzon L, et al. Postoperative cognitive function following general versus regional anesthesia: a systematic review. J Neurosurg Anesthesiol. 2014;26(4):369–76.

57. Chen K, Wei P, Zheng Q, Zhou J, Li J. Neuroprotective effects of intravenous lidocaine on early postoperative cognitive dysfunction in elderly patients following spine surgery. Med Sci Monit. 2015;21:1402–7.
58. Qiao Y, Feng H, Zhao T, Yan H, Zhang H, Zhao X. Postoperative cognitive dysfunction after inhalational anesthesia in elderly patients undergoing major surgery: the influence of anesthetic technique, cerebral injury and systemic inflammation. BMC Anesthesiol. 2015;15:154.

Chapter 5
Spinal Prehab/Rehab in the Elderly

Leroy R. Lindsay, Heidi Chen, and Jaspal R. Singh

Back pain is the largest contributor to disability, impaired function, and decreased quality of life reported by older adults [1, 2]. While the ubiquitous nature of back pain has led to a myriad of treatment interventions, there remains an opportunity to optimize patients before surgery and assist with their recovery [3]. Notably, elective surgeries for degenerative spine pathology are still associated with lengthy hospital stays, increased rate of repeat surgery, and increased risk for developing postsurgical complications [4]. Moreover, many patients having elective procedures have modifiable risk factors that contribute to these complication rates and increased "episode-of-care" spending [3]. Lastly, many older adult patients do not achieve the level of function expected due to a confluence of factors. These elements underscored the importance of preoperative optimization and specific postoperative rehabilitation pathways [3, 4].

Many rehabilitation outcome measures attempt to standardize the reporting of an individual's functional status. The metrics aim to assess functional deficits commonly related to low back pain. These assessments help therapists identify physical deficiencies and tailor treatment plans for every patient. Despite the complex nature

L. R. Lindsay (✉)
Department of Clinical Rehabilitation Medicine, Weill Cornell Medical College, Cornell University, Ithaca, NY, USA
e-mail: lel9053@med.cornell.edu

H. Chen
Department of Rehabilitation and Regenerative Medicine, New York Presbyterian, New York, NY, USA
e-mail: hec9065@nyp.org

J. R. Singh
Department of Clinical Rehabilitation Medicine, Weill Cornell medical college, New York, NY, USA
e-mail: jrs9012@med.Cornell.edu

K.-M. G. Fu et al. (eds.), *Treatment of Spine Disease in the Elderly*,
https://doi.org/10.1007/978-3-031-12612-3_5

of these tools, many of these measures fail to include nutrition, psychosocial factors, and other medical conditions, which also contribute to an individual's functional capacity [5].

In order to improve functional outcomes after spine surgery, healthcare delivery models must move away from physicians operating in silos to a more interdisciplinary construct [4, 6]. Typically, rehabilitative care for spine conditions attempts to maintain and improve function while avoiding more invasive interventions. However, if surgical intervention is necessary, the focus of rehabilitation shifts to regaining function. This problem-based approach has its limitations which are further amplified in older adults. Instead, pre-rehabilitation followed by a surgical intervention and continued rehabilitation services is being explored in an attempt to maximize function while decreasing cost, length of stay, morbidity, and mortality. This care model has been limited as it requires significant amounts of coordination of care, and represents a paradigm shift in how healthcare is delivered. While this model has been considered in many surgical subspecialties (cardiac surgery, transplant surgery), little has been done to develop a dedicated pathway for spine care. The older adult is especially vulnerable as it is well-established that their assessments, interventions, and expectations are different from those of a younger healthier cohort. Providers should be aware of changes to body systems that may render older adults susceptible to persistent pain, physical activity decline, and physical function decline. Spine pre-rehabilitation and early rehabilitation after surgery for older adults must consist of appropriate assessments, optimization, and appropriate interventions [7].

With these concepts in mind, we return to the paradigm shift of incorporating prehabilitation to the early recovery after surgery protocol (ERAS) following spine surgery. Carli and Zavorksy presented a multimodal prehabilitation program for the elderly prior to any surgery including endurance, strength, flexibility, and nutrition for a minimum of 4 weeks up to 3 months. Specific recommendations regarding endurance and strength training are delineated in Table 5.1. They advocate for an endurance program duration of 3 months as it has been shown to provide a clinically meaningful increase in VO2max, reduction in blood pressure, and increase in vagal tone. Additionally, progressive increase from moderate to vigorous exercise intensity encourages angiogenesis in fast-twitch muscle fibers which subsequently improves oxygen transport. Nutrition recommendations call for consumption of ~560 kcal of carbohydrates approximately 3 h prior to exercise to improve glycogen storage and immediate consumption of ~200 kcal protein-carbohydrate within 30 min of weight training to promote muscle hypertrophy via protein synthesis.

Currently there is dearth of research on the benefits of prehabilitation on patients undergoing spinal surgeries. In a study by Nielsen et al., 28 patients underwent a prehabilitation program consisting of a 30-min home exercise routine focused on muscular strength for back and abdomen and cardiovascular conditioning daily for 6–8 weeks prior to lumbar surgery which resulted in improved function measured by the Roland-Morris scale, reached postoperative milestones quicker than the control patients, and had shorter length of stays in the hospital. However, objectively sit to stand and timed up and go scores did not significantly differ between the

Table 5.1 Recommendations for a 3-month endurance and strength training program prior to surgery

		Intensity	Duration	Considerations
Endurance	Aerobic exercises (walking, jogging, swimming, cycling, rowing, dancing)	Moderate intensity (45–65% of maximum heart rate)	30–50 min, four times a week	
		Periodic high-intensity interval training (~90% of maximum heart rate)		
Strength	8–10 exercises for major muscle groups	Four sets per exercise with vigorous intensity (80% maximal resistance)	2 nonconsecutive days per week with at least 72 h between sessions	Use weight machines before progressing to free weights
		For the more frail adult: four sets of exercise with moderate intensity (60% maximal resistance)		

intervention and control groups. A more recent single-blinded, randomized control trial (PREPARE) evaluated the effects of prehabilitation program with physical therapy intervention two times per week for 9 weeks in addition to a recommended home exercise program prior to spine surgery compared to a group who awaited surgery. Each program was customized to each patient's ailment with physical therapy, a supervised exercise program, and a behavioral approach to reduce fear and improve activity level. The exercise program included 10-min intervals of cardiovascular exercise in the beginning, middle, and end of each session in addition to 5–6 exercises based on the patients' function, posture, and functional status with the posology of 15 repetitions in three sets. The goal intensity level was moderate [8]. Both groups followed a post-surgery rehabilitation program which included postural and gait training. Following outpatient therapy, home exercise program as well as a walking program was continued after discharge and advanced after 6 weeks [8]. Initial results from the PREPARE trial showed improvement in patient-reported outcomes including back pain, decreased anxiety, fear avoidance behavior, and physical activity prior to spine surgery; however, outcomes post-surgery were no different except for continued increased physical activity [8]. Secondary results and analysis from the PREPARE showed that individuals in the intervention group who underwent at least 12 treatments had significantly improved gait speeds, quadriceps femoris strength measured by dynamometer just prior to surgery, and self-reported level of physical activity and walking distances (Fors).

At present, prehabilitation shows some evidence of measurable improvement prior to surgery and in postsurgical outcomes. With that said, there is not enough evidence to definitively state that prehabilitation can be used to promote ERAS following spinal surgery. More research is required at this time regarding prehabilitation studies in the elderly undergoing spine surgery.

A battery of assessments can evaluate the modifiable mobility, balance, strength, and endurance deficits commonly found with spine pathology in the older adult population. The following are commonly used outcomes measures used in both the prehabilitation and postoperative groups.

The timed up and go (TUG) assesses mobility, balance, walking ability, and fall risk in the elderly. A score is created by measuring the time it takes for an individual to rise from an upright seated position in a chair, ambulate 3 m, and return to their starting position. While TUG is sensitive to detecting decreasing mobility in the elderly, it is nonspecific regarding which aspect of mobility is lacking in the tested individual limiting its utility in designing a rehabilitation program for an individual. There is however evidence that geriatric rehabilitation can improve mean TUG score from 31.9 to 21.2 [9].

The Berg Balance Scale is a battery of 14 items that assesses static balance in the adult population. Each item is scored on a scale 0–4 for a total of 0–56 points. Various studies have found different cutoffs for scores that may indicate a greater risk of falling with one studying finding a score <40 was associated with a near 100% fall risk and another found that within a nursing home population, a score <47 was associated with increased risk for falling [10, 11]. Limitations include no clear consensus in the interpretation of the BBS scores and the amount of time it takes to administer the test.

The handheld dynamometer is a device used to measure the strength produced in the hand and forearm by measuring force production in pounds or kilograms; this is measured as a mean of three trials. However, limitations include use of a standardized test position to avoid alteration of grip strength, and there is some evidence that grip strength does not correlate with lower limb strength and functional capacity particularly in elderly women [12].

While the dynamometer provides a direct measurement of upper limb strength, the five times sit to stand evaluates lower extremity strength by measuring the time that it takes for a patient to rise to a standing position from a seated position five times. This has been used as a screening tool to assess fall risk in the elderly with scores greater than or equal to 12 [13, 14]. Normative values for age-matched comparisons are available [15]. This test also has good test/retest reliability [13]. As this is not a direct measure of force production, Bohannon et al. showed in 2010 [16] that performance of this test is more reflective of lower limb strength particularly knee extension when compared to other variations of this test such as the 30-s sit to stand test.

Current methods for evaluating endurance during rehabilitation involve the 6-min walk test in which the total distance ambulated over 6 min is measured; individuals are allotted as many rest breaks as needed. The test is cost-effective and is simple to perform [5] with good test/retest reliability [17]. Score comparisons may be made with age-matched normative data [5]. In assessing functional improvements with the 6-min walk test, Perera et al. [7] found that small meaningful changes ranged from 19 to 22 m and substantial meaningful changes ranged from 47 to 49 m which is approximately half the length of a football field. The 2-min walk test is an abbreviated form of the 6-min walk test that was found to be better tolerated by geriatric inpatient rehabilitation patients [9] with excellent test/retest reliability. Normative data is available for age-matched groups (Connelly and Thomas 2009, [15]). However, it is important to note that these assessments are most suitable for the elderly with mild to moderate impairments and its utility may be more limited in healthier and more mobile elderly patients.

The ultimate long-term rehabilitation goals are congruent with the physical activity guidelines set forth by the American College of Sports Medicine and the United States Health and Human Services. For older adults, it is recommended to incorporate balance exercises in addition to resistance and endurance exercises already recommended for all adults. Intensity level of exercises can be measured in several ways (Table 5.2). This includes relative measurements of intensity in percentage of heart rate reserve (%HRR) which approximates percentage of oxygen consumption reserve (%VO2R), percentage of maximal heart rate (%MHR), and rating of perceived exertion either on a scale from 6 to 20 (BRPE) or 0 to 10 (RPE) as well as absolute measurements of intensity in metabolic equivalents (METs). %VO2R is the percentage of the difference between oxygen consumption at maximal effort versus at rest. MET is defined as the amount of oxygen consumed while sitting at rest and is equal to 3.5 mL O_2 per kg body weight × min.

Resistance exercises that build strength should be performed at least 2 days/week at either moderate or vigorous intensity; the scale is the same as above. The program should include progressive weight training or weight-bearing calisthenics, stair climbing, or other exercises that target major muscle groups. Regimens may include 8–10 exercises consisting of 8–12 repetitions each [18].

Table 5.2 Classification of physical activity intensity

	Endurance activities						Resistance-type exercises
	Relative intensity				Absolute intensity (METs) for age groups		Relative intensity
Intensity	VO2R (%), heart rate reserve (%)	Maximal heart rate (%)	RPE (scale of 0–10)	BRPE (scale of 6–20)	65–79 years old	80 years and older	Maximal voluntary contraction (%)
Very light	<20	<35	1–2	<10	<1.6	≤1.0	<30
Light	20–39	35–54	3–4	10–11	1.6–3.1	1.1–1.9	30–49
Moderate	40–59	55–69	5–6	12–13	3.2–4.7	2.0–2.9	50–69
Vigorous	60–84	70–89	7–8	14–16	4.8–6.7	3.0–4.25	70–84
Very vigorous	≥85	≥90	9	17–19	≥6.8	≥4.25	≥85
Maximal	100	100	10	20	8.0	5.0	100

RPE revised Borg rating of perceived exertion, *BRPE* Borg rating of perceived exertion, *%VO2R* percent of oxygen consumption reserve, METs metabolic equivalents
Adapted from [18]

Regarding endurance exercises, adults should aim to accumulate 150 min/week of moderate-intensity activities or 75 min/week of vigorous-intensity activities. Duration of physical activity is further delineated by type of activity. For moderate-intensity exercises, adults should aim to perform 30 min/day in at least 10-min intervals. For vigorous-intensity exercises, adults should aim to perform 20 min of continuous exercise daily [18].

Given the increased risk for falls in the elderly, it is recommended that balance exercises be incorporated for a multicomponent physical activity regimen. Despite this recommendation, there are no current specific guidelines regarding dosing or intensity at this time. Regimens should include progressively more challenging balance-oriented tasks that reduce base of support, stress support muscle groups in the lower leg and feet, incorporate dynamic movements that alter the center of gravity, and reduce sensory input [18]. There is some research that indicates a total of 50 h of balance training is needed to decrease fall risk [19].

A flexibility program in which major muscle groups undergo sustained stretch at a moderate intensity for 2 days/week is also recommended [18].

However, for the elderly functionally limited due to deconditioning, frailty, back pain, or other chronic conditions, a more conservative approach is recommended, and physical activity is performed as tolerated and progressed according to preference and tolerance. As such, a physical activity program should be custom-tailored to the individual at hand with protracted progression of difficulty [20–22].

Early Postoperative Rehabilitation

Postoperatively, rehabilitation begins within a day of undergoing surgery; there is growing evidence that early mobilization can decrease hospital length of stay, reduce readmissions, and reduce postoperative complications [23, 24]. Early mobilization has been variably defined as demonstrating independence in performing a log roll, moving out of bed to a chair several times a day, or participating with physical therapy and occupational therapy [24]. While it is clear that these are important functional activities, this lack of standardization in research has made it difficult to define the exact dosing and which physical activities are most beneficial to patients to promote mobility. Requirements for a safe discharge home postoperatively requires the ability to ambulate household distances, ascend or descend necessary stairs, and perform activities of daily living (ADLs) with relative independence or reasonable assistance provided by identified caretakers. If these goals are not attainable within the immediate perioperative period, alternative pathways prior to returning home are considered; these include acute rehabilitation or subacute rehabilitation depending on the patient's level of activity, ability to participate in therapy, and social support. In these settings, there is more time and resources to truly uncover the physical needs of an elderly patient. In general, there is no one-size-fits-all program that can adequately address the needs of the elderly when undergoing spine surgery.

Conclusion

Preoperative optimization should consist of more than managing modifiable risk factors. Pre-rehabilitation may be the necessary complement to risk factor management that leads to even lower incidence of postoperative complications. While crafting a surgery-specific prehabilitation program may not be necessary, directed functional assessment for the older adult population can provide insights and inform the postoperative recovery process. More high-quality studies are needed to validate pathology-specific functional assessments and targeted therapies. Ultimately, a multitiered approach is required to change behaviors and implement evidence-based practice. Healthcare provider and institutional-based protocols are the most logical next step. Additional attention must also be given to the psychological, cognitive, and social influences that are impediments to care.

References

1. Prince MJ, Wu F, Guo Y, Gutierrez Robledo LM, O'Donnell M, Sullivan R, et al. The burden of disease in older people and implications for health policy and practice. Lancet. 2015;385: 549–62. https://doi.org/10.1016/S0140-6736(14)61347-7.
2. Hoy D, Bain C, Williams G, et al. A systematic review of the global prevalence of low back pain. Arthritis Rheum. 2012;64(6):2028–37. https://doi.org/110.1002/art.34347.
3. General Surgery News. 2020. https://www.generalsurgerynews.com/In-the-News/Article/12-20/Surgeons-Can-Do-More-to-Prehab-Rehab-Patients/61398.
4. Nielsen PR, Jørgensen LD, Dahl B, Pedersen T, Tønnesen H. Prehabilitation and early rehabilitation after spinal surgery: randomized clinical trial. Clin Rehabil. 2010;24(2):137–48. https://doi.org/10.1177/0269215509347432.
5. Steffen TM, Hacker TA, Mollinger L. Age- and gender-related test performance in community-dwelling elderly people: Six-Minute Walk Test, Berg Balance Scale, Timed Up & Go Test, and gait speeds. Phys Ther. 2002;82(2):128–37. https://doi.org/10.1093/ptj/82.2.128. PMID: 11856064.
6. Carli F, Zavorsky GS. Optimizing functional exercise capacity in the elderly surgical population. Curr Opin Clin Nutr Metab Care. 2005;8(1):23–32. https://doi.org/10.1097/00075197-200501000-00005.
7. Perera S, Mody SH, Woodman RC, Studenski SA. Meaningful change and responsiveness in common physical performance measures in older adults. J Am Geriatr Soc. 2006;54(5):743–9. https://doi.org/10.1111/j.1532-5415.2006.00701.x. PMID: 16696738.
8. Lindbäck Y, Tropp H, Enthoven P, Abbott A, Öberg B. PREPARE: pre-surgery physiotherapy for patients with degenerative lumbar spine disorder: a randomized controlled trial protocol. BMC Musculoskelet Disord. 2016;17:270. https://doi.org/10.1186/s12891-016-1126-4.
9. Brooks D, Davis AM, Naglie G. The feasibility of six-minute and two-minute walk tests in in-patient geriatric rehabilitation. Can J Aging. 2007;26(2):159–62. https://doi.org/10.3138/cja.26.2.009. PMID: 17613447.
10. Shumway-Cook A, Baldwin M, Polissar NL, Gruber W. Predicting the probability for falls in community-dwelling older adults. Phys Ther. 1997;77(8):812–19. https://doi.org/10.1093/ptj/77.8.812.

11. Viveiro LAP, Gomes GCV, Bacha JMR, et al. Reliability, validity, and ability to identity fall status of the berg balance scale, balance evaluation systems test (BESTest), Mini-BESTest, and Brief-BESTest in older adults who live in nursing homes. J Geriatr Phys Ther. 2019;42(4):E45–E54. https://doi.org/10.1519/JPT.0000000000000215.
12. Rodacki ALF, Boneti Moreira N, Pitta A, et al. Is handgrip strength a useful measure to evaluate lower limb strength and functional performance in older women? Clin Interv Aging. 2020;15:1045–56. https://doi.org/10.2147/CIA.S253262.
13. Tiedemann A, Shimada H, Sherrington C, Murray S, Lord S. The comparative ability of eight functional mobility tests for predicting falls in community-dwelling older people. Age Ageing. 2008;37(4):430–35. https://doi.org/10.1093/ageing/afn100.
14. Buatois S, Perret-Guillaume C, Gueguen R, et al. A simple clinical scale to stratify risk of recurrent falls in community-dwelling adults aged 65 years and older. Phys Ther. 2010;90(4):550–60. https://doi.org/10.2522/ptj.20090158.
15. Bohannon RW. Normative reference values for the two-minute walk test derived by meta-analysis. J Phys Ther Sci. 2017;29(12):2224–7. https://doi.org/10.1589/jpts.29.2224.
16. Bohannon RW, Bubela DJ, Magasi SR, Wang YC, Gershon RC. Sit-to-stand test: performance and determinants across the age-span. Isokinet Exerc Sci. 2010;18(4):235–40. https://doi.org/10.3233/IES-2010-0389.
17. Steffens D, Maher CG, Pereira LS, et al. Prevention of low back pain: a systematic review and meta-analysis. JAMA Intern Med. 2016;176(2):199–208. https://doi.org/10.1001/jamainternmed.2015.7431.
18. American College of Sports Medicine, Chodzko-Zajko WJ, Proctor DN, Fiatarone Singh MA, Minson CT, Nigg CR, Salem GJ, Skinner JS. FACSM exercise and physical activity for older adults. Med Sci Sports Exerc. 2009;41(7):1510–30. https://doi.org/10.1249/MSS.0b013e3181a0c95c.
19. Shubert TE. Evidence-based exercise prescription for balance and falls prevention: a current review of the literature. J Geriatr Phys Ther. 2011;34(3):100–8. https://doi.org/10.1519/JPT.0b013e31822938ac.
20. Cadore EL, Pinto RS, Bottaro M, Izquierdo M. Strength and endurance training prescription in healthy and frail elderly. Aging Dis. 2014;5(3):183–95. https://doi.org/10.14336/AD.2014.0500183.
21. Piercy KL, Troiano RP, Ballard RM, Carlson SA, Fulton JE, Galuska DA, George SM, Olson RD. The physical activity guidelines for Americans. JAMA. 2018;320(19):2020–8. https://doi.org/10.1001/jama.2018.14854. PMID: 30418471.
22. Pauwels C, Roren A, Gautier A, Linières J, Rannou F, Poiraudeau S, Nguyen C. Home-based cycling program tailored to older people with lumbar spinal stenosis: barriers and facilitators. Ann Phys Rehabil Med. 2018;61(3):144–50. https://doi.org/10.1016/j.rehab.2018.02.005. Epub 2018 Feb 27. PMID: 29499383.
23. Epstein N. A review article on the benefits of early mobilization following spinal surgery and other medical/surgical procedures. Surg Neurol Int. 2014;5(4):S66–73.
24. Tong Y, Fernandez L, Bendo JA, Spivak JM. Enhanced recovery after surgery trends in adult spine surgery: a systematic review. Int J Spine Surg. 2020;14(4):623–40. https://doi.org/10.14444/7083. Epub 2020 Jul 31. PMID: 32986587; PMCID: PMC7477993.

Chapter 6
ERAS and Spine Surgery

Michael D. Staudt, Xiaofei Zhou, Olindi Wijesekera, Jonathan P. Miller, and Jennifer A. Sweet

Introduction

A patient's surgical experience is comprised of different facets of perioperative care, including the preoperative, intraoperative, and postoperative phases, and is overseen by a multitude of practitioners. As such, postoperative recovery is a complex process that is not only influenced by a technically successful operation but also depends on the quality of perioperative care as coordinated by a multidisciplinary team. Such coordinated efforts are essential in reducing pain, morbidity, and recovery time. Indeed, a significant proportion of patients undergoing surgery will experience postoperative pain, with the majority reporting moderate or extreme pain [1]. Inadequate postoperative pain control has numerous adverse effects on the patient and healthcare system, including unwanted and harmful physiological side effects, poor patient satisfaction, and an increased overall cost of healthcare resource utilization [2].

Enhanced Recovery After Surgery (ERAS) protocols have thus been developed as a conceptual framework of optimizing surgical recovery. The core philosophy of ERAS consists of a multimodal approach to perioperative management, with the implementation of evidence-based approaches to treatment using a

M. D. Staudt
Department of Neurosurgery, Oakland University William Beaumont School of Medicine, Rochester, MI, USA

Michigan Head and Spine Institute, Southfield, MI, USA

X. Zhou · O. Wijesekera · J. P. Miller · J. A. Sweet (✉)
Department of Neurosurgery, University Hospitals Cleveland Medical Center, Case Western Reserve University, Cleveland, OH, USA
e-mail: Xiaofei.zhou@uhhospitals.org; Olindi.Wijesekera@uhhospitals.org; Jonathan.Miller@uhhospitals.org; jennifer.sweet@uhhospitals.org

K.-M. G. Fu et al. (eds.), *Treatment of Spine Disease in the Elderly*, https://doi.org/10.1007/978-3-031-12612-3_6

multidisciplinary team [3]. In 2001, the ERAS study group was founded by a group of European academic surgeons, who first developed a multimodal recovery protocol for colonic surgery based on the published literature [4]. Previously, the concept of "fast-track" surgery had been described in different specialties such as cardiac and general surgery [5–7] with an initial focus on expediting the speed of recovery, which then developed into a protocol for optimizing perioperative management to reduce complications and enhance recovery [8]. Subsequently, the ERAS Society was founded with a mission to "develop perioperative care and to improve recovery through research, education, audit and implementation of evidence-based practice" (http://www.erassociety.org).

Although the ERAS Society has published numerous guidelines and consists of multiple specialties, there is no neurosurgical representation, and no guidelines exist regarding the perioperative management of spinal surgeries; however, the Congress of Neurological Surgeons is currently developing perioperative spine surgery guidelines, which are expected to be published in 2021. Until recently, the literature lacked detailed studies outlining ERAS protocols and outcomes for spine surgery [9], and the past few years have seen a newfound enthusiasm in ERAS development for a variety of spinal procedures and pathologies [10, 11]. The purpose of this chapter is to outline the components of ERAS protocols as they relate to spine surgery, and to review the process of ERAS development and published outcomes in the literature.

Rationale for the Use of ERAS in Spinal Surgery

There is a compelling case for the implementation of ERAS into the routine management of spinal surgery. Some spine procedures are associated with long operative duration, extensive muscle retraction and dissection, and the implantation of hardware, which can lead to prolonged recovery, delayed mobilization, and significant pain. In particular, both lumbar fusion and complex spinal reconstruction procedures have been rated by patients as having the most significant pain on the first postoperative day [12]. Accordingly, postoperative pain influences several outcome measures, including length of hospitalization, time to mobilization, readmission rates, and opioid tolerance and dose escalation [13].

The complexity of pain management for spinal pathologies is derived from the diverse pain etiologies arising from nociceptive, neuropathic, and inflammatory mechanisms, with potential anatomical sources of pain including the paraspinal muscles, bone, facet joints, and the intervertebral discs [14]. In addition to delaying recovery and prolonging a patient's initial hospital admission, the intensity of pain experienced in the early postoperative period may lead to the development of chronic postsurgical pain [15]. Pain can also be associated with kinesiophobia, or the "fear of movement" following spine surgery, which can impair early mobilization, leading to even greater pain, disability, and adverse psychological effects [16, 17].

Previously, the liberal use of opioids was favored in the treatment of acute postoperative pain; however, the rise in morbidity and mortality associated with acute and chronic opioid therapy has encouraged the development of multimodal analgesia (MMA) paradigms to both reduce perioperative opioid use and improve postoperative pain control and patient recovery [18, 19]. It is important to recognize that a majority of patients presenting for major spine surgery are taking opioids and that higher utilization of preoperative opioid use and higher pain scores are associated with chronic postoperative opioid use [20]. Interestingly, the preoperative use of high-potency opioids has also been associated with an increased reoperation rate following lumbar decompression or fusion surgeries [21]. Furthermore, opioid use in the elderly can be fraught with complications, as these patients are at an elevated risk of developing complications due to their comorbidities and higher likelihood of polypharmacy [22]. In particular, one must take into account a potentially elevated fall and fracture risk [23]. Although data on opioid abuse for adults aged 65 years and older are largely lacking [24], a number of studies have reported increasing rates of misuse and addiction [25, 26].

In the United States, the rates of surgical procedures for degenerative spine disease have rapidly increased over the past few decades, in particular the use of fusion for lumbar stenosis and spondylolisthesis [27–29]. The increasing complexity of cases necessitating fusion has also been associated with increased cost and risk of major complications and mortality [30]. Interestingly, some studies have suggested that postoperative, but not intraoperative, events are more predictive of increased length of stay (LOS) following lumbar fusion [31]. There is significant diversity in the nature of postoperative care among institutions and individual surgeons, with differing practices regarding the prescribing of medications, mobilization, and instructions for return to activity or work. As such, implementation of an ERAS protocol following spine surgery could potentially streamline postoperative care and improve outcomes.

ERAS Components

A multimodal ERAS management strategy focuses on optimizing the preoperative, intraoperative, and postoperative periods (Fig. 6.1). The foundation of these strategies is in minimizing stressors from a variety of physiological, psychological, and economic sources [32, 33].

Preoperative Period

Preoperative optimization begins even before the patient presents to the hospital for their procedure. Preparation begins with education, which can include the basic details of the surgical procedure, expected length of the procedure and LOS,

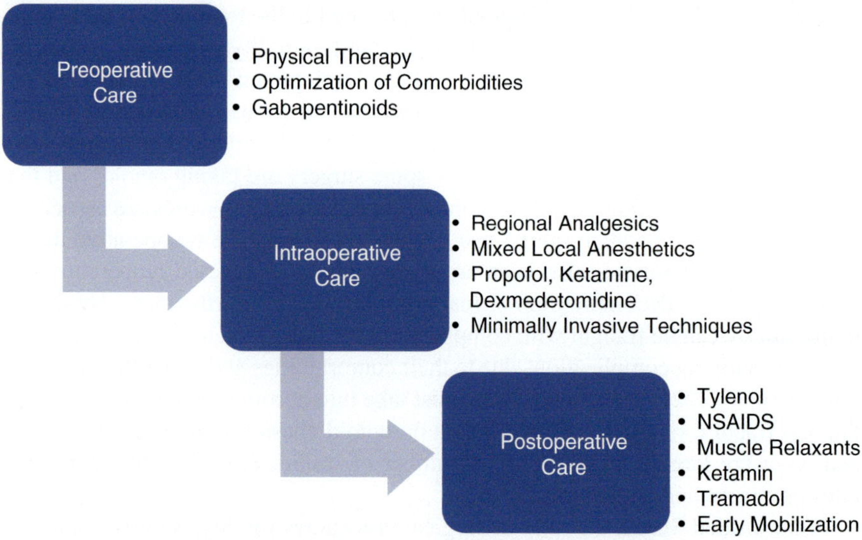

Fig. 6.1 Typical components of an ERAS pathway

postoperative expectations for discharge, potential restrictions on mobility and activity, and expected course of postoperative recovery. Despite the seemingly basic nature of this information, having a structured approach to providing education can empower patients. Indeed, there is evidence that such preoperative education sessions improve pain, function, and psychological outcomes following spine surgery [34, 35]. "Prehabilitation," or the process of enhancing functional capacity prior to elective surgery, has also been researched in spine surgery [36]; however, there are few studies addressing this topic, and it is not clear if their implementation results in significant improvements in pain or function.

Additional preoperative considerations include the management and optimization of comorbidities, particularly in an elderly population with a higher incidence of heart disease and diabetes. The rising rates of obesity are concerning, and there is often an association with diabetes. Multiple studies have shown that patients with poorly controlled diabetes have a higher incidence of postoperative complications following spine surgery, including infection and poor wound healing [37, 38]. Similarly, tobacco use is associated with a higher rate of adverse events following spine surgery, including infection, fusion failure, and cardiopulmonary complications [39, 40]. Screening for such factors is essential to optimize preoperative health and function. Other considerations include the identification of nutritional insufficiency or malnutrition—this often unrecognized risk factor has been independently associated with adverse events following spine surgery including infection, increased LOS, and mortality [41, 42]. In addition to these modifiable factors, non-modifiable factors such as the use of anticoagulation medications may also contribute to the development of perioperative complications and should be managed appropriately.

As discussed, infection is an important complication in spine surgery. In addition to optimizing comorbidities, other critical considerations include the use of preoperative antibiotics, and appropriate sterile preparation and surgical technique. Preoperative bathing with chlorhexidine gluconate has received recent attention in the orthopedic literature as a means of reducing surgical site infections [43]. A recent analysis of 4266 spine surgeries reported that the implementation of a protocol requiring patients to shower at least 3 times prior to surgery with chlorhexidine significantly decreased the risk of developing an infection [44]. Interestingly, this decreased risk was only observed in patients undergoing spine surgery without fusion in univariate analysis, perhaps as a result of the increased complexity of cases requiring fusion [44].

"Preemptive" analgesia refers to the preoperative administration of pain medications to prevent postoperative pain. Mechanistically these medications inhibit or reduce autonomic reactivity and nociceptive signals generated through tissue damage and inflammation [13]. The use of gabapentinoids, including gabapentin and pregabalin in the preoperative setting, has been demonstrated to decrease opioid consumption and improve pain scores following lumbar surgery [45, 46], and both drugs may be equally efficacious [47]. The use of nonsteroidal anti-inflammatory drugs (NSAIDs) has also been demonstrated to improve pain scores and reduce opioid use in the postoperative period [48]. Although there have been concerns regarding the use of NSAIDs and the development of pseudoarthrosis or nonunion, numerous studies have reported their safety in the postoperative period when judiciously dosed [49, 50]. Many ERAS protocols will combine different agents based on institutional or provider preference, and common combinations include a gabapentinoid, NSAID, and/or acetaminophen [51–53]. Another consideration is timing of medication administration, as different protocols may initiate therapy on the morning of surgery and/or the night before surgery. For gabapentinoids, this may include administration of a single or divided oral dose of 300–1200 mg, 2–24 h before surgery [54]; one meta-analysis of multiple inpatient surgical procedures identified an association between the cumulative gabapentin dose and a total reduction in morphine consumption [54].

Intraoperative Period

There are numerous intraoperative considerations for ERAS implementation, including the choice of anesthetic agent, MMA with a focus on opioid-sparing medications, antimicrobial prophylaxis, and the maintenance of both normothermia and normovolemia.

A number of different anesthetic regimens have been described in conjunction with ERAS protocols. When general anesthesia is desired, propofol tends to be the agent of choice in multiple ERAS paradigms [52, 53, 55, 56]. The use of ketamine as both a pre-incisional bolus and intraoperative infusion has been reported to reduce opioid consumption and incisional hyperalgesia, and also improve the efficacy of neurophysiologic monitoring by reducing inhalational anesthetic requirements [14, 57]. Dexmedetomidine has also been investigated as a sedative and analgesic adjuvant in spine surgery, with notable reductions in both intraoperative and postoperative opioid use reported [58]. Intravenous glucocorticoids have been reported to reduce postoperative pain as well as nausea and vomiting [59], although some studies have reported a higher rate of postoperative infection [60]. The use of regional (neuraxial) anesthesia in spine surgery has also been described in a number of studies, commonly employing the use of spinal bupivacaine [61]. Compared to a general anesthetic, regional anesthesia may be associated with decreased blood loss, a lower incidence of nausea and vomiting, and reduced pain scores and LOS [61].

Infiltration of the incision with local anesthetic is a widely utilized and efficacious technique [62], and is routinely infiltrated underneath the skin prior to incision and into the muscle prior to closure. Such measures may reduce postoperative pain scores and opioid use [63]. Although local anesthetics are generally limited by their relatively short duration of action, there has been recent enthusiasm in the use of multivesicular liposomes containing bupivacaine, which allows for sustained drug release that can last for a few days. Recent studies assessing the use of liposomal bupivacaine suggest improved mobility and reduced opioid consumption when either used as a sole intervention [64] or in conjunction with an ERAS protocol [65]. The use of intrathecal morphine has also been reported to reduce pain scores and postoperative opioid use following spine surgery [66]. Complications including pruritus and respiratory depression have been reported in some studies [66]. Although pain is improved in the immediate postoperative period, the efficacy tends not to persist after 48–72 h, and is not associated with a decreased LOS [66–68].

Spine operations can be associated with numerous homeostatic insults, particularly in those of longer duration and requiring more exposure and/or instrumentation. Longer operations are associated with potentially extended periods of hypothermia, which has been reported to increase the incidence of infection [69]; as such, maintaining overall normothermia and targeting a core temperature of 36 °C is considered essential. Major spine surgery can also be associated with elevated blood loss, resulting in hypotension and an increased risk of end-organ damage. In one study, patients requiring a blood transfusion during lumbar fusion were significantly more likely to develop a complication, including sepsis, pulmonary embolus, or infection [70]. The maintenance of normovolemia in spine surgery is therefore essential, and has been associated with reduced blood loss and lower rates of transfusion, as well as improved respiratory and bowel function [71]. The use of tranexamic acid has been reported to be effective in reducing perioperative blood loss and the need for transfusion [72], and may provide an especially useful adjunct when used in conjunction with thorough surgical hemostasis techniques [73].

An additional consideration is the avoidance or early removal of urinary catheters and surgical drains. Urinary catheters are associated with development of urinary tract infections, and there is mixed evidence in their association with the development of a surgical site infection following spine surgery [74]. The prolonged use of surgical drains has similarly been reported as an independent risk factor for developing a surgical site infection [75]. Minimally invasive surgeries (MIS) may be able to avoid the use of catheters and drains, although they may be necessary following major spine surgery with longer durations and larger exposures. Accordingly, many ERAS protocols specify early removal to facilitate mobilization [11].

Postoperative Period

The key postoperative considerations following spine surgery focus on pain control, mobilization and the path to discharge. Whereas early "fast-track" protocols may have focused exclusively on the speed of recovery and discharge, ERAS places greater emphasis on optimizing the patient experience.

One of the most important postoperative considerations is that of pain control and the appropriate medication regimen. If implemented judiciously, the use of pre-emptive and intraoperative MMA as described in previous sections can improve postoperative pain control through an opioid-sparing approach. Different agents are used in combination to synergistically treat pain, and common postoperative drugs include acetaminophen, gabapentin or pregabalin, NSAIDs, and muscle relaxants. The use of scheduled NSAIDs, as opposed to the as-needed administration, may act synergistically with opioids in the postoperative period [18]. This may enable an overall decreased dose of opioids, indirectly reducing postoperative nausea and sedation [18]. Such benefits may be of particular use to the elderly population, who are particularly susceptible to opioid-related side effects [22, 76]. Of course the use of perioperative NSAIDs must be measured with the risk of potential platelet dysfunction, gastrointestinal irritation, and/or renal impairment [18].

The use of NMDA agonists, such as ketamine, in the perioperative period may also be an effective approach to surgical pain. Different administration protocols have been described, including its use as a pre-incisional bolus, an intraoperative infusion, and postoperative use in combination with a patient-controlled analgesia (PCA) pump [77]. Given as infusions, they can lower the use of opioid therapy and decrease nausea and vomiting [18, 57, 77]. However, the administration of the agent in this manner may require a coordinated effort from pharmacy, the recovery unit nursing staff, and anesthesia, who will likely ultimately be overseeing its delivery. Furthermore, ketamine is a psychoactive drug, which could potentially contribute to the development of postoperative cognitive side effects in a vulnerable elderly population [78]. In a multicenter randomized trial of patients aged 60 years or older undergoing major surgery, the use of a subanesthetic ketamine dose during surgery did not reduce the incidence of postoperative delirium, and instead increased the incidence of postoperative nightmares and hallucinations [79].

It is difficult if not impossible to avoid the use of opioids altogether, and the judicious administration of short-acting opioids and/or tramadol may be necessary. Tramadol acts weakly at the μ-opioid receptors, but also acts at non-opioid receptors, resulting in inhibition of norepinephrine and serotonin reuptake. Consequently, there is a multimodal benefit of this single agent [18]. Tramadol's weak action at the opioid receptor also diminishes the risk of addiction and other systemic side effects seen with traditional opioids use [18]. One novel treatment strategy involves administration of pain medications based on NRS scores, with non-opioids administered for scores 4 or less, tramadol for scores between 5 and 7, and oxycodone for scores between 8 and 10 [55]. In this protocol, assessment by an anesthesiologist is required if pain is refractory and dose escalation is required [55].

PCA pumps are commonly used as postoperative adjuncts in the first 12–24 h. Following this initial period, the patient is transitioned to oral medications with dosing determined by the amount and frequency of PCA use [14]. However, PCA usage has been reported to be associated with increased total opioid use and increased adverse events [80]. Interestingly, PCA use has also been associated with equivalent or even worse postoperative pain control compared to MMA [80, 81], which suggests careful consideration for their inclusion in an ERAS protocol. When implemented, there should always be a plan for early discontinuation and transition to oral therapy [82].

An essential component of ERAS protocols is early mobilization, referring to mobilization on the day of surgery or the first postoperative day thereafter. The adverse effects of bed rest and immobilization are well-documented, in particular the elevated risk of deconditioning, cardiopulmonary events, and thromboembolism [83–85]. Across multiple disciplines, the benefits of early mobilization are apparent in reducing the postoperative LOS, and also as measured by an overall reduction in rates of infection, respiratory compromise, thromboembolic events, and sepsis [86]. Few studies have specifically investigated the impact of early mobilization following spine surgery; however, these studies have uniformly identified improvements in rates of perioperative complications and LOS [87–90]. Accordingly, they have been adopted with enthusiasm into spine ERAS protocols [91]. Equally important considerations are involvement with physical and occupational therapy during an inpatient admission [52, 55, 92], and to continue physical therapy on an outpatient basis.

Outcomes by Type of Spine Surgery

Few publications on ERAS and spine surgery were available prior to 2018, and the past few years have seen an exponential increase in interest and published protocols. These protocols are highly variable and tend to be institutional-specific, but have generally focused on providing improved education, early nutrition and mobilization, multimodal pain management, and a general trend toward a transition to minimally invasive techniques. These protocols have been studied in a variety of spine surgeries, from simple decompressive laminectomies to more extensive tumor and fusion surgeries. The majority of currently reported protocols are focused on lumbar surgeries. Regardless of the specific ERAS elements, nearly all studies have reported beneficial effects, often related to decreased LOS and reduced opioid usage, without an increase in complications or readmissions [93]. Table 6.1 comprehensively outlines selected studies that evaluate ERAS protocols compared to cohorts with conventional care.

Table 6.1 Selected ERAS studies in spine surgery with comparison to conventional care pathways

Author, year	Type of study	Study size	Open or MIS	Type of spine surgery	ERAS components	LOS (vs. traditional)	Pain	Complications/ readmissions	Cost reduction
Fletcher, 2014 [94]	Retrospective	ERAS 279, control 86	Open	AIS undergoing PSF	Postoperative: early oral meds, drain removal, PT, nutrition	2.92 days vs. 4.28 days			$1885 vs. $2779
Gornitzky, 2016 [95]	Prospective	ERAS 58, control 81	Open	AIS undergoing PSF	Perioperative: MMA Postoperative: early ambulation, nutrition	LOS 31% shorter	Decreased pain at POD 0,1,2	No difference	
Muhly, 2016 [96]	Prospective	ERAS 84, transition period 104, historic controls 134	Open	AIS undergoing PSF	Postoperative: MMA, early mobilization, nutrition, transition to oral medications, drain removal	4 days vs. 5.7 days	Decreased pain at POD 0 and POD 1	No difference	
Fletcher, 2017 [97]	Retrospective	ERAS 105, control 45	Open	AIS undergoing PSF	Postoperative: early mobilization, nutrition, transition to oral medications, drain removal	48% shorter LOS		No difference	

(continued)

Table 6.1 (continued)

Author, year	Type of study	Study size	Open or MIS	Type of spine surgery	ERAS components	LOS (vs. traditional)	Pain	Complications/ readmissions	Cost reduction
Rao, 2017 [98]	Retrospective	Pre-ERAS 51, first protocol 100, second protocol 39	Open	AIS undergoing PSF	First: early PCA discontinuation, epidural pain infusion until POD 3, full nutrition POD 2, drain removed on POD 2, cefazolin until drain removal, d/c Foley after epidural catheter is pulled, up to chair on POD 2 with short walks	84.3 h (second protocol) vs. 98.4 h (first protocol)	No difference		
					Second: full nutrition POD 0, d/c Foley if epidural drain still in place if able to stand				

Li, 2018 [99]	Retrospective	ERAS 114, control 110	Open	Cervical (laminoplasty)	Preoperative: education, antimicrobial prophylaxis Perioperative: reduced fasting time, MMA Postoperative: MMA, early drain/catheter removal, nutrition, mobilization	5.75 days vs. 7.67 days	POD 3 VAS score 2.72 vs. 3.35 (no difference in frequency of breakout pain)	Lower rate of urinary tract infections Higher rate of nausea and vomiting	
Debono, 2020 [100]	Retrospective	ERAS 202, control 202	Open	Cervical (ACDF)	Preoperative: patient education Perioperative: disinfection protocol, preemptive analgesia, no routine drain, seated in recovery room without brace, early PT Posthospitalization: trained nurse available for phone fast tracking, satisfaction survey, outcome metrics	1.40 days vs. 2.96 days	No difference in levels of satisfaction	No difference	

(continued)

Table 6.1 (continued)

Author, year	Type of study	Study size	Open or MIS	Type of spine surgery	ERAS components	LOS (vs. traditional)	Pain	Complications/ readmissions	Cost reduction
Carr, 2019 [53]	Retrospective	ERAS 620, traditional 183, non-ERAS after ERAS implemented 129	Open	Cervical, thoracic, lumbar	Preoperative: education, carbohydrate loading, MMA, temperature control, nasal povidone-iodine swab	LOS: 5.4 days vs. 8.2 days			Savings of $19.344 between traditional and ERAS pathways
					Perioperative: temperature control, MMA, TXA	ICU LOS: 1.8 days vs. 3.1 days			
					Postoperative: MMA, early nutrition, drain removal, mobilization				

Dagal, 2019 [101]	Controlled before and after study	ERAS 267, traditional 183, non-ERAS after ERAS implemented 108	Open	Cervical, thoracic, lumbar	Preoperative: optimization of comorbidities, patient education, carbohydrate loading, MMA, temperature control, nasal povidone-iodine swab	LOS: 6.1 days vs. 8.2 days		No difference	$62,429 vs. $53,355
					Perioperative: temperature control, antibiotic and antiemetic prophylaxis, MMA, fluid management	ICU LOS: 1.9 days vs. 3.1 days			
					Postoperative: MMA, early nutrition, mobilization catheter/drain removal				

(continued)

Table 6.1 (continued)

Author, year	Type of study	Study size	Open or MIS	Type of spine surgery	ERAS components	LOS (vs. traditional)	Pain	Complications/ readmissions	Cost reduction
Debono, 2019 [102]	Retrospective	ERAS 1920, control 1563	Both	Cervical and lumbar	Preoperative: patient education, reduced fasting time	ALIF: 3.33 days vs. 6.06 days		ALIF: no difference	
					Perioperative: MIS, limited drain/brace usage	ACDF: 1.3 days vs. 3.08 days		ACDF: no difference	
					Postoperative: MMA, RN on call for questions and mobile app (48 h pre-op to POD 15)	Posterior lumbar fusion: 4.8 days vs. 6.7 days		Posterior lumbar fusion: 10.9% vs. 14.8%	
Sivaganesan, 2019 [103]	Prospective	ERAS 151, control 1596	Open	Cervical and lumbar	Perioperative: MMA	Cervical: no difference		Lower overall complication rate (4.6% vs. 11.3%)	
					Postoperative: early mobilization	Lumbar: 2.5 days vs. 2.9 days		Cervical: no difference	
								Lumbar: lower complication (3.8% vs. 12.8%)	

Ifrach, 2020 [104]	Prospective	ERAS 504, control 60	Open	Cervical, thoracic, lumbar (small cohort of peripheral nerve surgeries)	Preoperative: education, consults (e.g., pain management, sleep, endocrine, nutrition) Perioperative: carb load, MMA Postoperative: early ambulation, meals OOB in chair, limited Foley, dispo on oxycodone 5 mg, PCP follow-up within 2 weeks	3.7 days vs. 4.3 days	Reduced 1 month (36.2% vs. 71.7%) and 3 month (33.0% vs. 80%) opioid use with no significant increase in pain scores		
Bradywood, 2017 [82]	Controlled before and after study	ERAS 244, control 214	Open	Lumbar	Use of order sets (postoperative care/ medications, mobility/therapy, patient education), patient education with milestones/ expectations, multidisciplinary rounds with providers/nursing	3.4 days vs. 3.9 days, with greater discharge to home (75% vs. 64%)	No difference	No difference	

(continued)

Table 6.1 (continued)

Author, year	Type of study	Study size	Open or MIS	Type of spine surgery	ERAS components	LOS (vs. traditional)	Pain	Complications/ readmissions	Cost reduction
Wang, 2018 [105]	Retrospective	ERAS 38, control 15	MIS	Lumbar	endoscopic decompression, liposomal bupivacaine, no intubation	1.23 days vs. 3.9 days			\$19,212 vs. \$22,656
Ali, 2019 [106]	Controlled before and after study	ERAS 201, control 74	Open	Lumbar (small cohort of peripheral nerve surgeries)	Preoperative: patient education, consults (e.g., pain management, sleep medicine, primary care, endocrine, nutrition), phone app Perioperative: carb load, MMA	No difference	No difference in pain scores (1 month decrease in use of opioids 38.8% vs. 52.7%)	No difference	

Tarikci Kilic, 2019 [107]	Retrospective	ERAS 60, control 60	MIS	Lumbar	Preoperative: counseling/ education, reduced fasting time	26.52 h vs. 30.10 h	Pre-op: no difference	Decreased nausea (15% vs. 63.3%)	Anesthesia: ₺73.00 vs. ₺270.42
					Perioperative: MIS technique, prophylactic nausea prevention, temperature control, euvolemia, local bupivacaine		6 h: 1.68 vs. 4.03 (VAS)		
					Postoperative: early mobilization/ nutrition, MMA		12 h: 1.12 vs. 3.08 (VAS)		Surgery: ₺1,258.67 vs. ₺1,991.67

(continued)

Table 6.1 (continued)

Author, year	Type of study	Study size	Open or MIS	Type of spine surgery	ERAS components	LOS (vs. traditional)	Pain	Complications/ readmissions	Cost reduction
Soffin, 2019 [55]	Retrospective	ERAS 18, control 18	MIS	Lumbar	Preoperative: premedication with acetaminophen and gabapentin, education on NRS pain scale	No statistical difference	No difference in NRS pain scores or PACU opioid consumption, but a decrease in total perioperative opioid consumption in ERAS patients (2.43 vs. 38.125 oral morphine equivalents)		
					Perioperative: MIS, opioid-free anesthesia				
					Postoperative: early nutrition, MMA				
Angus, 2019 [108]	Controlled before and after study	ERAS 214, control 412	Open	Lumbar	Preoperative: prehabilitation, vit D replacement, smoking cessation	Scoliosis: 8 days vs. 11 days		Reduced 30-day readmission (1.9% vs. 2.1% but not statistically significant)	
					Perioperative: carbohydrate load, MMA	Complex fixation: 5.2 days vs. 7 days			
					Postoperative: MMA, post-discharge day 1.3 phone call, post-op check at 6 days				

Brusko, 2019 [65]	Prospective	ERAS 57, control 40	Both	Lumbar	Perioperative: bupivacaine Postoperative: 1 g IV acetaminophen infusion, daily ERAS team visits	2.9 days vs. 3.8 days	POD 1 pain decreased: 4.2 vs. 6		
Smith, 2019 [109]	Retrospective	ERAS 96, control 123	Open	Lumbar	Preoperative: patient education, anesthesia consult, diabetes optimization Perioperative: MMA, prophylactic antiemetic regimen Postoperative: early mobilization, early removal of catheter	No difference	No difference in pain scores (reduction in use of long-acting opioids—5.2% vs. 14.6%)		
Feng, 2019 [110]	controlled, before and after	ERAS 30, control 44	MIS	Lumbar	Preoperative: patient education Perioperative: MMA, TXA Postoperative: early mobilization, nutrition support	5 days vs. 7 days		No difference	¥71,426 vs. ¥70,467

(continued)

Table 6.1 (continued)

Author, year	Type of study	Study size	Open or MIS	Type of spine surgery	ERAS components	LOS (vs. traditional)	Pain	Complications/ readmissions	Cost reduction
Grasu, 2018 [52]	Retrospective, controlled, before and after	ERAS 41, control 56	MIS	Tumor	Preoperative: education, anxiety management, pain consult if patient on >5 opioid tablets/day with preoperative tramadol/gabapentin, reduced fasting time	No difference	Trend toward better pain scores and decreased opioid consumption (no statistical significance)	No difference	
					Perioperative: temperature management, MIS when able, IV anesthesia maximization				
					Postoperative: MMA, early mobilization/ nutrition, pain management consult				

ACDF anterior cervical discectomy and fusion, *AIS* adolescent idiopathic scoliosis, *LOS* length of stay, *MIS* minimally invasive surgery, *MMA* multimodal analgesia, *NRS* numeric rating scale, *POD* postoperative day, *PSF* posterior spinal fusion, *PT* physical therapy, *TXA* tranexamic acid, *VAS* visual analog scale

Surgery by Anatomical Level

ERAS protocols have been studied in cervical spine patients [53, 99–104], although many studies report their outcomes in mixed cohorts with other spine surgery procedures. In the study described by Soffin et al., 33 patients underwent with anterior cervical discectomy and fusion or cervical arthroplasty, with each receiving an average of 18 ERAS elements. Patients were found to have minimal complications and no readmissions after 90 days [114]. In another study reported by Debono et al., two groups of patients undergoing anterior cervical discectomy and fusion were compared before and after ERAS implementation, without increased complications and with a significantly decreased LOS [100]. Sivaganesan et al. reported on pre- and post-protocol implementation results in elective degenerative spine surgeries; although there was a significant reduction in LOS with fewer 90-day complications, a subgroup analysis of cervical spine patients showed no significant changes [103]. Venkata and van Dellen also described the implementation of an ERAS protocol centered on early mobilization, opioid use reduction, patient counseling, and reduction of drains. This was a mixed cohort of lumbar and cervical patients, with the majority having undergone non-instrumented lumbar decompression surgeries. Logistic regression models showed no influence on LOS by the type of surgery performed [115]. Other similar studies with mixed cohorts of anatomical levels reported overall cost reductions or improvements in LOS [53, 101].

Lumbar spine surgery accounts for the majority of published ERAS protocols [55, 65, 82, 105–113]. An early fast-track protocol for lumbar spine surgery was reported by Scanlon and Richards in 2004 [116]. In this "same day laminectomy program," patients aged 55 years or less without chronic comorbidities were subjected to a protocol that primarily involved a change in anesthesia from propofol for pentathol, the omission of long-acting muscle relaxants, and early postoperative mobilization. No preoperative changes were made. With their sample of 27 patients that were able to be discharged on the same day of surgery, they estimated an elimination of 54 hospital days and cost savings of $111,420 in costs for the hospital [116]. ERAS protocols have also been evaluated specifically in lumbar fusion surgeries. In a retrospective study, Bradywood et al. found that lumbar fusion patients who entered into a standardized care pathway had significantly decreased median LOS, with a higher percentage of patients discharged home compared to prior to implementation (75% vs. 64%) [82]. No significant differences were identified in pain scores, readmission rates, or falls between groups. In another retrospective study, Wang et al. evaluated their ERAS protocol in elderly patients undergoing one- or two-level lumbar fusions and also found an overall decreased LOS [68].

Opioid consumption following spine surgery is an important consideration that has been evaluated in a few studies. In a prospective controlled study of predominantly thoracolumbar elective spine surgery, Ali et al. compared opioid consumption, pain scores, LOS, and readmission rates [106]. The ERAS protocol that was used involved preoperative education and a carbohydrate load, as well as evaluation by various consultants including nutrition, endocrinology, sleep medicine, and pain management for evaluation and optimization if necessary. Although there was no change in the LOS, the ERAS group had significantly less opioid use immediately postoperatively and at 1 month [106]. This reduction was seen at 3 and 6 months in a follow-up publication [117]. Patients with opioid use disorders undergoing open lumbar surgery have been reported to have increased complications and overall hospitals costs, suggesting that this patient population could benefit from specialized ERAS protocols [118].

Some studies have looked at removing opioids entirely from the intraoperative period. This strategy, known as opioid-free anesthesia, does not allow for systemic, neuraxial, or tissue infiltration with opioids. In a single-surgeon series of MIS lumbar surgeries, patients who underwent such a protocol within an established ERAS pathway did not demonstrate an increase in postoperative pain compared to patients who were treated with a standard ERAS pathway using opioids [55]. Although this study is limited by its sample size, it represents a promising avenue for research and treatment.

Minimally Invasive Surgery

One of the most important innovations in spine surgery has been the proliferation of MIS techniques. Compared to conventional open spinal surgery, MIS techniques often involve smaller incisions, the use of the microscope, endoscope or tubular working channels, and implantation of expandable cages and percutaneous screws. Previous studies have demonstrated that posterior lumbar interbody fusion or transforaminal lumbar interbody fusion (TLIF) procedures done in a MIS fashion reduce both blood loss and LOS compared to open surgery [119, 120]. Despite these apparent benefits, clinical outcomes following MIS procedures are generally equivalent to open procedures [9, 121, 122]. However, multiple studies have reported clear advantages with MIS techniques including fewer postoperative infections [123], reduced opioid consumption [124], improved mobilization [125], and reduced hospital costs [105, 121, 122, 126]. As such, the true value of MIS techniques may be seen when incorporated into a rigorous ERAS framework.

Chang et al. compared endoscopic discectomy with an expandable cage to a standard MIS dissection using a microscope, and reported reduced opioid utilization and LOS in the endoscopic ERAS group [127]. Other major components of this ERAS protocol included IV sedation without intubation, and injection of liposomal bupivacaine. Similarly, Wang et al. found decreased LOS and blood loss in patients undergoing endoscopic MIS TLIF as compared to standard MIS TLIF [105]. There was also a significant cost reduction in the endoscopic ERAS group of 15.2%, approximately $3444, compared to the traditional group [105].

In ERAS protocols where MIS techniques are employed, much of the benefit is attributed to the change in surgical technique; however, that is not to say other ERAS elements are less influential. Feng et al. compared the implementation of an ERAS protocol for MIS TLIF to a historical cohort without an ERAS protocol, and without modification of the surgical technique used between groups [110]. Based on the implementation of 11 ERAS components, there was a significant reduction in LOS, blood loss, cost, and complications [110].

Deformity Surgery

ERAS pathways in fusion for the treatment of adolescent idiopathic scoliosis (AIS) have been studied by multiple groups [94–98]. These complex surgeries often lead to prolonged hospital courses, which is why ERAS protocols may be especially useful in this population. Muhly et al. formalized an accelerated recovery pathway with a focus on MMA, early mobilization and nutrition, and studied outcomes prior to protocol initialization, during the time of transition, and post-protocol [96]. Compared with pre-protocol patients, the LOS was significantly reduced without an increase in readmission rates, and pain in the early postoperative period was significantly reduced. Gornitzky et al. also emphasized the utilization of MMA in the perioperative and postoperative period, demonstrating a 31% reduction in inpatient hospitalization and a 34% decrease in PCA usage [95].

Sanders et al. employed a comprehensive ERAS protocol for AIS and noted a decrease in postoperative hospitalization costs [128]. This protocol utilized preoperative education, early mobilization, drain removal, and nutrition, along with early transition to oral pain medications. With this decrease in hospital usage, there was a decrease in average cost decrease by 22%, from $23,640 to $18,360. There was no increase in rate of complications despite the early discharge [128]. Fletcher et al. also emphasized early mobilization, nutrition, and drain removal following AIS surgery, and reported earlier discharge with a 33% decrease in average costs, and without an increase in the rate of complications [94]. However, the accelerated and standard discharge groups had some notable differences, including a significantly higher utilization of implants and pedicle screws in the standard group. The same group evaluated their pathway in a subsequent publication, reporting a 48% reduction in LOS [97].

Tumor Surgery

ERAS programs lend themselves to improving outcomes in high-risk populations, such as patients with cancer. Grasu et al. devised an ERAS protocol that focused on preconditioning, decreased fasting time, MMA, MIS surgical techniques, and early postoperative mobilization for patients with metastatic spinal tumors [52]. Surgeries ranged from simple decompressions to vertebrectomies. All surgeries were done in an elective manner, and emergency cases were excluded. Both control and ERAS groups had similar preoperative characteristics with similar pain scores, although the tumor location and primary tumor origin were heterogeneous. Patients in the

ERAS group trended toward better postoperative pain control and a decrease in opioid consumption; however, there was no difference in LOS, readmission rates, or complications between the two groups [52].

Outcomes in Elderly Patients

Spine surgery in the aging population is becoming an increasingly relevant topic for neurosurgery as the global population of geriatric adults increases. The United Nation's 2017 World Population Aging Report found that, from 1980 to 2017, the number of adults above age 60 doubled, to increase to an estimated 2.1 billion adults by 2050 [129]. These population trends are starting to be seen in elective spine surgery as well; population data from 2004 to 2015 indicate that the number of elective lumbar fusions increased by 138.7% in patients older than 65 years [27]. Though the literature is sparse, there are definite considerations and potential for specialized protocols, including ERAS protocols, to better address the needs of elderly patients undergoing spine surgery.

Important initial considerations when considering spine surgery in the elderly are to clarify the goal of surgery and perform the proper preoperative evaluation. It has been reported that the goals of the elderly patient are more focused on being pain-free, maintaining mobility, and maintaining the ability to live independently [130]. The preoperative evaluation of geriatric patients should take into consideration patient quality of life and the various "geriatric syndromes," and how they contribute to the overall health and ability to undergo spine surgery. Geriatric syndrome is a term used to describe a set of diseases that are common to geriatric patients although are not necessarily linked physiologically to a specific organ system [131], and include diverse pathologies such as osteoporosis, sarcopenia, malnutrition, disability, decubitus ulcers, delirium, cognitive impairment, and a propensity for falls [129].

There have been several attempts to provide a comprehensive geriatric assessment that incorporates geriatric syndromes and frailty, and can be used to aid preoperative assessment. One such assessment is the Canadian Study of Health and Aging Frailty Index (CSHA-FI) [132], which evaluates 70 variables to measure the accumulative deficits with regard to physical, cognitive, functional, and social domains—this is a comprehensive assessment and is thus time-consuming to administer. A modified version of the CSHA-FI assessment using less variables has been termed the "modified frailty index" [133], and has been applied to predicting morbidity and mortality from spine surgery [134, 135]. In the study reported by Leven et al., patients in the oldest age group (mean of 72 ± 8.3 years) were more likely to have a higher frailty index than younger patients—this was an independent predictor of postoperative complications (need for blood transfusions, thromboembolic events, etc.), mortality, LOS, and reoperations in patients that underwent spinal fusion procedures [134]. As such, it is clear from these studies that the elderly are a vulnerable surgical population and that the development of protocols geared toward their needs is increasingly necessary in spine surgery.

The goals of ERAS protocols are to reduce the surgical stress response and minimize postoperative complications for patients. Although the role of geriatric risk factors in spinal surgery is understudied, most data on elderly patients are intermixed with younger patients, and studies evaluating the effects of ERAS protocols on elderly spine surgery patients are lacking. Few such studies have been published [104, 112]; although the protocols have different specifications, there are many commonalities geared toward meeting the needs of geriatric patients, such as preoperative education and counseling, minimizing prolonged preoperative fasting, early ambulation and oral feedings, and using multimodal perioperative analgesia.

Ifrach et al. examined the efficacy of an ERAS pathway in elderly patients undergoing elective laminectomy, discectomy, foraminotomy, thoracolumbosacral fusion, cervicothoracic fusion, and anterior cervical discectomy and fusion [104]. Relevant pain outcomes included self-reported opioid use at 1 and 3 months and patient-reported pain scores. The preoperative ERAS phase included written educational materials, smoking cessation, and the incorporation consults focused on nutrition, sleep medicine, pain, and endocrinology. Perioperative initiatives included a carbohydrate drink and gabapentin therapy. Postoperative medications included acetaminophen, ketorolac, and muscle relaxants, and limiting opioids for breakthrough pain to only postoperative day 1. Other initiatives included early ambulation, starting thromboembolism prophylaxis on day 1, and follow-up with the patient's primary care physician within 2 weeks. These patients had a significant reduction in 1-month and 3-month self-reported narcotic use without an increase in patient-reported pain scores. Reduction of opioid use in elderly patients is an important topic, as these patients are often subject to polypharmacy due to their multiple medical comorbidities.

Wang et al. studied the efficacy of an ERAS protocol in patients 65 years and older who had lumbar disc herniations or spinal stenosis, requiring one- or two-level lumbar fusion [112]. This retrospective study examined whether such protocols affected complications, LOS, postoperative pain scores, and 30-day readmission rates, compared to a historical cohort of patients who did not receive an ERAS protocol. Preoperative initiatives included patient education and counseling, limiting preoperative fasting, fluid and carbohydrate loading, antibiotic therapy, and antithrombotic stocking. Intraoperative initiatives included the use of tranexamic acid to decrease blood loss, maintaining normothermia, and the use of local analgesia. Postoperative initiatives included early ambulation, transition to oral feeding, early removal of urinary catheters, and multimodal analgesia. Compliance rates to the ERAS protocol were 92.1%, with the poorest compliance reported with discontinuation of the urinary catheter (52.6% of patients). Overall, no differences were identified between ERAS and non-ERAS protocol patients in the number of complications or mortality rates, nor were there differences in validated outcome metrics including the Japanese Orthopaedic Association score, visual analog scale, or Oswestry Disability Index. However, there was a significant decrease in the LOS for patients in the ERAS group (12.30 ± 3.03 days vs. 15.50 ± 1.88 days). Compliance with an

ERAS protocol is closely associated with prognosis; in one retrospective study of elderly patients undergoing lumbar fusion, older patients were less compliant with the protocol, and had a higher incidence of complications and a longer LOS [136].

Elderly patients represent an increasing proportion of patients with degenerative spine disease who will require surgical treatment when conservative measures fail. Their goals of surgery are often different than their younger counterparts, and are focused on their ability to maintain independence and mobility. Chakravarty et al. described an ERAS protocol used at Cleveland Clinic that included referral of all elective spine surgery patients over the age of 75 to geriatricians for frailty assessment and adequate time for optimization and prehabilitation [92]. Further study into the benefits of tailored preoperative optimization and surgical treatments aimed toward the geriatric population is needed, such as MIS procedures which generally have less blood loss and shorter LOS. Elderly patients are a vulnerable population that could benefit from tailored, multidisciplinary ERAS protocols to optimize their surgical treatment, including involvement of geriatricians, nutritionists, pain management specialists, and anesthesiologists.

ERAS Implementation

Ultimately, thoughtful delivery of an ERAS protocol for perioperative spinal surgery requires a multidisciplinary, team-based approach. This should be specific to each institution to appropriately address the needs of the patient population by incorporating readily available resources. For instance, employing a preoperative ERAS protocol with "prehabilitation," optimization of medical comorbidities, and timely administration of gabapentinoids may necessitate the involvement of departmental nurses, nurse practitioners, physical therapists, and referring physicians. Similarly, open dialogue with the anesthesia team and operating room staff may be critical for intraoperative ERAS strategies. Postoperative ERAS implementation using pain management algorithms and early mobilization may require the development of a detailed postoperative order sets for residents, physician extenders, and hospitalists. Additionally educational materials, team-based meetings, and open communication with patients, nurses, nutritionists, physical therapists, and consulting physicians will reduce errors and unify messaging. All of this is essential to enhance both recovery after surgery and the patient experience.

Despite the general consensus that ERAS protocols are beneficial in spine surgery, they are not universally embraced. In a multinational survey of spine surgeons, less than half of respondents were familiar with ERAS as a concept, with only about one-third utilizing ERAS protocols in their own practice [137]. Spine surgery is heterogeneous and multiple options are available for even a single pathology; therefore, no single protocol is universally applicable, making widespread utilization difficult to achieve. As the spine-specific ERAS literature becomes more robust, protocols will become more established and utilization will undoubtedly increase.

Conclusion

Due to the high level of variability and the number of simultaneous changes made in implementing ERAS protocols, the direct effect of any specific change is difficult to ascertain. A recent systematic review of the published literature from 2004 to 2019 regarding multimodality ERAS in adult elective spine surgery identified a variety of protocols, with the most common implementation being preoperative education and peri- and postoperative MMA [11]. Half of the included studies found a significant reduction in LOS, with no study identifying a worse outcome after implementation of an ERAS protocol [11].

The principle of ERAS is based on the synergistic effects of a multimodal approach in caring for a patient from the preoperative to the postoperative phase, with a focus on a multidisciplinary approach in improving surgical outcome and patient satisfaction. A single change alone would not necessarily qualify as an ERAS framework. In general, despite the wide variability in protocol elements and patient populations, ERAS protocols are associated with decreased LOS without any additional complications or readmission rates. Future research and implementation should focus on optimizations that may benefit specific surgical procedures or patient populations.

References

1. Gan TJ, Habib AS, Miller TE, White W, Apfelbaum JL. Incidence, patient satisfaction, and perceptions of post-surgical pain: results from a US national survey. Curr Med Res Opin. 2014;30(1):149–60. Epub 2013/11/19.
2. Joshi GP, Beck DE, Emerson RH, Halaszynski TM, Jahr JS, Lipman AG, et al. Defining new directions for more effective management of surgical pain in the United States: highlights of the inaugural Surgical Pain Congress. Am Surg. 2014;80(3):219–28. Epub 2014/03/29.
3. Ljungqvist O, Scott M, Fearon KC. Enhanced recovery after surgery: a review. JAMA Surg. 2017;152(3):292–8. Epub 2017/01/18.
4. Fearon KC, Ljungqvist O, Von Meyenfeldt M, Revhaug A, Dejong CH, Lassen K, et al. Enhanced recovery after surgery: a consensus review of clinical care for patients undergoing colonic resection. Clin Nutr. 2005;24(3):466–77. Epub 2005/05/18.
5. Engelman RM, Rousou JA, Flack JE III, Deaton DW, Humphrey CB, Ellison LH, et al. Fast-track recovery of the coronary bypass patient. Ann Thorac Surg. 1994;58(6):1742–6. Epub 1994/12/01.
6. Bardram L, Funch-Jensen P, Jensen P, Crawford ME, Kehlet H. Recovery after laparoscopic colonic surgery with epidural analgesia, and early oral nutrition and mobilisation. Lancet. 1995;345(8952):763–4. Epub 1995/03/25.
7. Kehlet H, Mogensen T. Hospital stay of 2 days after open sigmoidectomy with a multimodal rehabilitation programme. Br J Surg. 1999;86(2):227–30. Epub 1999/04/01.
8. Kehlet H. Multimodal approach to control postoperative pathophysiology and rehabilitation. Br J Anaesth. 1997;78(5):606–17. Epub 1997/05/01.
9. Wainwright TW, Immins T, Middleton RG. Enhanced recovery after surgery (ERAS) and its applicability for major spine surgery. Best Pract Res Clin Anaesthesiol. 2016;30(1):91–102. Epub 2016/04/03.

10. Elsarrag M, Soldozy S, Patel P, Norat P, Sokolowski JD, Park MS, et al. Enhanced recovery after spine surgery: a systematic review. Neurosurg Focus. 2019;46(4):E3. Epub 2019/04/02.
11. Tong Y, Fernandez L, Bendo JA, Spivak JM. Enhanced recovery after surgery trends in adult spine surgery: a systematic review. Int J Spine Surg. 2020;14(4):623–40. Epub 2020/09/29.
12. Gerbershagen HJ, Aduckathil S, van Wijck AJ, Peelen LM, Kalkman CJ, Meissner W. Pain intensity on the first day after surgery: a prospective cohort study comparing 179 surgical procedures. Anesthesiology. 2013;118(4):934–44. Epub 2013/02/09.
13. Devin CJ, McGirt MJ. Best evidence in multimodal pain management in spine surgery and means of assessing postoperative pain and functional outcomes. J Clin Neurosci. 2015;22(6):930–8. Epub 2015/03/15.
14. Puvanesarajah V, Liauw JA, Lo SF, Lina IA, Witham TF, Gottschalk A. Analgesic therapy for major spine surgery. Neurosurg Rev. 2015;38(3):407–18; discussion 19. Epub 2015/02/15.
15. Kehlet H, Jensen TS, Woolf CJ. Persistent postsurgical pain: risk factors and prevention. Lancet. 2006;367(9522):1618–25. Epub 2006/05/16.
16. Svensson GL, Lundberg M, Ostgaard HC, Wendt GK. High degree of kinesiophobia after lumbar disc herniation surgery: a cross-sectional study of 84 patients. Acta Orthop. 2011;82(6):732–6. Epub 2011/11/10.
17. Archer KR, Seebach CL, Mathis SL, Riley LH III, Wegener ST. Early postoperative fear of movement predicts pain, disability, and physical health six months after spinal surgery for degenerative conditions. Spine J. 2014;14(5):759–67. Epub 2013/11/12.
18. Wick EC, Grant MC, Wu CL. Postoperative multimodal analgesia pain management with nonopioid analgesics and techniques: a review. JAMA Surg. 2017;152(7):691–7. Epub 2017/06/01.
19. Bartels K, Mayes LM, Dingmann C, Bullard KJ, Hopfer CJ, Binswanger IA. Opioid use and storage patterns by patients after hospital discharge following surgery. PLoS One. 2016;11(1):e0147972. Epub 2016/01/30.
20. Dunn LK, Yerra S, Fang S, Hanak MF, Leibowitz MK, Tsang S, et al. Incidence and risk factors for chronic postoperative opioid use after major spine surgery: a cross-sectional study with longitudinal outcome. Anesth Analg. 2018;127(1):247–54. Epub 2018/03/24.
21. Samuel AM, Lovecchio FC, Premkumar A, Louie PK, Vaishnav AS, Iyer S, et al. Preoperative use of higher-strength opioids has a dose-dependent association with reoperations after lumbar decompression and interbody fusion surgery. Spine. 2020;46:E203. Epub 2020/10/21.
22. Chau DL, Walker V, Pai L, Cho LM. Opiates and elderly: use and side effects. Clin Interv Aging. 2008;3(2):273–8. Epub 2008/08/09.
23. Becker WC, O'Connor PG. The safety of opioid analgesics in the elderly: new data raise new concerns: comment on "The comparative safety of opioids for nonmalignant pain in older adults". Arch Intern Med. 2010;170(22):1986–8. Epub 2010/12/15.
24. Le Roux C, Tang Y, Drexler K. Alcohol and opioid use disorder in older adults: neglected and treatable illnesses. Curr Psychiatry Rep. 2016;18(9):87. Epub 2016/08/05.
25. Carter MW, Yang BK, Davenport M, Kabel A. Increasing rates of opioid misuse among older adults visiting emergency departments. Innov Aging. 2019;3(1):igz002. Epub 2019/03/14.
26. Cublier M, Menecier P, von Gunten A, Lepetit A, Dorey JM, Rolland B. Mesusage d'antalgiques opioides chez le sujet age : une mise au point [Analgesic opioids misuse in the elderly: a review]. Geriatr Psychol Neuropsychiatr Vieil. 2020;18(3):343–9. Epub 2020/08/08.
27. Martin BI, Mirza SK, Spina N, Spiker WR, Lawrence B, Brodke DS. Trends in lumbar fusion procedure rates and associated hospital costs for degenerative spinal diseases in the United States, 2004 to 2015. Spine. 2019;44(5):369–76. Epub 2018/08/04.
28. Rajaee SS, Bae HW, Kanim LE, Delamarter RB. Spinal fusion in the United States: analysis of trends from 1998 to 2008. Spine. 2012;37(1):67–76. Epub 2011/02/12.
29. Yoshihara H, Yoneoka D. National trends in the surgical treatment for lumbar degenerative disc disease: United States, 2000 to 2009. Spine J. 2015;15(2):265–71. Epub 2014/10/05.

30. Deyo RA, Mirza SK, Martin BI, Kreuter W, Goodman DC, Jarvik JG. Trends, major medical complications, and charges associated with surgery for lumbar spinal stenosis in older adults. JAMA. 2010;303(13):1259–65. Epub 2010/04/08.
31. Gruskay JA, Fu M, Bohl DD, Webb ML, Grauer JN. Factors affecting length of stay after elective posterior lumbar spine surgery: a multivariate analysis. Spine J. 2015;15(6):1188–95. Epub 2013/11/05.
32. Wang MY, Chang P, Grossman J. Development of an Enhanced Recovery After Surgery (ERAS) approach for lumbar spinal fusion. J Neurosurg Spine. 2017;26(4):411–8. Epub 2016/12/24.
33. Ren L, Zhu D, Wei Y, Pan X, Liang L, Xu J, et al. Enhanced Recovery After Surgery (ERAS) program attenuates stress and accelerates recovery in patients after radical resection for colorectal cancer: a prospective randomized controlled trial. World J Surg. 2012;36(2):407–14. Epub 2011/11/22.
34. Burgess LC, Arundel J, Wainwright TW. The effect of preoperative education on psychological, clinical and economic outcomes in elective spinal surgery: a systematic review. Healthcare. 2019;7(1):48. Epub 2019/03/25.
35. Fleege C, Arabmotlagh M, Almajali A, Rauschmann M. Pra- und postoperative Fast-track-Behandlungskonzepte in der Wirbelsaulenchirurgie : Patienteninformation und Patientenkooperation [Pre- and postoperative fast-track treatment concepts in spinal surgery: patient information and patient cooperation]. Der Orthopade 2014;43(12):1062–4, 6–9. Epub 2014/11/13.
36. Gometz A, Maislen D, Youtz C, Kary E, Gometz EL, Sobotka S, et al. The effectiveness of prehabilitation (Prehab) in both functional and economic outcomes following spinal surgery: a systematic review. Cureus. 2018;10(5):e2675. Epub 2018/07/28.
37. Golinvaux NS, Varthi AG, Bohl DD, Basques BA, Grauer JN. Complication rates following elective lumbar fusion in patients with diabetes: insulin dependence makes the difference. Spine. 2014;39(21):1809–16. Epub 2014/07/11.
38. Klemencsics I, Lazary A, Szoverfi Z, Bozsodi A, Eltes P, Varga PP. Risk factors for surgical site infection in elective routine degenerative lumbar surgeries. Spine J. 2016;16(11):1377–83. Epub 2016/08/16.
39. Durand WM, DePasse JM, Bokshan SL, Eltorai AEM, Daniels AH. Tobacco use and complications following spinal fusion: a comparison of the national surgical quality improvement program and national inpatient sample datasets. World Neurosurg. 2019;123:e393–407. Epub 2018/12/01.
40. Wilson JRF, Jiang F, Badhiwala JH, Shaffrey CI, Carreon LY, Cheung KMC, et al. The effect of tobacco smoking on adverse events following adult complex deformity surgery: analysis of 270 patients from the prospective, multicenter scoli-RISK-1 study. Spine. 2020;45(1):32–7. Epub 2019/08/16.
41. Klein JD, Hey LA, Yu CS, Klein BB, Coufal FJ, Young EP, et al. Perioperative nutrition and postoperative complications in patients undergoing spinal surgery. Spine. 1996;21(22):2676–82. Epub 1996/11/15.
42. Phan K, Kim JS, Xu J, Di Capua J, Lee NJ, Kothari P, et al. Nutritional insufficiency as a predictor for adverse outcomes in adult spinal deformity surgery. Glob Spine J. 2018;8(2):164–71. Epub 2018/04/18.
43. Cai Y, Xu K, Hou W, Yang Z, Xu P. Preoperative chlorhexidine reduces the incidence of surgical site infections in total knee and hip arthroplasty: a systematic review and meta-analysis. Int J Surg. 2017;39:221–8. Epub 2017/02/13.
44. Chan AK, Ammanuel SG, Chan AY, Oh T, Skrehot HC, Edwards CS, et al. Chlorhexidine showers are associated with a reduction in surgical site infection following spine surgery: an analysis of 4266 consecutive surgeries. Neurosurgery. 2019;85(6):817–26. Epub 2018/12/28.
45. Pandey CK, Navkar DV, Giri PJ, Raza M, Behari S, Singh RB, et al. Evaluation of the optimal preemptive dose of gabapentin for postoperative pain relief after lumbar diske-

ctomy: a randomized, double-blind, placebo-controlled study. J Neurosurg Anesthesiol. 2005;17(2):65–8. Epub 2005/04/21.

46. Khurana G, Jindal P, Sharma JP, Bansal KK. Postoperative pain and long-term functional outcome after administration of gabapentin and pregabalin in patients undergoing spinal surgery. Spine. 2014;39(6):E363–8. Epub 2014/01/05.
47. Yu L, Ran B, Li M, Shi Z. Gabapentin and pregabalin in the management of postoperative pain after lumbar spinal surgery: a systematic review and meta-analysis. Spine. 2013;38(22):1947–52. Epub 2013/08/08.
48. Rivkin A, Rivkin MA. Perioperative nonopioid agents for pain control in spinal surgery. Am J Health Syst Pharm. 2014;71(21):1845–57. Epub 2014/10/17.
49. Sucato DJ, Lovejoy JF, Agrawal S, Elerson E, Nelson T, McClung A. Postoperative ketorolac does not predispose to pseudoarthrosis following posterior spinal fusion and instrumentation for adolescent idiopathic scoliosis. Spine. 2008;33(10):1119–24. Epub 2008/05/02.
50. Dodwell ER, Latorre JG, Parisini E, Zwettler E, Chandra D, Mulpuri K, et al. NSAID exposure and risk of nonunion: a meta-analysis of case-control and cohort studies. Calcif Tissue Int. 2010;87(3):193–202. Epub 2010/06/17.
51. Kim SI, Ha KY, Oh IS. Preemptive multimodal analgesia for postoperative pain management after lumbar fusion surgery: a randomized controlled trial. Eur Spine J. 2016;25(5):1614–9. Epub 2015/09/02.
52. Grasu RM, Cata JP, Dang AQ, Tatsui CE, Rhines LD, Hagan KB, et al. Implementation of an Enhanced Recovery After Spine Surgery program at a large cancer center: a preliminary analysis. J Neurosurg Spine. 2018;29(5):588–98. Epub 2018/08/18.
53. Carr DA, Saigal R, Zhang F, Bransford RJ, Bellabarba C, Dagal A. Enhanced perioperative care and decreased cost and length of stay after elective major spinal surgery. Neurosurg Focus. 2019;46(4):E5. Epub 2019/04/02.
54. Arumugam S, Lau CS, Chamberlain RS. Use of preoperative gabapentin significantly reduces postoperative opioid consumption: a meta-analysis. J Pain Res. 2016;9:631–40. Epub 2016/09/28.
55. Soffin EM, Wetmore DS, Beckman JD, Sheha ED, Vaishnav AS, Albert TJ, et al. Opioid-free anesthesia within an enhanced recovery after surgery pathway for minimally invasive lumbar spine surgery: a retrospective matched cohort study. Neurosurg Focus. 2019;46(4):E8. Epub 2019/04/02.
56. Staartjes VE, de Wispelaere MP, Schroder ML. Improving recovery after elective degenerative spine surgery: 5-year experience with an enhanced recovery after surgery (ERAS) protocol. Neurosurg Focus. 2019;46(4):E7. Epub 2019/04/02.
57. Loftus RW, Yeager MP, Clark JA, Brown JR, Abdu WA, Sengupta DK, et al. Intraoperative ketamine reduces perioperative opiate consumption in opiate-dependent patients with chronic back pain undergoing back surgery. Anesthesiology. 2010;113(3):639–46. Epub 2010/08/10.
58. Tsaousi GG, Pourzitaki C, Aloisio S, Bilotta F. Dexmedetomidine as a sedative and analgesic adjuvant in spine surgery: a systematic review and meta-analysis of randomized controlled trials. Eur J Clin Pharmacol. 2018;74(11):1377–89. Epub 2018/07/17.
59. Wang F, Shi K, Jiang Y, Yang Z, Chen G, Song K. Intravenous glucocorticoid for pain control after spinal fusion: a meta-analysis of randomized controlled trials. Medicine. 2018;97(20):e10507. Epub 2018/05/17.
60. Nielsen RV, Siegel H, Fomsgaard JS, Andersen JD, Martusevicius R, Mathiesen O, et al. Preoperative dexamethasone reduces acute but not sustained pain after lumbar disk surgery: a randomized, blinded, placebo-controlled trial. Pain. 2015;156(12):2538–44. Epub 2015/08/14.
61. Zorrilla-Vaca A, Healy RJ, Mirski MA. A Comparison of regional versus general anesthesia for lumbar spine surgery: a meta-analysis of randomized studies. J Neurosurg Anesthesiol. 2017;29(4):415–25. Epub 2016/08/27.

62. Ong CK, Lirk P, Seymour RA, Jenkins BJ. The efficacy of preemptive analgesia for acute postoperative pain management: a meta-analysis. Anesth Analg. 2005;100(3):757–73, table of contents. Epub 2005/02/25.
63. Perera AP, Chari A, Kostusiak M, Khan AA, Luoma AM, Casey ATH. Intramuscular local anesthetic infiltration at closure for postoperative analgesia in lumbar spine surgery: a systematic review and meta-analysis. Spine. 2017;42(14):1088–95. Epub 2016/01/13.
64. Roh MS, Kucher OA, Shick KM, Knolhoff DR, McGarvey JS, Peterson SC. Intramuscular liposomal bupivacaine decreases length of stay and opioid usage following lumbar spinal fusion. Clin Spine Surg. 2020;33(8):E359–E63. Epub 2020/05/20.
65. Brusko GD, Kolcun JPG, Heger JA, Levi AD, Manzano GR, Madhavan K, et al. Reductions in length of stay, narcotics use, and pain following implementation of an enhanced recovery after surgery program for 1- to 3-level lumbar fusion surgery. Neurosurg Focus. 2019;46(4):E4. Epub 2019/04/02.
66. Pendi A, Acosta FL, Tuchman A, Movahedi R, Sivasundaram L, Arif I, et al. Intrathecal morphine in spine surgery: a meta-analysis of randomized controlled trials. Spine. 2017;42(12):E740–E7. Epub 2017/04/20.
67. Dhaliwal P, Yavin D, Whittaker T, Hawboldt GS, Jewett GAE, Casha S, et al. Intrathecal morphine following lumbar fusion: a randomized, placebo-controlled trial. Neurosurgery. 2019;85(2):189–98. Epub 2018/09/29.
68. Wang Y, Guo X, Guo Z, Xu M. Preemptive analgesia with a single low dose of intrathecal morphine in multilevel posterior lumbar interbody fusion surgery: a double-blind, randomized, controlled trial. Spine J. 2020;20(7):989–97. Epub 2020/03/18.
69. Guest JD, Vanni S, Silbert L. Mild hypothermia, blood loss and complications in elective spinal surgery. Spine J. 2004;4(2):130–7. Epub 2004/03/16.
70. Basques BA, Anandasivam NS, Webb ML, Samuel AM, Lukasiewicz AM, Bohl DD, et al. Risk factors for blood transfusion with primary posterior lumbar fusion. Spine. 2015;40(22):1792–7. Epub 2015/07/15.
71. Bacchin MR, Ceria CM, Giannone S, Ghisi D, Stagni G, Greggi T, et al. Goal-directed fluid therapy based on stroke volume variation in patients undergoing major spine surgery in the prone position: a cohort study. Spine. 2016;41(18):E1131–7. Epub 2016/04/06.
72. Hui S, Xu D, Ren Z, Chen X, Sheng L, Zhuang Q, et al. Can tranexamic acid conserve blood and save operative time in spinal surgeries? A meta-analysis. Spine J. 2018;18(8):1325–37. Epub 2017/12/17.
73. Mikhail C, Pennington Z, Arnold PM, Brodke DS, Chapman JR, Chutkan N, et al. Minimizing blood loss in spine surgery. Glob Spine J. 2020;10(1 Suppl):71S–83S. Epub 2020/01/15.
74. Yao R, Zhou H, Choma TJ, Kwon BK, Street J. Surgical site infection in spine surgery: who is at risk? Glob Spine J. 2018;8(4 Suppl):5S–30S. Epub 2018/12/24.
75. Pennington Z, Lubelski D, Molina C, Westbroek EM, Ahmed AK, Sciubba DM. Prolonged post-surgical drain retention increases risk for deep wound infection after spine surgery. World Neurosurg. 2019;130:e846–e53. Epub 2019/07/12.
76. Weesie YM, Hek K, Schermer TRJ, Schellevis FG, Leufkens HGM, Rook EJ, et al. Use of opioids increases with age in older adults: an observational study (2005-2017). Front Pharmacol. 2020;11:648. Epub 2020/06/02.
77. Park PJ, Makhni MC, Cerpa M, Lehman RA, Lenke LG. The role of perioperative ketamine in postoperative pain control following spinal surgery. J Spine Surg. 2020;6(3):591–7. Epub 2020/10/27.
78. Chou R, Gordon DB, de Leon-Casasola OA, Rosenberg JM, Bickler S, Brennan T, et al. Management of postoperative pain: a clinical practice guideline from the American Pain Society, the American Society of Regional Anesthesia and Pain Medicine, and the American Society of Anesthesiologists' Committee on Regional Anesthesia, Executive Committee, and Administrative Council. J Pain. 2016;17(2):131–57. Epub 2016/02/02.
79. Avidan MS, Maybrier HR, Abdallah AB, Jacobsohn E, Vlisides PE, Pryor KO, et al. Intraoperative ketamine for prevention of postoperative delirium or pain after major surgery

in older adults: an international, multicentre, double-blind, randomised clinical trial. Lancet. 2017;390(10091):267–75. Epub 2017/06/04.
80. Rajpal S, Gordon DB, Pellino TA, Strayer AL, Brost D, Trost GR, et al. Comparison of perioperative oral multimodal analgesia versus IV PCA for spine surgery. J Spinal Disord Tech. 2010;23(2):139–45. Epub 2010/04/09.
81. Patel AA, Walker CT, Prendergast V, Radosevich JJ, Grimm D, Godzik J, et al. Patient-controlled analgesia following lumbar spinal fusion surgery is associated with increased opioid consumption and opioid-related adverse events. Neurosurgery. 2020;87(3):592–601. Epub 2020/05/02.
82. Bradywood A, Farrokhi F, Williams B, Kowalczyk M, Blackmore CC. Reduction of inpatient hospital length of stay in lumbar fusion patients with implementation of an evidence-based clinical care pathway. Spine. 2017;42(3):169–76. Epub 2016/05/24.
83. Allen C, Glasziou P, Del Mar C. Bed rest: a potentially harmful treatment needing more careful evaluation. Lancet. 1999;354(9186):1229–33. Epub 1999/10/16.
84. Haines KJ, Skinner EH, Berney S. Association of postoperative pulmonary complications with delayed mobilisation following major abdominal surgery: an observational cohort study. Physiotherapy. 2013;99(2):119–25. Epub 2012/12/12.
85. Aissaoui N, Martins E, Mouly S, Weber S, Meune C. A meta-analysis of bed rest versus early ambulation in the management of pulmonary embolism, deep vein thrombosis, or both. Int J Cardiol. 2009;137(1):37–41. Epub 2008/08/12.
86. Epstein NE. A review article on the benefits of early mobilization following spinal surgery and other medical/surgical procedures. Surg Neurol Int. 2014;5(Suppl 3):S66–73. Epub 2014/05/21.
87. Rupich K, Missimer E, O'Brien D, Shafer G, Wilensky EM, Pierce JT, et al. The benefits of implementing an early mobility protocol in postoperative neurosurgical spine patients. Am J Nurs. 2018;118(6):46–53. Epub 2018/05/26.
88. Adogwa O, Elsamadicy AA, Fialkoff J, Cheng J, Karikari IO, Bagley C. Early ambulation decreases length of hospital stay, perioperative complications and improves functional outcomes in elderly patients undergoing surgery for correction of adult degenerative scoliosis. Spine. 2017;42(18):1420–5. Epub 2017/09/14.
89. Nielsen PR, Jorgensen LD, Dahl B, Pedersen T, Tonnesen H. Prehabilitation and early rehabilitation after spinal surgery: randomized clinical trial. Clin Rehabil. 2010;24(2):137–48. Epub 2010/01/28.
90. Qvarfordh P, Olsen KS, Bendix T, Esbensen BA. Should patients walk from the postanesthesia care unit to the general ward after a lumbar discectomy? A randomized study. J Perianesth Nurs. 2014;29(5):377–84. Epub 2014/09/28.
91. Burgess LC, Wainwright TW. What is the evidence for early mobilisation in elective spine surgery? A narrative review. Healthcare. 2019;7(3):92. Epub 2019/07/22.
92. Chakravarthy VB, Yokoi H, Coughlin DJ, Manlapaz MR, Krishnaney AA. Development and implementation of a comprehensive spine surgery enhanced recovery after surgery protocol: the Cleveland Clinic experience. Neurosurg Focus. 2019;46(4):E11. Epub 2019/04/02.
93. Dietz N, Sharma M, Adams S, Alhourani A, Ugiliweneza B, Wang D, et al. Enhanced recovery after surgery (ERAS) for spine surgery: a systematic review. World Neurosurg. 2019;130:415–26. Epub 2019/07/06.
94. Fletcher ND, Shourbaji N, Mitchell PM, Oswald TS, Devito DP, Bruce RW. Clinical and economic implications of early discharge following posterior spinal fusion for adolescent idiopathic scoliosis. J Child Orthop. 2014;8(3):257–63. Epub 2014/04/29.
95. Gornitzky AL, Flynn JM, Muhly WT, Sankar WN. A rapid recovery pathway for adolescent idiopathic scoliosis that improves pain control and reduces time to inpatient recovery after posterior spinal fusion. Spine Deform. 2016;4(4):288–95. Epub 2016/12/09.
96. Muhly WT, Sankar WN, Ryan K, Norton A, Maxwell LG, DiMaggio T, et al. Rapid recovery pathway after spinal fusion for idiopathic scoliosis. Pediatrics. 2016;137(4):e20151568. Epub 2016/03/25.

97. Fletcher ND, Andras LM, Lazarus DE, Owen RJ, Geddes BJ, Cao J, et al. Use of a novel pathway for early discharge was associated with a 48% shorter length of stay after posterior spinal fusion for adolescent idiopathic scoliosis. J Pediatr Orthop. 2017;37(2):92–7. Epub 2015/07/28.
98. Rao RR, Hayes M, Lewis C, Hensinger RN, Farley FA, Li Y, et al. Mapping the road to recovery: shorter stays and satisfied patients in posterior spinal fusion. J Pediatr Orthop. 2017;37(8):e536–e42. Epub 2016/05/04.
99. Li J, Li H, Xv ZK, Wang J, Yu QF, Chen G, et al. Enhanced recovery care versus traditional care following laminoplasty: a retrospective case-cohort study. Medicine. 2018;97(48):e13195. Epub 2018/12/05.
100. Debono B, Sabatier P, Boniface G, Bousquet P, Lescure JP, Garnaud V, et al. Implementation of enhanced recovery after surgery (ERAS) protocol for anterior cervical discectomy and fusion: a propensity score-matched analysis. Eur Spine J. 2020;30:560. Epub 2020/05/16.
101. Dagal A, Bellabarba C, Bransford R, Zhang F, Chesnut RM, O'Keefe GE, et al. Enhanced perioperative care for major spine surgery. Spine. 2019;44(13):959–66. Epub 2019/06/18.
102. Debono B, Corniola MV, Pietton R, Sabatier P, Hamel O, Tessitore E. Benefits of enhanced recovery after surgery for fusion in degenerative spine surgery: impact on outcome, length of stay, and patient satisfaction. Neurosurg Focus. 2019;46(4):E6. Epub 2019/04/02.
103. Sivaganesan A, Wick JB, Chotai S, Cherkesky C, Stephens BF, Devin CJ. Perioperative protocol for elective spine surgery is associated with reduced length of stay and complications. J Am Acad Orthop Surg. 2019;27(5):183–9. Epub 2018/09/08.
104. Ifrach J, Basu R, Joshi DS, Flanders TM, Ozturk AK, Malhotra NR, et al. Efficacy of an enhanced recovery after surgery (ERAS) pathway in elderly patients undergoing spine and peripheral nerve surgery. Clin Neurol Neurosurg. 2020;197:106115. Epub 2020/08/26.
105. Wang MY, Chang HK, Grossman J. Reduced Acute Care Costs With the ERAS(R) minimally invasive transforaminal lumbar interbody fusion compared with conventional minimally invasive transforaminal lumbar interbody fusion. Neurosurgery. 2018;83(4):827–34 Epub 2017/09/26.
106. Ali ZS, Flanders TM, Ozturk AK, Malhotra NR, Leszinsky L, McShane BJ, et al. Enhanced recovery after elective spinal and peripheral nerve surgery: pilot study from a single institution. J Neurosurg Spine. 2019;30:1–9. Epub 2019/01/27.
107. Tarikci Kilic E, Demirbilek T, Naderi S. Does an enhanced recovery after surgery protocol change costs and outcomes of single-level lumbar microdiscectomy? Neurosurg Focus. 2019;46(4):E10. Epub 2019/04/02.
108. Angus M, Jackson K, Smurthwaite G, Carrasco R, Mohammad S, Verma R, et al. The implementation of enhanced recovery after surgery (ERAS) in complex spinal surgery. J Spine Surg. 2019;5(1):116–23. Epub 2019/04/30.
109. Smith J, Probst S, Calandra C, Davis R, Sugimoto K, Nie L, et al. Enhanced recovery after surgery (ERAS) program for lumbar spine fusion. Perioper Med. 2019;8:4. Epub 2019/06/01.
110. Feng C, Zhang Y, Chong F, Yang M, Liu C, Liu L, et al. Establishment and implementation of an enhanced recovery after surgery (ERAS) pathway tailored for minimally invasive transforaminal lumbar interbody fusion surgery. World Neurosurg. 2019;129:e317–e23. Epub 2019/05/28.
111. Heo DH, Park CK. Clinical results of percutaneous biportal endoscopic lumbar interbody fusion with application of enhanced recovery after surgery. Neurosurg Focus. 2019;46(4):E18. Epub 2019/04/02.
112. Wang P, Wang Q, Kong C, Teng Z, Li Z, Zhang S, et al. Enhanced recovery after surgery (ERAS) program for elderly patients with short-level lumbar fusion. J Orthop Surg Res. 2020;15(1):299. Epub 2020/08/09.
113. Yang Y, Wu X, Wu W, Liu Z, Pang M, Chen Y, et al. Enhanced recovery after surgery (ERAS) pathway for microendoscopy-assisted minimally invasive transforaminal lumbar interbody fusion. Clin Neurol Neurosurg. 2020;196:106003. Epub 2020/06/20.

Part II
Spine Disease in the Elderly

Chapter 7
Surgical Treatment of Cervical Spondylotic Myelopathy

Ilyas Eli and Zoher Ghogawala

Introduction

Cervical spondylotic myelopathy (CSM) is a degenerative cervical spine disease caused by progressive compression of the spinal cord that typically occurs in older adults (average age 60 years) [1]. CSM is a major cause of neurological impairment associated with disability and has a negative effect on overall health-related quality of life. As the size of the aging population continues to grow, a higher incidence of CSM will be seen in the US population. Currently, degenerative spine disease has an incidence of 76 per million persons, making it the most common cause of non-traumatic spinal cord injury in North America [2]. Without intervention, it is estimated that 20–62% of patients with mildly symptomatic CSM will have further deterioration [3, 4].

Surgical treatment is often used to prevent further deterioration and permit neurological recovery in symptomatic cases. The goal of surgery for CSM is to decompress the spinal cord, restore alignment, and treat any instability that is present [5]. Nearly 19% of cervical spine surgeries are performed to treat CSM [6], and hospital charges for treating CSM in the USA exceed $2 billion/year [7]. Trends from the Nationwide Inpatient Sample (NIS) showed that the number of cervical spine

I. Eli
Department of Neurosurgery, Clinical Neurosciences Center, University of Utah, Salt Lake City, UT, USA

Department of Neurosurgery, Lahey Hospital and Medical Center, Tufts University School of Medicine, Burlington, MA, USA

Z. Ghogawala (✉)
Department of Neurosurgery, Lahey Hospital and Medical Center, Tufts University School of Medicine, Burlington, MA, USA
e-mail: zoher.ghogawala@lahey.org

K.-M. G. Fu et al. (eds.), *Treatment of Spine Disease in the Elderly*,
https://doi.org/10.1007/978-3-031-12612-3_7

procedures increased from 150,372 procedures in 2002 to 186,679 procedures in 2009, and the average age of patients was 52.6 years [8]. Surgical intervention entails a ventral, dorsal, or combined approach, all of which are common in the USA with the exception of cervical laminoplasty. Despite the growing number of cases, the optimal approach (with special considerations for the elderly) has yet to be determined.

Pathophysiology

CSM is associated with direct physical compression of the spinal cord. The stress on the spinal cord results in injury and dysfunction that manifests as physical symptoms and signs of myelopathy. CSM is a result of both static and dynamic factors that result in repetitive injury to the spinal cord. Static factors include canal stenosis due to protruding intervertebral disc and hypertrophy of ligamentum flavum [9]. Dynamic factors result from further compression during active neck extension due to the invagination of ligamentum flavum and intervertebral disc resulting in dynamic shearing and stretch injury to the spinal cord [9, 10]. The pathogenesis underlying the mechanism results in neuronal damage as well as impaired function of oligodendrocytes, astrocytes, and microglia resulting in apoptosis, inflammation, and vascular compromise. Impairment of microcirculation by compression of vascular structures has also been postulated to lead to CSM [11, 12]. The corticospinal and spinocerebellar tracts are initially affected, resulting in fine motor difficulties and gait imbalance. On examination at this stage, patients may demonstrate lower motor neuron signs at the level of the injury and upper motor signs such as the Hoffman sign, Babinski reflex, and clonus below the affected level. Additional findings include neck pain, shoulder pain, radiculopathy, bladder dysfunction, and hand numbness [13]. The overall natural history of CSM is variable, and symptoms can present in a gradual fashion, with some patients exhibiting periods of stability or absence of symptoms. Studies suggest that 20–62% of patients with CSM managed conservatively will have worsening neurological function by 3–6 years after diagnosis [4]. Surgery treats the underlying cause and can result in neurological recovery in many cases.

Elderly Perioperative Considerations

Advanced age alone is typically not a contraindication for surgical treatment of patients with symptomatic CSM, and in fact the need for treatment can become urgent in elderly patients with CSM because symptoms can result in rapid deterioration and can be associated with falls [14]. There may be some reluctance to offer surgery to the elderly population because of the concern around surgical complications. However, care can be directed toward optimizing patient comorbidities and focusing on improvement of preoperative status to increase chances for a better surgical outcome. In the elderly, a comprehensive preoperative workup is important. The workup should include a cardiac evaluation to rule out unstable coronary syndromes, heart failure, arrhythmias, and severe valvular disease [15]. Pulmonary workup should evaluate for the presence of pneumonia, chronic obstructive pulmonary disease (COPD), and respiratory failure [15]. Additionally, hepatic and renal dysfunction should be assessed using routine blood work. Nutritional status is relevant in the elderly because age >60 years is a risk factor for poor nutritional status [16]. Nutritional optimization is essential because it may support improved surgical outcome and decrease the rates of complications.

Preoperative identification of patient comorbidities to allow for optimization can result in better surgical outcome and decreased intraoperative complications. In particular, an estimated 26% of women >65 years of age and 50% of those >85 years have osteoporosis, making assessment of bone density a priority for patients who are being considered for CSM surgery [17, 18]. As it relates to patients older than 50 years of age undergoing elective spine surgery, 14.5% of men and 51.3% of women have osteoporosis [19]. Diagnosis can be made by measuring the bone mineral density using a dual-energy X-ray absorptiometry (DEXA) scanner. Presence of osteoporosis can also be estimated by obtaining a cervical spine computed tomography scan and measuring the Hounsfield units [20]. If osteoporosis is diagnosed, then treatment can be initiated by the primary care physician or endocrinologist. Treatment involves calcium and vitamin D supplementations in most patients. Additionally, bisphosphonates, calcitonin, parathyroid hormones (PTHs), and estrogen receptor modulators are second-line treatments in patients with concerning osteoporosis. Bisphosphonates encourage apoptosis of osteoclasts, which results in slower bone remodeling, and PTHs promote bone formation by their anti-apoptotic effect on osteoblasts [21]. Selective estrogen receptor modulators (SERMs) are another option used to treat osteoporosis in the elderly because they stimulate an estrogen-mediated response in bone resulting in increased bone mass. SERMs have been shown to reduce vertebral fracture rates by 50% compared with placebo, but are not considered first-line treatment because of the cardiovascular risks associated with estrogen [22, 23]. Calcitonin is an intranasal medication that directly inhibits osteoclasts, with studies showing reduction of spine fractures by 33% compared with placebo [24, 25]. Diagnosis of osteoporosis and adequate treatment can prevent surgical complications such as hardware failure, nonunion, and adjacent-level fractures.

Surgical Management

The goal of surgery is to expand and restore the canal diameter to 12 mm by decompression, allowing for improvement of blood supply and of spinal cord morphology to aid in neurological recovery and halting progression of disease. Surgery for CSM can be effective by either a ventral or a dorsal approach, depending on patient factors and imaging characteristics. Ventral approaches include anterior cervical discectomy and fusion (ACDF) and anterior corpectomy and fusion (ACCF). Dorsal approaches involve laminectomy, laminectomy and fusion, and laminoplasty. The chosen approach is based on factors such as the levels of disease involved, sagittal alignment, location of the compression (ventral vs. dorsal), previous surgeries, and age [26–28].

Overall, surgical intervention results in improvement in two-thirds of patients; however, results 15–30% of cases end with no improvement [29]. Additionally, 10–20% of cases result in a clinically worse outcome [29]. In an effort to evaluate the role of age in patient outcomes after surgery for cervical myelopathy, Grodzinski et al. conducted a systematic review of the literature [30]. Older patients were more likely to undergo a posterior surgery. Age was also a predictor of the number of levels decompressed. Advanced age was not a contraindication for surgical treatment for CSM, but age remains a significant concern for surgeons in performing interventions on the elderly.

Ventral Approaches

Anterior approaches allow for the resection of compressive lesions located in the anterior spine such as disc herniation and disc-osteophyte complex. One advantage to the anterior approach is the ability to treat and often correct cervical kyphosis. Anterior approaches are also associated with lower risk of infection, less postoperative pain, and shorter hospital stay when compared with posterior approaches [31]. Anterior approaches thus may result in lower hospital costs. Additionally, anterior surgery is also associated with a lower 5-year reoperation rate compared with posterior approaches (12.1% vs. 17.7%) [32]. A prospective comparative trial by Ghogawala et al. demonstrated that ACDFs resulted in greater improvement in health-related QOL, shorter hospital stay, and lower costs when compared with dorsal approaches [33].

ACDF

An anterior cervical approach is often used for patients with 1–2 levels of cervical spondylosis with anterior cord compression especially related to disc-osteophyte that is amenable to removal with an anterior approach. The procedure is well

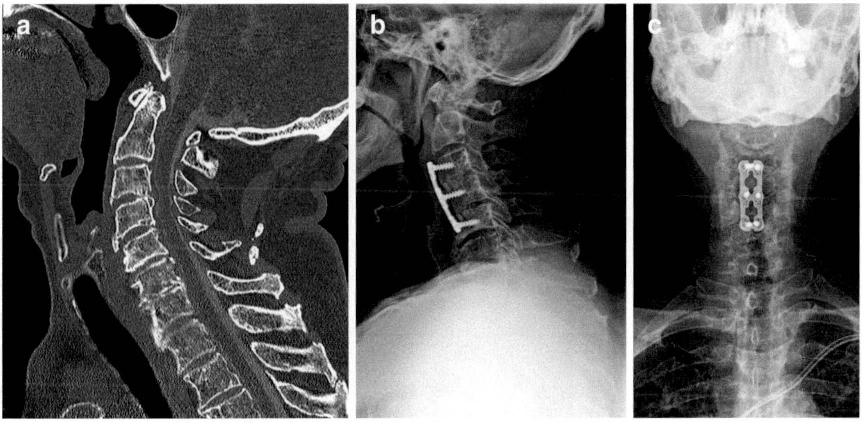

Fig. 7.1 (**a**) Preoperative sagittal CT myelogram demonstrating ventral compression at C3–C4 and C4–C5. (**b**) Postoperative lateral plain cervical radiograph showing C4–C5 and C5–C6 anterior cervical discectomy and fusion (ACDF). (**c**) Postoperative anteroposterior plain cervical radiograph showing C4–C5 and C5–C6 ACDF hardware

described elsewhere [34]. The presence of kyphosis in addition to CSM makes the anterior approach more attractive because lordotic grafts can be used with this approach to correct the kyphosis. Surgeons typically use allograft or titanium spacers at each disc space after removing all compressive disc and disc-osteophyte complexes. Fixation is then achieved with titanium plates unless a stand-alone spacer is used (Fig. 7.1).

Corpectomy

ACCF is an ideal surgical approach when there is ventral compression from the dorsal part of the vertebral body that cannot be decompressed with a discectomy approach alone. Factors that might influence the decision to perform an ACCF include the degree of cervical deformity, the anatomy of compression, and the presence of focal ossification of posterior longitudinal ligament (OPLL). The details of an ACCF have been well described in the literature [35]. A 15- to 20-mm-wide vertebral body resection is planned for the decompression after the uncinate processes are identified. The vertebral body, osteophyte, and posterior longitudinal ligament are removed. After adequate decompression, a titanium cage or bone graft is placed and fixed with a plate and screws for anterior fixation (Fig. 7.2).

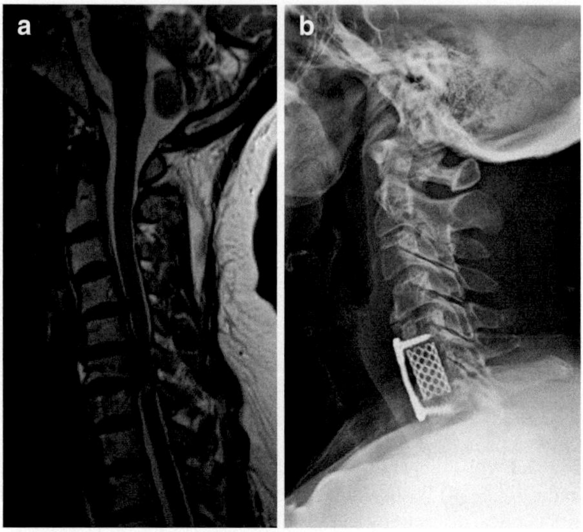

Fig. 7.2 (**a**) Preoperative sagittal T2-weighted MRI demonstrating stenosis and kyphosis in a patient with CSM. (**b**) Lateral plain cervical radiograph demonstrating decompression and correction of kyphosis with C6 corpectomy with anterior plate fixation from C5 to C7

Dorsal Approaches

There are several reasons to consider a dorsal approach for surgical treatment of CSM, including the presence of OPLL or rostral disease involving the C2–C3 level, older age, and stenosis involving three more levels. Posterior approaches include laminectomy alone, laminectomy and fusion, or laminoplasty. The AOSpine CSM study showed that the majority of posterior approaches to treat CSM were via a laminectomy and fusion (58%) followed by laminoplasty (35%), and only 7% had laminectomy alone [36]. The NIS database showed an increase in posterior fusion procedures by 0.3% and a decline in laminectomies alone because of concerns around the development of delayed kyphotic deformities following laminectomy alone [7]. However, fixed cervical kyphotic deformity is considered a contraindication for posterior approach, and typically is treated with a ventral or sometimes a combined approach [37].

Laminectomy

Cervical laminectomy involves removing the lamina along with the interspinous and supraspinous ligaments, followed by resection of the ligamentum flavum of the affected levels posteriorly until an adequate decompression is achieved. One downside of performing a laminectomy alone is the development of kyphotic deformity over time, which can occur in 21–42% of cases [4]. Risk factors for postoperative kyphosis in CSM include wide laminectomies, presence of preoperative kyphosis or loss of lordosis, hypermobile spine, laminectomy involving C2, and laminectomy at the junctional level (C7) [38–40]. Additionally, recurrent stenosis and segmental instability can also occur. A small randomized study by Bartels et al. comparing laminectomy ($n = 9$) with laminectomy and fusion ($n = 9$) showed no difference in outcome and quality of life in the short term with follow-up of 18.3 months [41]. Laminectomy alone thus can be reserved for select patients with preserved lordosis who are not ideal candidates for fusion.

Laminectomy and Fusion

To prevent the development of post laminectomy kyphotic deformity, a fusion can be added to the decompression. In cases where kyphosis and instability are present in combination with multilevel stenosis, a laminectomy with instrumentation is often used. When performed to increase lordosis and improve alignment, laminectomy and fusion are associated with improved outcomes [42]. Surgery entails placing the patient in the prone position with a Mayfield head holder attached to the patient's skull for immobilization. The patient is placed in a neutral head position. The decompression is followed by instrumentation, which is completed by inserting the screw and rod construct, achieving arthrodesis, and placing bilateral autograft/allograft for fusion. Many techniques and trajectories have been described for screw placement, such as pars or pedicle screws at C2, lateral mass screws at C3–C6, pedicle screw or lateral mass screws at C7, and pedicle screws at T1 and T2. The different screw techniques and trajectories are typically left to the surgeon's discretion and familiarity with various approaches (Fig. 7.3).

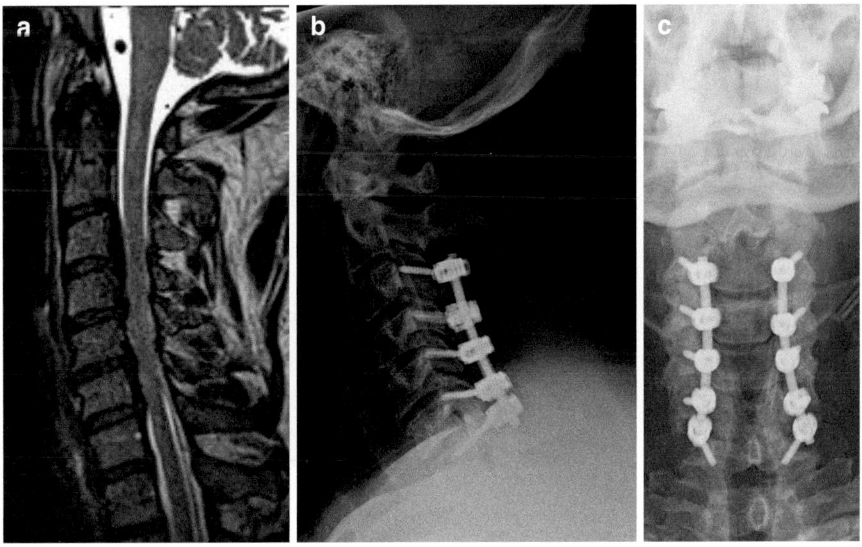

Fig. 7.3 (**a**) Preoperative sagittal T2-weighted MRI demonstrating compression at C3–C7. (**b**) Postoperative lateral plain cervical radiograph showing C3–C7 posterior laminectomy and fusion. (**c**) Postoperative anteroposterior plain cervical radiograph demonstrating C3–C7 hardware

Laminoplasty

Laminoplasty is another dorsal surgical approach that results in decompression without the need for fusion. Laminoplasty allows for expanding the spinal canal by lifting and restructuring the lamina into a new position. Laminoplasty does not destabilize the posterior elements, and it preserves motion. Laminoplasty was initially described in the Japanese literature and performed via an open-door technique detailed by Heller and colleagues [43]. The surgery involves placing the patient prone in a Mayfield three-pin fixation or resting the head on a foam headrest. A small laminotomy is performed on one side, and a hinge is drilled on the contralateral side; then, a titanium plate is affixed to widen the cervical canal (Fig. 7.4). Several laminoplasty techniques have been described, such as the Z-plasty, the French door, and the open-door approach [44]. Hinge plates are also available in cases where there is concern about fracture on the hinge side. The plate is typically secured with a 4- to 6-mm self-tapping screw to fix the plate onto the lamina and lateral mass at each level. Laminoplasty is indicated for multilevel compression with preserved lordosis. It is contraindicated in patients with kyphosis and instability and also may be inappropriate for patients with significant preoperative neck pain [45].

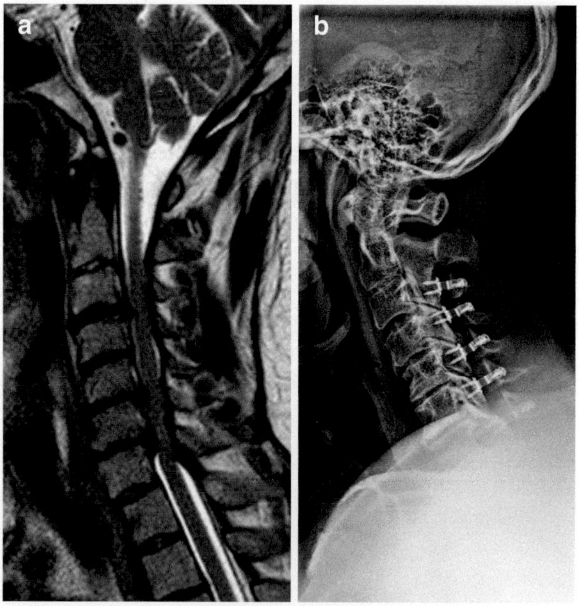

Fig. 7.4 (**a**) Preoperative sagittal T2-weighted MRI demonstrating multilevel stenosis from C3 to C7. (**b**) Postoperative lateral plain cervical radiograph showing placement of C3–C7 laminoplasty plates

Combined Approach

Combined anterior and posterior surgery is performed mainly to treat fixed kyphotic deformity or instability, but is also used in patients in whom there is poor bone quality. The presence of three or more levels of disease in addition to a fixed kyphotic deformity where a corpectomy is contemplated is an ideal indication to perform a combined approach to achieve the desired decompression of the spinal cord and correction of the deformity and to maximize the chances of a successful fusion [46]. Depending on the availability of surgical time as well as consideration of patient comorbidities, the surgery can be staged or performed all in 1 day.

Complications

Age

Numerous studies have demonstrated that surgery for CSM is associated with high rates of surgical complications particularly in elderly patients. Age has been identified as an independent predictor of outcome in a study by Nakashima et al. [47], who showed that patients ≥65 years had worse outcome on modified Japanese Orthopedic Association (mJOA) scores and Nurick scores when compared with patients <65 years of age. Not all studies have identified age >65 years as a predictor of poorer outcomes. For example, Son et al. demonstrated no significant difference in mJOA scores (a validated disease-specific outcome measurement) between patients ≥65 years and<65 years of age [48]. Wang et al. reported that age >74 years was an independent predictor for complications using the NIS database from 1992 through 2001 when considering hospital discharges associated with cervical spine surgery [6]. Another study showed that the complication rate in patients older than 75 years was significantly higher compared with that of younger patients (38% vs. 6%) [49].

Approach

Complications associated with the anterior approach involve injury to the anterior vascular structures (carotid artery and jugular vein), recurrent laryngeal nerve, trachea, and esophagus; postoperative hematoma; and development of Horner syndrome, which can lead to hoarseness, difficulty breathing, and dysphagia [50]. Complications associated with performing a laminectomy alone include recurrent stenosis and development of kyphotic deformity over time. Overall complications associated with the placement of instrumentation include adjacent-segment disease, hardware failure, pseudoarthrosis, nonunion, and adjacent-level fracture.

When comparing dorsal and ventral approaches, Boayke et al. examined 58,115 admissions in the NIS database from 1993 to 2002 and demonstrated that the complication rates were higher in dorsal fusion compared with ventral surgery (16.4% vs. 11.9%) [51]; however, complications can be more frequent with ACCF than with ACDF. Yonenobu et al. also showed that even though treatment of CSM with either corpectomy or laminoplasty yielded good outcomes, corpectomy was associated with a higher complication rate compared with laminoplasty (29.3% vs. 7.1%) [52]. Similar findings were also demonstrated by Edwards et al.; they observed similar surgical outcomes but higher complications with corpectomy than with laminoplasty [53].

Common Complications

The two most commonly encountered complications with surgical treatment of CSM are dysphagia and C5 nerve root palsy. Dysphagia is reported at a rate that ranges from 7.1% to 31% after anterior surgery [27, 54]. Common risk factors that are associated with dysphagia include older age, female sex, multilevel surgery, and revision surgery [55]. C5 palsy is characterized by the development of delayed-onset deltoid and biceps weakness in a unilateral or bilateral fashion 1–2 days after surgery [56]. The published rate of C5 palsy ranges from 12% in ventral surgeries to 30% in posterior surgeries [57]; however, there have been no direct comparisons of the rate of C5 palsies after ventral and dorsal approaches. Risk factors that most strongly correlate with development of C5 palsy include posterior surgery and surgery at the C4–C5 level [58]. The risk of developing C5 palsy is lower in anterior surgery, but there is a higher incidence of C5 palsy with corpectomies than with ACDF [58]. Over time, both C5 palsy and dysphagia tend to improve, even though in the short term there is temporary disability and negative effects on health-related quality of life. Delayed complications include the development of progressive kyphotic deformity after cervical laminectomy [48, 49] the reported rate of which ranges from 21% to 42% [4].

Future Research

Randomized studies regarding surgical approaches for CSM will help patients and physicians choose among the various procedures based on high-quality data. In the near future, the results of a randomized clinical trial (CSM-S; ClinicalTrials.gov identifier: NCT02076113) comparing ventral and dorsal surgery will be available. In this trial, health-related quality of life is the primary outcome, and differences in complications and health resource utilization are being measured as well. Another important feature of the trial will be comparisons of return to productivity rates among various surgical options.

Conclusions

CSM is the most common form of nontraumatic spinal cord injury in adults. With an aging population, CSM will be seen more frequently in the elderly. Surgical treatment of CSM in the elderly may improve quality of life for these patients. Preoperative workup and optimization of comorbidities including osteoporosis may result in reduced intraoperative and postoperative complications. Surgery for the treatment of CSM can be performed either by an anterior, posterior, or a combined approach. Common complications encountered in the treatment of CSM include dysphagia and C5 palsy, both of which often improve over time. Upcoming randomized trials will expand our understanding of which surgical approach is most effective in specific types of patients with CSM.

Disclosure Statement The authors have no relationship with any commercial company that has direct financial interest in the subject matter or materials discussed.

References

1. Karadimas SK, Gatzounis G, Fehlings MG. Pathobiology of cervical spondylotic myelopathy. Eur Spine J. 2015;24(Suppl 2):132–8. Epub 2014/03/15.
2. New PW, Cripps RA, Bonne LB. Global maps of non-traumatic spinal cord injury epidemiology: towards a living data repository. Spinal Cord. 2014;52(2):97–109. Epub 2013/01/16.
3. Badhiwala JH, Wilson JR. The natural history of degenerative cervical myelopathy. Neurosurg Clin N Am. 2018;29(1):21–32. Epub 2017/11/28.
4. Karadimas SK, Erwin WM, Ely CG, Dettori JR, Fehlings MG. Pathophysiology and natural history of cervical spondylotic myelopathy. Spine. 2013;38(22 Suppl 1):S21–36. Epub 2013/08/22.
5. Fehlings MG, Wilson JR, Kopjar B, Yoon ST, Arnold PM, Massicotte EM, et al. Efficacy and safety of surgical decompression in patients with cervical spondylotic myelopathy: results of the AOSpine North America prospective multi-center study. J Bone Joint Surg Am. 2013;95(18):1651–8. Epub 2013/09/21.
6. Wang MC, Chan L, Maiman DJ, Kreuter W, Deyo RA. Complications and mortality associated with cervical spine surgery for degenerative disease in the United States. Spine. 2007;32(3):342–7. Epub 2007/02/03.
7. Patil PG, Turner DA, Pietrobon R. National trends in surgical procedures for degenerative cervical spine disease: 1990-2000. Neurosurgery. 2005;57(4):753–8; discussion 8.
8. Oglesby M, Fineberg SJ, Patel AA, Pelton MA, Singh K. Epidemiological trends in cervical spine surgery for degenerative diseases between 2002 and 2009. Spine. 2013;38(14):1226–32. Epub 2013/02/14.
9. Akter F, Kotter M. Pathobiology of degenerative cervical myelopathy. Neurosurg Clin N Am. 2018;29(1):13–9. Epub 2017/11/28.
10. Nishida N, Kato Y, Imajo Y, Kawano S, Taguchi T. Biomechanical analysis of cervical spondylotic myelopathy: the influence of dynamic factors and morphometry of the spinal cord. J Spinal Cord Med. 2012;35(4):256–61. Epub 2012/08/29.
11. Al-Mefty O, Harkey HL, Marawi I, Haines DE, Peeler DF, Wilner HI, et al. Experimental chronic compressive cervical myelopathy. J Neurosurg. 1993;79(4):550–61.

12. Baron EM, Young WF. Cervical spondylotic myelopathy: a brief review of its pathophysiology, clinical course, and diagnosis. Neurosurgery. 2007;60(1 Suppl 1):S35–41.
13. Iyer A, Azad TD, Tharin S. Cervical spondylotic myelopathy. Clin Spine Surg. 2016;29(10):408–14. Epub 2016/06/29.
14. Suzuki A, Misawa H, Simogata M, Tsutsumimoto T, Takaoka K, Nakamura H. Recovery process following cervical laminoplasty in patients with cervical compression myelopathy: prospective cohort study. Spine. 2009;34(26):2874–9. Epub 2009/12/02.
15. Halpin RJ, Sugrue PA, Gould RW, Kallas PG, Schafer MF, Ondra SL, et al. Standardizing care for high-risk patients in spine surgery: the Northwestern high-risk spine protocol. Spine. 2010;35(25):2232–8. Epub 2010/11/26.
16. Qureshi R, Rasool M, Puvanesarajah V, Hassanzadeh H. Perioperative nutritional optimization in spine surgery. Clin Spine Surg. 2018;31(3):103–7. Epub 2018/03/30.
17. Park SB, Chung CK. Strategies of spinal fusion on osteoporotic spine. J Korean Neurosurg Soc. 2011;49(6):317–22. Epub 2011/09/03.
18. Glassman SD, Polly DW, Bono CM, Burkus K, Dimar JR. Outcome of lumbar arthrodesis in patients sixty-five years of age or older. J Bone Joint Surg Am. 2009;91(4):783–90. Epub 2009/04/03.
19. Chin DK, Park JY, Yoon YS, Kuh SU, Jin BH, Kim KS, et al. Prevalence of osteoporosis in patients requiring spine surgery: incidence and significance of osteoporosis in spine disease. Osteoporos Int. 2007;18(9):1219–24. Epub 2007/03/28.
20. Colantonio DF, Saxena SK, Vanier A, Rodkey D, Tintle S, Wagner SC. Cervical spine computed tomography hounsfield units accurately predict low bone mineral density of the femoral neck. Clin Spine Surg. 2020;33(2):E58–62. Epub 2019/09/10.
21. Jilka RL, Weinstein RS, Bellido T, Roberson P, Parfitt AM, Manolagas SC. Increased bone formation by prevention of osteoblast apoptosis with parathyroid hormone. J Clin Invest. 1999;104(4):439–46. Epub 1999/08/17.
22. Gardner MJ, Demetrakopoulos D, Shindle MK, Griffith MH, Lane JM. Osteoporosis and skeletal fractures. HSS J. 2006;2(1):62–9. Epub 2008/08/30.
23. Lane JM. Osteoporosis. Medical prevention and treatment. Spine. 1997;22(24 Suppl):32S–7S. Epub 1998/02/07.
24. Lane JM, Gardner MJ, Lin JT, van der Meulen MC, Myers E. The aging spine: new technologies and therapeutics for the osteoporotic spine. Eur Spine J. 2003;12(Suppl 2):S147–54. Epub 2003/10/10.
25. Chesnut CH III, Silverman S, Andriano K, Genant H, Gimona A, Harris S, et al. A randomized trial of nasal spray salmon calcitonin in postmenopausal women with established osteoporosis: the prevent recurrence of osteoporotic fractures study. PROOF Study Group. Am J Med. 2000;109(4):267–76. Epub 2000/09/21.
26. Fehlings MG, Barry S, Kopjar B, Yoon ST, Arnold P, Massicotte EM, et al. Anterior versus posterior surgical approaches to treat cervical spondylotic myelopathy: outcomes of the prospective multicenter AOSpine North America CSM study in 264 patients. Spine. 2013;38(26):2247–52. Epub 2013/10/11.
27. Lawrence BD, Jacobs WB, Norvell DC, Hermsmeyer JT, Chapman JR, Brodke DS. Anterior versus posterior approach for treatment of cervical spondylotic myelopathy: a systematic review. Spine. 2013;38(22 Suppl 1):S173–82. Epub 2013/08/22.
28. Abduljabbar FH, Teles AR, Bokhari R, Weber M, Santaguida C. Laminectomy with or without fusion to manage degenerative cervical myelopathy. Neurosurg Clin N Am. 2018;29(1):91–105. Epub 2017/11/28.
29. Rowland LP. Surgical treatment of cervical spondylotic myelopathy: time for a controlled trial. Neurology. 1992;42(1):5–13.
30. Grodzinski B, Durham R, Mowforth O, Stubbs D, Kotter MRN, Davies BM. The effect of ageing on presentation, management and outcomes in degenerative cervical myelopathy: a systematic review. Age Ageing. 2020;50:705. Epub 2020/11/22.

31. Wang T, Tian XM, Liu SK, Wang H, Zhang YZ, Ding WY. Prevalence of complications after surgery in treatment for cervical compressive myelopathy: a meta-analysis for last decade. Medicine. 2017;96(12):e6421. Epub 2017/03/23.
32. King JT Jr, Abbed KM, Gould GC, Benzel EC, Ghogawala Z. Cervical spine reoperation rates and hospital resource utilization after initial surgery for degenerative cervical spine disease in 12,338 patients in Washington State. Neurosurgery. 2009;65(6):1011–22; discussion 22–3.
33. Ghogawala Z, Martin B, Benzel EC, Dziura J, Magge SN, Abbed KM, et al. Comparative effectiveness of ventral vs dorsal surgery for cervical spondylotic myelopathy. Neurosurgery. 2011;68(3):622–30; discussion 30–1. Epub 2010/12/18.
34. Stewart TJ, Schlenk RP, Benzel EC. Multiple level discectomy and fusion. Neurosurgery. 2007;60(1 Suppl 1):S143–8.
35. Douglas AF, Cooper PR. Cervical corpectomy and strut grafting. Neurosurgery. 2007;60(1 Suppl 1):S137–42.
36. Fehlings MG, Santaguida C, Tetreault L, Arnold P, Barbagallo G, Defino H, et al. Laminectomy and fusion versus laminoplasty for the treatment of degenerative cervical myelopathy: results from the AOSpine North America and International prospective multicenter studies. Spine J. 2017;17(1):102–8. Epub 2016/09/07.
37. Winestone JS, Farley CW, Curt BA, Chavanne A, Dollin N, Pettigrew DB, et al. Laminectomy, durotomy, and piotomy effects on spinal cord intramedullary pressure in severe cervical and thoracic kyphotic deformity: a cadaveric study. J Neurosurg Spine. 2012;16(2):195–200. Epub 2011/11/15.
38. Mikawa Y, Shikata J, Yamamuro T. Spinal deformity and instability after multilevel cervical laminectomy. Spine. 1987;12(1):6–11. Epub 1987/01/01.
39. Guigui P, Benoist M, Deburge A. Spinal deformity and instability after multilevel cervical laminectomy for spondylotic myelopathy. Spine. 1998;23(4):440–7.
40. Kaptain GJ, Simmons NE, Replogle RE, Pobereskin L. Incidence and outcome of kyphotic deformity following laminectomy for cervical spondylotic myelopathy. J Neurosurg. 2000;93(2 Suppl):199–204. Epub 2000/09/30.
41. Bartels RH, Groenewoud H, Peul WC, Arts MP. Lamifuse: results of a randomized controlled trial comparing laminectomy with and without fusion for cervical spondylotic myelopathy. J Neurosurg Sci. 2017;61(2):134–9. Epub 2015/06/18.
42. Sielatycki JA, Armaghani S, Silverberg A, McGirt MJ, Devin CJ, O'Neill K. Is more lordosis associated with improved outcomes in cervical laminectomy and fusion when baseline alignment is lordotic? Spine J. 2016;16(8):982–8. Epub 2016/04/16.
43. Heller JG, Edwards CC II, Murakami H, Rodts GE. Laminoplasty versus laminectomy and fusion for multilevel cervical myelopathy: an independent matched cohort analysis. Spine. 2001;26(12):1330–6.
44. Patel CK, Cunningham BJ, Herkowitz HN. Techniques in cervical laminoplasty. Spine J. 2002;2(6):450–5. Epub 2003/11/01.
45. Tetreault L, Goldstein CL, Arnold P, Harrop J, Hilibrand A, Nouri A, et al. Degenerative cervical myelopathy: a spectrum of related disorders affecting the aging spine. Neurosurgery. 2015;77(Suppl 4):S51–67. Epub 2015/09/18.
46. Mummaneni PV, Haid RW, Rodts GE Jr. Combined ventral and dorsal surgery for myelopathy and myeloradiculopathy. Neurosurgery. 2007;60(1 Suppl 1):S82–9.
47. Nakashima H, Tetreault LA, Nagoshi N, Nouri A, Kopjar B, Arnold PM, et al. Does age affect surgical outcomes in patients with degenerative cervical myelopathy? Results from the prospective multicenter AOSpine International study on 479 patients. J Neurol Neurosurg Psychiatry. 2016;87(7):734–40. Epub 2015/10/01.
48. Son DK, Son DW, Song GS, Lee SW. Effectiveness of the laminoplasty in the elderly patients with cervical spondylotic myelopathy. Korean J Spine. 2014;11(2):39–44. Epub 2014/08/12.
49. Holly LT, Moftakhar P, Khoo LT, Shamie AN, Wang JC. Surgical outcomes of elderly patients with cervical spondylotic myelopathy. Surg Neurol. 2008;69(3):233–40.

50. Sugawara T. Neurologic complications in managing degenerative cervical myelopathy: pathogenesis, prevention, and management. Neurosurg Clin N Am. 2018;29(1):129–37. Epub 2017/11/28.
51. Boakye M, Patil CG, Santarelli J, Ho C, Tian W, Lad SP. Cervical spondylotic myelopathy: complications and outcomes after spinal fusion. Neurosurgery. 2008;62(2):455–61; discussion 61-2.
52. Yonenobu K, Hosono N, Iwasaki M, Asano M, Ono K. Laminoplasty versus subtotal corpectomy. A comparative study of results in multisegmental cervical spondylotic myelopathy. Spine. 1992;17(11):1281–4. Epub 1992/11/01.
53. Edwards CC II, Heller JG, Murakami H. Corpectomy versus laminoplasty for multilevel cervical myelopathy: an independent matched-cohort analysis. Spine. 2002;27(11):1168–75. Epub 2002/06/05.
54. Edwards CC II, Karpitskaya Y, Cha C, Heller JG, Lauryssen C, Yoon ST, et al. Accurate identification of adverse outcomes after cervical spine surgery. J Bone Joint Surg Am. 2004;86A(2):251–6.
55. Joaquim AF, Murar J, Savage JW, Patel AA. Dysphagia after anterior cervical spine surgery: a systematic review of potential preventative measures. Spine J. 2014;14(9):2246–60. Epub 2014/03/26.
56. Radcliff KE, Limthongkul W, Kepler CK, Sidhu GD, Anderson DG, Rihn JA, et al. Cervical laminectomy width and spinal cord drift are risk factors for postoperative C5 palsy. J Spinal Disord Tech. 2014;27(2):86–92. Epub 2012/03/20.
57. Bose B, Sestokas AK, Schwartz DM. Neurophysiological detection of iatrogenic C-5 nerve deficit during anterior cervical spinal surgery. J Neurosurg Spine. 2007;6(5):381–5.
58. Bydon M, Macki M, Kaloostian P, Sciubba DM, Wolinsky JP, Gokaslan ZL, et al. Incidence and prognostic factors of c5 palsy: a clinical study of 1001 cases and review of the literature. Neurosurgery. 2014;74(6):595–604; discussion 5. Epub 2014/02/25.

Chapter 8
Atlantoaxial Fracture Management

Ellina Hattar, Thiago S. Montenegro, Tyler D. Alexander, Glenn A. Gonzalez, and James S. Harrop

Introduction

The geriatric population is at especially high risk of atlantoaxial fractures. The two mechanisms responsible for these injuries are predominantly due to a ground-level fall followed by high-velocity injuries secondary to motor vehicle accidents [1–3]. The population above 65 years of age is the fastest growing demographic group in the United States estimated to account for 20% of the population by 2030 [4]. As the number of geriatric patients rises, cervical and specifically atlantoaxial injuries are expected to become more prevalent in trauma and emergency centers. The management of such injuries in the elderly is a challenge due to the presence of medical comorbidities, poor bone quality secondary to osteopenia, low tolerance to halo immobilization, higher prevalence of preexisting cognitive impairment or dementia, and reduced potential for bony union [2].

Anatomy and Mechanical Properties of the Atlantoaxial Complex

The articulation between the atlas and axis is the most mobile segment of the spine and allows for three-dimensional movement. The atlantoaxial complex is responsible for 40° of unilateral rotation at the C1–2 joint, accounting for 40% of the total

E. Hattar (✉) · T. S. Montenegro · T. D. Alexander · G. A. Gonzalez · J. S. Harrop
Department of Neurological Surgery, Thomas Jefferson University, Philadelphia, PA, USA
e-mail: ellina.hattar@jefferson.edu; thiago.scharthmontenegro@jefferson.edu; tyler.alexander@students.jefferson.edu; glennarturo.gonzalezozuna@jefferson.edu; james.harrop@jefferson.edu

K.-M. G. Fu et al. (eds.), *Treatment of Spine Disease in the Elderly*, https://doi.org/10.1007/978-3-031-12612-3_8

rotation in the cervical spine, 10–13° of flexion-extension, and 5° of lateral bending [5]. Translation is limited to 2 mm, primarily due to the limitation afforded by the transverse-atlantal ligament that maintains the odontoid process against the anterior arch of C1 [6]. The atlantoaxial complex not only provides a large component of the mobility of the cervical spine but also protects the upper cervical spine and the vertebral arteries. These traversing structures may thus be injured in atlantoaxial fractures and could lead to significant morbidity and mortality [7].

Epidemiology

Fractures of the atlantoaxial complex and the odontoid process in particular are the most prevalent spine injury in the elderly [1, 8, 9]. The number of spine injury-related hospital admissions among the elderly has increased fivefold since the 1980s, increasing the prevalence of these fractures [10]. Several epidemiologic studies have demonstrated that the risk of fractures of the odontoid process increases with age [1, 11]. There is a female predominance among patients with fractures of the atlantoaxial complex, perhaps due to a greater prevalence of osteopenia and osteoporosis in this population [2]. Moreover, geriatric patients have a tendency toward combined C1–2 fractures as well as a higher likelihood for concurrent injuries including intracranial trauma [2, 8, 12]. Cervical spine fractures among patients over 70 years of age are associated with an 8.1% 30-day mortality. Moreover, geriatric patients with spinal cord injuries have a mortality approaching 28% [10].

Odontoid Fractures

Odontoid fractures are the most common type of cervical spine fracture in patients over 65 years of age as they represent 5–29% of cervical spine fractures [3, 13, 14] with Anderson and D'Alonzo type II fractures accounting for 8–15% of cervical spine fractures [15, 16]. Several classifications have been created for the description of odontoid fractures. The most widely accepted is the Anderson and D'Alonzo classification [17]. Type I describes an oblique fracture at the tip of the odontoid process. This fracture pattern may have an association with atlanto-occipital dislocation [18]. Type II is a horizontally oriented fracture at the base of the odontoid process disconnecting it from the vertebral body of the axis. It results from hyperextension injuries as the anterior aspect of the ring of the atlas exerts pressure on and fractures the odontoid. It is thought that with age, the subaxial cervical spine is affected by spondylosis at a greater degree than the atlantoaxial segment and stiffens, resulting in a lever arm effect on the upper cervical spine during even low-velocity traumas [19]. Due to poor vascularity, the small surface area of the fracture, and the predominance of cortical bone, the type II odontoid fracture is at higher risk of non-union than other odontoid fractures [20, 21]. Other risk factors for non-union

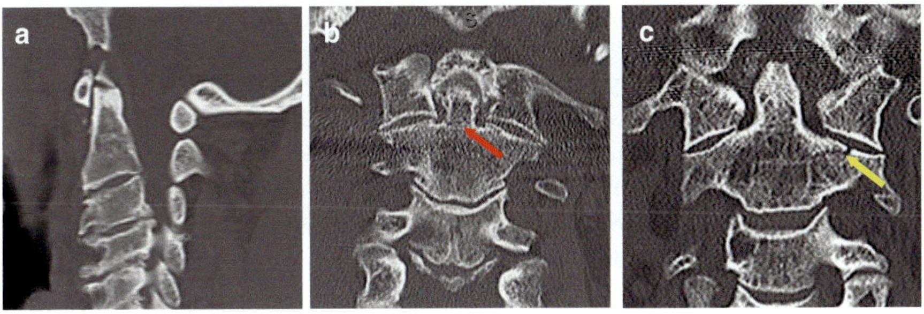

Fig. 8.1 Anderson and D'Alonzo classification of odontoid fractures. (**a**) Sagittal cervical spine CT showing a type I odontoid fracture across the tip of the odontoid without evidence of atlanto-occipital dislocation. (**b**) Coronal cervical spine CT of a type II odontoid fracture of the base of the odontoid (red arrow). (**c**) Coronal cervical spine CT of a type III odontoid fracture of the body of the axis with extension into the left atlantoaxial facet joint (yellow arrow)

include posterior displacement greater than 5 mm, or angulation greater than 10°, comminution of the fracture, and tobacco use [13, 21–24]. The type III is one that extends to the body of the axis and the facet joints (Fig. 8.1).

Due to its prevalence in the geriatric population, the next section will in large part focus on the evidence-based medicine pertaining to the management of type II odontoid fractures. To date, there is no class I evidence on the subject, and most literature on the subject consists of retrospective reviews and limited case series.

Diagnosis

In addition to a thorough neurologic examination, an adequate radiographic workup is necessary to evaluate for cervical injuries in elderly patients. Clinical symptoms of atlantoaxial and especially odontoid fractures are usually nonspecific as patients often present with poorly localized posterior neck pain, paravertebral muscle spasms, tenderness, and decreased range of motion of the neck [21]. Although there is a subset of patients who die prior to reaching the hospital following an odontoid injury, those who survive often do not have a neurologic deficit [25]. If neurologic injury is present, it may range from occipital neuralgia from irritation of the greater occipital nerve to monoplegia with sensory deficits to high tetraplegia with respiratory depression [21]. Furthermore, delayed symptoms attributable to posterior displacement of the odontoid can lead to cervical myelopathy with symptoms of neck pain, hand wasting and weakness, and gait dysfunction [25]. Even in the absence of a neurologic deficit, however, a high index of suspicion for atlantoaxial and odontoid injury must be present for the geriatric patient following even a seemingly innocuous fall.

Few studies exist describing the long-term natural history of odontoid fractures. A study by Hart et al. revealed no evidence of myelopathy among five patients over the age of 70 followed for a minimum of 16 months [22]. In this last study, however, patients may have not been followed long enough to properly identify the eventual development of myelopathy. In fact, in another study by Crockard et al., among patients managed without surgical stabilization, 69% of patients were diagnosed with myelopathy over a year after the initial injury, while 38% were diagnosed over 5 years following [25]. Finally, not much is known on the eventual cause of mortality in this population and whether death could be related to the development of a high cervical spinal cord injury (SCI).

Imaging

Radiographs are insufficient in ruling out cervical fractures in the elderly. It is estimated that 35% of C1 and 14% of C2 fractures are missed on plain lateral radiographs [26]. Computed tomography (CT) scan is the most cost-effective study for patients with high likelihood of cervical fracture. Magnetic resonance imaging (MRI) can further identify ligamentous damage in the upper cervical spine [27]. On plain radiographs, the atlantodental interval (ADI), which is commonly considered abnormal when greater than 3 mm in men and 2.5 mm in women, can suggest incompetence of the transverse-atlantal ligament and thus indicate atlantoaxial instability [28, 29].

Morbidity and Mortality

In a study by Muller et al., the overall complication rate of odontoid fractures in the elderly was 52% as compared to 33% among younger patients, while mortality was 35% as compared to 4% [3]. Most of these patients were treated conservatively. The two most common causes of death among older patients were pneumonia and cardiac and pulmonary arrest. Furthermore, halo-vest immobilization in the elderly has been shown to have a significantly higher rate of morbidity and mortality than in younger patients with a mortality rate of 40% in a study by Majercik et al. [30].

Management

The management strategy for the type II odontoid fracture has been a topic of debate. Treatment options include external fixation with rigid cervical orthoses, halo-vest immobilization, and atlantoaxial fusion. It has been shown that immobilization either through external immobilization or surgical fixation is required as the rate of non-union likely approaches 100% in patients not managed with immobilization [21].

External Immobilization

Conservative treatment for type II odontoid fractures generally involves the use of either halo vests or cervical orthoses. Among patients over the age of 65 years, mortality associated with halo-vest immobilization was published at 42%, while major complications were observed in 66% of patients in the group [2, 31]. Furthermore, external immobilization is not as effective in promoting bony fusion in the geriatric population as it is in younger patients. Polin et al. showed that patients over the age of 60 with type II odontoid fractures who were managed with external immobilization with halo vests or collars had a lower rate of bony fusion at 38%, while younger patients had a fusion rate of 82% [20]. In another study by Smith et al., there was a significantly higher incidence of airway complications among octogenarians with odontoid fractures managed with halo-vest immobilization (31%) as compared to cervical orthoses (4%) [32]. The type III odontoid fracture in the elderly patient may be managed with hard cervical collar with bony fusion rates previously reported at 100% in nondisplaced fractures.

Operative Management

Several studies support the surgical management of type II odontoid fractures in the elderly. In a study by Muller et al., 5 of 11 patients with nondisplaced type II odontoid fractures experienced non-union; all 5 were initially treated with a cervical orthoses alone [3]. The group recommended either surgical fixation or halo-vest immobilization for type II odontoid fractures among elderly patients with the consideration that halo fixation may be poorly tolerated by the population (Fig. 8.2).

Mortality rate among patients with type II odontoid fractures may be lower in geriatric patients undergoing surgery than those who are conservatively managed. In a study by Smith et al., mortality was 12.5% in elderly patients undergoing surgical treatment as compared to 15% of patients who were conservatively managed [33]. Chapman et al. had similar results with a 7% mortality rate in the surgical group and 22% mortality rate in the nonoperative group at 30 days [34]. Woods et al. also found a statistically reduced mortality in their surgical subgroup as compared to those managed conservatively [35]. These collective findings on mortality rate suggest that surgically managed patients may have a survival benefit as they may be able to be mobilized sooner than conservatively managed patients.

Type II odontoid fractures may be treated with several surgical options including an anterior approach with an odontoid screw and posterior approaches with lateral mass fusion or transarticular screw placement [36]. The rate of union in a study by Omeis et al. was greater than 30% for both anterior and posterior approaches [36]. Furthermore, of the 29 surgically treated patients in the study, 86% were ultimately

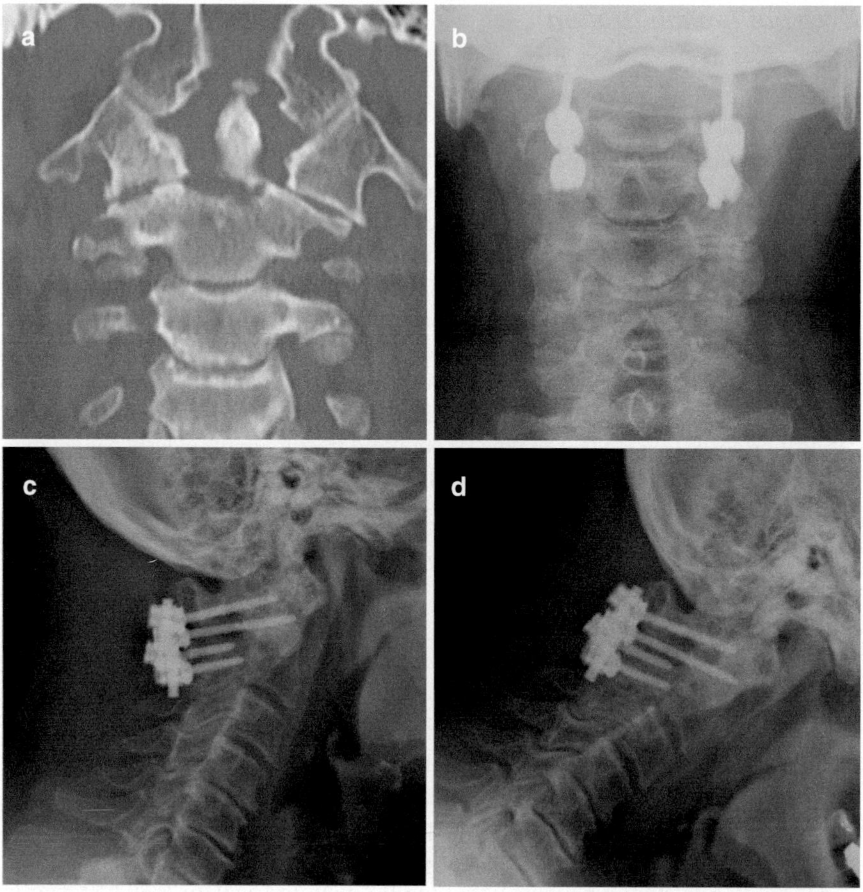

Fig. 8.2 (**a**) Coronal cervical spine CT showing a type II odontoid fracture. (**b**) Anteroposterior postoperative cervical spine X-ray showing a posterior construct was performed with C1 lateral mass and C2 pars screw. (**c**, **d**) Lateral X-rays of the C1–2 fusion construct showing no displacement of the dens and a solid fusion on flexion X-rays (**d**). These images were obtained 2 years following fusion

able to return to their previous residential environment. Although results appeared to be comparable in this last study, another study by Andersson et al. suggested that posterior fixation may have superior results with a non-union rate approaching 0% as compared to that of the odontoid screw yielding a non-union rate of 9% and conservative treatment associated with a rate of 54% [37]. This may be due to the fact that the cortical bone, in which posterior fixation is secured, is less affected by degenerative changes than cancellous bone. Also, the odontoid screw may further create a larger lever arm in the spondylitic geriatric cervical spine. Furthermore, the anterior odontoid screw approach may be associated with higher rates of pneumonia and dysphagia [33].

Fractures of the Atlas

Fractures of the atlas are relatively rare and represent approximately 2% of all spine fractures [14]. A classification system of C1 fractures has been proposed by Landells et al. with type I involving a single arch, type II involving both the anterior and posterior arches of the atlas with two or more fragments, and a type III fractures involving the lateral mass of the atlas [38]. The classically described Jefferson fracture is a subtype of the type II fracture in which an axial loading force results in a four-point burst fracture of the C1 ring (Fig. 8.3).

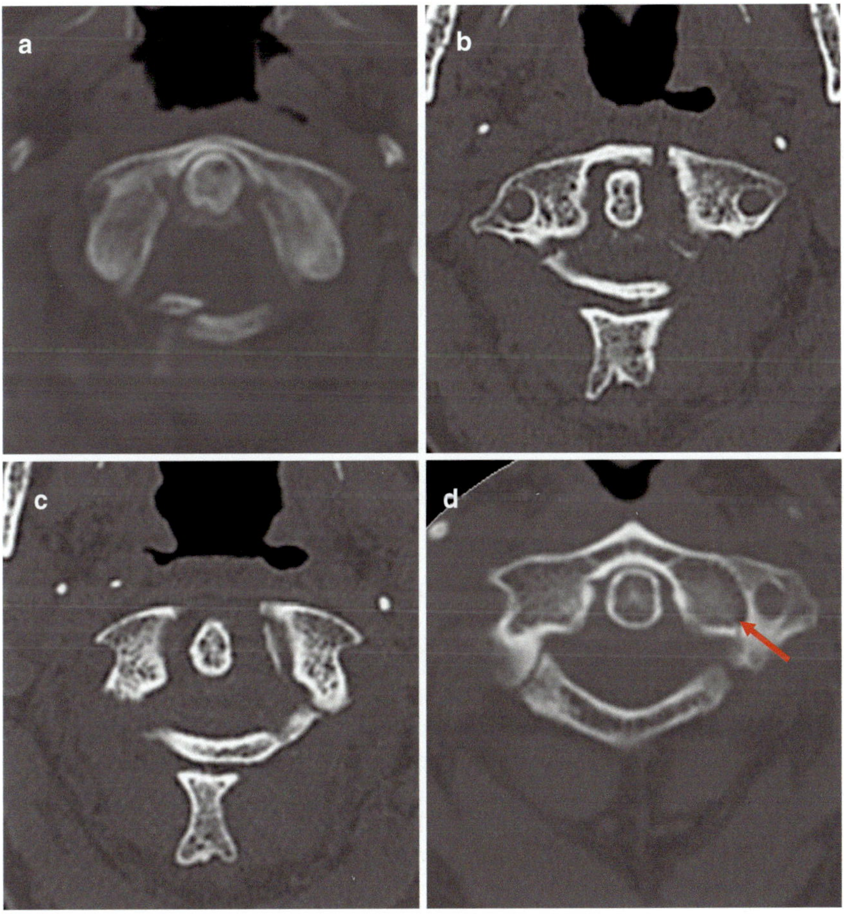

Fig. 8.3 Fractures of the atlas according to the Landells classification as shown on axial cervical spine CT imaging. (**a**) Type I C1 fracture of the posterior arch only. (**b**, **c**) Type II fracture involving the anterior and posterior arches of the atlas. (**d**) Type III fracture showing extension into the left C1 lateral mass (red arrow)

Diagnosis and Treatment

Neurologic deficits have historically been thought to be rare due to the relatively large spinal canal diameter at this level and due to the tendency of fractured fragments to be forced outward away from the spinal canal. In the geriatric population, however, these fractures may not be as benign as once thought as this specific population is at higher risk of poor outcomes including death [39]. As with other upper cervical injuries, plain radiographs, CT, angiography, and MRI are essential during evaluation. The transverse ligament is considered to be the most important determinant of stability for fractures of the atlas. The rule of Spence may be used to determine stability of the injury as it can suggest injury to the transverse ligament when the C1 on C2 lateral mass total overhang equals or exceeds 7 mm on open-mouth odontoid view radiographs [40]. Type I, stable type II (with an intact transverse ligament), and type III fractures of the atlas can all be managed in a rigid cervical collar. In cases of transverse ligament disruption, sagittal split lateral mass fractures, or in the presence of concomitant fractures of the atlantoaxial complex or other cervical segments, surgical fixation may be necessary. Fractures of the atlas are associated with additional fractures of the cervical spine in 30–70% of cases [41, 42]. Occipitocervical fusion to C2 may be necessary in cases of atlanto-occipital dissociation or concurrent fractures of the occipital condyles [39]. Posterior atlantoaxial fusion is the gold standard either with lateral mass screw and rod fixation or transarticular fixation, with or without the addition of wiring. Although the reduction of the C1 ring is feasible through the transoral approach, it is not as commonly performed at most institutions. In addition to the halo vest being poorly tolerated in the elderly, the device may also be insufficient in stabilizing and reducing unstable fractures of the atlas.

C1–2 Dislocation and Subluxation

Atlantoaxial instability is a serious condition that can present with symptoms ranging from greater occipital nerve irritation to tetraplegia and death. The odontoid process itself prevents hyperextension at the joint, but the majority of motion about the atlantoaxial joint is dictated by ligamentous and capsular attachments [6].

Atlantoaxial subluxation in the geriatric population is often related to cervical rheumatoid arthritis (RA) [43]. Atlantoaxial instability is the most common presentation of cervical rheumatoid disease, occurring in greater than 70% of patients with RA [44]. Joints and ligaments affected by RA will determine the direction of subluxation [43]:

- Involvement of the synovial joint on the dorsal surface of the odontoid process will lead to laxity of the transverse ligament and ventral subluxation of C1 on C2.

- Involvement and osteomalacia of the odontoid process may lead to dorsal subluxation.
- Involvement of the synovial apophyseal joints of C1–2 may lead to lateral rotary subluxation.
- Further facet destruction may lead to collapse of the occiput on C1 and vertical displacement of the odontoid process. This is also known as basilar invagination, atlantoaxial impaction, vertical subluxation, and cranial settling. It is thought to occur at more advanced stages of the disease.

Other inflammatory conditions such as ankylosing spondylitis (AS) may also lead to atlantoaxial instability, however far less commonly. Atlantoaxial dislocation (AAD) is associated with a high likelihood of morbidity and mortality. While it can occur in the pediatric population as a result of infection, in the geriatric population, AAD is typically caused by trauma [7].

Subluxation can be broadly grouped into four main categories: anterior, rotary subluxation, vertical subluxation, and lateral subluxation. Rotary subluxation, also known as atlantoaxial rotatory fixation (AARF), can be subdivided into four main types according to a classification system created by Fielding and Hawkins [45]. In type I, the atlas is rotated on the odontoid with no displacement. In type II, there is 3–5 mm of anterior displacement of the atlas with slight rotation. In type III, there is greater than 5-mm anterior displacement. Type IV is defined by posterior displacement of the atlas with rotation. Type III and IV rotary subluxations are considered unstable and warrant fixation.

Imaging and Diagnosis

Symptoms typically include neck pain, along with headache, torticollis, and reduced rotation of the cervical region. The contralateral chin and sternocleidomastoid will be spastic; for example, a right-sided subluxation will present with spasm of the left sternocleidomastoid muscle.

Lateral radiographs may be used to determine the stability of the atlantoaxial complex. The ADI can again be used. When the ADI is greater than 3 mm in men and 2.5 mm in women, it suggests rupture of the transverse ligament. Additionally, an ADI greater than 10 mm indicates total ligamentous damage [46]. Radiographic assessments of transverse ligament integrity can also be inferred by the rule of Spence. CT is the gold standard of imaging for suspected subluxation or dislocation. CT angiography can identify vascular injury to the vertebral arteries. Finally, MRI is essential in further characterizing extent of spinal cord injury when present and may aid in the diagnosis of ligamentous injury (Fig. 8.4) [7].

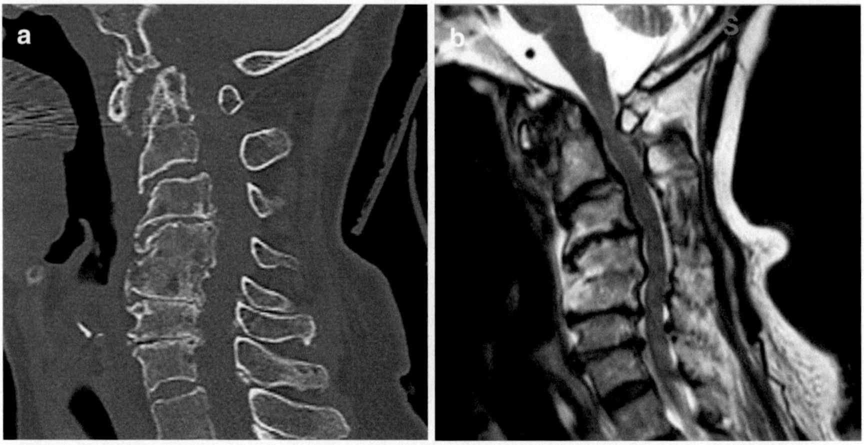

Fig. 8.4 (**a**) Sagittal cervical spine CT showing anterior atlantoaxial subluxation with widened atlantodental interval to 6.5 mm and basilar invagination. (**b**) Sagittal T2 cervical spine MRI showing multilevel central stenosis with severe C1–2 stenosis

Treatment

Surgical treatment is considered if the anterior displacement is greater than 5 mm in adults. Acute atlantoaxial dislocation has a high morbidity and mortality, while subluxation, which is a chronic progressive pathology, has a better prognosis. Acute atlantoaxial dislocations are rare in adults and are often accompanied by neurovascular dysfunction. Reduction and fixation of such injuries is necessary in the majority of cases [7]. In cases of symptomatic atlantoaxial subluxation secondary to RA, occipitocervical fusion has been shown to decrease nuchal pain and improve symptoms of myelopathy [47, 48]. Management of these pathologies remains a topic of debate as no large-scale randomized studies exist on the subject.

Hangman's Fractures

Hangman's fractures consist of a traumatic spondylolisthesis of the axis with bilateral fractures of the C2 pars interarticularis [49]. This fracture coined its name from injuries thought to be produced by judicial hangings, although it was later realized that only a minority of hanging victims had this fracture type [50, 51]. These injuries account for 4–7% of all cervical spine fractures and occur as a solitary lesions in up to 74% of patients and associated with other fractures in 9% of patients [9, 52–54]. In the elderly population, Hangman's fractures usually result from relatively low-energy injuries due to bone fragility, and its incidence has been growing in the past decades [55, 56]. The first classification system uses the mechanism of injury to classify this type of fracture and was developed by Effendi et al. and subsequently modified by Levine and Edwards, which is currently the most commonly used classification [57, 58].

The Modified Effendi Classification System

Type I fractures are the only nondisplaced fractures without evidence of angulation or C2–3 disc involvement and result from a hyperextension-axial loading force. These are considered stable and can be managed conservatively in a cervical collar. Type II fractures result from a combined hyperextension-axial loading force, with a rebound flexion and compression force, causing a significant angulation (>11°) and translation (>3 mm) of C2. Type IIA and type III fractures are caused by the same injury pattern, a flexion-distraction mechanism. In the former, there is a very severe angulation without translation of C2, while the later results in not only a fracture of the lamina or the pedicle but also bilateral facet dislocation. Type II, IIA, and III usually involve rupture of the C2 and C3 disc and anterior and posterior longitudinal ligament involvement [49, 52, 58]. Furthermore, there is an atypical presentation of Hangman's fractures where canal compromise can result from traumatic spondylolisthesis of the axis, instead of canal expansion (Fig. 8.5) [59].

Diagnosis

In order to establish the diagnosis, measuring both angulation and translation of C2 is important. The standard measurement technique is the endplate method for which a lateral cervical radiograph or midsagittal CT reconstruction can be used. Lines are drawn perpendicular to the inferior endplate of C2 and C3 to measure angulation. The posterior vertebral body tangent method can also be used With this method, lines are drawn along the posterior aspect of C2 vertebral body and odontoid to enable measurement of angulation and displacement [60].

Management and Operative Technique

The management strategies and the surgical indications for Hangman's fractures are still a topic of debate, particularly for type II and type III. A systematic review demonstrated that 62.5% of publications advocated that the primary therapy for all Hangman's fractures should be conservative, 22% suggested that conservative treatment was acceptable to some stable fractures, and only one manuscript claimed that surgery would be the best primary approach to type II, IIa and III fractures [61, 62].

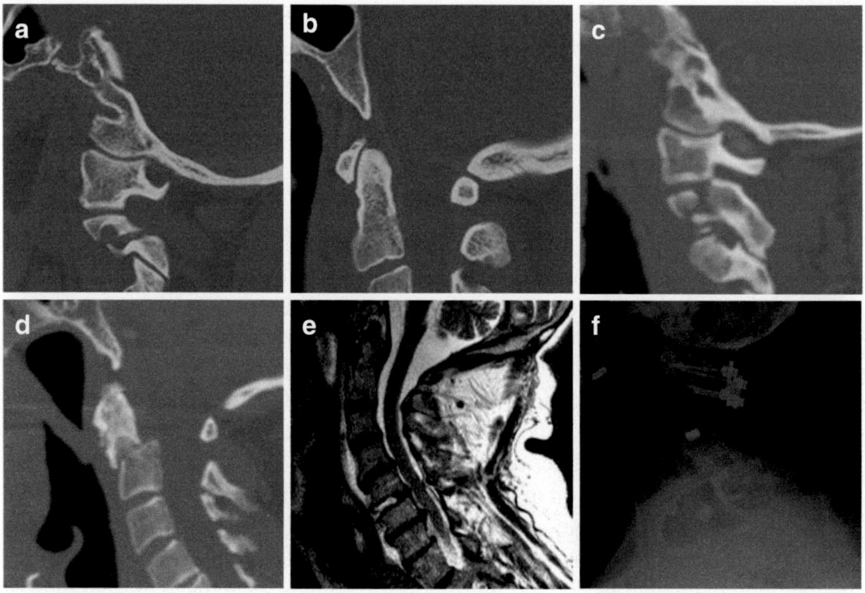

Fig. 8.5 (**a**, **b**) Sagittal cervical CT showing Effendi type I fracture with a nondisplaced pars fracture without displacement of C2 on C3 vertebral bodies. Images (**c**–**f**) belong to the same patient. (**c**) Sagittal CT angiogram of the neck showing a fracture through the pars interarticularis of the atlas. (**d**) The same patient had a concurrent odontoid fracture with associated angulation of the posterior aspect of the C2 odontoid on the remaining C2 and C3 vertebral bodies. (**e**) T2 sagittal cervical spine MRI showing an associated rupture of the C5–6 intervertebral disc. (**f**) The patient underwent a staged C5–6 ACDF followed by a posterior C1–2 fusion

The conservative management of the fractures can be conducted with either a hard collar or rigid immobilization. [49] The operative management of Hangman's fracture is usually conducted using an anterior approach with a C2–3 graft and plate fusion, which has the advantage of having a relative short fusion construct, although the approach would not address the detached posterior arch of C2 [63]. Other posterior techniques are also feasible, including the direct fixation with C2 pars interarticularis screws, or posterior C2–3 fixation connecting C2 pars screws to C3 lateral mass screws, with the advantages of preserving the axis motion, but not addressing the instability secondary to disc disruption [62, 64–66].

Conclusions

The management of atlantoaxial injuries in the elderly is challenging and only growing in importance with the aging population. Although no class I evidence exists to guide management of such injuries, the literature provides management suggestions for the optimal treatment of atlantoaxial pathologies in the elderly.

Management is complicated by suboptimal bone quality, intolerance to immobilization, presence of concurrent injuries, and preexisting medical conditions. Through careful consideration of these factors as well as the clinical and radiographic characteristics, favorable patient outcomes may be achieved.

References

1. Tarawneh A, Taqvi S, Salem K, Sahota O. Cervical spine fragility fractures in older people: 5-year experience at a regional spine centre. Age Ageing. 2020;49(6):1102–4.
2. Weller SJ, Malek AM, Rossitch E Jr. Cervical spine fractures in the elderly. Surg Neurol. 1997;47(3):274–80; discussion 280–271.
3. Müller EJ, Wick M, Russe O, Muhr G. Management of odontoid fractures in the elderly. Eur Spine J. 1999;8(5):360–5.
4. Roberts AW OS, Blakeslee L, Rabe MA. The population 65 years and older in the United States. Am Commu Survey Rep. 2018;38.
5. Maiman DJYN. Biomechanics of cervical spine trauma. Clin Neurosurg. 1991;37:543–70.
6. Yoganandan NDC, Benzel CE. Practical anatomy and fundamental biomechanics. In: Spine surgery, vol. 1. Elsevier Saunders; 2012. p. 55–83.
7. Meyer C, Eysel P, Stein G. Traumatic atlantoaxial and fracture-related dislocation. Biomed Res Int. 2019;2019:1–9.
8. Wang H. Geriatric trauma patients with cervical spine fractures due to ground level fall: five years experience in a level one trauma center. J Clin Med Res. 2013;5(2):75–83.
9. Ryan MD, Henderson JJ. The epidemiology of fractures and fracture-dislocations of the cervical spine. Injury. 1992;23(1):38–40.
10. Fassett DR, Harrop JS, Maltenfort M, et al. Mortality rates in geriatric patients with spinal cord injuries. J Neurosurg Spine. 2007;7(3):277–81.
11. Frakturen des Atlas und Axis bei älteren Patienten: Untersuchung des Radiologischen Spektrums der Frakturen und bedeutsamer Faktoren für die Bildgebende Diagnostik. 2004;176(2):222–8.
12. Guiot B, Fessler RG. Complex atlantoaxial fractures. J Neurosurg. 1999;91(2 Suppl):139–43.
13. Pepin JW, Bourne RB, Hawkins RJ. Odontoid fractures, with special reference to the elderly patient. Clin Orthop Relat Res. 1985;193:178–83.
14. Marcon RM, Cristante AF, Teixeira WJ, Narasaki DK, Oliveira RP, de Barros Filho TE. Fractures of the cervical spine. Clinics (Sao Paulo). 2013;68(11):1455–61.
15. Chapman J, Bransford R. Geriatric spine fractures: an emerging healthcare crisis. J Trauma. 2007;62(6 Suppl):S61–2.
16. Wagner SC, Schroeder GD, Kepler CK, et al. Controversies in the management of geriatric odontoid fractures. J Orthop Trauma. 2017;31(Suppl 4):S44–s48.
17. Anderson LD, D'Alonzo RT. Fractures of the odontoid process of the axis. 1974. J Bone Joint Surg Am. 2004;86(9):2081.
18. Eismont FJ, Bohlman HH. Posterior atlanto-occipital dislocation with fractures of the atlas and odontoid process. J Bone Joint Surg Am. 1978;60(3):397–9.
19. Ryan MD, Taylor TK. Odontoid fractures in the elderly. J Spinal Disord. 1993;6(5):397–401.
20. Polin RS, Szabo T, Bogaev CA, Replogle RE, Jane JA. Nonoperative management of types II and III odontoid fractures: the Philadelphia collar versus the halo vest. Neurosurgery. 1996;38(3):450–6; discussion 456–457.
21. Clark CR, White AA III. Fractures of the dens. A multicenter study. J Bone Joint Surg Am. 1985;67(9):1340–8.
22. Hart R, Saterbak A, Rapp T, Clark C. Nonoperative management of dens fracture nonunion in elderly patients without myelopathy. Spine (Phila Pa 1976). 2000;25(11):1339–43.

23. Dunn ME, Seljeskog EL. Experience in the management of odontoid process injuries: an analysis of 128 cases. Neurosurgery. 1986;18(3):306–10.
24. Greene KA, Dickman CA, Marciano FF, Drabier JB, Hadley MN, Sonntag VK. Acute axis fractures. Analysis of management and outcome in 340 consecutive cases. Spine (Phila Pa 1976). 1997;22(16):1843–52.
25. Crockard HA, Heilman AE, Stevens JM. Progressive myelopathy secondary to odontoid fractures: clinical, radiological, and surgical features. J Neurosurg. 1993;78(4):579–86.
26. Blahd WH Jr, Iserson KV, Bjelland JC. Efficacy of the posttraumatic cross table lateral view of the cervical spine. J Emerg Med. 1985;2(4):243–9.
27. Andrews CEFE, Montenegro TS, Gonzalez GA, Harrop JS. Upper cervical spine MRI. In: Atlas of spinal imaging: phenotypes, measurements and classification systems; 2020.
28. Hinck VC, Hopkins CE. Measurement of the atlanto-dental interval in the adult. Am J Roentgenol Radium Therapy, Nucl Med. 1960;84:945–51.
29. Rojas CA, Bertozzi JC, Martinez CR, Whitlow J. Reassessment of the craniocervical junction: normal values on CT. Am J Neuroradiol. 2007;28(9):1819–23.
30. Majercik S, Tashjian RZ, Biffl WL, Harrington DT, Cioffi WG. Halo vest immobilization in the elderly: a death sentence? J Trauma. 2005;59(2):350–6; discussion 356–358.
31. Tashjian RZ, Majercik S, Biffl WL, Palumbo MA, Cioffi WG. Halo-vest immobilization increases early morbidity and mortality in elderly odontoid fractures. J Trauma. 2006;60(1):199–203.
32. Smith HE, Kerr SM, Maltenfort M, et al. Early complications of surgical versus conservative treatment of isolated type II odontoid fractures in octogenarians: a retrospective cohort study. J Spinal Disord Tech. 2008;21(8):535–9.
33. Smith HE, Vaccaro AR, Maltenfort M, et al. Trends in surgical management for type II odontoid fracture: 20 years of experience at a regional spinal cord injury center. Orthopedics. 2008;31(7):650.
34. Chapman J, Smith JS, Kopjar B, et al. The AOSpine North America geriatric odontoid fracture mortality study. Spine. 2013;38(13):1098–104.
35. Woods BI, Hohl JB, Braly B, Donaldson W III, Kang J, Lee JY. Mortality in elderly patients following operative and nonoperative management of odontoid fractures. J Spinal Disord Tech. 2014;27(6):321–6.
36. Omeis I, Duggal N, Rubano J, et al. Surgical treatment of C2 fractures in the elderly: a multicenter retrospective analysis. J Spinal Disord Tech. 2009;22(2):91–5.
37. Andersson S, Olerud C, Rodrigues M. Odontoid fractures: high complication rate associated with anterior screw fixation in the elderly. Eur Spine J. 2000;9(1):56–9.
38. Landells CD, Van Peteghem PK. Fractures of the atlas: classification, treatment and morbidity. Spine (Phila Pa 1976). 1988;13(5):450–2.
39. Smith RM, Bhandutia AK, Jauregui JJ, Shasti M, Ludwig SC. Atlas fractures: diagnosis, current treatment recommendations, and implications for elderly patients. Clin Spine Surg. 2018;31(7):278–84.
40. Spence KF Jr, Decker S, Sell KW. Bursting atlantal fracture associated with rupture of the transverse ligament. J Bone Joint Surg Am. 1970;52(3):543–9.
41. Fowler JL, Sandhu A, Fraser RD. A review of fractures of the atlas vertebra. J Spinal Disord. 1990;3(1):19–24.
42. Gleizes V, Jacquot FP, Signoret F, Feron JM. Combined injuries in the upper cervical spine: clinical and epidemiological data over a 14-year period. Eur Spine J. 2000;9(5):386–92.
43. Porensky PTN, Rea GL, Weinstein PR. Anatomy and pathophysiology of acquired spinal disorders. In: Spine surgery, vol. 1. Elsevier Saunders; 2012. p. 146–08.
44. Zygmunt SSH, Brattstrom H, et al. Reduction of rheumatoid periodontoid pannus following posterior occipito-cervical fusion visualised by magnetic resonance imaging. Br J Neurosurg. 1988;2:315–20.
45. Fielding JW, Hawkins RJ. Atlanto-axial rotatory fixation. (Fixed rotatory subluxation of the atlanto-axial joint). J Bone Joint Surg Am. 1977;59(1):37–44.

46. Fielding JWHR, Ratzan SA. Spine fusion for atlanto-axial instability. J Bone Joint Surg Am. 1976;58:400–7.
47. Matsunaga S, Ijiri K, Koga H. Results of a longer than 10-year follow-up of patients with rheumatoid arthritis treated by occipitocervical fusion. Spine (Phila Pa 1976). 2000;25(14):1749–53.
48. Wasserman BR, Moskovich R, Razi AE. Rheumatoid arthritis of the cervical spine—clinical considerations. Bull NYU Hosp Jt Dis. 2011;69(2):136–48.
49. Murphy H, Schroeder GD, Shi WJ, et al. Management of hangman's fractures: a systematic review. J Orthop Trauma. 2017;31:S90–5.
50. Schneider RC, Livingston KE, Cave A, Hamilton G. "Hangman's fracture" of the cervical spine. J Neurosurg. 1965;22(2):141–54.
51. James R, Nasmyth-Jones R. The occurrence of cervical fractures in victims of judicial hanging. Forensic Sci Int. 1992;54(1):81–91.
52. Al-Mahfoudh R, Beagrie C, Woolley E, et al. Management of typical and atypical hangman's fractures. Global Spine J. 2016;6(3):248–56.
53. Ge C, Hao D, He B, Mi B. Anterior cervical discectomy and fusion versus posterior fixation and fusion of C2–3 for unstable hangman's fracture. Clin Spine Surg. 2015;28(2):E61–6.
54. Gehweiler JA Jr, Clark WM, Schaaf RE, Powers B, Miller MD. Cervical spine trauma: the common combined conditions. Radiology. 1979;130(1):77–86.
55. Zusman NL, Ching AC, Hart RA, Yoo JU. Incidence of second cervical vertebral fractures far surpassed the rate predicted by the changing age distribution and growth among elderly persons in the United States (2005–2008). Spine. 2013;38(9):752–6.
56. Kannus P, Parkkari J, Koskinen S, et al. Fall-induced injuries and deaths among older adults. JAMA. 1999;281(20):1895–9.
57. Effendi B, Roy D, Cornish B, Dussault R, Laurin C. Fractures of the ring of the axis. A classification based on the analysis of 131 cases. J Bone Joint Surg. 1981;63(3):319–27.
58. Levine AM, Edwards C. The management of traumatic spondylolisthesis of the axis. J Bone Joint Surg Am. 1985;67(2):217–26.
59. Starr JK, Eismont FJ. Atypical hangman's fractures. Spine. 1993;18(14):1954–7.
60. Bono CM, Vaccaro AR, Fehlings M, et al. Measurement techniques for upper cervical spine injuries: consensus statement of the Spine Trauma Study Group. Spine. 2007;32(5):593–600.
61. Li X-F, Dai L-Y, Lu H, Chen X-D. A systematic review of the management of hangman's fractures. Eur Spine J. 2006;15(3):257–69.
62. Verheggen R, Jansen J. Hangman's fracture: arguments in favor of surgical therapy for type II and III according to Edwards and Levine. Surg Neurol. 1998;49(3):253–62.
63. Tuite GF, Papadopoulos SM, Sonntag VK. Caspar plate fixation for the treatment of complex hangman's fractures. Neurosurgery. 1992;30(5):761–4.
64. Duggal N, Chamberlain RH, Perez-Garza LE, Espinoza-Larios A, Sonntag VK, Crawford NR. Hangman's fracture: a biomechanical comparison of stabilization techniques. Spine. 2007;32(2):182–7.
65. Borne GM, Bedou GL, Pinaudeau M. Treatment of pedicular fractures of the axis: a clinical study and screw fixation technique. J Neurosurg. 1984;60(1):88–93.
66. Bristol R, Henn JS, Dickman CA. Pars screw fixation of a hangman's fracture: technical case report. Oper Neurosurg. 2005;56(suppl_1):ONS-E204-ONS-E204.

Chapter 9
MIS Cervical Approaches in the Elderly

Jacob L. Goldberg, Alexandra Giantini Larsen, Fabian Sommer, Joseph A. Carnevale, Sertac Kirnaz, Branden Medary, Lynn McGrath, and Roger Hartl

Introduction

In the United States, as a result of increasing life expectancy and the current population structure, the number of elderly patients seeking medical care is increasing [1]. Specifically, more elderly patients will continue to need spine surgery given the fact that degenerative spinal pathology increases with age [2]. While the elderly population face increased risks associated with surgery, it is important to find strategies to perform surgery in the elderly as untreated spinal pathology can have a profoundly negative impact on overall health and quality of life [3, 4]. In patients with symptoms refractory to medical or conservative management, severe pain, myelopathy, and/or other neurological deficits, surgical intervention is discussed. In select surgical candidates with amenable pathology, minimally invasive techniques potentially offering less muscle dissection, blood loss, and recovery time pose attractive alternatives to open surgery (Fig. 9.1).

Minimally invasive spine (MIS) surgery has seen relatively fewer cervical applications compared to its use in the thoracic and lumbar spine. In part, this is due to the increased risk associated with cervical spine surgery given the proximity to the cervical spinal cord and owing to its unique anatomy including the presence of the vertebral arteries and their course through the vertebrae. Anteriorly, the vertebral

Jacob L. Goldberg and Alexandra Giantini Larsen co-first authors.

J. L. Goldberg · A. G. Larsen · F. Sommer · J. A. Carnevale · S. Kirnaz · B. Medary · L. McGrath · R. Hartl (✉)
New York Presbyterian/Weill Cornell Medical Center, New York, NY, USA
e-mail: jag9177@nyp.org; amg9084@nyp.org; fjv4001@med.cornell.edu; joc3003@nyp.org; sek2024@med.cornell.edu; brm4011@med.cornell.edu; lbm90092@med.cornell.edu; Roh9005@med.cornell.edu

K.-M. G. Fu et al. (eds.), *Treatment of Spine Disease in the Elderly*, https://doi.org/10.1007/978-3-031-12612-3_9

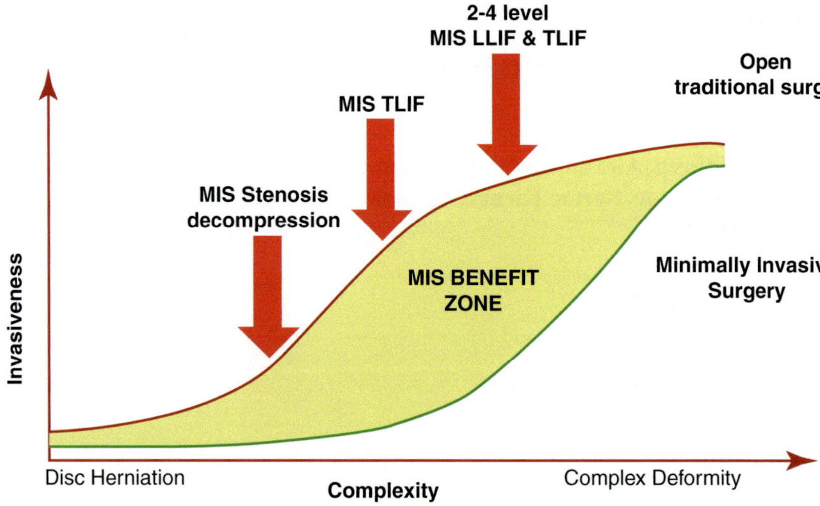

Fig. 9.1 Comparison between level of complexity and invasiveness in minimally invasive spine surgery versus open surgery

bodies are in close proximity to the trachea, esophagus, and other vital structures. In addition, the overall smaller size of vertebrae and intervertebral discs make surgery in this region more challenging. However, advances in intraoperative navigation have forged a path forward for several MIS cervical techniques [5]. In this chapter, we discuss several minimally invasive posterior cervical approaches which are important surgical options in elderly patients. For each technique we outline benefits, contraindications, and key operative considerations.

MIS Posterior Fusion via Facet Joint Arthrodesis

The placement of cages posteriorly into the cervical facet joints was first described as part of a procedure for atlantoaxial joint fusion in patients with basilar invagination [6]. In this setting, placement of facet cages was noted to confer a high degree of stability and promote arthrodesis [7]. Since that time, this concept has evolved as an alternative to the traditional lateral mass screw fixation and can be placed via a posterior percutaneous approach [8, 9]. In elderly patients at high risk for periprocedural complication after traditional open lateral mass fusion, posterior percutaneous facet cage-based fusion provides an alternative (Fig. 9.2). Through a cadaveric study, it was elucidated that bilateral facet cage placement conferred similar stability as compared to lateral mass screw fixation [10]. In addition to providing stability/fusion, these procedures can potentially address some of the facet-mediated pain observed in degenerative disease. This can be performed as a stand-alone procedure in situations requiring

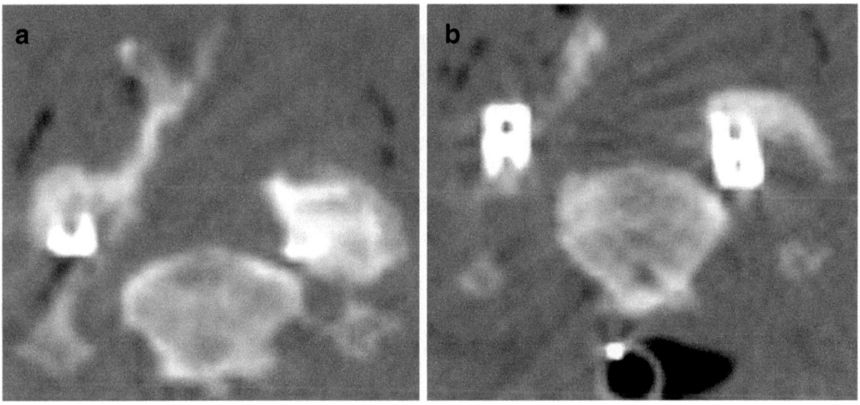

Fig. 9.2 Intraoperative CT demonstrates bilateral cervical decompression through the unilateral approach with good decompression and facet cages in adequate position. (**a**, **b**) show different planes of the intraoperative image

posterior-only fusion or used to further stabilize/augment anterior decompression and/or fusion. Compared with data reported for similar techniques, facet cage arthrodesis may offer less blood loss, decreased length of hospital stay, and overall faster recovery time [11]. Facet cage-based fusion is contraindicated in disease states that alter the stability around the facet joint such as neoplastic involvement of the facet joint or facet joint disruption due to trauma. In addition, patients with significant listhesis are not candidates for fusion via this approach [12, 13]. Outcomes assessments reveal significant improvements as assessed by the Neck Disability Index (NDI), visual analog pain scores (VAS), and SF12 on a 2-week follow-up and at 1 year postoperatively [9, 13]. Long-term follow-up data in one small reported case series found no recurrent radicular symptoms at a 5-year follow-up [14]. Radiographic findings have been encouraging with fusion at 2 years noted in 98% of cases. Further, there were no findings of development in a significant kyphotic deformity, device failures, or need for surgical reintervention [9].

The complications associated with this procedure are low. In a retrospective review of 89 patients (average age 58 ± 12) with cervical radiculopathy, the rate of periprocedural complication related to surgery was 3.4%, and all experienced full recovery [11]. Blood loss was negligible and the average length of stay was 29 h [11]. These two factors are important considerations for surgery in the geriatric population as they are potentially modifiable risk factors for postoperative delirium [15–17].

Several surgical considerations and key technical steps are notable in the successful performance of this procedure. We prefer to perform this procedure with 3D intraoperative navigation though it can be performed with fluoroscopy alone. As with other elective cervical fusion cases, neuromonitoring including SSEP and MEP is a useful operative adjunct when available. The patient is positioned prone with rigid head fixation to ensure immobilization of the cervical spine which is important both for procedural safety and to ensure navigational accuracy (if using intraoperative navigation). The medial and lateral aspects of the facet joint are identified using navigation or fluoroscopy (Fig. 9.3). The joint space is entered with an access tool in a colinear (medial to lateral) trajectory. Care must be taken to avoid nerve root injury as can occur with medially positioned implants. Decortication is performed with a trephine which slides over the chisel onto the joint capsule. The inner aspect of the facet joint is addressed with a decortication burr. The facet cage is inserted after decortication. Screws are used to affix the implant to the inferior

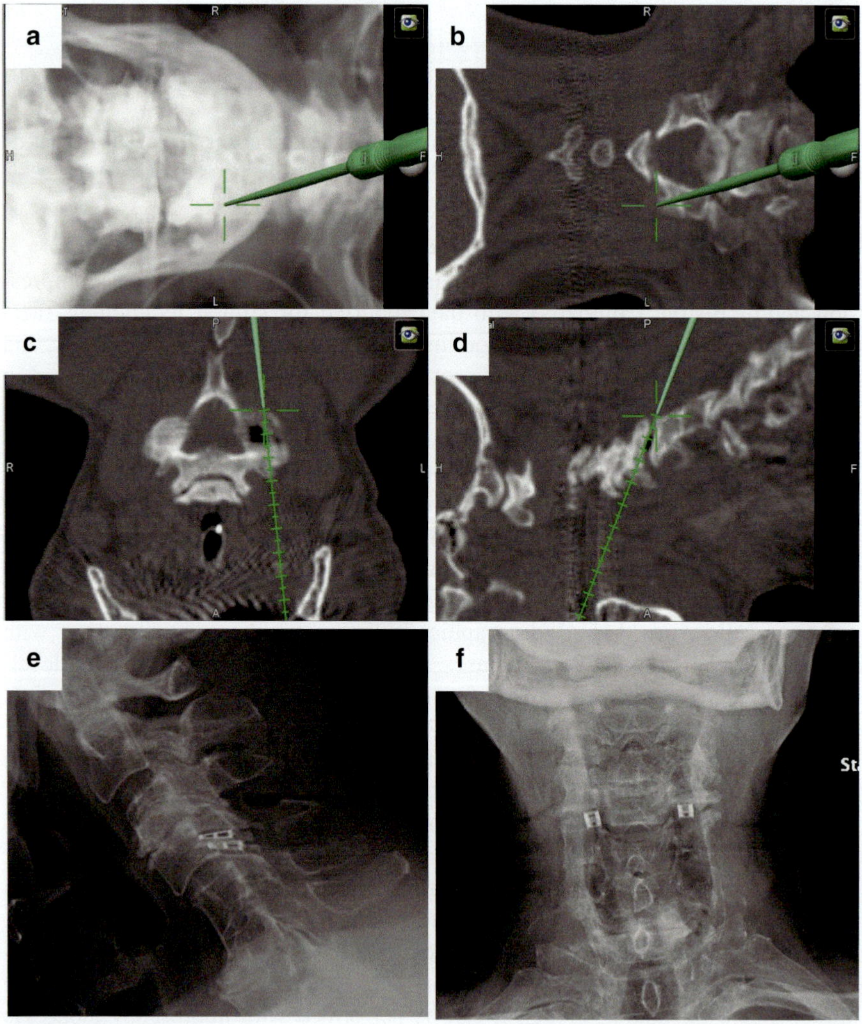

Fig. 9.3 (**a**–**d**) Intraoperative 3D navigation pictures showing the trajectory and position of the interfacet cage. Postoperative (**e**) lateral and (**f**) anteroposterior radiographs after bilateral interfacet joint cage implantation

facet. After all instruments are removed (with exception of the guide tube), bone graft is injected into the joint space. After inspection for hemostasis and antibiotic irrigation, the incision is closed in the usual manner.

MIS Posterior Cervical Foraminotomy (PCF)

Minimally invasive techniques for posterior cervical foraminotomy were first described in 2001 and remain an excellent surgical option in patients with unilateral radiculopathy due to foraminal pathology [18]. These techniques have been applied successfully to a range of pathology encroaching on exiting nerve roots including synovial cysts, bone spurs, and soft foraminal disc fragments [19, 20]. PCF avoids morbidity related to the anterior approach and permanent device implantation, preserves mobility, and can be performed on an outpatient basis. In addition, should the patient require an anterior approach surgery in the future, initial posterior approach means that the anterior corridor will be easier to navigate in the future. Regarding patient selection, this procedure is contraindicated in patients primarily symptomatic from central stenosis (with resultant myelopathy), cervical kyphotic deformity, or instability as these symptoms will not be addressed and may be made worse. In addition to the standard preoperative workup, careful assessment for dynamic instability and/or contralateral facet pathology should be evaluated with flexion/extension radiographs, MRI, and CT when necessary.

When evaluating pathology amenable to PCF, there is often consideration given to an anterior approach such as anterior cervical discectomy and fusion (ACDF). ACDF, given the approach, carries higher risk of esophageal injury, dysphagia, recurrent laryngeal nerve injury, or dysfunction. Notably, the geriatric population can have a more complicated recovery from ACDF with postoperative dysphagia being particularly concerning. It is in this population that a PCF may offer advantages in avoiding potential dysphagia. Comparative analyses between ACDF and PCF have found similar 1–3-year postoperative outcomes with respect to arm pain and neck pain [21–23]. In addition, compared with ACDF in patients with unilateral radiculopathy, PCF was found to offer cost savings [24]. A separate study evaluating outcomes of PCF noted 1.1% and 0.9% annualized risks of requiring a fusion at the index-level and adjacent-level disease, respectively [25]. Important in the postoperative management of all populations but especially geriatric, investigators comparing open cervical foraminotomy with minimally invasive techniques found less blood loss, analgesic use, and time to hospital discharge [26]. To the contrary, while both anterior and posterior foraminotomies carry a risk of C5 palsy, this risk is highest in older patients undergoing PCF [27]. Of note, 86% of the patients with PCF who developed C5 palsy had complete recovery [27].

Several surgical nuances and key procedural steps are worth noting. For this procedure, the patient is placed in rigid head fixation and positioned prone. After fluoroscopic or 3D navigation is used to verify the level (Fig. 9.4), a skin incision is made, and sequential dilation is performed until an appropriately sized tubular

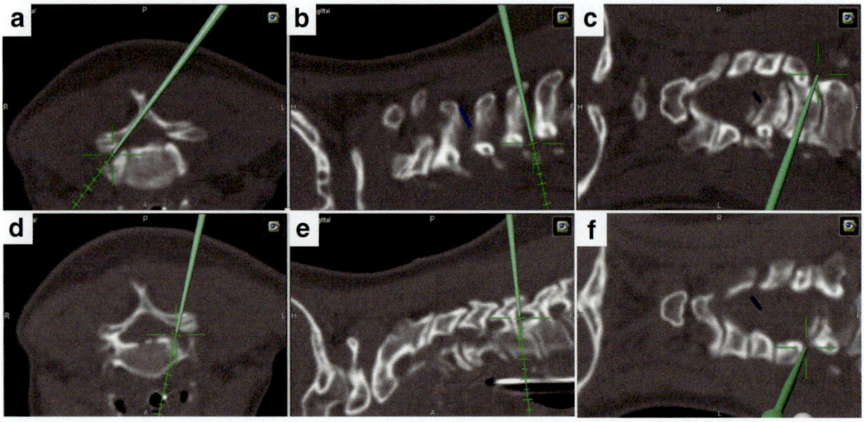

Fig. 9.4 (**a**–**f**) Intraoperative 3D navigation pictures presenting a posterior cervical foraminotomy case highlighting the trajectory of the contralateral decompression and the anatomy around the facets

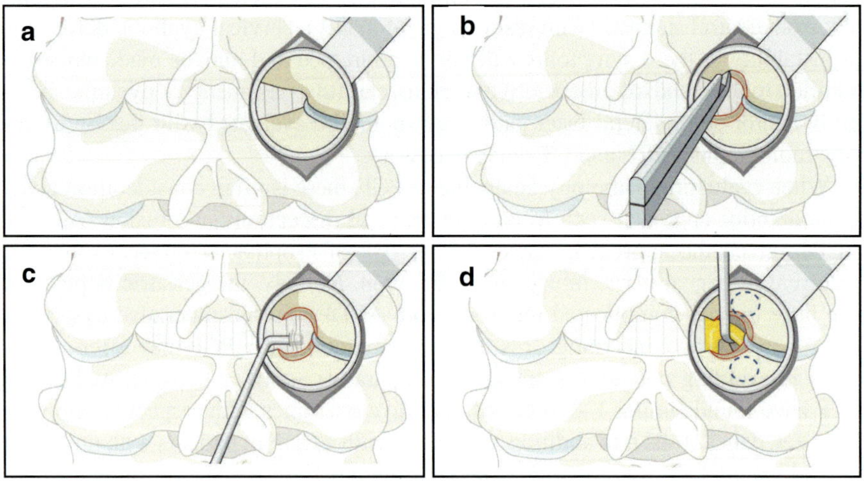

Fig. 9.5 (**a**) Tubular retractor in position over lateral aspect of canal and medial aspect of facet joint. (**b**) Removal of the thinned-out hemilamina with a Kerrison punch. (**c**) The ligamentum flavum bluntly dissected with nerve hook under direct visualization. (**d**) Cranial retraction of the nerve root. The pedicle above and below should be palpable with a nerve hook. The position of the pedicles is indicated

retractor is able to be placed. Though preference varies by surgeon, an approximately 16-mm tubular retractor is adequate for the performance of this procedure (Fig. 9.5). At this time, the operative microscope is brought into the field. If 3D navigation is being used, it can provide a helpful confirmation of the docking site, defining safe boundaries for resection, or locating specific foraminal pathology. A high-speed burr is used to remove the medial third of the facet joint and the lateral aspect of the lamina. Along the path of the exiting nerve root, Kerrison rongeurs are used to remove bone to widen the area of decompression. Patient-specific pathology can be addressed at this time. For example, if symptoms are predominately due to a foraminal disc fragment, it can be accessed and carefully removed at this time. After adequate decompression is achieved and hemostasis obtained, the tubular retractor is removed, antibiotic irrigation applied, and the incision closed in the usual fashion. In terms of complication avoidance, it should be noted that while foraminotomy carries a risk of destabilization leading to a mechanical failure, this is seen more often when 50% or more of the medial facet joint is removed [28].

Tubular Cervical Unilateral Laminotomy for Bilateral Decompression

Open cervical laminectomy is an effective procedure for decompression but involves a relatively long recovery time due to the pain associated with the muscular dissection in the posterior neck and risks including delayed instability and kyphotic deformity development [29, 30]. In elderly patients, significant pain impairing the ability to walk safely can be associated with high morbidity. The use of a unilateral approach to achieve bilateral decompression was first described in open lumbar surgery, subsequently modified with a minimally invasive technique, and now routinely used at all spinal levels [31–34]. Ideal candidates are symptomatic from central compression and have no evidence of instability or segmental kyphosis (Fig. 9.6). Compared with open laminotomy, the unilateral laminotomy for bilateral decompression (ULBD) technique is associated with less muscle injury, bone removal, and blood loss. While studies comparing open to MIS cervical laminotomy have not been performed, this comparison in other spinal segments suggests a reduced rate of infections, narcotic use, and shorter length of hospital stay. This is of particular benefit in the elderly population where an added level of invasiveness would be more risky [35].

Several key surgical steps and operative nuances are notable. For this procedure, the patient is in prone position with neck in a neutral position. The patient should be well padded and secured to the bed (as the bed will be rotated to perform "over-the-top" decompression). At this point, the entry site can be determined with fluoroscopic guidance or 3D navigation. An approximately 3-cm incision is made at the surgical level. A combination of sharp dissection and electrocautery can be used until the fascia is visualized. Dilators are sequentially placed until an appropriately sized tubular retractor (~16 mm) can be placed. Beginning at the caudal aspect of the lamina and moving cranially, a high-speed drill is used to remove bone to expose the ligamentum flavum. To perform the contralateral decompression, the operating room table is rotated away from the surgeon (Fig. 9.7). The spinous process is then undercut, and the anterior aspect of the contralateral lamina is removed with the high-speed drill. The ligamentum flavum is left in place as much as possible during

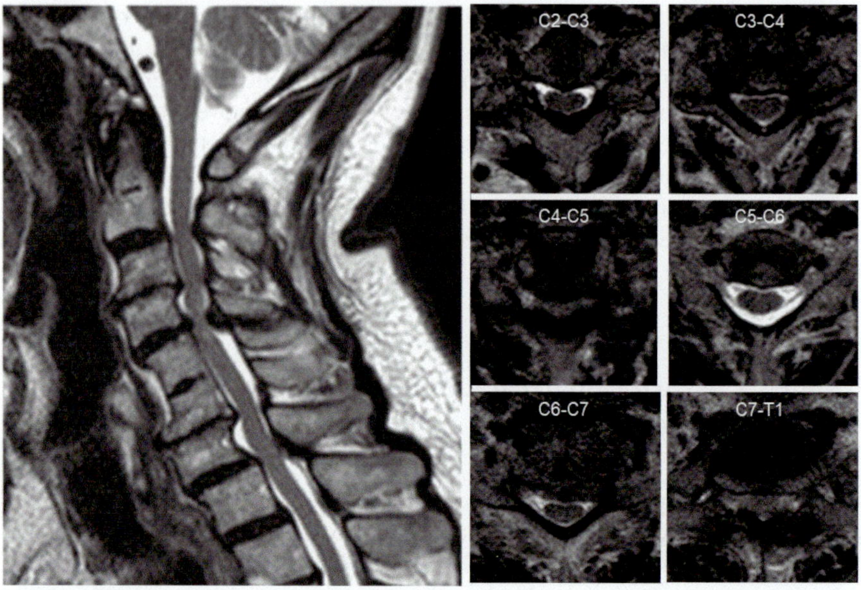

Fig. 9.6 A 65-year-old female patient presenting with multilevel cervical degenerative with degenerative disc disease at multiple levels but most notably severe central stenosis at C4–5 due mainly to ligamentous hypertrophy. This pathology was amenable to tubular decompression via unilateral approach for bilateral decompression

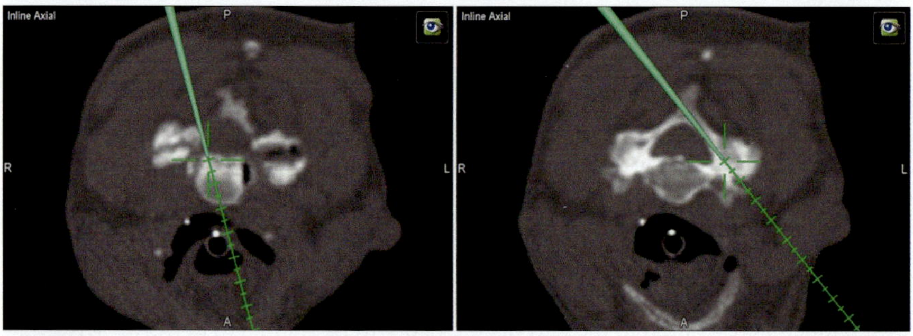

Fig. 9.7 Intraoperative 3D navigation pictures showing adequate unilateral and over-the-top contralateral decompression

this step to protect against incidental durotomy. A Frazier suction tip is used to gently depress the ligamentum flavum to allow for efficient bony removal. At this point, care must be taken not to exert excess force on the spinal cord with the Frazier suction tip. A ball tip probe is used to carefully remove the ligament where it remains attached to bone. Next, a Kerrison rongeur is used to resect the remaining ligament. Finally, the laminotomy bed is inspected and meticulous hemostasis obtained. After antibiotic irrigation, the incision is closed in the usual fashion.

Conclusion

The number of elderly patients seeking medical care for spinal disorders is increasing and will continue to increase. Given the dramatic improvement in functional status and quality of life that can accompany surgical treatment of debilitating spine disorders, it is important to have pathology-specific options in this higher-risk population. When patient-specific pathology and surgical readiness are favorable, minimally invasive options offer several potential advantages over open approaches including decreased risk of blood loss, infection, and postoperative narcotic requirements. While anterior surgery in the elderly can be unavoidable in some cases, several posterior MIS approaches are worth noting. Posterior percutaneous facet cages can offer an MIS alternative to traditional lateral mass screws or used to augment anterior procedures. In cases of unilateral radiculopathy due to foraminal pathology without contraindications, MIS posterior foraminotomy is a great option allowing the surgeon to avoid placement of a permanent implant, avoid the anterior approach, and allow for motion preservation. Lastly in cases of central stenosis, MIS tubular unilateral laminectomy for bilateral decompression has proven safe and effective. While all of these procedures can be performed with fluoroscopy, they are all well suited to be performed with the aid of 3D navigation.

References

1. Fehlings MG, Tetreault L, Nater A, Choma T, Harrop J, Mroz T, Santaguida C, Smith JS. The aging of the global population: the changing epidemiology of disease and spinal disorders. Neurosurgery. 2015;77(Suppl 4):S1–5.
2. Schwab F, Dubey A, Gamez L, El Fegoun AB, Hwang K, Pagala M, Farcy JP. Adult scoliosis: prevalence, SF-36, and nutritional parameters in an elderly volunteer population. Spine. 2005;30:1082–5.
3. Bess S, Line B, Fu K-M, et al. The health impact of symptomatic adult spinal deformity: comparison of deformity types to United States population norms and chronic diseases. Spine. 2016;41:224–33.
4. Smith JS, Line B, Bess S, et al. The health impact of adult cervical deformity in patients presenting for surgical treatment: comparison to United States population norms and chronic disease states based on the EuroQuol-5 Dimensions Questionnaire. Neurosurgery. 2017;80:716–25.
5. Hussain I, Schmidt FA, Kirnaz S, Wipplinger C, Schwartz TH, Härtl R. MIS approaches in the cervical spine. J Spine Surg. 2019;5:S74–83.
6. Goel A. Treatment of basilar invagination by atlantoaxial joint distraction and direct lateral mass fixation. J Neurosurg Spine. 2004;1:281–6.
7. Goel A. Interfacetal intra-articular spacers: emergence of a concept. J Craniovertebr Junction Spine. 2016;7:72–4.
8. Siemionow K, Janusz P, Glowka P. Cervical cages placed bilaterally in the facet joints from a posterior approach significantly increase foraminal area. Eur Spine J. 2016;25:2279–85.
9. Siemionow K, Janusz P, Phillips FM, Youssef JA, Isaacs R, Tyrakowski M, McCormack B. Clinical and radiographic results of indirect decompression and posterior cervical fusion for single-level cervical radiculopathy using an expandable implant with 2-year follow-up. J Neurol Surg A, Cent Eur Neurosurg. 2016;77:482–8.

10. Voronov LI, Siemionow KB, Havey RM, Carandang G, Patwardhan AG. Biomechanical evaluation of DTRAX(®) posterior cervical cage stabilization with and without lateral mass fixation. Med Devices (Auckl). 2016;9:285–90.
11. Siemionow KB, Glowka P, Blok RJ, Gillespy MC, Gundanna MI, Smith WD, Hyder Z, McCormack BM. Perioperative complications in patients treated with posterior cervical fusion and bilateral cages. J Craniovertebr Junction Spine. 2017;8:342–9.
12. Goel A. Facet distraction spacers for treatment of degenerative disease of the spine: rationale and an alternative hypothesis of spinal degeneration. J Craniovertebr Junction Spine. 2010;1:65–6.
13. McCormack BM, Bundoc RC, Ver MR, Ignacio JMF, Berven SH, Eyster EF. Percutaneous posterior cervical fusion with the DTRAX Facet System for single-level radiculopathy: results in 60 patients. J Neurosurg Spine. 2013;18:245–54.
14. Goel A, Shah A, Patni N, Ramdasi R. Immediate postoperative reversal of disc herniation following facetal distraction-fixation surgery: report of 4 cases. World Neurosurg. 2016;94:339–44.
15. Wang C-G, Qin Y-F, Wan X, Song L-C, Li Z-J, Li H. Incidence and risk factors of postoperative delirium in the elderly patients with hip fracture. J Orthop Surg Res. 2018;13:186.
16. Wu X, Sun W, Tan M. Incidence and risk factors for postoperative delirium in patients undergoing spine surgery: a systematic review and meta-analysis. Biomed Res Int. 2019;2019:2139834.
17. Robinson TN, Eiseman B. Postoperative delirium in the elderly: diagnosis and management. Clin Interv Aging. 2008;3:351–5.
18. Adamson TE. Microendoscopic posterior cervical laminoforaminotomy for unilateral radiculopathy: results of a new technique in 100 cases. J Neurosurg. 2001;95:51–7.
19. Henderson CM, Hennessy RG, Shuey HM, Shackelford EG. Posterior-lateral foraminotomy as an exclusive operative technique for cervical radiculopathy: a review of 846 consecutively operated cases. Neurosurgery. 1983;13:504–12.
20. Zeidman SM, Ducker TB. Posterior cervical laminoforaminotomy for radiculopathy: review of 172 cases. Neurosurgery. 1993;33:356–62.
21. Dunn C, Moore J, Sahai N, Issa K, Faloon M, Sinha K, Hwang KS, Emami A. Minimally invasive posterior cervical foraminotomy with tubes to prevent undesired fusion: a long-term follow-up study. J Neurosurg Spine. 2018;29:358–64.
22. Selvanathan SK, Beagrie C, Thomson S, Corns R, Deniz K, Derham C, Towns G, Timothy J, Pal D. Anterior cervical discectomy and fusion versus posterior cervical foraminotomy in the treatment of brachialgia: the Leeds spinal unit experience (2008-2013). Acta Neurochir. 2015;157:1595–600.
23. Foster MT, Carleton-Bland NP, Lee MK, Jackson R, Clark SR, Wilby MJ. Comparison of clinical outcomes in anterior cervical discectomy versus foraminotomy for brachialgia. Br J Neurosurg. 2019;33:3–7.
24. Lewandrowski K-U. Incidence, management, and cost of complications after transforaminal endoscopic decompression surgery for lumbar foraminal and lateral recess stenosis: a value proposition for outpatient ambulatory surgery. Int J Spine Surg. 2019;13:53–67.
25. Skovrlj B, Gologorsky Y, Haque R, Fessler RG, Qureshi SA. Complications, outcomes, and need for fusion after minimally invasive posterior cervical foraminotomy and microdiscectomy. Spine J. 2014;14:2405–11.
26. Winder MJ, Thomas KC. Minimally invasive versus open approach for cervical laminoforaminotomy. Can J Neurol Sci. 2011;38:262–7.
27. Bydon M, Macki M, Kaloostian P, Sciubba DM, Wolinsky J-P, Gokaslan ZL, Belzberg AJ, Bydon A, Witham TF. Incidence and prognostic factors of c5 palsy: a clinical study of 1001 cases and review of the literature. Neurosurgery. 2014;74:595–604; discussion 604.
28. Zdeblick TA, Zou D, Warden KE, McCabe R, Kunz D, Vanderby R. Cervical stability after foraminotomy. A biomechanical in vitro analysis. J Bone Joint Surg Am. 1992;74:22–7.
29. Oppenheimer JH, DeCastro I, McDonnell DE. Minimally invasive spine technology and minimally invasive spine surgery: a historical review. Neurosurg Focus. 2009;27:E9.

30. Geck MJ, Eismont FJ. Surgical options for the treatment of cervical spondylotic myelopathy. Orthop Clin North Am. 2002;33:329–48.
31. Abbas SF, Spurgas MP, Szewczyk BS, Yim B, Ata A, German JW. A comparison of minimally invasive posterior cervical decompression and open anterior cervical decompression and instrumented fusion in the surgical management of degenerative cervical myelopathy. Neurosurg Focus. 2016;40:E7.
32. Guiot BH, Khoo LT, Fessler RG. A minimally invasive technique for decompression of the lumbar spine. Spine. 2002;27:432–8.
33. Palmer S, Turner R, Palmer R. Bilateral decompressive surgery in lumbar spinal stenosis associated with spondylolisthesis: unilateral approach and use of a microscope and tubular retractor system. Neurosurg Focus. 2002;13:E4.
34. Spetzger U, Bertalanffy H, Naujokat C, von Keyserlingk DG, Gilsbach JM. Unilateral laminotomy for bilateral decompression of lumbar spinal stenosis. Part I: anatomical and surgical considerations. Acta Neurochir. 1997;139:392–6.
35. Avila MJ, Walter CM, Baaj AA. Outcomes and complications of minimally invasive surgery of the lumbar spine in the elderly. Cureus. 2016;8:e519.

Chapter 10
Subaxial Spinal Trauma

Asdrubal Falavigna and Charles André Carazzo

Introduction

The expected number of people over 65 years of age in the American population in 2030 is 88.5 millions [1]. Consequently the incidence of cervical spine fractures in the elderly will increase at the same rate [2]. In those cases, the association of severe neurological injuries and incidence of complications and high mortality are observed [1, 3, 4].

Cervical spine traumatic fractures are common in the elderly [5]. Upper cervical spine fractures are more frequent due to the anatomical and biomechanical conditions of these patients, but subaxial spine injuries are also common, with an incidence of injury even higher than C0–C2 fractures in the 65–75 age group [6]. More than half of the injuries occur in C5–C7 segments [5, 6]. Low-energy trauma can lead to unstable and complex fractures in the elderly population due to senescence-associated changes of osteopenia and degeneration [6].

Early diagnosis and individualized treatments are essential to improve survival in these patients, who generally have significant comorbidities which increase the risk of an unfavorable outcome [7]. Protocols for radiographic investigation in elderly patients with the highest probability of fracture/luxation reported the importance of computed tomography in identifying the injuries [7–9].

A. Falavigna (✉)
Department of Neurosurgery, University of Caxias do Sul,
Caxias do Sul, Rio Grande do Sul, Brazil

C. A. Carazzo
Department of Neurosurgery, University of Passo Fundo, São Vicente de Paulo Hospital,
Passo Fundo, Rio Grande do Sul, Brazil
e-mail: carazzo@upf.br

K.-M. G. Fu et al. (eds.), *Treatment of Spine Disease in the Elderly*,
https://doi.org/10.1007/978-3-031-12612-3_10

AO Spine Classification is one of the classifications used to categorize the injuries with a high degree of reliability [10]. The decision-making process and treatment planning depend on injury morphology, neurological impairment, and the patient's comorbidity, frailty index, and general health conditions [11]. Unstable subaxial cervical spine injuries should be treated surgically by anterior, posterior, or combined approach, unless the patient's condition contraindicates the procedure [11]. Conservative treatment with a cervical collar or halo vest is reserved for minor, stable fractures without risk of neurological injuries, or in special situations of patients who do not present the clinical conditions for surgical treatment [12, 13].

Epidemiology

The elderly population is growing worldwide with a major risk for traumatic musculoskeletal injuries [14]. The proportion of major trauma patients aged over 75 years rose sharply from 8.1% to 26.9% between 1990 and 2013 in the UK and 12% of elderly Americans go to emergency departments annually for injury [14, 15]. The most common location of fractures includes the hip, radius, humerus, and cervical spine [4].

The incidence of traumatic cervical spine fractures demonstrates a bimodal class, between 15–54 and 65–80 years of age [14]. The prevalence of cervical fracture is 2.6–4.7% in patients older than 65 years, and the great majority of injuries occur from lower-energy traumas such falling from a standing position [16]. The incidence of fractures in the subaxial spine is approximately 30%, usually related to high-intensity trauma [17].

Etiology

The causes of a higher incidence of cervical spine fractures in elderly people have been attributed to the increasing number of falls, greater risk of motor vehicle accidents, and the biochemical attrition associated with senile osteopenia and tissue degeneration [1, 18]. Cervical fractures in elderly patients usually occur as a consequence of low-energy trauma from standing or seated height, related to reduced visual acuity, peripheral neuropathies, reduction of reaction time, and blunting of reflexes [19].

Spivak et al. (1994) retrospectively studied 2059 patients with cervical trauma and divided their analysis according to age (<40 and >65 years) [17]. He found a significant difference in etiology between these two groups of patients. Adults under 40 years of age presented traumas related mainly to automobile accidents and diving (40.9% and 19.1%), while in patients over 65 years of age, fall injuries were responsible for 71.5% [17]. The main injuries in elderly patients due to falls occurred in the high cervical spine (69.8%) and the minority in the subaxial spine (30.2%), inferring that for lesions in the subaxial spine, they would probably need more energy trauma [17].

Asemota et al. (2010) collected data from the Nationwide Inpatient Sample (NIS) that represents 20% of the stratified sample of all US inpatients [2]. They analyzed 167,278 older adults with a median age of 81 years, whose main cause of injury in 51.2% was a fall. Isolated cervical fracture was observed in 91.3% and associated with spinal cord injury in 8.7% [2].

Lomoschitz et al. (2002) evaluated 225 cervical traumas and analyzed them according to two age groups (65–75 years and >75 years) [6]. The main etiology of spinal injuries in patients aged 65–75 years was high-energy trauma, like car accidents and falls from a greater than standing height, and usually located in the subaxial spine. On the other hand, the injuries in patients over 75 years of age occurred mostly due to lower-energy trauma, like falls from standing or seated height, and the majority are located in the upper cervical region [6].

Under normal conditions, C3–C7 segments are more mobile and predisposed to injury, but with advancing age, these segments become stiffer, and C1–C2 become the most mobile portion of the cervical spine. The biomechanical changes in the spine of the elderly population are associated with osteoporosis and degeneration of muscle, ligaments, and intervertebral disc, which determines the higher incidence of fractures in these patients with low-energy traumas [3].

Although the upper cervical spine (C0–C2) is more affected, the multiple level fractures have a 30–40% incidence of multiple fractures, which may be adjacent to or distant from the injured vertebrae (Fig. 10.1) [1, 6].

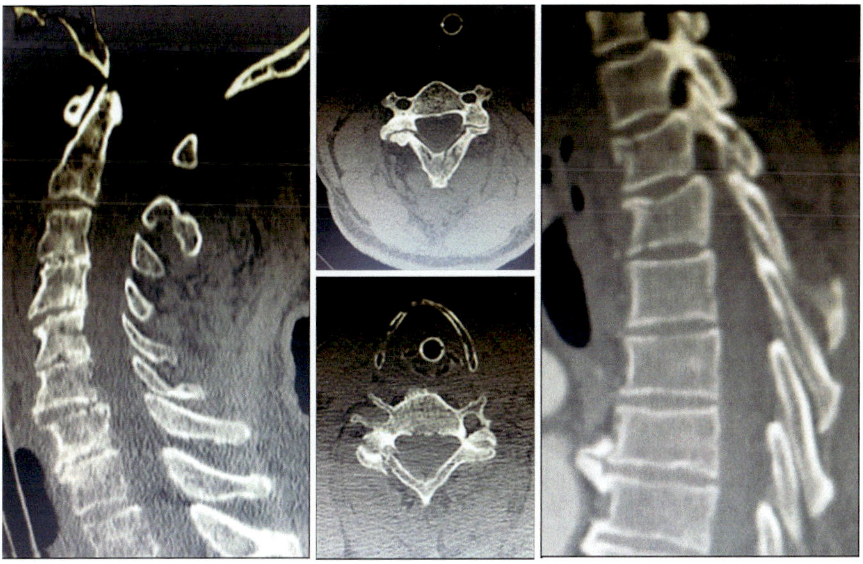

Fig. 10.1 A 75-year-old male with 2 ft fall and multiple fractures: fracture in lamina of C3, right facet joint C5, and vertebral body of T3 and T4

Diagnosis

The main difficulties to diagnose subaxial cervical fractures in the elderly are the poor visualization on plain films and the specific anatomical alterations like osteopenia and osteoarthritis. The majority of the guidelines suggest that decision-making for radiography should be based on the Canadian C-spine Rule and NEXUS (National Emergency X-radiography Utilization Study) [8, 9, 20].

The NEXUS rules were described in 1998 by Hoffman et al. [8] to select low risk for spine injuries of patients based on five criteria: (1) absence of intoxication, (2) absence of posterior midline neck tenderness, (3) no distracting painful injury, (4) without altered level of alertness, and (5) without altered neurologic function (Table 10.1). A validation study of NEXUS rules in 34,069 patients with cervical spine injury showed 99.6% sensitivity and 12.9% specificity [21]. Nevertheless, its use is questionable in elderly patients over 65 years, because the data is very contradictory, with sensitivity ranging from 89% to 100% [22, 23]. The difficulties and confounding factors related to the NEXUS rules leading to missed injury are (1) no pain on initial presentation and denied tenderness on palpation, (2) subjective criteria of absence of distracting painful injury, and (3) different interpretation of altered level of alertness [7, 24].

The Canadian C-spine Rule is based on three high-risk criteria, five low-risk criteria, and the ability of patients to rotate their necks (Fig. 10.2) [20]. The study was conducted in 8924 patients with cervical spine fracture, with 100% sensitivity and 42.5% specificity to identify the injuries. Unfortunately, little benefit from the Canadian C-spine Rule was observed for elderly patients, as it requires a Glasgow Coma Score (GCS) of 15 and images for any patient over 65 years old [20].

The decision should be made based on individualized clinical aspects, the neurologic examination, patient's comorbidity, type of injury, and the energy of the trauma. The appropriate diagnostic test for this scenario is the computed tomography, despite considerations regarding cost and high exposure to ionizing radiation. The question to be asked is: Which elderly patients with trauma should be exposed to CT? High-quality plain radiographs of the cervical spine, including an open-mouth and dens vision, remain a valuable screening tool for a low probability of injury in elderly patients up to 75 years old [3]. Above 75 years old, the probability of injury increases substantially, and CT should be performed if there is a clinical suspicion of spine fracture [3].

Table 10.1 NEXUS (National Emergency X-radiography Utilization Study)

1. Absence of intoxication
2. Absence of posterior midline neck tenderness
3. No distracting painful injury
4. Without altered level of alertness
5. Without altered neurologic function

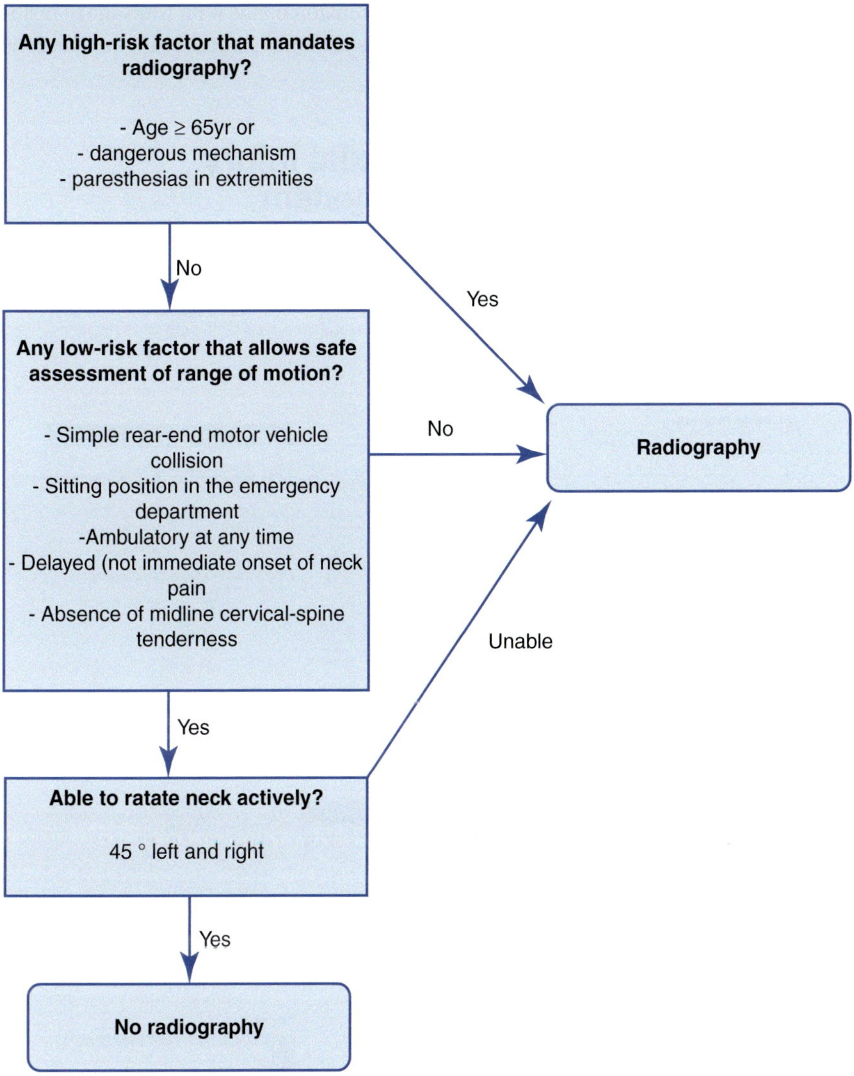

Fig. 10.2 Canadian C-spine Rule: high-risk criteria, low-risk criteria, and the ability of patients to rotate their necks

Classification

Classifications have been proposed to standardize the diagnosis and management: Holdsworth [25], Allen and Fergusson [26], Magerl [27], Subaxial Injury Classification System (SLIC) [28], and AOSpine Classifications [10]. The AOSpine Classifications of subaxial spine fracture combine the clinical, neurological, and morphologic parameters. The fractures were classified as vertebral compression (type A), disruption of either the anterior or the posterior tension band (type B), and disruption of both the anterior and the posterior tension bands with translatory instability (type C). In addition, facet joint injury, neurologic status, and comorbidities were also evaluated (Fig. 10.3) [10, 29].

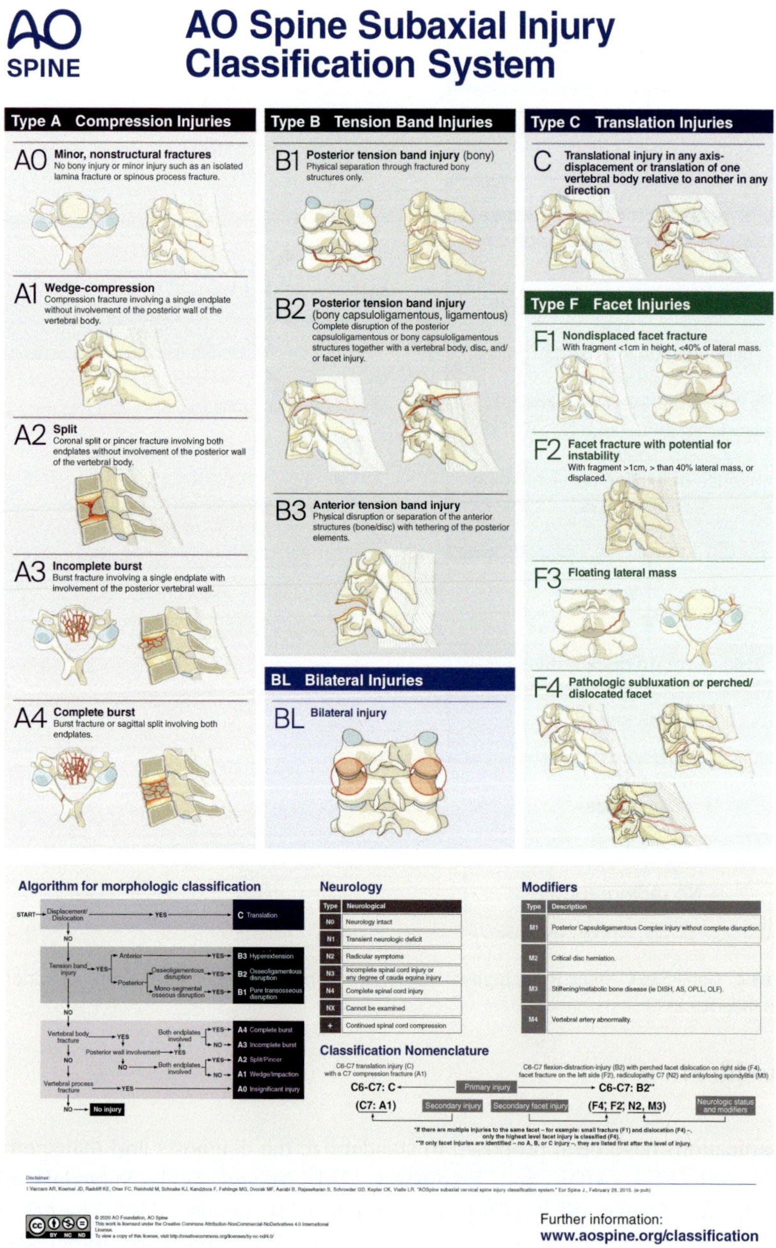

Fig. 10.3 AOSpine subaxial classification

Treatment

Treatment of subaxial spine injuries in elderly patients is challenging. They require several comorbidities, disabilities, low physiologic reserve, and osteoporosis [19]. Patient requires a personalization of the management and precision medicine to deal safely with different and concomitant variables presented, making the standardization of guidelines difficult and controversial [30].

Therapeutic strategies are generally based on the injury morphology, neurological deficit, and time of trauma. In elderly patients, close attention should be given to pre-existing pathologies, bone quality, healing potential, medications taken, and capacity to tolerate a surgical intervention (Table 10.2) [11].

Table 10.2 Operative and nonoperative treatment according to AO Spine cervical spine classifications

Type of fracture	Nonoperative treatment	Operative treatment
A		
A0	Soft cervical collar for a short period (maximum 6 weeks)	Not indicated
A1	Soft cervical collar for a short period (maximum 6 weeks)	If kyphotic angulation >15°: Anterior monosegmental fusion
A2	Soft cervical collar for a short period (maximum 6 weeks)	If kyphotic angulation >15°: Anterior bisegmental fusion
A3	If kyphotic angulation <15° and no relevant narrowing of the spinal canal: Rigid cervical collar for 6 weeks	Anterior fusion is recommended either in a mono- or bisegmental manner, depending on the degree of vertebral destruction
A4	Not indicated	Anterior bisegmental fusion
B		
B1	Hyperextended cervical orthesis in specific cases	Posterior bisegmental instrumentation
B2	Not indicated	Surgical stabilization is recommended: Anterior, posterior, or combined approach and the decision for fusion length (mono- or bisegmental) mainly depends on the A-component (degree of vertebral body destruction)
B3	Not indicated	Anterior monosegmental fusion
C		
C	Not indicated	Surgical stabilization is recommended: Anterior, posterior, or combined approach and the decision for fusion length (mono- or bisegmental) mainly depends on the A-component (degree of vertebral body destruction)

(continued)

Table 10.2 (continued)

Type of fracture	Nonoperative treatment	Operative treatment
F		
F1	Cervical collar may be used for pain relief for a short period (maximum 6 weeks)	Not indicated
F2	If isolated F2 fracture can be treated with rigid cervical collar for 6 weeks	Usually components of unstable B- or C-injuries, which dictate the surgical strategy. Possible nerve root compression by the facet fragment may therefore require an additional posterior approach in case of an anterior stabilization
F3	Not indicated	Usually components of unstable B- or C-injuries, which dictate the surgical strategy. Possible nerve root compression by the facet fragment may therefore require an additional posterior approach in case of an anterior stabilization
F4	Not indicated	– Usually components of unstable B- or C-injuries, which dictate the surgical strategy. Possible nerve root compression by the facet fragment may therefore require an additional posterior approach in case of an anterior stabilization – Unilateral or bilateral locked facets require a differentiated concept in order to ensure safe reduction without neurologic involvement and the anterior, posterior, or combined approach can be indicated
M		
M3	Not indicated	Ankylosing disease (e.g., ankylosing spondylitis, DISH) is an indication for posterior multilevel stabilization reduction of the preinjury sagittal profile is not mandatory; instead correction of a pre-existing kyphotic deformity is often possible

Cervical collar treatment with different degrees of stiffness or a halo vest can be used for external immobilization. The orthoses are usually indicated for patients with type A0, A1, and A2 AO Spine fractures. The type A3 injuries occur in oligo-symptomatic patients with <15° kyphosis without spinal cord compression. In those cases, a Philadelphia collar for a period of 6–12 weeks is indicated. Halo vest is an option for cases with greater instability in patients with contraindications for surgery. Patients should be followed and imaging studies performed 8–12 weeks after immobilization, looking for possible neurological deterioration, secondary displacement of the fracture, or post-traumatic deformity. Physical therapy should be started after radiographic bone healing.

Surgical treatment is indicated in type A4, B, and C AO Spine fractures. The goals of surgical treatment are to treat the spine instability, reduce the risk of late deformities, and revert neurological injury (see Fig. 10.4).

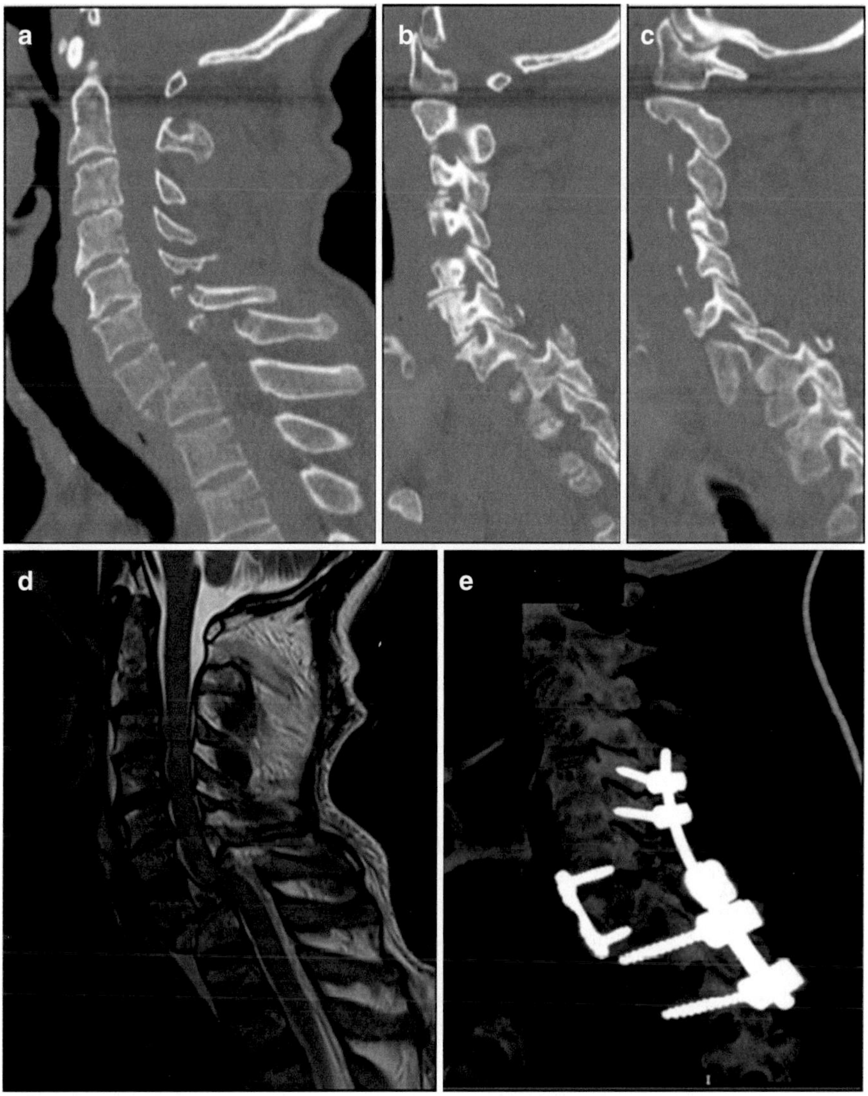

Fig. 10.4 A 68-year-old man with a roof fall and tetraparesia. (**a**) AO Spine fractures type C, C7–T1; A1, T1; F4 bilateral. (**b**) Locked right facet. (**c**) Locked left facet. (**d**) MRI image showing spinal cord compression. (**e**) Surgical treatment (anterior and posterior fixation)

Facet injuries need to be analyzed individually. F1 injuries are stable and should be treated with a cervical collar. Type F2, F3, and F4 facet injuries are usually seen in unstable type B or C lesions, which require surgical intervention for fixation. The type of surgical approaches, anterior, posterior, or combined, depends on the degree of kyphosis, bone dislocation, bone density, and associated neurological deficit [11].

Special attention should be given to the M3 modifier in elderly patients with ankylosing spondylitis and diffuse idiopathic skeletal hyperostosis (DISH). The combination of trauma and ankylosis creates long lever arms acting on a hard and stiff spine, which usually results in highly unstable fractures, even with low-energy traumas.

The spinal cord has an increased risk of bruising or transection due to the natural degenerative cervical stenosis observed in elderly patients, leading to a high rate of neurological deficits directly related to the trauma or secondary to spine instability. The surgical treatment for this group of patients is the posterior approach using long instrumentation construction. A combined approach is indicated in some cases [3, 11].

Outcomes, Mortality and Complications

The main objectives of treatment in patients with cervical spine trauma are the biomechanical restructuring of the spine, reduction of the fracture, realignment, stabilization, neural decompression, and bone fusion. Although spine surgeons are aware of those surgical indications, the rate of complications and mortality in elderly patients is not clear because a significant proportion of them have different comorbidities that affect surgical risk, complications rate, and the incidence of mortality.

There are studies that attempt to improve prediction and management in elderly patients with cervical spine fracture, but the majority of them are retrospective series with little evidence [17, 31].

In 1994, Spivak et al. reported a retrospective study of 2059 patients with spine injury [17]. Cervical spine trauma was observed in 1174 cases (57%) with a general mortality rate of 25.9% in patients over 65 years old, and in 80% of the cases, the fracture was located in the subaxial region [17]. The main causes of death were cardiac arrest (38%), pneumonia (14%), and sepsis (14%) [17].

In 1999, Olerud et al. published a retrospective series of 65 elderly patients with cervical spine trauma [31]. The mortality rate was 38.5%, and the main factors associated with higher mortality were the presence of preinjury diseases, severe neurological injury, increased age, and the presence of ankylosing spondylitis [31]. The conclusion of those papers was that high mortality is expected in elderly patients with cervical spine trauma, independently of the treatment performed, conservative or operative.

A study conducted in 2005 by Jackson et al. evaluated 458 patients aged 18–94 years who underwent operative treatment of cervical spine trauma. Upper cervical spine fracture was observed in 12.2% of cases, and 87.8% of patients had subaxial spine fractures. Of these, 74 patients (16%) were over 65 years old. In this group there was a mortality rate of 12.2%. Important risk factors for mortality were the presence of neurologic involvement (20% mortality in a complete neurological injury × 16.7% in incomplete injury × 0.0% in neurologically intact) and injury level (40% mortality in C7, 18.2% in C6, 3.6% in C5, 21.4% in C4, 16.7 in C3, and

0.0% in C1–C2). The main complications were cardiac arrhythmia (12.6%), pneumonia (10.8%), and urinary tract infection (5.4%) [32].

Conservative treatment was evaluated for two studies. In 2019, Nakanishi et al. reported that a retrospective series of 1154 older cervical trauma patients treated with cervical collars showed 5.1% of collar-related complications when used for more than 24 h. The main complications were pressure ulcer (12.2%) and hospital- or ventilator-associated pneumonia (11.1%) [12]. In 2015, Sharpe et al. evaluated the impact of a halo vest on outcomes in patients with cervical spine fractures without spinal cord injury. The mortality in halo vest patients older than 54 years was 13% vs. 0% in those younger than 54 years, and the unit length of stay was significantly increased in older patients despite less severe injury. They concluded that treatment with a halo vest in older patients is a potential risk for complications and mortality and should be strongly considered before placement in this patient age group [13].

Comparative studies between conservative and surgical treatment regarding morbidity and mortality showed variable results. In 2007, Sokolowski et al. evaluated 193 elderly patients of a series of 979 cervical trauma patients. The mortality of operated and non-operated patients was similar (12% vs. 15%). In 2010, Harris et al. published a retrospective series of 640 patients above and 64 years old that showed a mortality of 19% in 3 months and 28% in 1 year. Of these, surgical treatment was associated with a lower mortality in the first 3 months compared to conservative treatment (18% vs. 20%), but 1-year mortality was similar between the two treatment groups (27% vs. 28%) [4]. In 2018, Godat et al. reported a study that evaluated 10,938 patients and showed a mortality rate of 10% at initial admission, 28% at 1 year and 50% at 15 years. The initial mortality was 7% in the patients treated with a halo vest and 6% in those treated surgically, but at the end of 1 year, it increased to 26% and 19%, respectively. They concluded that the surgical treatment is associated with improved survival in this group of patients [30]. In 2010, Middentorp et al. published a systematic review that included 26 studies in elderly patients with cervical spine fractures. As regards mortality, an overall mean of 22% was reported, and the cause of death was not reported in 46% of the studies. The most frequent cause of death was myocardial infarction (16%), cerebral disorder, and head injury (5.2%). The overall conclusion was that pre-existing comorbidities, concomitant injuries, follow-up, and cause of death need to be reported more clearly in the studies to strengthen the validity of risk factors for mortality in older patients.

References

1. Malik SA, Murphy M, Connolly P, O'Byrne J. Evaluation of morbidity, mortality and outcome following cervical spine injuries in elderly patients. Eur Spine J. 2008;17(4):585–91.
2. Asemota AO, Ahmed AK, Purvis TE, Passias PG, Goodwin CR, Sciubba DM. Analysis of cervical spine injuries in elderly patients from 2001 to 2010 using a nationwide database: increasing incidence, overall mortality, and inpatient hospital charges. World Neurosurg. 2018;120:e114–e30.

3. Sandstrom CK, Nunez DB. Head and neck injuries: special considerations in the elderly patient. Neuroimaging Clin N Am. 2018;28(3):471–81.
4. Harris MB, Reichmann WM, Bono CM, Bouchard K, Corbett KL, Warholic N, et al. Mortality in elderly patients after cervical spine fractures. J Bone Joint Surg Am. 2010;92(3):567–74.
5. Aebi M. Surgical treatment of upper, middle and lower cervical injuries and non-unions by anterior procedures. Eur Spine J. 2010;19(Suppl 1):S33–9.
6. Lomoschitz FM, Blackmore CC, Mirza SK, Mann FA. Cervical spine injuries in patients 65 years old and older: epidemiologic analysis regarding the effects of age and injury mechanism on distribution, type, and stability of injuries. AJR Am J Roentgenol. 2002;178(3):573–7.
7. Healey CD, Spilman SK, King BD, Sherrill JE, Pelaez CA. Asymptomatic cervical spine fractures: current guidelines can fail older patients. J Trauma Acute Care Surg. 2017;83(1):119–25.
8. Hoffman JR, Wolfson AB, Todd K, Mower WR. Selective cervical spine radiography in blunt trauma: methodology of the National Emergency X-Radiography Utilization Study (NEXUS). Ann Emerg Med. 1998;32(4):461–9.
9. Stiell IG, Clement CM, McKnight RD, Brison R, Schull MJ, Rowe BH, et al. The Canadian C-spine rule versus the NEXUS low-risk criteria in patients with trauma. N Engl J Med. 2003;349(26):2510–8.
10. Vaccaro AR, Koerner JD, Radcliff KE, Oner FC, Reinhold M, Schnake KJ, et al. AOSpine subaxial cervical spine injury classification system. Eur Spine J. 2016;25(7):2173–84.
11. Schleicher P, Kobbe P, Kandziora F, Scholz M, Badke A, Brakopp F, et al. Treatment of injuries to the subaxial cervical spine: recommendations of the spine section of the German Society for Orthopaedics and Trauma (DGOU). Global Spine J. 2018;8(2 Suppl):25S–33S.
12. Nakanishi T, Mitra B, Ackland H, O'Reilly G, Cameron P. Time in collars and collar-related complications in older patients. World Neurosurg. 2019;129:e478–e84.
13. Sharpe JP, Magnotti LJ, Weinberg JA, Schroeppel TJ, Fabian TC, Croce MA. The old man and the C-spine fracture: impact of halo vest stabilization in patients with blunt cervical spine fractures. J Trauma Acute Care Surg. 2016;80(1):76–80.
14. Yadollahi M, Paydar S, Ghaem H, Ghorbani M, Mousavi SM, Taheri Akerdi A, et al. Epidemiology of cervical spine fractures. Trauma Mon. 2016;21(3):e33608.
15. Kehoe A, Smith JE, Edwards A, Yates D, Lecky F. The changing face of major trauma in the UK. Emerg Med J. 2015;32(12):911–5.
16. Golob JF, Claridge JA, Yowler CJ, Como JJ, Peerless JR. Isolated cervical spine fractures in the elderly: a deadly injury. J Trauma. 2008;64(2):311–5.
17. Spivak JM, Weiss MA, Cotler JM, Call M. Cervical spine injuries in patients 65 and older. Spine (Phila Pa 1976). 1994;19(20):2302–6.
18. Jawa RS, Singer AJ, Rutigliano DN, McCormack JE, Huang EC, Shapiro MJ, et al. Spinal fractures in older adult patients admitted after low-level falls: 10-year incidence and outcomes. J Am Geriatr Soc. 2017;65(5):909–15.
19. Damadi AA, Saxe AW, Fath JJ, Apelgren KN. Cervical spine fractures in patients 65 years or older: a 3-year experience at a level I trauma center. J Trauma. 2008;64(3):745–8.
20. Stiell IG, Wells GA, Vandemheen KL, Clement CM, Lesiuk H, De Maio VJ, et al. The Canadian C-spine rule for radiography in alert and stable trauma patients. JAMA. 2001;286(15):1841–8.
21. Hoffman JR, Mower WR, Wolfson AB, Todd KH, Zucker MI. Validity of a set of clinical criteria to rule out injury to the cervical spine in patients with blunt trauma. National Emergency X-Radiography Utilization Study Group. N Engl J Med. 2000;343(2):94–9.
22. Katelyn A, Young CLB, Walker CW, Dove JT, Widom KA, Torres DM, Wild JL. Cervical spine fracture in geriatric blunt trauma: are the NEXUS criteria sensitive enough? Int Surg J. 2019;6(9):3038–47.
23. Touger M, Gennis P, Nathanson N, Lowery DW, Pollack CV, Hoffman JR, et al. Validity of a decision rule to reduce cervical spine radiography in elderly patients with blunt trauma. Ann Emerg Med. 2002;40(3):287–93.
24. Goode T, Young A, Wilson SP, Katzen J, Wolfe LG, Duane TM. Evaluation of cervical spine fracture in the elderly: can we trust our physical examination? Am Surg. 2014;80(2):182–4.

25. Holdsworth F. Fractures, dislocations, and fracture-dislocations of the spine. J Bone Joint Surg Am. 1970;52(8):1534–51.
26. Allen BL, Ferguson RL, Lehmann TR, O'Brien RP. A mechanistic classification of closed, indirect fractures and dislocations of the lower cervical spine. Spine (Phila Pa 1976). 1982;7(1):1–27.
27. Magerl F, Aebi M, Gertzbein SD, Harms J, Nazarian S. A comprehensive classification of thoracic and lumbar injuries. Eur Spine J. 1994;3(4):184–201.
28. Vaccaro AR, Hulbert RJ, Patel AA, Fisher C, Dvorak M, Lehman RA, et al. The subaxial cervical spine injury classification system: a novel approach to recognize the importance of morphology, neurology, and integrity of the disco-ligamentous complex. Spine (Phila Pa 1976). 2007;32(21):2365–74.
29. Joaquim AF, Patel AA. Subaxial cervical spine trauma: evaluation and surgical decision-making. Global Spine J. 2014;4(1):63–70.
30. Godat LN, Kobayashi LM, Chang DC, Coimbra R. Improving life expectancy: a 'broken neck' doesn't have to be a terminal diagnosis for the elderly. Trauma Surg Acute Care Open. 2018;3(1):e000174.
31. Olerud C, Andersson S, Svensson B, Bring J. Cervical spine fractures in the elderly: factors influencing survival in 65 cases. Acta Orthop Scand. 1999;70(5):509–13.
32. Jackson AP, Haak MH, Khan N, Meyer PR. Cervical spine injuries in the elderly: acute post-operative mortality. Spine (Phila Pa 1976). 2005;30(13):1524–7.

Chapter 11
Anterior vs. Posterior Cervical Approaches for the Elderly

Nathan J. Lee, Andrei F. Joaquim, and K. Daniel Riew

Introduction

In recent decades, there has been a dramatic increase in the prevalence of cervical degenerative disease requiring surgery [1–5]. This is likely due to the aging population in the United States [6]. According to the United States Census Bureau, one in five Americans will be 65 years and older by 2030. Although various surgical options exist for the treatment of cervical degeneration, the ideal approach depends on a multitude of factors. This is further complicated in the elderly patient, who is known to be at significant risk for worse complications for both anterior and posterior cervical spine surgeries than their younger counterparts [7–11].

There is some controversy regarding the efficacy and safety of surgical decompression for cervical disease in elderly patients in comparison to younger patients. Numerous studies have identified age as a significant risk factor for complications. This may be attributed to the fact that older patients are associated with increased medical comorbidities, age-related changes to the spinal cord, more severe degenerative pathology requiring more complex surgery, and diminished physiologic reserve [12–15]. Another important factor is the bone quality of an aging spine. It has been shown that osteoporotic patients have slower and less reliable bone healing [16–18]. In a national study by Guzman et al., patients with osteoporosis were found to have significantly higher rates of revision surgery after an elective cervical spine procedure in comparison to those without osteoporosis [11]. Poor bone quality may increase the risk for bone-implant failure, interbody cage subsidence, screw pullout,

N. J. Lee (✉) · K. D. Riew
Department of Orthopaedics, Columbia University Medical Center, The Och Spine Hospital at New York-Presbyterian, New York, NY, USA
e-mail: njl2116@cumc.columbia.edu; kr2637@cumc.columbia.edu

A. F. Joaquim
Department of Neurosurgery, University of Campinas (Unicamp), Campinas, SP, Brazil

K.-M. G. Fu et al. (eds.), *Treatment of Spine Disease in the Elderly*,
https://doi.org/10.1007/978-3-031-12612-3_11

pseudarthrosis, adjacent level degeneration, compression fractures, and junctional kyphosis, which may necessitate revision surgery.

In a recent prospective, multicenter study, Nakashima et al. studied 479 patients with degenerative cervical myelopathy who underwent cervical decompression with or without fusion and compared the outcomes and complications between older ($\geq$65 years old, $n = 119$) and younger cohorts (<65 years old, $n = 360$) [19]. After controlling for a number of surgical factors (e.g., number of decompressed levels, surgical approach, corpectomy), older patients were found to be at significantly higher risk for worse neurological outcomes and reduced recovery rates than younger patients. This is likely to due to the changes in the composition of the spinal cord and diminished physiologic reserve in older patients. It is important to note that the absolute changes in functional scores were still substantial and in excess of the MCID in the older cohort. Furthermore, no differences were observed in specific perioperative complications, including C5 nerve root palsy, superficial or deep infection, dysphagia, and dural tear. However, older patients experienced greater rates of screw malposition and longer length of postoperative stay (older: 13 days vs. younger: 9.5 days, $p = 0.009$). Given that age is an independent predictor of functional status in patients with degenerative cervical disease, it is necessary to critically assess and discuss with the elderly patient the ideal surgical approach and options in order to ensure a successful outcome.

Patient Selection

Several surgical techniques exist for both anterior and posterior approaches to the cervical spine. The decision to choose one approach over the other may be based on the cervical alignment, number of levels requiring decompression, approach-related complications, and other factors, such as the presence of ossification of the posterior longitudinal ligament (OPLL), body habitus, short neck, and surgeon preference. In some cases, there may be a clear benefit of one approach over the other. For instance, an anterior approach is preferred for those with focal kyphosis with significant anterior cord compression. In situations where there is true equipoise between anterior and posterior-based surgeries, it is likely that a well-performed operation from either approach will achieve similar outcomes for the patient [20]. The following are important factors that should be considered when deciding the optimal surgical approach:

Cervical Spine Alignment

The cervical sagittal alignment is commonly measured as the Cobb angle from C2 to C7. Normally, the cervical alignment ranges from 20 to 35 degrees of lordosis [21]. Generally, non-instrumented posterior-based approaches (e.g., laminoplasty, laminectomy) should not be performed for a fixed, kyphotic cervical spine, especially when the focal kyphosis exceeds 13 degrees [22]. In a kyphotic cervical spine, the spinal cord is draped over the vertebral body and is compressed by anterior pathology (e.g., disc, osteophyte). If a posterior decompression is performed without any correction to the sagittal alignment, the spinal cord will not "float away" from the ventral compression. On the other hand, when the cervical spine is straight to lordotic, a posterior decompression will allow the spinal cord to drift dorsally and away from the anterior pathology, thus resulting in indirect ventral decompression.

Other relevant sagittal parameters to consider include C2-C7 sagittal vertical axis (SVA) (the deviation of the C2 plumb line from the centroid of the axis to the posterior/superior endplate of C7) and the T1 slope minus C2-C7 lordosis (T1S-CL) (Fig. 11.1). The T1 slope is the angle between the horizontal line and the upper endplate of T1 (Fig. 11.2). According to Hyun et al., both C2-C7 SVA and T1S-CL are positively correlated with worse neck disability index (NDI) scores. Specifically, a C2-C7 SVA value greater than 43.5 mm and a T1S-CL value greater than 22.2 degrees are statistically significant cutoffs for worse NDI scores (>25) at a minimum 2-year follow-up [23]. These parameters may be useful in determining whether a posterior approach without instrumentation or fusion would be appropriate, since

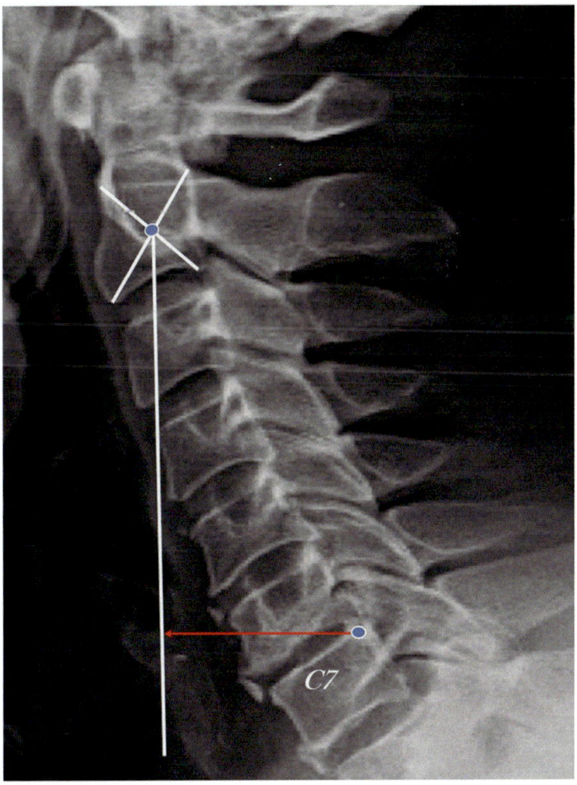

Fig. 11.1 C2-C7 sagittal vertical axis (SVA) is the deviation of the C2 plumb line from the centroid of the axis to the posterior/superior endplate of C7

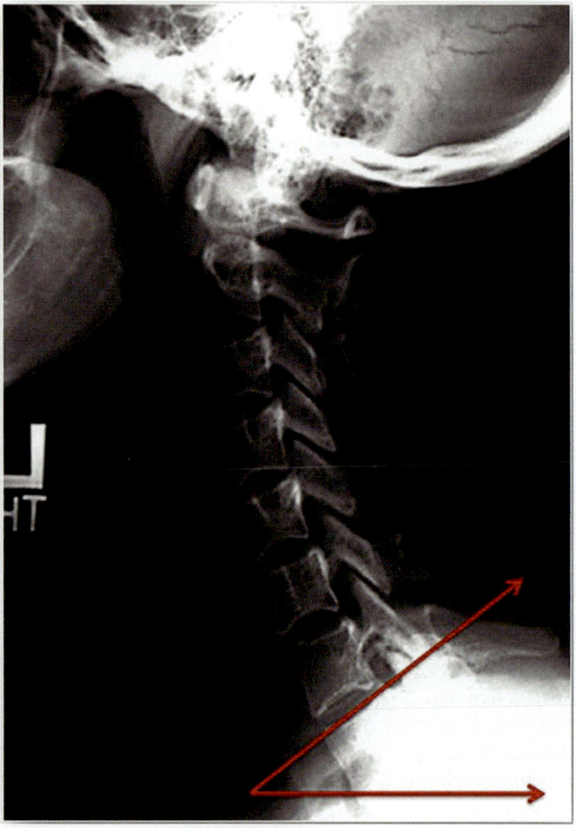

Fig. 11.2 The T1 slope is the angle between the horizontal line and the upper endplate of T1

inadequate correction and maintenance of sagittal balance will lead to worse outcomes [24, 25]. In elderly patients, correction of these sagittal parameters should be balanced with the medical risks of a more extensive procedure.

Number of Levels Requiring Decompression

The location of the compressive pathology and the number of levels involved are important factors in choosing the surgical approach. For instance, mechanical compression of the neural elements may be from facet joint hypertrophy, intervertebral discs, vertebral bodies, hypertrophy of the ligamentum flavum, and OPLL. A posterior approach can indirectly decompress the entire cervical spine, in comparison to an anterior approach, which is typically limited cranially to C2. Conversely, an anterior approach may be favored in the setting of focal kyphosis, significant anterior neuroforaminal compression, and large disc herniations compressing the ventral spinal cord, or short-segment disease with only one or two levels requiring decompression. When more than three levels are involved, anterior cervical fusions are known to be associated with significantly higher rates of pseudarthrosis particularly at the more caudal levels, postoperative hematoma requiring secondary surgery, and dysphagia attributed to greater soft tissue swelling [26–31]. Of note, dysphagia is commonly present in elderly patients preoperatively, and this should be taken into account. Therefore, an anterior approach is typically preferred for one- to three-level cases.

Approach-Related Complications to Consider

In a recent prospective multicenter study, Kato et al. compared the perioperative complications and the 2-year patient-reported outcomes between those who received an anterior and a posterior surgical approach for the treatment of degenerative cervical myelopathy [20]. These authors found that the overall complication rates and 2-year patient reported outcomes were not statistically different between cohorts. However, in the sub-analysis, they found that the complication profiles were significantly different based on surgical approach (e.g., anterior, dysphagia/dysphonia; posterior, surgical site infection, C5 radiculopathy).

Another recent large prospective, controlled multicenter study on myelopathy patients, by Ghogawala et al., found that laminoplasty had significantly better SF-36 Physical Component Summary scores (9.72) when compared with anterior procedures (5.2; $P = 0.04$) and posterior decompression and fusion (4.53; $P = 0.05$). Laminoplasty also had the lowest major complication rate of 7%, compared to 15% for anterior decompression and fusion and 20% for posterior decompression and fusion ($p = 0.04$) [32].

C5, C8, and T1 Nerve Root Injuries

C5 nerve root palsy is a common complication that has been observed after anterior and posterior cervical surgery. According to a recent meta-analysis, the prevalence of C5 nerve root palsy over the last decade is about 6.3% [33]. However, this is most commonly seen after posterior cervical approaches. It is thought that C5 palsy can result from stretch neuropraxia, when there is excessive cord shift posteriorly after decompression. The C5 nerve root has a relatively more horizontal and shorter trajectory, which may increase its vulnerability to traction, especially in severely degenerated spines, most commonly found in elderly patients. Furthermore, inadequate neuroforaminal decompression at the C4-C5 level can likely exacerbate the neuropraxia. If conservative management fails and advanced imaging confirms nerve root compression consistent with patient symptoms, then revision surgery involving an anterior based approach may be necessary. An anterior C4-C5 discectomy can increase foraminal height and perhaps decrease the risk for C5 palsy after an isolated posterior approach.

C8 and T1 nerve palsies are less frequent nerve root injuries. On exam, they are associated with weakness to the intrinsic muscles of the hand and ulnar-based numbness along the hand and forearm. A preoperative lordosis position test can be useful in determining the surgical approach. In this test, the patient is positioned supine with the neck extended for several minutes. If the patients begin to experience paresthesia, weakness, or pain in the arms, then it may be necessary for a combined anterior and posterior approach. In patients with significant disc height loss at the level of the foraminal stenosis, a foraminotomy alone will not fully address the stenotic level, since a foraminotomy increases the anterior-posterior dimension of the foramen and not its height. Furthermore, creating lordosis without restoring disc height may worsen the foraminal height. Therefore, an anterior approach may be necessary to restore disc height to distract the stenotic foramen.

Dysphagia

The most common complication after anterior cervical spine surgery is dysphagia. The incidence has been reported to be greater than 50% in the early postoperative period [34]. Fortunately, the symptoms typically improve within a few weeks in the majority of patients. Possible mechanisms include esophageal retraction, direct cervical plate irritation to the esophagus, hematoma, soft tissue swelling and edema, and nerve root injuries. Generally, the pharyngeal plexus may be injured in surgeries from C2-C5, the superior laryngeal nerves from C3-C4, the recurrent laryngeal nerves between C5 to T1 and the hypoglossal nerve in surgeries above C3 [35]. According to a prior randomized controlled trial, the approach may affect the incidence of dysphagia as well [36]. Fengben et al. found that a higher incidence of dysphagia occurred during C3-C4 level surgery, when dissection was made between the tracheoesophageal sheath and the omohyoid muscle. Anatomically, the internal branch of the superior laryngeal nerve is easier to identify in the plane between the sternocleidomastoid and omohyoid muscles at the level of C3-C4 than in the space between the tracheoesophageal sheath and the omohyoid muscle. On the other hand, for C6-C7 level surgery, they found that a more lateral approach (between the sternocleidomastoid and omohyoid muscles) was associated with a higher degree of dysphagia. Dissection lateral to the omohyoid muscle at this level may require more forceful retraction medially to obtain the necessary exposure.

Other known risk factors include multilevel surgeries, a combined anterior-posterior approach, female sex, older patients (age > 60 years old), revision procedures, and thicker plates [34, 37–40]. In order to decrease the risk for dysphagia, surgeons should avoid a prolonged operative time (or retractor time). If self-retaining retraction is used, the surgeon should be mindful of the retraction time and relax the retractors whenever possible (i.e., when obtaining x-rays or while cutting bone graft). If the retraction time of an anterior approach is more than 3 h, then the surgeon should consider keeping the patient intubated overnight to avoid airway compromise. In addition, the operative duration should be considered relative to the number of levels involved. For instance, a one-level surgery requiring 3 h of retraction will likely have more soft tissue swelling and edema than a five-level case with 3 h of total retraction time, since a shorter time of retraction is spent per level and the more extensive exposure allows for reduced retraction force to the operative area.

Retropharyngeal steroids have been shown to significantly reduce the risk for dysphagia in a prospective, randomized study and may be particularly beneficial when BMP is used [41–43]. However, retropharyngeal steroids should not be used, if there is prominent instrumentation as it can further erode an esophagus that may be thinned by steroids. Lee and Riew reported two cases of delayed esophageal perforation, which likely was related to the use of retropharyngeal steroids [44].

Dysphonia

Dysphonia is another complication observed after anterior cervical surgery. It is less common than dysphagia and has an incidence ranging from 2% to 30% [35]. Dysphonia is defined as a change in voice, and the severity can range from mild hoarseness to severe speaking problems. This complication can result from either direct or indirect injury to the recurrent or superior laryngeal nerves, vocal cord trauma, arytenoid dislocation, and laryngeal edema. Symptoms are most often transient with rates of persistent vocal cord paresis ranging from 0.33% to 2.5% [45, 46]; however, in cases where persistent vocal cord paresis exists, patients may need to be additionally assessed by an otolaryngologist.

Wound Complications

Wound infection following anterior cervical spine surgery is relatively rare with an estimated incidence of 0.2% to 1.6% [30]. Furthermore, among prospective studies, the incidence of postoperative cervical hematoma ranges from 0% to 0.7% [47]. This may be attributed to the fact that the anterior cervical anatomy is well vascularized and has substantial lymphatic drainage compared to a posterior approach. On the other hand, wound complications are known to be more common with a posterior approach. According to a national database study, the 30-day rate for surgical site infections after a posterior cervical surgery is about 3% [48]. Risk factors for wound complications include chronic steroid use, diabetes, prolonged operative time, and morbid obesity. Interestingly, older age does not appear to be a risk factor for wound issues [49]. It is possible that the anatomy in the posterior spine is less forgiving than the anterior approach and that the higher tensile forces that pull at the midline fascia along the backside of the neck may contribute to the higher risk for wound issues.

Other Surgical Considerations

Since being introduced by Smith and Robinson more than 60 years ago, ACDF surgery has evolved significantly [71]. With modified burring of the vertebral endplates, Bohlman et al. showed significantly higher rates of fusion than traditional approaches [72, 73]. The use of plates across a fusion construct was found to substantially decrease rates of nonunion, especially for multilevel ACDF [74–77].

There remains considerable debate between dynamic and static ACDF plates to maximize fusion and minimize complications (e.g., pseudoarthrosis, subsidence, kyphotic collapse). Static plates provide rigid fixation but may introduce graft stress shielding and reduce mechanical loads necessary for fusion. A dynamic plate can facilitate the load sharing but the allowed motion may be excessive and lead to inferior fusion rates, segmental kyphosis, or foraminal narrowing. Earlier biomechanical studies have demonstrated that dynamic plating allows for significantly more load transmission by the graft and comparable construct stiffness [78, 79]. A recent metanalysis reported that locked plating may improve fusion rates, decrease subsidence, and provide slightly better VAS neck pain scores [80]. Although dynamic plates were designed with theoretical advantages over rigid plates, there is currently a lack of evidence demonstrating clinical superiority of dynamic over rigid fixation.

In a recent study, screw length relative to the vertebral body (screw length less than 75% of the vertebral body depth) was found to be strongly correlated to radiographic pseudarthrosis in the early postoperative period [81]. As an intraoperative guide, spine surgeons can use the screw-vertebral body% threshold of <75% to avoid unnecessarily short screws. Once the disc space is prepared, a potential screw can be placed in the prepared space parallel to the endplate to ensure that the posterior cortex and spinal canal will not be violated. This may be a useful technique in maximizing screw length intraoperatively.

As described earlier, dysphagia is a common complication after ACDF. Some authors believe that a prominent plate can contribute to this [34]. Strategies to minimize plate-related dysphagia include a thorough removal of anterior osteophytes to allow the plate to sit flush on the ventral spine, contouring the plate into lordosis to follow the natural contour of the spine, and using a low-profile plate. Another known complication after ACDF is adjacent segment disease. According to Hilibrand et al., the incidence of symptomatic disease is about 3% per year [82]. However, he did not report on reoperation rates. In a more recent and larger study, Lee et al. found that adjacent segment surgery occurred at 2.3% per year with Kaplan-Meier analysis, predicting that 21.9% of patients would need adjacent segment surgery by 10 years postoperatively (Risk-Factor Analysis of Adjacent-Segment Pathology Requiring Surgery Following Anterior, Posterior, Fusion, and Nonfusion Cervical Spine Operations Survivorship Analysis of 1358 Patients: Lee, Lee, Peters, Riew: J Bone Joint Surg Am. 2014;96:1761–7). Degeneration occurs most commonly at C5-C6 and C6-C7 and occur more frequently after single-level than multilevel fusion. Park and Riew showed that there is a positive association between adjacent-level ossification following ACDF and the plate-to-disc distance [83]. Placing an anterior cervical plate more than 5 mm away from the adjacent disc space can reduce the risk of adjacent-level ossification. The assumption here is that ossification likely contributes to early degeneration.

Anterior Cervical Corpectomy and Fusion (ACCF)

An ACCF is typically indicated when the ventral spinal cord compression is at the level of the posterior vertebral body beyond the level of the disc space (e.g., large posterior osteophyte, disc fragment migrated to the vertebral body posteriorly, developmental stenosis). The surgical exposure is the same as that for an ACDF. Discectomies are performed above and below the level of the intended corpectomy. A Leksell rongeur and a high-speed burr can be used to remove the vertebral body between the uncovertebral joints as well as the most posterior part of the vertebral body. Resection of the PLL can allow for complete visualization of the thecal sac. Similar to ACDF, various interbody devices can be inserted, such as such as titanium mesh cages, allograft, autologous bone (iliac crest, fibula, rib grafts), and PEEK cages, among others. It is important to carefully inspect the depth of the graft placement to ensure it is clear from the spinal canal. Anterior cervical plating is necessary to not only encourage fusion but also avoid graft dislodgement.

Other Surgical Considerations

Some studies have indicated equipoise between ACDF and ACCF for the treatment of multilevel cervical spondylotic myelopathy [84, 85]. However, others argue that ACCF may be superior, since it minimizes the number of graft-host interfaces, allows for extensive decompression, and provides a source for bony autograft to promote fusion [86–88]. On the other hand, the morbidity of a corpectomy may be slightly greater than an ACDF, which may primarily be due to the prolonged operative time and greater blood loss. In a recent comparative analysis using national data, a one-level ACCF was found to be independently associated with longer length of stay, longer operative time, and a greater risk for 30-day complications in comparison to two-level ACCF [89]. Furthermore, two-level ACCF was found to be an independent predictor for longer length of stay and higher rates of 30-day complications compared to three-level ACDF for the treatment of cervical spondylotic myelopathy. In another study, Lau et al. compared outcomes between two-level ACCF and three-level ACDF (without any concomitant posterior cervical surgery) and found that perioperative complication rates were similar. Furthermore, both groups achieved similar postoperative cervical lordosis, adjacent segment disease rates, pseudarthrosis rates, neurological improvement, and pain relief [84].

For multilevel ACCF, it is advisable to use posterior supplementation to avoid graft extrusion or hardware failure, especially in elderly patients or those with poor bone conditions. Long strut grafts for multilevel corpectomies are mechanically unfavorable and prone to construct failure. Buttress plates have been used to prevent graft dislodgement; however, there have been reports that this can still result in airway obstruction if the graft dislodges and kicks out the plate at a 45-degree angle [90, 91]. Treatment should be individualized according to a patient's characteristics (radiological, comorbidities, bone mineral density). In selected cases with two-level disc disease in patients with increased risk for pseudoarthrosis, such as heavy smokers or diabetics, a single-level corpectomy may be advantageous compared to a two-level ACDF. The posterior vertebral body (about 2–3 mm) can be left intact to avoid graft retropulsion into the spinal cord, and fusion needs to only take place at two graft-bone interfaces, as opposed to four interfaces with a two-level ACDF. In addition to fewer graft-bone interfaces, the cancellous bone of the excised vertebral body is rich in osteoprogenitors and can be utilized as autogenous bone graft.

For two- or more level corpectomies, the senior author recommends both anterior plating and posterior supplementation to minimize graft extrusion. A two-level corpectomy may be performed as stand-alone procedures in selected cases; however, great care must be taken to achieve perfect graft press fit and to avoid edge-loading. Rigid immobilization and frequent radiographic evaluation are recommended. We feel that the safer alternative is to augment the construct with posterior instrumentation and arthrodesis.

A hybrid procedure, which involves a combination of a corpectomy and an ACDF, can be performed as an alternative to multilevel corpectomies [92]. The advantage of a hybrid procedure is greater mechanical stability since screws can be placed in all vertebral bodies to maintain fixation and alignment. For three-level disease, surgeons may choose to perform a one level corpectomy for the cranial two levels and an ACDF at the most caudal level, placing a plate across all three levels (Fig. 11.3). This technique was first described by the senior author in 1998 as a corpectomy-discectomy [93]. For four-level disease, two single level corpectomies separated by an intervening vertebra may be a very reasonable option. This was described as a corpectomy-corpectomy or skip-corpectomy [93]. Increasing the number of screws in the plate fixation may decrease the long-term risk of hardware fatigue and also improve construct rigidity necessary for bony fusion.

Anterior Cervical Hemi-Corpectomy and Fusion (ACHCF)

ACHCF involves the longitudinal removal of only half of the vertebral body [94] (Figs. 11.4 and 11.5). This technique differs from the traditional cervical corpectomy in which a corpectomy is performed from uncus to uncus. The preservation of one hemi-vertebral body can increase the surface area for fusion, provide bony autograft to promote fusion, and enable segmental screw fixation across the corpectomy site. This should only be appropriate in cases where the cord compression can be addressed by decompressing 50–80% of the width of the vertebral body. According to the senior author's experience, ACHCF has shown earlier fusion rates in

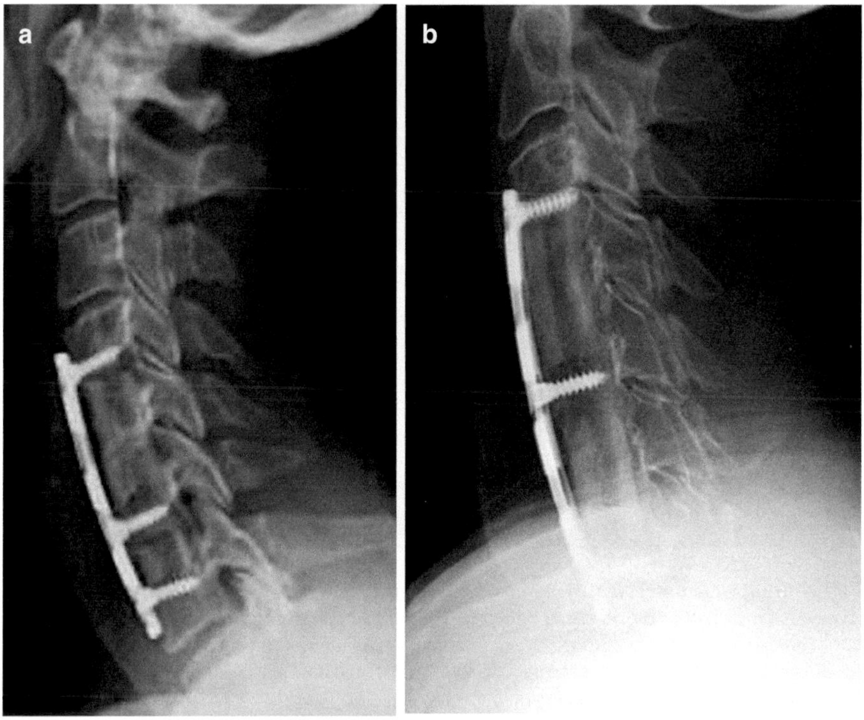

Fig. 11.3 (**a**) For three-level disease, surgeons may choose to perform a one-level corpectomy for the cranial two levels and an ACDF at the most caudal level, placing a plate across all three levels. This is described as a corpectomy-discectomy. (**b**) For four-level disease, two single-level corpectomies separated by an intervening vertebra may be a very reasonable option. This is described as a corpectomy-corpectomy or skip-corpectomy

three-level cases in comparison to traditional ACDF. This may be a viable alternative to standard corpectomies when appropriately indicated; however, further research examining both the short- and long-term risks and benefits over conventional ACCF are needed to further validate this technique.

Cervical Disc Arthroplasty (CDA)

CDA is a motion-preserving alternative to ACDF. One of the main drivers of CDA has been to reduce the risk for adjacent segment disease by preserving motion instead of fusing [82]. Since first being introduced to the United States in the early 1990s, there has been a substantial amount of literature investigating its safety and clinical outcomes compared to ACDF. There is certainly some controversy regarding the superiority of cervical arthroplasty over ACDF for patients with myelopathy. However, several high-quality studies have recently demonstrated that CDA, when

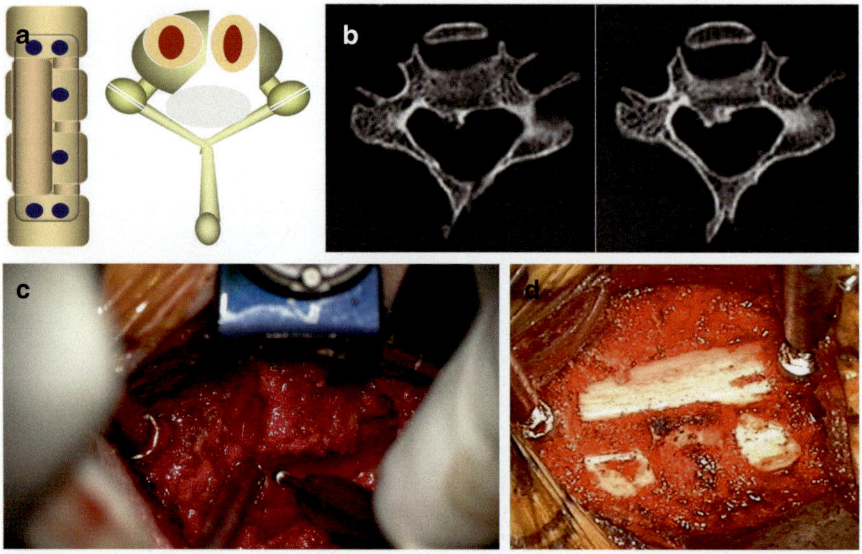

Fig. 11.4 (**a**) Anterior cervical hemi-corpectomy and fusion (ACHCF) involves the longitudinal removal of only half of the vertebral body. (**b**) This should only be appropriate in cases, where the cord compression can be addressed by decompressing 50–80% of the width of the vertebral body. (**c**) An intraoperative view of anterior cervical hemi-corpectomy. (**d**) The allograft is placed in hemi-corpectomy side after proper decompression

appropriately indicated and performed, can achieve similar or even slightly superior outcomes compared to ACDF [95–98].

The indications for cervical arthroplasty include patients with radiculopathy and/or myelopathy with one or two levels due to retro-discal cord compression. It would not be appropriate for those with retro-vertebral cord compression, which would require a corpectomy. Patients should also have a preserved disc height (at least 3 mm according to some authors), good bone density (no osteoporosis), and preserved motion. Contraindications include instability, inflammatory or metabolic disease, ossifying diseases (e.g., DISH, OPLL, ankylosing spondylitis), segmental kyphosis, severe disc degeneration, and severe facet joint arthritis. It should be emphasized that, because of the high prevalence of the contraindications to CDA listed above, practically no elderly patient is a candidate for CDA. However, age alone is not a contraindication to the procedure; if the patient is otherwise a good candidate, it can be performed.

Of note, CDA is technically more challenging than ACDF procedures. For CDA, it is imperative to aim for precise endplate preparation and positioning of the implant. For instance, misplacement of Caspar pins even a few millimeters off center can distract the disc space unevenly and compromise the biomechanics of the CDA and potentially increase the risk for implant failure, adjacent segment disease, pain, and revision surgery. Great care should be placed toward centering the implant

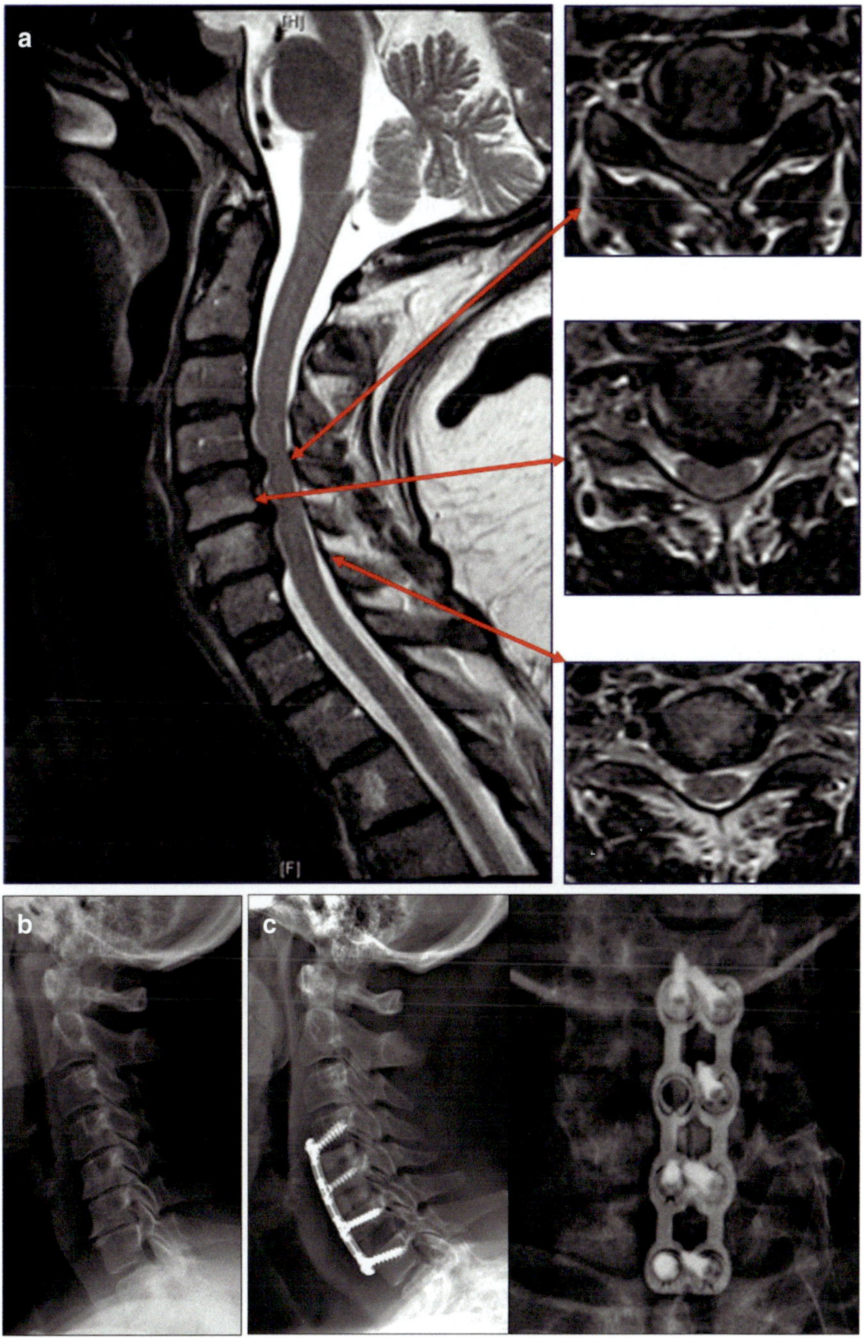

Fig. 11.5 Hemi-corpectomy-discectomy (**a**) the preoperative MRI demonstrating multilevel cervical disease at C4-C5, C5-C6, and C6-C7. (**b**) and (**c**) Show the pre-op and post-op radiographs, respectively

and ensuring it sits flush with the endplates. The CDA should be sized to fill the disc space anterior to posterior to optimize biomechanics.

The literature comparing outcomes after CDA in older versus young patients is somewhat limited. In a recent comparative study with a 2-year follow-up, older patients (≥65 years old) were found to have similar patient reported outcomes (VAS, NDI, JOA) to younger patients (≤40) [99]. The elderly group demonstrated a small reduction in cervical range of motion after CDA in comparison to the younger group, which experienced a small increase in mobility. Furthermore, the complications were not significantly different between groups. These results are promising, but it is important to note that the mean follow-up was about 28 months and long-term studies may be needed to compare the true incidence of outcomes and complications.

Posterior Cervical Approaches

Laminectomy and Fusion

A posterior approach to the cervical spine typically involves either a laminectomy with or without fusion or laminoplasty. A laminectomy/fusion can effectively decompress the cord but result in a significant loss of cervical range of motion [100]. In contrast, laminoplasty serves as a motion-preserving procedure that may obviate the risk of pseudoarthrosis, provide the option for future anterior procedures, and allow for effective indirect decompression, which may be safer than direct decompression. In some instances, a laminectomy/fusion may be more appropriate than laminoplasty (e.g., significant axial neck pain, cervical kyphosis >10–15 degrees, negative k-line, hill-shaped OPLL) [54, 101–104]. However, if a patient is a candidate for both, we prefer laminoplasty over laminectomy/fusion. New evidence supports this opinion: Ghogawala et al. found that, in the appropriate candidate, laminoplasty had better outcomes and lower major complication rates than laminectomy/fusion (7% versus 20%, respectively; $p = 0.04$).

During a posterior cervical approach, a meticulous midline dissection in the amuscular and avascular raphe should be performed (Figs. 11.6, 11.7, and 11.8). The nuchal ligament, which connect the external occipital protuberance to the spinous process of C2, is the only ligament that one encounters in the approach. Many surgeons are taught to dissect lateral to the nuchal and interspinous ligaments to preserve them. We would like to emphasize that there is no such thing as an interspinous ligament in the cervical spine. Websites showing pictures of this are simply wrong. In its place in the cervical spine is the interspinalis muscle, which gets its blood supply from either side of the spine. When surgeons cut on either side of the nuchal ligament and the interspinalis muscle in their misbegotten attempt to preserve the nuchal and the nonexistent interspinous ligament, all they are doing is devascularizing both the nuchal ligament and the interspinalis muscle. The

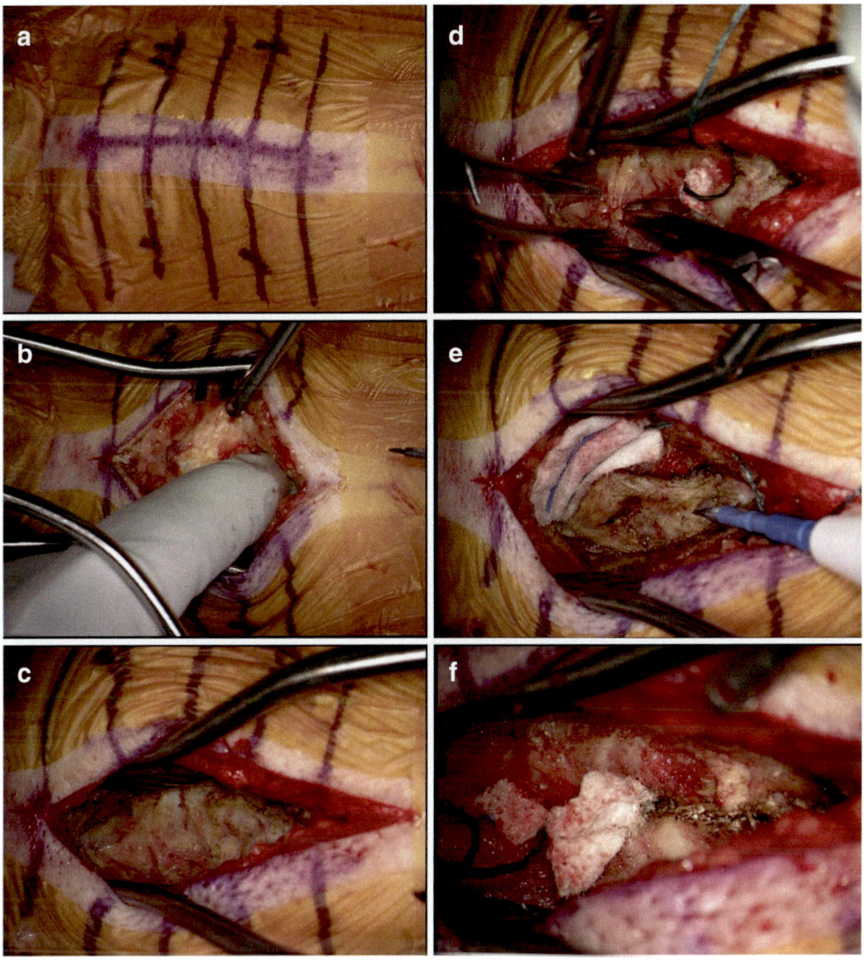

Fig. 11.6 Posterior cervical exposure. (**a**) The posterior cervical incision is marked along the spinous processes. (**b**) A midline dissection in the amuscular and avascular raphe should be performed. The nuchal ligament should be divided down the middle, leaving it attached to the lateral muscles that provide its blood supply. Thereafter, blunt dissection starting at the most distal spinous process and using a finger to palpate the spinous processes and rubbing cranially and caudally between the spinous processes will help to delineate the midline raphe. (**c–f**) Further dissection down to the midline of the bifid spinous processes is performed with meticulous dissection

devascularized ligament and muscle are then destined to die, becoming a potential nidus for a wound infection. Instead, the nuchal ligament should be divided down the middle, leaving it attached to the lateral muscles that provide its blood supply. Thereafter, blunt dissection starting at the most distal spinous process and using a finger to palpate the spinous processes and rubbing cranially and caudally between the spinous processes will help to delineate the midline raphe. The senior author prefers to divide the bifid spinous processes with a bone cutter, keeping the

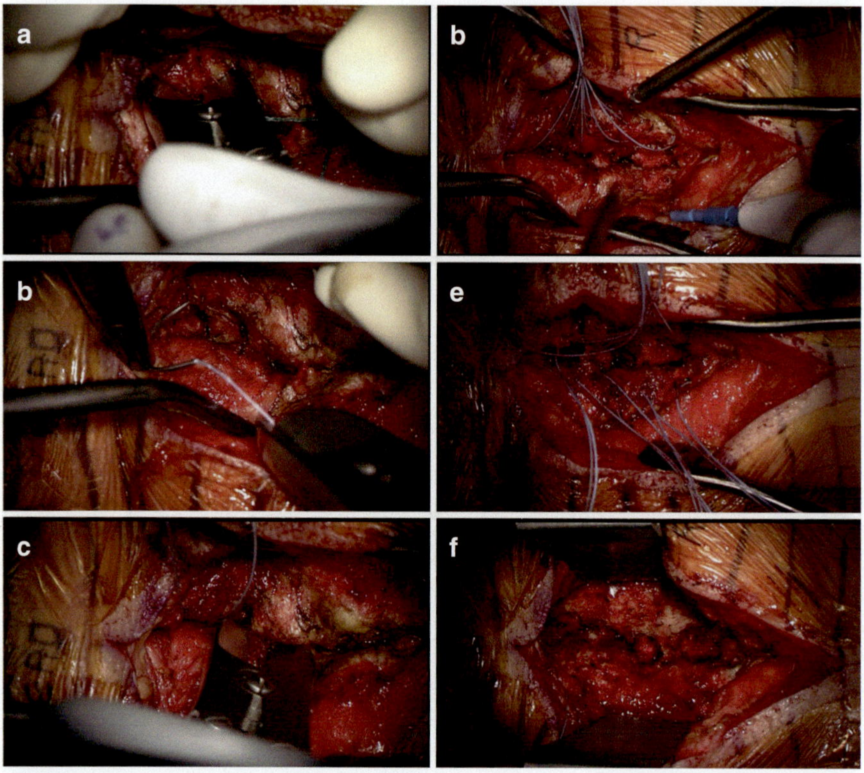

Fig. 11.7 (**a**) The senior author prefers to divide the bifid spinous processes with a bone cutter, keeping the interspinalis and other paraspinal muscles attached. (**b–e**) These are tagged and can facilitate bone-to-bone closure at the end of the operation. (**f**) This technique avoids suturing directly into the muscle, which can compromise vascular supply to the muscle and subsequently necrose the captured muscle

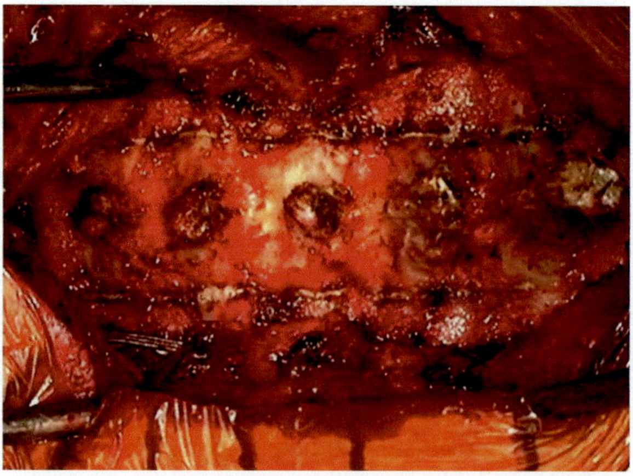

Fig. 11.8 Intraoperative exposure of posterior cervical spine. The interspinalis muscle is preserved, and all muscles and the nuchal ligament have been divided meticulously down the avascular and amuscular midline

interspinalis and other paraspinal muscles attached. These are tagged and can facilitate bone-to-bone closure at the end of the operation. This technique avoids suturing directly into muscle, which can compromise vascular supply to the muscle and subsequently necrose the captured muscle. Subperiosteal exposure of the lamina and lateral masses are performed, but care should be taken to only expose enough of the lateral masses to place lateral mass screws. Exposure beyond the lateral masses can increase the risk of encountering the venous plexus, which can bleed profusely. In addition, the dorsal nerves innervating the paraspinal muscles can be injured with excessive exposure and therefore result in substantial muscle atrophy. For posterior cervical fusion, the facet joints are exposed, and the joint cartilage is denuded with curettes or small rasps. The joint space is then packed with autologous bone chips. C2 fixation can be achieved by screws placed in the pars, pedicle, or lamina. For C3 to C6, standard lateral mass screws can be placed. Pedicle screws are typically used for fixation at T1 and T2. When extending the fusion to T1 or below, fixation into C7 is can be skipped to facilitate screw fixation into T1. Although rarely used these days, additional sublaminar hooks or translaminar screws can be used at the caudal part of the construct to reinforce the screw fixation if necessary. A better alternative is to supplement the fixation with laminar screws and a third rod or spinous process cables.

For the decompression, we prefer to perform laminoplasty and fusion, instead of laminectomy. This is because the retained lamina provides a protective cover over the cord and allows for bone grafting over the laminoplasty. Mini-laminoplasty plates can be used without fixation screws to prop up the laminae, or the holes can be enlarged with a bur and the lateral mass screws can be placed thru the hole (Fig. 11.9). An alternative technique to cover the decompression site is to do laminectomies and then place a strut allograft iliac crest to cover the defect.

Given the higher risk for wound complications compared to anterior approaches, meticulous closure should include smaller bites to avoid muscle necrosis and closure of multiple layers to avoid any dead space, which can serve as a nidus for infection.

Laminoplasty

Cervical laminoplasty was first described by Omaya et al. in 1973. Since then, this procedure has been further refined; however, the general concepts continue to include preservation of dorsal elements, expansion of the spinal canal through manipulation of the laminae, and preservation of segmental motion.

Laminoplasty is typically indicated for patients with cervical myelopathy or myeloradiculopathy, which may be due to multilevel disc herniation, OPLL, cervical spondylosis, and congenital stenosis. Furthermore, laminoplasty can be considered in patients who have neutral to lordotic alignment, a positive k-line, and a C2-C7 sagittal vertical axis (SVA) less than 40 mm and do not have substantial axial neck pain. Laminoplasty in the elderly patient is somewhat controversial. In a recent

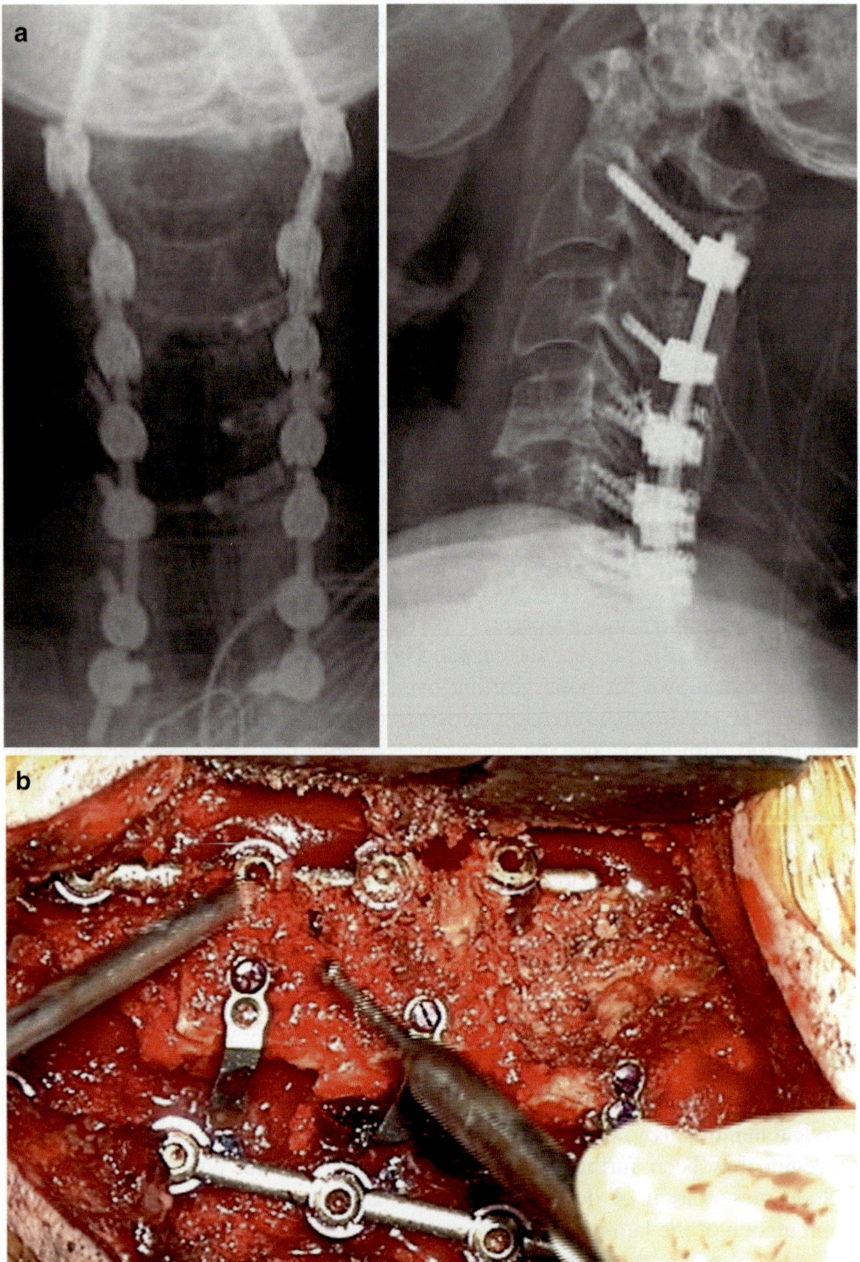

Fig. 11.9 (**a**) Radiograph images and (**b**) intraoperative depiction of how mini-laminoplasty plates can be used without fixation screws to prop up the laminae or the holes can be enlarged with a bur and the lateral mass screws can be placed thru the hole

meta-analysis on the surgical treatment of cervical spondylotic myelopathy in elderly versus non-elderly patients, older patients had poorer surgical outcomes (lower pre- and postoperative JOA scores) but no difference in complications (e.g., C5 nerve palsy) [105]. Despite these findings, laminoplasty has been shown to provide clinical benefit to even the very elderly (older than 80 years old) [106] . Older patients are likely to deteriorate more rapidly than their younger counterparts; therefore, earlier surgical intervention for the elderly patients with cervical spondylotic myelopathy should be considered.

Generally, laminoplasty techniques can be broadly categorized as either unilateral open-door laminoplasty or bilateral French-door laminoplasty. In open-door laminoplasty, which was originally described by Hirabayashi et al. in 1978, the spinal canal is expanded by hinging the posterior arch on one side of the lamina-facet junction and completing an osteotomy on the contralateral side, which has greater compression and symptoms. Door reclosure has been a concern and resulted in several modifications, such as suture anchor fixation, and the use of bony spacers enhanced with rigid fixation [107–109]. In French-door laminoplasty, which was originally described by Kurokawa et al. in 1982, symmetrical decompression is created by opening the midline spinous processes and hinging this opening on both laminae. Bilateral gutters are created on each lamina to create the "double-door" or "French-door" opening. Meta-analyses comparing these two techniques suggest that neither is superior based on radiological and complication data [110]. Some studies suggest that open-door laminoplasty may result in higher functional outcome and recovery rates [111].

Shiraishi developed a less invasive surgical approach to laminoplasty that takes advantage of intermuscular planes in comparison to the subperiosteal dissection used in the conventional approach, which can result in complete detachment of muscles from the posterior elements of the spine [112]. This approach uses the interval between the tips of adjacent spinous processes in order to expose and divide the right and left interspinales, semispinalis cervicis, and multifidus muscles. According to Kotani et al., the Shiraishi technique can result in considerably less axial neck pain, less range of motion loss, preserved muscle volume, and improved quality of life at a follow-up of 2 years [113].

We prefer to perform a C3 laminectomy instead of a laminoplasty, along with laminoplasties of *C4, C5, and C6 as Takeuchi reported less neck pain, compared to including the C3 level as a laminoplasty [114] (Fig. 11.10). This is because in order get adequate exposure to do a laminoplasty of C3, one has to detach much of the semispinalis cervicis muscle off of its major insertion onto the spinous process of C2. Since the semispinalis cervicis is the major neck extensor muscle, detaching it can lead to cervical kyphosis. Much less exposure is required to perform a C3 laminectomy than a laminoplasty. In addition, a laminoplasty of C3 elevates that lamina in close proximity to the large spinous process of C2, limiting extension at that level. This also has the added benefit.

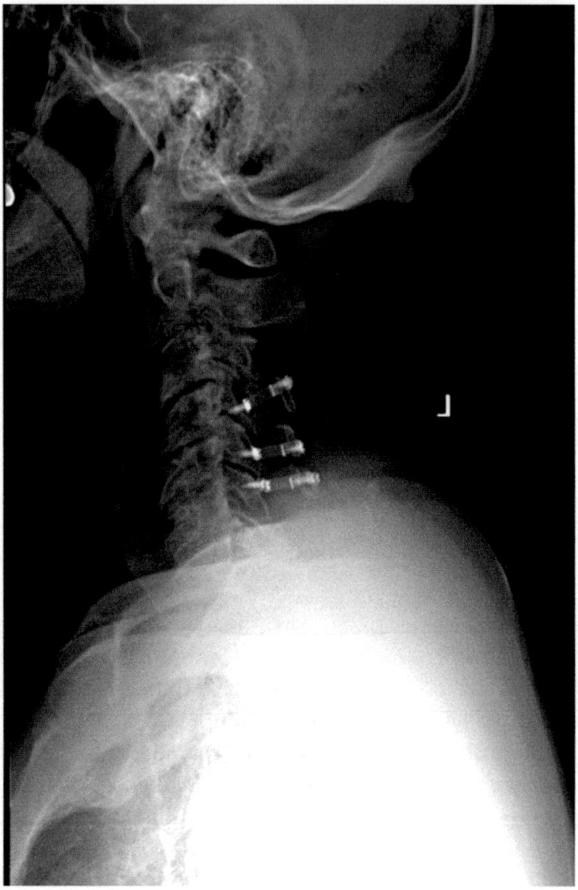

Fig. 11.10 We prefer to perform a C3 laminectomy instead of a laminoplasty, along with laminoplasties of C4, C5, and C6, as Takeuchi reported less neck pain, compared to including the C3 level as a laminoplasty [114]. This is because in order get adequate exposure to do a laminoplasty of C3, one has to detach much of the semispinalis cervicis muscle off of its major insertion onto the spinous process of C2. Since the semispinalis cervicis is the major neck extensor muscle, detaching it can lead to cervical kyphosis. Much less exposure is required to perform a C3 laminectomy than a laminoplasty. In addition, a laminoplasty of C3 elevates that lamina in close proximity to the large spinous process of C2, limiting extension at that level. This also has the added benefit

Laminoplasty Versus ACDF

A number of studies have demonstrated that laminoplasty can achieve similar patient reported outcomes to ACDF, a greater range of cervical motion, and possibly lower complications [115–117]. Liu et al. compared these approaches for those with multilevel cervical spondylotic myelopathy and found that both groups reached similar JOA recovery rates. However, these authors reported that there was a decrease in cervical range of motion and higher complication rates with those who underwent ACDF. In a prospective study, Hirai et al. reported similar JOA scores at 1-year follow-up, but significantly higher JOA scores for the ACDF group at 2-, 3-, and 5-year follow-up. Complications, including dysphagia, dysphonia, and pseudarthrosis, were higher in the ACDF group. The incidence of C5 nerve palsy was higher for laminoplasty. As noted previously, the recent large prospective, controlled multicenter study on myelopathy patients by Ghogawala et al. found that laminoplasty had significantly better SF-36 Physical Component Summary scores

(9.72) when compared with anterior procedures (5.2; $P = 0.04$). Laminoplasty also had a lower major complication rate of 7%, compared to 15% for anterior decompression ($p = 0.04$) [32].

Laminoplasty Versus Laminectomy and Fusion

There is more evidence that support the superiority of laminoplasty over laminectomy and fusion in appropriate candidates. As noted above, the recent large prospective, controlled multicenter study on myelopathy patients by Ghogawala et al. found that laminoplasty had significantly better SF-36 Physical Component Summary scores (9.72) when compared to laminectomy and fusion (4.53; $P = 0.05$). Laminoplasty also had the lowest major complication rate of 7%, compared to 20% for laminectomy and fusion ($p = 0.04$) [32]. In a prior national database study, Varthi et al. reviewed 779 patients who underwent cervical laminoplasty versus posterior decompression and fusion [118, 119]. These authors found that laminectomy/fusion increased LOS, any adverse events (19.7% vs. 11.1%), and readmission risk (7.9% vs. 3.3%).

In a single-surgeon retrospective matched cohort analysis, Woods et al. compared laminoplasty to laminectomy/fusion in 121 patients over a 5-year period with a minimum 6.7 month follow-up period [120]. They found that subjective clinical improvements occurred in both cohorts in regard to gait and pain. Interestingly, laminoplasty patients trended toward a higher overall complication rate (13% vs. 9%) and revision rate (5% vs. 2%); however, there was no statistical significance associated with these differences. This may also be related to surgeon experience and technique. In a meta-analysis, Lee et al. reported similar improvements in JOA scores, VAS scores, and loss of lordosis between those who underwent laminoplasty (302 patients) and those who underwent laminectomy and fusion (290 patients). However, in the sub-analysis of studies with >18 months of follow-up, these authors noted a better lordosis preservation in patients with laminectomy and fusion than those in the laminoplasty cohort. Therefore, it's generally recommended that patients with >10 to 15 degrees of C2-C7 kyphosis should undergo laminectomy and fusion instead of laminoplasty. It's possible that the variability in outcomes depend, at least in part, by the surgical techniques employed. Although laminoplasty is a motion-sparing procedure, some patients report some loss of range of motion after surgery. Some even report a loss of lordosis, but this may be technique dependent. For example, disruption of the semispinalis cervicis attachments to the spinous processes, especially to C2, during a posterior cervical approach can result in kyphosis, and possibly worse axial neck pain [121]. Loss of the C7 spinous process, which serves as an important structure for the extensor muscle complex, may also result in worse cervical kyphosis and axial neck pain. Therefore, it is important to preserve the semispinalis cervicis muscle attachments to C2 and avoid a C7 laminoplasty, if possible.

Conclusion

Overall, there are several good surgical options for treating cervical disease in the elderly spine. We reviewed a number of important considerations including cervical alignment, the location of pathology, the number of levels involved, the presence of OPLL, revision surgery, and several common approach-related complications. The main advantage of the anterior approach is the direct decompression of anterior pathology, restoration of sagittal alignment, and lower risk for wound complications. As we have described, there are a number of options with the anterior approach including ACDF, ACCF, HCCF, hybrid fusions, and cervical disc arthroplasty. These surgeries offer some significant advantages over posterior-based operations in properly selected patients with amenable pathology. Posterior-based surgeries can effectively provide indirect decompression and achieve similar outcomes to an anterior-based surgery. Posterior cervical surgeries include laminoplasty and laminectomy with or without fusion. In comparison to anterior fusion cases for multilevel disease, laminoplasty may offer a viable, motion-preserving option for patients. In cases where there is true equipoise between an anterior and posterior surgical approach, a well-preformed procedure with meticulous surgical technique can achieve comparable outcomes with either approach. The expert spine surgeon should be aware of the risks and benefits of each surgical technique in order to best address the patient's their goals and expectations for surgery.

References

1. Fehlings MG, Tetreault LA, Riew KD, Middleton JW, Aarabi B, Arnold PM, et al. A clinical practice guideline for the Management of Patients with Degenerative Cervical Myelopathy: recommendations for patients with mild, moderate, and severe disease and nonmyelopathic patients with evidence of cord compression. Global Spine J. 2017;7(3 Suppl):70s–83s.
2. Badhiwala JH, Ahuja CS, Akbar MA, Witiw CD, Nassiri F, Furlan JC, et al. Degenerative cervical myelopathy—update and future directions. Nat Rev Neurol. 2020;16(2):108–24.
3. Marquez-Lara A, Nandyala SV, Fineberg SJ, Singh K. Current trends in demographics, practice, and in-hospital outcomes in cervical spine surgery: a national database analysis between 2002 and 2011. Spine. 2014;39(6):476–81.
4. Oglesby M, Fineberg SJ, Patel AA, Pelton MA, Singh K. Epidemiological trends in cervical spine surgery for degenerative diseases between 2002 and 2009. Spine. 2013;38(14):1226–32.
5. Passias PG, Marascalchi BJ, Boniello AJ, Yang S, Bianco K, Jalai CM, et al. Cervical spondylotic myelopathy: national trends in the treatment and peri-operative outcomes over 10 years. J Clin Neurosci. 2017;42:75–80.
6. Ortman SLCaJM. Projections of the Size and Composition of the U.S. Population: 2014 to 2060. Population Estimates and Projections. In: Administration USDoCEaS, editor.: United States Census Bureau; 2015. p. 25–1143.
7. Jalai CM, Worley N, Marascalchi BJ, Challier V, Vira S, Yang S, et al. The impact of advanced age on peri-operative outcomes in the surgical treatment of cervical Spondylotic myelopathy: a Nationwide study between 2001 and 2010. Spine. 2016;41(3):E139–47.

8. Shin JI, Kothari P, Phan K, Kim JS, Leven D, Lee NJ, et al. Frailty index as a predictor of adverse postoperative outcomes in patients undergoing cervical spinal fusion. Spine. 2017;42(5):304–10.
9. Di Capua J, Somani S, Kim JS, Phan K, Lee NJ, Kothari P, et al. Elderly age as a risk factor for 30-day postoperative outcomes following elective anterior cervical discectomy and fusion. Global Spine J. 2017;7(5):425–31.
10. Medvedev G, Wang C, Cyriac M, Amdur R, O'Brien J. Complications, readmissions, and reoperations in posterior cervical fusion. Spine. 2016;41(19):1477–83.
11. Guzman JZ, Feldman ZM, McAnany S, Hecht AC, Qureshi SA, Cho SK. Osteoporosis in cervical spine surgery. Spine. 2016;41(8):662–8.
12. Terao S, Sobue G, Hashizume Y, Li M, Inagaki T, Mitsuma T. Age-related changes in human spinal ventral horn cells with special reference to the loss of small neurons in the intermediate zone: a quantitative analysis. Acta Neuropathol. 1996;92(2):109–14.
13. Terao S, Sobue G, Hashizume Y, Shimada N, Mitsuma T. Age-related changes of the myelinated fibers in the human corticospinal tract: a quantitative analysis. Acta Neuropathol. 1994;88(2):137–42.
14. Polanczyk CA, Marcantonio E, Goldman L, Rohde LE, Orav J, Mangione CM, et al. Impact of age on perioperative complications and length of stay in patients undergoing noncardiac surgery. Ann Intern Med. 2001;134(8):637–43.
15. Daubs MD, Lenke LG, Cheh G, Stobbs G, Bridwell KH. Adult spinal deformity surgery: complications and outcomes in patients over age 60. Spine. 2007;32(20):2238–44.
16. Pang J, Ye M, Gu X, Cao Y, Zheng Y, Guo H, et al. Ovariectomy-induced osteopenia influences the middle and late periods of bone healing in a mouse femoral osteotomy model. Rejuvenation Res. 2015;18(4):356–65.
17. Giannoudis PV, Schneider E. Principles of fixation of osteoporotic fractures. J Bone Joint Surg. 2006;88(10):1272–8.
18. Hao YJ, Zhang G, Wang YS, Qin L, Hung WY, Leung K, et al. Changes of microstructure and mineralized tissue in the middle and late phase of osteoporotic fracture healing in rats. Bone. 2007;41(4):631–8.
19. Nakashima H, Tetreault LA, Nagoshi N, Nouri A, Kopjar B, Arnold PM, et al. Does age affect surgical outcomes in patients with degenerative cervical myelopathy? Results from the prospective multicenter AOSpine international study on 479 patients. J Neurol Neurosurg Psychiatry. 2016;87(7):734–40.
20. Kato S, Nouri A, Wu D, Nori S, Tetreault L, Fehlings MG. Comparison of anterior and posterior surgery for degenerative cervical myelopathy: An MRI-based propensity-score-matched analysis using data from the prospective multicenter AOSpine CSM North America and international studies. J Bone Joint Surg Am. 2017;99(12):1013–21.
21. Borden AG, Rechtman AM, Gershon-Cohen J. The normal cervical lordosis. Radiology. 1960;74:806–9.
22. Suda K, Abumi K, Ito M, Shono Y, Kaneda K, Fujiya M. Local kyphosis reduces surgical outcomes of expansive open-door laminoplasty for cervical spondylotic myelopathy. Spine. 2003;28(12):1258–62.
23. Hyun SJ, Kim KJ, Jahng TA, Kim HJ. Clinical impact of T1 slope minus cervical lordosis after multilevel posterior cervical fusion surgery: a minimum 2-year follow up data. Spine. 2017;42(24):1859–64.
24. Tang JA, Scheer JK, Smith JS, Deviren V, Bess S, Hart RA, et al. The impact of standing regional cervical sagittal alignment on outcomes in posterior cervical fusion surgery. Neurosurgery. 2015;76(Suppl 1):S14–21; discussion S
25. Tang JA, Scheer JK, Smith JS, Deviren V, Bess S, Hart RA, et al. The impact of standing regional cervical sagittal alignment on outcomes in posterior cervical fusion surgery. Neurosurgery. 2012;71(3):662–9; discussion 9

26. Bolesta MJ, Rechtine GR 2nd, Chrin AM. Three- and four-level anterior cervical discectomy and fusion with plate fixation: a prospective study. Spine. 2000;25(16):2040–4; discussion 5-6
27. De la Garza-Ramos R, Bydon A. Erratum: Long-term clinical outcomes following 3- and 4-level anterior cervical discectomy and fusion. J Neurosurg Spine. 2016;24(6):996.
28. Lee DH, Cho JH, Hwang CJ, Lee CS, Cho SK, Kim C, et al. What is the fate of pseudarthrosis detected 1 year after anterior cervical discectomy and fusion? Spine. 2018;43(1):E23–e8.
29. Wang M, Chou D, Chang CC, Hirpara A, Liu Y, Chan AK, et al. Anterior cervical discectomy and fusion performed using structural allograft or polyetheretherketone: pseudarthrosis and revision surgery rates with minimum 2-year follow-up. Journal of neurosurgery. Spine. 2019:1–8.
30. Epstein NE. A review of complication rates for anterior cervical diskectomy and fusion (ACDF). Surg Neurol Int. 2019;10:100.
31. De la Garza-Ramos R, Xu R, Ramhmdani S, Kosztowski T, Bydon M, Sciubba DM, et al. Long-term clinical outcomes following 3- and 4-level anterior cervical discectomy and fusion. J Neurosurg Spine. 2016;24(6):885–91.
32. Edward C. Benzel ZG, Adam Kanter, Praveen V. Mummaneni, Erica Bisson, James Harrop, Robert F. Heary, Michael P. Steinmetz, Michael G. Fehlings, Todd J. Albert, Paul M. Arnold, K. Daniel Riew, Marjorie C. Wang, Jong G. Heller, Fred G. Barker II. A randomized controlled multi-center trial comparing ventral and dorsal surgery for CSM: 2-year results. Cervical Spine Research Society; December 10–12, 2020; Las Vegas, Nevada2020.
33. Wang T, Wang H, Liu S, Ding WY. Incidence of C5 nerve root palsy after cervical surgery: a meta-analysis for last decade. Medicine. 2017;96(45):e8560.
34. Joaquim AF, Murar J, Savage JW, Patel AA. Dysphagia after anterior cervical spine surgery: a systematic review of potential preventative measures. Spine J. 2014;14(9):2246–60.
35. Daniels AH, Riew KD, Yoo JU, Ching A, Birchard KR, Kranenburg AJ, et al. Adverse events associated with anterior cervical spine surgery. J Am Acad Orthop Surg. 2008;16(12):729–38.
36. Fengbin Y, Xinwei W, Haisong Y, Yu C, Xiaowei L, Deyu C. Dysphagia after anterior cervical discectomy and fusion: a prospective study comparing two anterior surgical approaches. Eur Spine J. 2013;22(5):1147–51.
37. Orlando ER, Caroli E, Ferrante L. Management of the cervical esophagus and hypofarinx perforations complicating anterior cervical spine surgery. Spine. 2003;28(15):E290–5.
38. Chen CJ, Saulle D, Fu KM, Smith JS, Shaffrey CI. Dysphagia following combined anterior-posterior cervical spine surgeries. J Neurosurg Spine. 2013;19(3):279–87.
39. Lee MJ, Bazaz R, Furey CG, Yoo J. Risk factors for dysphagia after anterior cervical spine surgery: a two-year prospective cohort study. Spine J. 2007;7(2):141–7.
40. Lee MJ, Bazaz R, Furey CG, Yoo J. Influence of anterior cervical plate design on dysphagia: a 2-year prospective longitudinal follow-up study. J Spinal Disord Tech. 2005;18(5):406–9.
41. Lee SH, Kim KT, Suk KS, Park KJ, Oh KI. Effect of retropharyngeal steroid on prevertebral soft tissue swelling following anterior cervical discectomy and fusion: a prospective, randomized study. Spine. 2011;36(26):2286–92.
42. Vaidya R, Carp J, Sethi A, Bartol S, Craig J, Les CM. Complications of anterior cervical discectomy and fusion using recombinant human bone morphogenetic protein-2. Eur Spine J. 2007;16(8):1257–65.
43. Shields LB, Raque GH, Glassman SD, Campbell M, Vitaz T, Harpring J, et al. Adverse effects associated with high-dose recombinant human bone morphogenetic protein-2 use in anterior cervical spine fusion. Spine. 2006;31(5):542–7.
44. Lee SH, Mesfin A, Riew KD. Delayed esophageal perforation after anterior cervical fusion and retropharyngeal steroid use: a report of two cases. Spine J. 2015;15(10):e75–80.
45. Jung A, Schramm J, Lehnerdt K, Herberhold C. Recurrent laryngeal nerve palsy during anterior cervical spine surgery: a prospective study. J Neurosurg Spine. 2005;2(2):123–7.
46. Apfelbaum RI, Kriskovich MD, Haller JR. On the incidence, cause, and prevention of recurrent laryngeal nerve palsies during anterior cervical spine surgery. Spine. 2000;25(22):2906–12.

47. Yee TJ, Swong K, Park P. Complications of anterior cervical spine surgery: a systematic review of the literature. J Spine Surg. 2020;6(1):302–22.
48. Sebastian A, Huddleston P 3rd, Kakar S, Habermann E, Wagie A, Nassr A. Risk factors for surgical site infection after posterior cervical spine surgery: an analysis of 5,441 patients from the ACS NSQIP 2005-2012. Spine J. 2016;16(4):504–9.
49. Vonck CE, Tanenbaum JE, Bomberger TT, Benzel EC, Savage JW, Kalfas IH, et al. Short-term outcomes following posterior cervical fusion among octogenarians with cervical spondylotic myelopathy: a NSQIP database analysis. Spine J. 2018;18(9):1603–11.
50. Boakye M, Patil CG, Santarelli J, Ho C, Tian W, Lad SP. Cervical spondylotic myelopathy: complications and outcomes after spinal fusion. Neurosurgery. 2008;62(2):455–61; discussion 61–2
51. Yue JK, Upadhyayula PS, Deng H, Sing DC, Ciacci JD. Risk factors for 30-day outcomes in elective anterior versus posterior cervical fusion: a matched cohort analysis. J Craniovertebr Junction Spine. 2017;8(3):222–30.
52. Chen YC, Kuo CH, Cheng CM, Wu JC. Recent advances in the management of cervical spondylotic myelopathy: bibliometric analysis and surgical perspectives. J Neurosurg Spine. 2019;31(3):299–309.
53. Zhang J, Liang Q, Qin D, Song J, An Q, Wang X, et al. The anterior versus posterior approach for the treatment of ossification of the posterior longitudinal ligament in the cervical spine: a systematic review and meta-analysis. J Spinal Cord Med. 2019:1–10.
54. Kim DH, Lee CH, Ko YS, Yang SH, Kim CH, Park SB, et al. The clinical implications and complications of anterior versus posterior surgery for multilevel cervical ossification of the posterior longitudinal ligament; An updated systematic review and meta-analysis. Neurospine. 2019;16(3):530–41.
55. Fraser JF, Härtl R. Anterior approaches to fusion of the cervical spine: a metaanalysis of fusion rates. J Neurosurg Spine. 2007;6(4):298–303.
56. Leven D, Cho SK. Pseudarthrosis of the cervical spine: risk factors, diagnosis and management. Asian Spine J. 2016;10(4):776–86.
57. Koller H, Schmidt R, Mayer M, Hitzl W, Zenner J, Midderhoff S, et al. The stabilizing potential of anterior, posterior and combined techniques for the reconstruction of a 2-level cervical corpectomy model: biomechanical study and first results of ATPS prototyping. Eur Spine J. 2010;19(12):2137–48.
58. Koller H, Schmoelz W, Zenner J, Auffarth A, Resch H, Hitzl W, et al. Construct stability of an instrumented 2-level cervical corpectomy model following fatigue testing: biomechanical comparison of circumferential antero-posterior instrumentation versus a novel anterior-only transpedicular screw-plate fixation technique. Eur Spine J. 2015;24(12):2848–56.
59. Fernyhough JC, White JI, LaRocca H. Fusion rates in multilevel cervical spondylosis comparing allograft fibula with autograft fibula in 126 patients. Spine. 1991;16(10 Suppl):S561–4.
60. Yonenobu K, Fuji T, Ono K, Okada K, Yamamoto T, Harada N. Choice of surgical treatment for multisegmental cervical spondylotic myelopathy. Spine. 1985;10(8):710–6.
61. Reinard KA, Cook DM, Zakaria HM, Basheer AM, Chang VW, Abdulhak MM. A cohort study of the morbidity of combined anterior-posterior cervical spinal fusions: incidence and predictors of postoperative dysphagia. Eur Spine J. 2016;25(7):2068–77.
62. Wewel JT, Brahimaj BC, Kasliwal MK, Traynelis VC. Perioperative complications with multilevel anterior and posterior cervical decompression and fusion. J Neurosurg Spine. 2019:1–6.
63. Farey ID, McAfee PC, Davis RF, Long DM. Pseudarthrosis of the cervical spine after anterior arthrodesis. Treatment by posterior nerve-root decompression, stabilization, and arthrodesis. J Bone Joint Surg Am. 1990;72(8):1171–7.
64. Phillips FM, Carlson G, Emery SE, Bohlman HH. Anterior cervical pseudarthrosis. Natural history and treatment. Spine. 1997;22(14):1585–9.
65. Carreon L, Glassman SD, Campbell MJ. Treatment of anterior cervical pseudoarthrosis: posterior fusion versus anterior revision. Spine J. 2006;6(2):154–6.

66. Kuhns CA, Geck MJ, Wang JC, Delamarter RB. An outcomes analysis of the treatment of cervical pseudarthrosis with posterior fusion. Spine. 2005;30(21):2424–9.
67. Elder BD, Sankey EW, Theodros D, Bydon M, Goodwin CR, Lo SF, et al. Successful anterior fusion following posterior cervical fusion for revision of anterior cervical discectomy and fusion pseudarthrosis. J Clin Neurosci. 2016;24:57–62.
68. Lowery GL, Swank ML, McDonough RF. Surgical revision for failed anterior cervical fusions. Articular pillar plating or anterior revision? Spine. 1995;20(22):2436–41.
69. Gillis CC, Kaszuba MC, Traynelis VC. Cervical radiographic parameters in 1- and 2-level anterior cervical discectomy and fusion. J Neurosurg Spine. 2016;25(4):421–9.
70. Tan LA, Riew KD, Traynelis VC. Cervical spine deformity-part 2: management algorithm and anterior techniques. Neurosurgery. 2017;81(4):561–7.
71. Robinson RASG. Anterolateral cervical disk removal and interbody fusion for cervical disk syndrome. Bull Johns Hopkins Hosp. 1955;96:223–4.
72. Bohlman HH, Emery SE, Goodfellow DB, Jones PK. Robinson anterior cervical discectomy and arthrodesis for cervical radiculopathy. Long-term follow-up of one hundred and twenty-two patients. J Bone Joint Surg Am. 1993;75(9):1298–307.
73. Emery SE, Bolesta MJ, Banks MA, Jones PK. Robinson anterior cervical fusion comparison of the standard and modified techniques. Spine. 1994;19(6):660–3.
74. Wang JC, McDonough PW, Endow KK, Delamarter RB. Increased fusion rates with cervical plating for two-level anterior cervical discectomy and fusion. Spine. 2000;25(1):41–5.
75. Wang JC, McDonough PW, Endow K, Kanim LE, Delamarter RB. The effect of cervical plating on single-level anterior cervical discectomy and fusion. J Spinal Disord. 1999;12(6):467–71.
76. Coric D, Branch CL Jr, Jenkins JD. Revision of anterior cervical pseudoarthrosis with anterior allograft fusion and plating. J Neurosurg. 1997;86(6):969–74.
77. Connolly PJ, Esses SI, Kostuik JP. Anterior cervical fusion: outcome analysis of patients fused with and without anterior cervical plates. J Spinal Disord. 1996;9(3):202–6.
78. van Eck CF, Regan C, Donaldson WF, Kang JD, Lee JY. The revision rate and occurrence of adjacent segment disease after anterior cervical discectomy and fusion: a study of 672 consecutive patients. Spine. 2014;39(26):2143–7.
79. Laratta JL, Reddy HP, Bratcher KR, McGraw KE, Carreon LY, Owens RK 2nd. Outcomes and revision rates following multilevel anterior cervical discectomy and fusion. J Spine Surg. 2018;4(3):496–500.
80. Oliver JD, Goncalves S, Kerezoudis P, Alvi MA, Freedman BA, Nassr A, et al. Comparison of outcomes for anterior cervical discectomy and fusion with and without anterior plate fixation: a systematic review and meta-analysis. Spine. 2018;43(7):e413–e22.
81. Lee NJ, Vulapalli M, Park P, Kim JS, Boddapati V, Mathew J, et al. Does screw length for primary two-level ACDF influence pseudarthrosis risk? Spine J. 2020;20(11):1752–60.
82. Hilibrand AS, Carlson GD, Palumbo MA, Jones PK, Bohlman HH. Radiculopathy and myelopathy at segments adjacent to the site of a previous anterior cervical arthrodesis. J Bone Joint Surg Am. 1999;81(4):519–28.
83. Park JB, Cho YS, Riew KD. Development of adjacent-level ossification in patients with an anterior cervical plate. J Bone Joint Surg Am. 2005;87(3):558–63.
84. Lau D, Chou D, Mummaneni PV. Two-level corpectomy versus three-level discectomy for cervical spondylotic myelopathy: a comparison of perioperative, radiographic, and clinical outcomes. J Neurosurg Spine. 2015;23(3):280–9.
85. Jiang SD, Jiang LS, Dai LY. Anterior cervical discectomy and fusion versus anterior cervical corpectomy and fusion for multilevel cervical spondylosis: a systematic review. Arch Orthop Trauma Surg. 2012;132(2):155–61.
86. Gore DR. The arthrodesis rate in multilevel anterior cervical fusions using autogenous fibula. Spine. 2001;26(11):1259–63.

87. Fountas KN, Kapsalaki EZ, Nikolakakos LG, Smisson HF, Johnston KW, Grigorian AA, et al. Anterior cervical discectomy and fusion associated complications. Spine. 2007;32(21):2310–7.
88. Oh MC, Zhang HY, Park JY, Kim KS. Two-level anterior cervical discectomy versus one-level corpectomy in cervical spondylotic myelopathy. Spine. 2009;34(7):692–6.
89. Banno F, Zreik J, Alvi MA, Goyal A, Freedman BA, Bydon M. Anterior cervical corpectomy and fusion versus anterior cervical discectomy and fusion for treatment of multilevel cervical Spondylotic myelopathy: insights from a National Registry. World Neurosurg. 2019;132:e852–e61.
90. Riew KD, Sethi NS, Devney J, Goette K, Choi K. Complications of buttress plate stabilization of cervical corpectomy. Spine. 1999;24(22):2404–10.
91. Emery SE, Bohlman HH, Bolesta MJ, Jones PK. Anterior cervical decompression and arthrodesis for the treatment of cervical spondylotic myelopathy. Two to seventeen-year follow-up. J Bone Joint Surg Am. 1998;80(7):941–51.
92. Riew KD. Microscope-assisted anterior cervical decompression and plating techniques for multilevel cervical spondylosis. Oper Tech Orthop. 1998;8(1):22–3.
93. Riew KD. Microscope-Assisted Anterior Cervical Decompression and Plating Techniques for Multilevel Cervical Spondylosis. In: Operative Techniques in Orthopaedics, vol. 8. Amsterdam: Elsevier; 1998. p. 22–33.
94. Joaquim A, Sielatycki J, Riew K. Anterior surgical options for cervical spondylotic myelopathy. Indian Spine J. 2019;2(1):33–41.
95. Findlay C, Ayis S, Demetriades AK. Total disc replacement versus anterior cervical discectomy and fusion: a systematic review with meta-analysis of data from a total of 3160 patients across 14 randomized controlled trials with both short- and medium- to long-term outcomes. Bone Joint J. 2018;100-B(8):991–1001.
96. Coric D, Guyer RD, Nunley PD, Musante D, Carmody C, Gordon C, et al. Prospective, randomized multicenter study of cervical arthroplasty versus anterior cervical discectomy and fusion: 5-year results with a metal-on-metal artificial disc. J Neurosurg Spine. 2018;28(3):252–61.
97. Riew KD, Buchowski JM, Sasso R, Zdeblick T, Metcalf NH, Anderson PA. Cervical disc arthroplasty compared with arthrodesis for the treatment of myelopathy. J Bone Joint Surg Am. 2008;90(11):2354–64.
98. Buchowski JM, Anderson PA, Sekhon L, Riew KD. Cervical disc arthroplasty compared with arthrodesis for the treatment of myelopathy. Surgical technique. J Bone Joint Surg Am. 2009;91(Suppl 2):223–32.
99. Wu JC, Chang HK, Huang WC, Tu TH, Fay LY, Kuo CH, et al. Radiological and clinical outcomes of cervical disc arthroplasty for the elderly: a comparison with young patients. BMC Musculoskelet Disord. 2019;20(1):115.
100. Manzano GR, Casella G, Wang MY, Vanni S, Levi AD. A prospective, randomized trial comparing expansile cervical laminoplasty and cervical laminectomy and fusion for multilevel cervical myelopathy. Neurosurgery. 2012;70(2):264–77.
101. Cho SK, Kim JS, Overley SC, Merrill RK. Cervical laminoplasty: indications, surgical considerations, and clinical outcomes. J Am Acad Orthop Surg. 2018;26(7):e142–e52.
102. Koda M, Mochizuki M, Konishi H, Aiba A, Kadota R, Inada T, et al. Comparison of clinical outcomes between laminoplasty, posterior decompression with instrumented fusion, and anterior decompression with fusion for K-line (−) cervical ossification of the posterior longitudinal ligament. Eur Spine J. 2016;25(7):2294–301.
103. Yoon ST, Raich A, Hashimoto RE, Riew KD, Shaffrey CI, Rhee JM, et al. Predictive factors affecting outcome after cervical laminoplasty. Spine. 2013;38(22 Suppl 1):S232–52.
104. Fujiyoshi T, Yamazaki M, Kawabe J, Endo T, Furuya T, Koda M, et al. A new concept for making decisions regarding the surgical approach for cervical ossification of the posterior longitudinal ligament: the K-line. Spine. 2008;33(26):E990–3.

105. Takeshima Y, Matsuoka R, Nakagawa I, Nishimura F, Nakase H. Surgical outcome of laminoplasty for cervical Spondylotic myelopathy in an elderly population - potentiality for effective early surgical intervention: a meta-analysis. Neurol Med Chir. 2017;57(7):366–73.
106. Notani N, Miyazaki M, Kanezaki S, Ishihara T, Tsumura H. Surgical outcomes of laminoplasty for cervical spondylotic myelopathy in very elderly patients (older than 80 years): time from symptom onset to surgery and changes in spinal cord signal intensity on MRI. Clin Neurol Neurosurg. 2017;160:78–82.
107. Lee DH, Park SA, Kim NH, Hwang CJ, Kim YT, Lee CS, et al. Laminar closure after classic Hirabayashi open-door laminoplasty. Spine. 2011;36(25):E1634–40.
108. Wang JM, Roh KJ, Kim DJ, Kim DW. A new method of stabilising the elevated laminae in open-door laminoplasty using an anchor system. J Bone Joint Surg. 1998;80(6):1005–8.
109. Yang SC, Niu CC, Chen WJ, Wu CH, Yu SW. Open-door laminoplasty for multilevel cervical spondylotic myelopathy: good outcome in 12 patients using suture anchor fixation. Acta Orthop. 2008;79(1):62–6.
110. Luo W, Li Y, Zhao J, Gu R, Jiang R, Lin F. Open-versus French-door laminoplasty for the treatment of cervical multilevel compressive myelopathy: a meta-analysis. World Neurosurg. 2018;117:129–36.
111. Wiguna I, Magetsari R, Noor Z, Suyitno S, Nindrea RD. Comparative effectiveness and functional outcome of open-door versus French-door laminoplasty for multilevel cervical myelopathy: a meta-analysis. Open Access Maced J Med Sci. 2019;7(19):3348–52.
112. Shiraishi T. A new technique for exposure of the cervical spine laminae. Technical note. J Neurosurg. 2002;96(1 Suppl):122–6.
113. Kotani Y, Abumi K, Ito M, Sudo H, Takahata M, Ohshima S, et al. Minimum 2-year outcome of cervical laminoplasty with deep extensor muscle-preserving approach: impact on cervical spine function and quality of life. Eur Spine J. 2009;18(5):663–71.
114. Takeuchi K, Yokoyama T, Aburakawa S, Saito A, Numasawa T, Iwasaki T, et al. Axial symptoms after cervical laminoplasty with C3 laminectomy compared with conventional C3-C7 laminoplasty: a modified laminoplasty preserving the semispinalis cervicis inserted into axis. Spine. 2005;30(22):2544–9.
115. Fang Z, Tian R, Sun TW, Yadav SK, Hu W, Xie SQ. Expansion open-door laminoplasty with foraminotomy versus anterior cervical discectomy and fusion for coexisting multilevel cervical myelopathy and unilateral radiculopathy. Clin Spine Surg. 2016;29(1):E21–7.
116. Seng C, Tow BP, Siddiqui MA, Srivastava A, Wang L, Yew AK, et al. Surgically treated cervical myelopathy: a functional outcome comparison study between multilevel anterior cervical decompression fusion with instrumentation and posterior laminoplasty. Spine J. 2013;13(7):723–31.
117. Montano N, Ricciardi L, Olivi A. Comparison of anterior cervical decompression and fusion versus laminoplasty in the treatment of multilevel cervical Spondylotic myelopathy: a meta-analysis of clinical and radiological outcomes. World Neurosurg. 2019;130:530–6.e2.
118. Varthi AG, Basques BA, Bohl DD, Golinvaux NS, Grauer JN. Perioperative outcomes after cervical laminoplasty versus posterior decompression and fusion: analysis of 779 patients in the ACS-NSQIP database. Clin Spine Surg. 2016;29(5):E226–32.
119. Boniello A, Petrucelli P, Kerbel Y, Horn S, Bortz CA, Brown AE, et al. Short-term outcomes following cervical laminoplasty and decompression and fusion with instrumentation. Spine. 2019;44(17):E1018–e23.
120. Woods BI, Hohl J, Lee J, Donaldson W 3rd, Kang J. Laminoplasty versus laminectomy and fusion for multilevel cervical spondylotic myelopathy. Clin Orthop Relat Res. 2011;469(3):688–95.
121. Riew KD, Raich AL, Dettori JR, Heller JG. Neck pain following cervical laminoplasty: does preservation of the C2 muscle attachments and/or C7 matter? Evid Based Spine Care J. 2013;4(1):42–53.

Chapter 12
Cervical Spine Disease in Elderly Patients with Ankylosing Spondylitis

Johnson Ku, Jason Ku, Chieh-Yi Chen, Hsuan-Kan Chang, and Jau-Ching Wu

Background and Etiology

Ankylosing spondylitis (AS), also known as Bechterew's disease, is a type of peripheral or axial spondyloarthropathy (a heterogeneous group of rheumatic diseases with common clinical and genetic features). It is a common inflammatory, rheumatic autoimmune disease that affects the axial skeleton via chronic inflammation in the spine. These inflammations can lead to fibrosis and calcification, resulting in loss of flexibility, and fusion of the spine into an immobile element with a "bamboo" appearance. Inflammation of the sacroiliac joint also occurs [1].

Idiopathic seronegative involvement of the cervical and lumbar spine remains a pressing issue and complicates early radiographic and OPD diagnoses [2]. Main clinical manifestations include back pain and progressive spinal rigidity as well as inflammation of the hips, shoulders, peripheral joints, and fingers/toes. In addition, there are extra-articular manifestations, such as acute anterior uveitis, psoriasis, and inflammatory bowel disease (IBD). However, AS progression in the cervical spine

J. Ku · J. Ku
University of California, Los Angeles, CA, USA
e-mail: jajousa@ucla.edu; jjj357@g.ucla.edu

C.-Y. Chen · J.-C. Wu (✉)
School of Medicine, National Yang Ming Chiao Tung University, Taipei City, Taiwan

Department of Neurosurgery, Taipei Veterans General Hospital, Taipei City, Taiwan

H.-K. Chang
School of Medicine, National Yang Ming Chiao Tung University, Taipei City, Taiwan

Department of Neurosurgery, Taipei Veterans General Hospital, Taipei City, Taiwan

Department of Biomedical Imaging and Radiological Sciences, National Yang Ming Chiao Tung University, Taipei City, Taiwan

K.-M. G. Fu et al. (eds.), *Treatment of Spine Disease in the Elderly*,
https://doi.org/10.1007/978-3-031-12612-3_12

remains inadequately addressed, as involvement is typically late but can predominate existing pain and other symptoms [3]. Ankylosing spondylitis of the cervical spine is associated with stiff kyphosis and increased risk of transversal unstable fracture. A spine surgeon may be involved mainly in the management of trauma cases, but in some situations, corrective surgery of a kyphotic cervical deformity is needed [3].

Immune cells and innate cytokines have been suggested to be crucial to the pathogenesis of AS, especially the human leukocyte antigen and the interleukin axis; however, the pathogenesis of AS remains unclear. Etiology of AS can be grouped into several categories, with main genetic factors being key areas of recent interest. One of the most important genetic factors is major histocompatibility complex (MHC) class I allele HLA-B27, which was discovered in 1973 [4]. Despite the unclear pathomechanism, HLA-B27 has been associated with the prevalence of AS in different populations around the world [5]. Studies have shown that 90–95% of AS patients are HLA-B27 positive, while 1–2% of HLA-B27-positive populations develop AS. This number increased to 15–20% for those with an affected first-degree relative [6]. The familial tendency of AS was remarkable with relative risks of 94, 25, and 4 for first-, second-, and third-degree relatives, respectively [6]. In addition to the association with the genesis of AS, HLA-B27-positive patients showed a significantly lower average onset age and a higher prevalence of acute anterior uveitis than did HLA-B27-negative patients [6].

Epidemiology and Risk Factors

Variations in AS prevalence depend on geography, demographics, and database information that represent diverse cohorts and study groups. A cross-sectional survey in 2012 estimated the prevalence of AS in the United States to be 0.9 to 1.4% of the adult population, similar to that of rheumatoid arthritis [7].

A more recent 2018 analysis of currently published epidemiological data, conducted by the Department of Rheumatology at Columbia University, on AS prevalence found a range of between 9 and 30 individuals per 10,000 persons [7]. Variations across different countries were reported as ranging from 9 individuals per 10,000 persons in a study conducted on two indigenous Oaxaca Mexican populations [8] to 14 to 48 individuals per 10,000 persons in two randomly selected Shantou Chinese populations [9].

In addition to established genetic risk factors involving more than 100 loci and the HLA B-27 marker, two additional studies mentioned in the 2018 review found significant factors associated with increased or decreased AS development later on in life.

Montoya et al. reported decreased AS incidence among breastfed individuals compared to their non-breastfed siblings. Of 203 study patients with AS, 57% were breastfed, compared with 72% of 293 unaffected siblings, indicating that breastfeeding was protective (odds ratio 0.53; 95% CI 0.36, 0.77) among candidates.

These findings suggest that early life gut microbiota cultivation may have protective benefits against AS development [10].

More research with long-term follow-up data is needed to better understand non-genetic factor effects on AS development across diverse demographic groups and geographic regions.

Medical Treatments for AS

Pharmacologic interventions focus on alleviating symptoms while reducing chronic inflammation and reducing radiographic progression rates. Traditional drugs aimed at treating AC have mainly revolved around the utilization of nonsteroidal anti-inflammatory drugs (NSAIDs), anti-TNF-α (TNFi) factors, and monoclonal antibody target therapies. However, recent developments in the realm of nanotechnology-driven drug delivery systems and in AI and technological modeling have shown promising results for AS management.

Tumor necrosis factors (TNF) belong to a group of pro-inflammatory cytokines with roles in AS pathways. Inhibiting TNF-mediated inflammatory pathways therefore prevent radiographic progression and alleviate symptoms even among cervically involved AS patients. Maas and colleagues investigated how TNF inhibitors (TNFi) affect the C-spine, with their results indicating that cervical facet joints and vertebral bodies decreased the ankylosing rate [11]. For nonresponsive NSAID patients, TNF inhibitor (TNFi) therapy not only effectively inhibits AS progression but also decreases inflammation via binding and blocking TNF cytokines, which recent studies have shown improves spinal mobility, pain, and fatigue. Common TNFi's used in late-stage AS to treat radiological cervical changes include adalimumab, etanercept, golimumab, and infliximab.

Infliximab is now approved in Europe for the treatment of AS patients with severe axial symptoms, elevated serological markers of inflammatory activity, and an inadequate response to conventional therapy. The first study to assess the effects of infliximab in AS patients was an open pilot trial of 11 individuals who were treated with 3 infusions of infliximab (at weeks 0, 2, and 6), in a dosage of 5 mg/kg. This study found improvement of ≥50% in activity, function, and pain scores in 9 of 10 patients. After 4 weeks, the median improvement in the Bath Ankylosing Spondylitis Disease Activity Index (BASDAI) was 70%. These benefits lasted for at least 6 weeks [12].

Cervical Spine Fracture in the Elderly

Manifestations of AS typically begin before the third decade and present slow but steady progression [13]. Compared to the general population, patients with AS are at higher risk of spinal fracture and subsequent spinal cord injury (SCI) [14]. Spine fractures in AS patients result in poorer outcomes due to systemic organ involvement of AS, with increased incidence of hypertension, cardiovascular mortality, and pulmonary disease. There is a fourfold increase in fracture risk among AS patients compared to the general population, with lifetime incidences of 5–15% [15]. The estimated vertebral fracture prevalence ranges from 4% to 18%, with annual an incidence up to 1.3% [16].

It is proposed that AS patients are prone to falling due to poor sagittal balance, pelvic retroversion, and altered knee bending and gait while walking. These conditions coupled with the compromised horizontal gaze due to kyphotic deformity, and other risk factors including old age, advanced disease, kyphosis and alcohol-use negatively impact balance [15]. Fusion of the cervical spine renders it vulnerable to trauma [17]. In a recent study using the nationwide inpatient sample (NIS) database from 2005 to 2011, 53% of fractures were located in the cervical spine, 41.9% were thoracic, 18.2% in the lumbar, and 1.5% in sacrum [18]. Most fractures were located on the vertebral level. Osteoporosis is another well-known complication of AS systemic involvement. Ligamentous ossification may occur on disc and joint capsules in AS patients. Weakened mechanical strength, especially on the vertebral level and the fracture on the vertebral level, should be considered as a combined result of osteoporosis and ligamentous ossification.

Unstable cervical fractures can still occur even after minor trauma or low energy impacts [17]. Low energy impacts such as falls from a standing or sitting position are a major cause of fractures (65.8%) in AS. Fractures mostly occur in the intervertebral disc (IVD) due to degradation of the IVD and chondroid metaplasia and loss of elasticity due to calcification of the annulus fibrosis, making IVD the weakest point of the AS spine [17]. Due to ligamentous ossification, injury often occurs as three-column injuries with unstable status [15]. Combined unstable fractures of the cervical spine and esophageal injuries have been reported in AS patients, even after minor trauma. A case report found during surgery the esophagus entrapped within the fracture, a relatively unusual presentation in AS-related fractures [19].

Neurological complications are common in AS-related fractures. AS with spinal fractures is highly associated with spinal cord injury (SCI). According to a large systemic review, SCI is present in 67.2% of spinal fractures within AS patients, with accompanying diverse neurologic function impairment [17]. SCI can be caused by dislocation, cord contusion or compression by fractured bone segments, ossified posterior ligamentum, herniated disc, or an epidural hematoma in AS patients with cervical spine fractures [15]. Secondary deterioration from collar usage, transportation, or manipulation in the posttreatment phase (after admission to posttreatment 3 months) is not uncommon, with a prevalence of 13.9% being reported in a corresponding systemic review [17]. Prognosis in AS patients with cervical fractures is relatively poor, with 6.4% and 11.3% mortality in surgically treated and conservatively treated patients, respectively, after short-term follow-up posttreatment. Also, the most relevant cause of mortality is pneumonia or respiratory failure [17].

Cervical fractures in AS patients can be easily overlooked due to chronic neck pain, or visual obfuscation by a humping shoulder on X-ray film, especially should the fracture take place at the lower cervical spine or cervicothoracic junction. Moreover, it is usually difficult to interpret the X-ray film due to distorted anatomy and osteoporosis in AS cases [15]. More than half of the cervical fractures were not discernible on C-spine X-ray film alone. Computed tomography (CT) scans should be routinely examined for any AS patient suspected of spinal fracture, while MRI can serve as an adjunct in evaluating soft tissue and spinal cord status, especially in patients suffering from neurological deficits [16].

There is an issue of delayed cervical fracture diagnoses in AS patients. Studies indicate that 17.1% of fractures are identified within 24 h following trauma. These fractures remain unnoticed until delayed development of neurological deficits present [17]. Delayed diagnosis may result from a history of rather minor trauma and difficulty in the interpretation of spinal radiographs.

The standard management of cervical fractures in AS patients include conservative and surgical treatments. Conservative treatments involve bed rest, Halo vests, collars, and orthosis. Most of the patients who undergo conservative management are mainly those at high surgical risk or who refuse aggressive management [17]. However, C-spine immobilization in unstable fractures is important in initial management. Careful evaluation of the preexisting spinal configuration is mandatory before applying a traditional collar, whereas inappropriate outfitting of traditional collars may cause hyperextension and further malpositioning of the fracture site, which in turn increases the risk of SCI [15]. Traction should be gentle, starting from low weight traction (<5 to 10 pounds), with force vectors directed anteriorly and superiorly [15]. Traction should be due to weakness of the paraspinal muscle and high instability. The head and upper back need to be supported by pillows or rolls in kyphotic cases [15]. The aim of traction is to restore previous alignment, which is usually kyphosis in AS patients, and to prevent secondary deterioration and facilitate fracture healing [15].

Surgery is usually inevitable in AS patients with cervical fractures. Surgical indications involve deterioration of neurological status, unstable fracture configurations, presence of epidural hematoma, or bony fragment compression that cause neurologic deterioration. Surgical choices vary according to patient condition. In an acute injury without significant deformity, one should consider treatment through anterior fusion or posterior fusion alone, depending on the fracture site. Acute and chronic injuries with deformities could first undergo light cervical traction for reduction. If the patient can remain prone, posterior fusion may be performed. Open reduction should be performed if close reduction with traction fails [20]. Sufficient decompressive laminectomy should be performed with a posterior approach if spinal cord compression is evident. Local bone harvesting for bone fusion is optional, while iliac crest bone grafts remain the gold standard for fusion material. The additional wound, however, may cause pain and immobilization that could lead to further complications. Thus, local bone harvesting from the spinous process for posterior approach cases, and allograft bone or cage with bone extenders for anterior approach cases, is also a viable option [20].

Anterior approaches can be difficult due to chin-on-chest deformities and potential blockage of surgical corridors. However, an anterior approach may be a viable choice if the patient cannot tolerate a prone position due to an AS-related cardiac-pulmonary condition [18]. Anterior fixation alone may result in implant loosening due to forces from the posterior column. A 50% failure rate for initial anterior fixation has been reported [18]. For posterior approaches, the number of fixations should be carried out at least two levels above and below. Long segment fixation provides the strongest stability [21]. Cervical pedicle screws allow the most powerful forces biomechanically, but are technically demanding. According to most studies, lateral mass screw fixation is strong enough. However, the construct should be extended below the cervicothoracic junction with thoracic pedicle screws in cases of lower cervical fractures, which are most of the cases where cervical fractures take place.

A combined anterior and posterior approach may be necessary when the spinal vertebral structure is significantly compromised, especially with marked kyphotic deformities at the fracture site (Fig. 12.1) [21]. However high pulmonary-related complication risks, probably due to longer surgical time and immobilization period, should be noted [18]. Some authors advocate circumferential fixation and fusion due to cervical fractures in AS always extending across anterior to posterior elements. A single approach may not be able to offer enough stability in most of the cases [21]. Poor bone quality in AS patients is also a

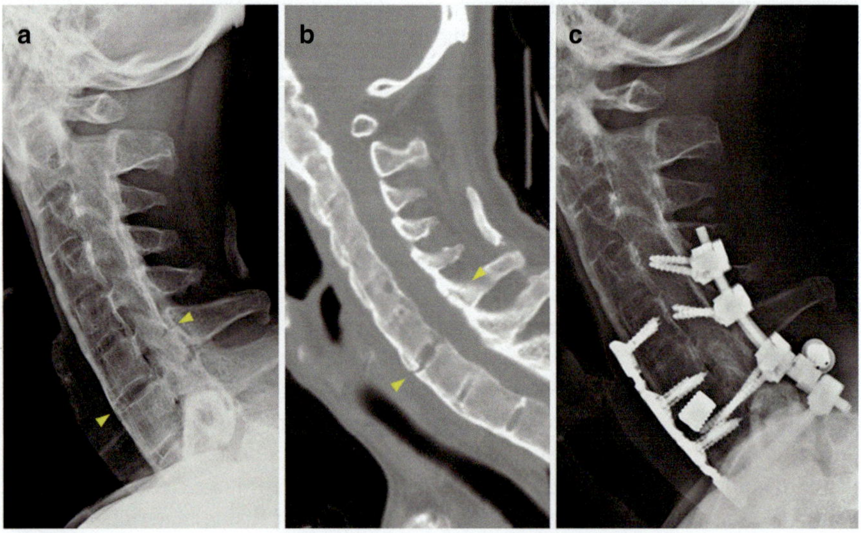

Fig. 12.1 A 54-year-old AS patient with a falling accident and severe neck pain. (**a**) Plain lateral film showed a subtle fracture over C6-C7 (arrow heads), which can be easily missed. (**b**) CT showed a three-column fracture from the C6-C7 intervertebral disc space to the C6 posterior column (arrow heads). (**c**) Plain lateral film after C6-C7 ACDF and C4-T1 posterior fixation. A long construct is often necessary for cervical fractures among AS patients

consideration for circumferential fixation. Etka et al. reviewed the NIS database from 2003 to 2014 and recognized a shift in surgical approaches from combined anterior and posterior fusion to posterior or anterior fusion alone, with posterior fusion being the most commonly performed option. In summary, the selected approach should be individualized, depending on fracture location and patient characteristics.

Overall, surgically treated patients are likely to have more neurologic improvements and less complications compared to nonsurgically treated ones. Surgical treatment is highly suggested for patients with unstable fractures or with neurological symptoms. A large retrospective review showed a mortality rate of 51% in the nonoperative group versus 23% in the operative group, with age >70 being a major risk factor [15]. Conservative treatments may lead to worse fracture healing with pseudoarthrodesis [18]. Surgical treatment for cervical fractures in AS patients remains challenging for spine surgeons. Osteoporosis and long lever length in such cases are more likely to result in instrument failure [20]. Comorbidity of AS, including aortic insufficiency, cardiac conduction abnormalities, uveitis and pulmonary disease, increase the surgical risk and lead to a higher complication rate postoperatively [15].

Cervical Deformity in the Elderly

Cervical kyphotic deformities in AS may be the result of prolonged and progressive postural flexion from spondylitic facet pain and auto-fusion in fixed flexion deformities. With the nature of osteoporosis, AS kyphotic deformities can also be aggravated by subtle cervical fractures that heal with poor alignment [22]. The kyphotic deformity can cause sagittal imbalance with general soreness and fatigue. In extreme cases a large chin-brow vertical angle (CBVA), so-called chin-on-chest deformities, difficulty of forward/upward vision and swallowing can further compromise patients' quality of life.

Flexion and extension radiographic films are often taken for the evaluation of remaining flexibility in fused AS spines or evaluation of subtle fractures with instabilities. AS disease progression and the ability to compensate should also be taken into consideration when making treatment plans. In general, treatment for AS deformity works under the same thinking processes, with treatment for adult spinal deformity taking precedence, along with taking global sagittal and coronal balance into consideration. Generally, AS patients with universal kyphosis and sagittal imbalances that need surgical correction and corrective hip surgery are first considered, followed by thoracolumbar deformity correction patients. Improvement in thoracic and lumbar alignment may significantly improve the T1 slope, C2-C7 SVA, and CBVA, thereby potentially sparing the need for further cervical kyphotic deformity surgery. However, correction of cervical kyphosis may still be indicated in AS patients without thoracolumbar (TL) deformities.

CBVA is the most important parameter for correcting AS cervical kyphotic deformity. Song et al. suggest a CBVA between 10° and 20° for optimal daily function and appearance [23]. Overcorrection of CBVA may also affect downward gaze and therefore compromise walking ability. However, the optimal CBVA should be tailored to meet individual needs. In addition to cervical/thoracic CT and MRI for preoperative planning, CT angiography is arranged for evaluation of vertebral artery courses in the evaluation of aggressive osteotomies. Cardiopulmonary function evaluation should also be considered throughout the procedure, due to the patient being placed in a prolonged prone or concord position.

For surgical correction of kyphotic deformities, a three-column osteotomy through a posterior approach is usually performed over the C7 level for better C2-C7 SVA and CBVA correction. Anatomically, the vertebral artery (VA) usually enters the transverse foramen at C6. Selecting C7 as the osteotomy level not only avoids injury to the VA but also could be beneficial due to a wider spinal canal and sparing of upper extremity function in case of spinal cord injury [22].

During the operation, wide exploration of the cervicothoracic junction is first done following insertion of screws. While lateral mass screws may be used in correction surgery, it is better to use both cervical and thoracic pedicle screws for their stronger pullout strength. A construct at least three levels above and below the osteotomy site is suggested due to general osteoporosis and the long auto-fused AS spine. O-arm navigation can be very helpful, especially as anatomical landmarks are often difficult to identify.

The posterior osteotomy is first done with a C7 laminectomy and bilateral C6-T1 facetectomy. The anterior column osteotomy can be done either using a pedicle subtraction osteotomy (PSO) or Smith-Peterson osteotomy (SPO). Once all three-column osteotomies are done, the rods can be contoured with the desired configuration, and thoracic nuts are tightened. The patient's head, which remains fixed to the Mayfield system, can be unlocked and adjusted to a more extended position gradually, and kyphosis can be corrected until satisfied positioning is reached. Neuromonitoring, especially motor evoke potential (MEP), should be closely monitored, as translation injury, cord compression from the osseous component, or excessive dura impingement may occur at this stage of correction.

Several osteotomy techniques are mentioned throughout current literature. SPO was first adapted to treat cervical kyphosis patients by Mason et al. [24] and Urist et al. [25] in the 1950s. With the SPO technique came the advantage of larger degrees of correction with less posterior element and spinal canal shortening. Some authors suggested an additional anterior approach osteotomy prior to the SPO procedure for anterior release [22]. Recently, Maciejczak et al. [26] reported a case of the modified SPO procedure using a crosswise osteotomy over the pedicles, reaching the anterior vertebral body to prevent aberrant osteoclasis. A downside to the technique is that it is very technically demanding.

All corrective surgeries for AS kyphotic deformities are very challenging. Complications may include spinal cord injury, C8 root injury during osteotomy, or neural foramen stenosis after correction. Other complications include postoperative dysphagia, or nonunion with pseudarthrosis [22].

Navigation Technology for the Surgical Treatment of Ankylosing Spondylitis

There is a scarcity of studies investigating the application of navigation technologies for surgical treatment in AS cases. Screw placement can be challenging in AS patients due to distorted anatomy. Guided imaging technology provides real-time orientation and device implant accuracy, which may decrease postoperative complications and/or failed surgeries in AS cervical spine cases. A study demonstrated that surgical treatment of cervical spine fractures in AS patients via posterior stabilization using CT scanner-based navigation intraoperatively resulted in a 4.5% inadequate anatomical insertion rate. Neither screw malposition nor any other intraoperative events were complicated by any neural, vascular, or visceral injury, and follow-up indicated complete bone fusion of the anterior part of the spinal column and lateral masses at one year follow-up. CT-guided posterior cervical stabilization may be a reliable and safe method for addressing C-spine complications and fractures among AS patients [27]. However, the use of navigation technology in AS cases requires more studies and evidence.

Nanomedicine: A Novel Treatment

Recent advancements in the realm of nanomedicine allow for longer drug retention at the targeted delivery site. Although there is currently no standard nano-based drug therapy for AS, well-established nano-preparations, such as liposomes, polymeric nanoparticles, and hydrogels, have already been successfully incorporated in the treatment of other chronic inflammatory diseases, such as osteoarthritis, backache, and RA, and therefore show promise in being a potential alternative in treating AS [28].

Liposomes, which are normally prepared using biodegradable nontoxic lipids, have the ability to hold both hydrophilic and hydrophobic drugs. Liposomal nano-preparations also increase the half-life and retention time of certain liposome-based NSAIDs, such as indomethacin, ibuprofen, etc., which have already been successfully used in the treatments of RA and osteoarthritis. Elron-Gross et al. reported improved retention time of diclofenac after using collagen lipid conjugates to encapsulate the drug, which allowed for slow release in the synovial area [28]. In a more recent example, Rakeshchandra et al. synthesized a peptide ligand ART-1 and encapsulated it in an IL-27-coated liposome (ART-1-IL-27). These nano-prepared liposomes not only displayed significant binding to endothelial cells but also were better able to hone in on arthritic joints when compared to control liposomes in Lewis rat models [29].

Polymeric nanoparticles are prepared using chitosan, poly-lactic acid (PLA), poly-lactic glycolic acid (PLGA), among many others. These particles increase the clinical efficacy of certain NSAID medications like diclofenac, which are well tolerated by patients but have unnecessarily high dosage frequencies when compared to other common NSAIDs, like naproxen, ibuprofen, sulindac, and diflunisal. The use of a slow-release PLGA microparticle containing diclofenac by Tuncay et al. in the treatment of osteoarthritis, for example, has been shown to effectively reduce dosing frequency [30]. In another report, the successful delivery of leukemia inhibitory factors (LIF) conducted by Stephanie et al. utilized fabricated poly(ethylene glycol)-poly(lactic acid) (PEG-PLA) polymer backbone polymeric nanoparticles (NanoLIF), with modified CD-11b antibody surfaces to target peripheral macrophages, and significantly decreased inflammation by inhibiting M1-cell growth over 72 h [31].

AI and Technological Modeling

As first-line agents, nonsteroidal anti-inflammatory drugs (NSAIDS) are initially prescribed to AS patients; however, studies indicate that over 40% of them exhibit NSAID nonresponse. For these nonresponders, second-line drugs such as TNF inhibitors may be prescribed, but guidelines require trials of at least two NSAIDS for at least 3 months, causing delays in effective treatment.

Artificial neural networks (ANN) are modern machine learning models that aim to identify, analyze, and assign early anti-TNF user candidacy with better precision and diagnostic ability than conventional statistical models. The study by Samsung Health Center employed computer models that used demographic (age, sex, height, weight, HLA-B27 status) and laboratory data (white blood cell count, hemoglobin, platelet count, blood urea nitrogen (BUN), creatinine, aspartate transaminase (AST), alanine transaminase (ALT), ESR, and CRP) as baseline characteristics to train an ANN for predicting early TNFi candidate populations. By enrolling AS candidates in both early TNF and non-early TNF user groups, researchers constructed a clinical dataset matrix, which was used to construct the model architecture for the ANN 5 hidden layers and 60 hidden nodes per layer. The ANN model was then trained to predict TNFi user candidacy by combining the data into hyperparameters and then tested against the conventional logistic regression model along with SVM, RF, and XGBoost machine models. The study's ANN model more accurately predicted symptom progression, anti-TNF receptivity, and treatment appropriateness for these AS patients than any of the other models. Results of this ANN model indicates the possibility of training precise machine models using only laboratory data and demographic data recorded in an average clinical setting. Future AI and ANN machine learning model studies should explore expanded parameters from wider datasets beyond a single hospital system [32].

References

1. Zhu W, He X, Cheng K, et al. Ankylosing spondylitis: etiology, pathogenesis, and treatments. Bone Res. 2019;7:22.
2. Britto NMF, Renor BS, Ghizoni E, Tedeschi H, Joaquim AF. Spine surgery in patients with ankylosing spondylitis. Rev Assoc Med Bras (1992). 2018;64(4):379–83.
3. Taurog JD, Chhabra A, Colbert RA. Ankylosing spondylitis and axial Spondyloarthritis. N Engl J Med. 2016;374(26):2563–74.
4. Brewerton DA, Hart FD, Nicholls A, Caffrey M, James DC, Sturrock RD. Ankylosing spondylitis and HL-A 27. Lancet. 1973;1(7809):904–7.
5. Reveille JD. An update on the contribution of the MHC to AS susceptibility. Clin Rheumatol. 2014;33(6):749–57.
6. Reveille JD. The genetic basis of spondyloarthritis. Ann Rheum Dis. 2011;70(Suppl 1):i44–50.
7. Reveille JD, Witter JP, Weisman MH. Prevalence of axial spondylarthritis in the United States: estimates from a cross-sectional survey. Arthritis Care Res (Hoboken). 2012;64(6):905–10.
8. Julian-Santiago F, Garcia-Garcia C, Garcia-Olivera I, Goycochea-Robles MV, Pelaez-Ballestas I. Epidemiology of rheumatic diseases in Mixtec and Chontal indigenous communities in Mexico: a cross-sectional community-based study. Clin Rheumatol. 2016;35(Suppl 1):35–42.
9. Zeng SY, Gong Y, Zhang YP, et al. Changes in the prevalence of rheumatic diseases in Shantou, China, in the past three decades: a COPCORD study. PLoS One. 2015;10(9):e0138492.
10. Montoya J, Matta NB, Suchon P, et al. Patients with ankylosing spondylitis have been breast fed less often than healthy controls: a case-control retrospective study. Ann Rheum Dis. 2016;75(5):879–82.
11. Maas F, Spoorenberg A, Brouwer E, et al. Radiographic damage and progression of the cervical spine in ankylosing spondylitis patients treated with TNF-alpha inhibitors: facet joints vs. vertebral bodies. Semin Arthritis Rheum. 2017;46(5):562–8.
12. Davis JC Jr. Understanding the role of tumor necrosis factor inhibition in ankylosing spondylitis. Semin Arthritis Rheum. 2005;34(4):668–77.
13. Lee HS, Kim TH, Yun HR, et al. Radiologic changes of cervical spine in ankylosing spondylitis. Clin Rheumatol. 2001;20(4):262–6.
14. Lukasiewicz AM, Bohl DD, Varthi AG, et al. Spinal fracture in patients with ankylosing spondylitis: cohort definition, distribution of injuries, and hospital outcomes. Spine (Phila Pa 1976). 2016;41(3):191–6.
15. Chaudhary SB, Hullinger H, Vives MJ. Management of acute spinal fractures in ankylosing spondylitis. ISRN Rheumatol. 2011;2011:150484.
16. Werner BC, Samartzis D, Shen FH. Spinal fractures in patients with ankylosing spondylitis: etiology, diagnosis, and management. J Am Acad Orthop Surg. 2016;24(4):241–9.
17. Westerveld LA, Verlaan JJ, Oner FC. Spinal fractures in patients with ankylosing spinal disorders: a systematic review of the literature on treatment, neurological status and complications. Eur Spine J. 2009;18(2):145–56.
18. Kurucan E, Bernstein DN, Mesfin A. Surgical management of spinal fractures in ankylosing spondylitis. J Spine Surg. 2018;4(3):501–8.
19. Vonhoff CR, Scandrett K, Al-Khawaja D. Minor trauma in ankylosing spondylitis causing combined cervical spine fracture and esophageal injury. World Neurosurg. 2018;119:151–4.
20. Kanter AS, Wang MY, Mummaneni PV. A treatment algorithm for the management of cervical spine fractures and deformity in patients with ankylosing spondylitis. Neurosurg Focus. 2008;24(1):E11.

21. Lazennec JY, d'Astorg H, Rousseau MA. Cervical spine surgery in ankylosing spondylitis: review and current concept. Orthop Traumatol Surg Res. 2015;101(4):507–13.
22. Hoh DJ, Khoueir P, Wang MY. Management of cervical deformity in ankylosing spondylitis. Neurosurg Focus. 2008;24(1):E9.
23. Song K, Su X, Zhang Y, et al. Optimal chin-brow vertical angle for sagittal visual fields in ankylosing spondylitis kyphosis. Eur Spine J. 2016;25(8):2596–604.
24. Mason C, Cozen L, Adelstein L. Surgical correction of flexion deformity of the cervical spine. Calif Med. 1953;79(3):244–6.
25. Urist MR. Osteotomy of the cervical spine; report of a case of ankylosing rheumatoid spondylitis. J Bone Joint Surg Am. 1958;40-A(4):833–43.
26. Maciejczak A, Wolan-Nieroda A, Guzik A. C7 extension crosswise osteotomy: a novel osteotomy for correction of chin-on-chest deformity in a patient with ankylosing spondylitis. J Neurosurg Spine. 2020:1–6.
27. Barsa P, Frohlich R, Adamik J, Suchomel P. Surgical treatment of cervical spine fractures in ankylosing spondylitis patients: posterior stabilization using intraoperative CT scanner-based navigation. Rozhl Chir. 2020;99(5):212–8.
28. Chevalier X. Intraarticular treatments for osteoarthritis: new perspectives. Curr Drug Targets. 2010;11(5):546–60.
29. Meka RR, Venkatesha SH, Moudgil KD. Peptide-directed liposomal delivery improves the therapeutic index of an immunomodulatory cytokine in controlling autoimmune arthritis. J Control Release. 2018;286:279–88.
30. Tuncay M, Calis S, Kas HS, Ercan MT, Peksoy I, Hincal AA. Diclofenac sodium incorporated PLGA (50:50) microspheres: formulation considerations and in vitro/in vivo evaluation. Int J Pharm. 2000;195(1–2):179–88.
31. Davis SM, Reichel D, Bae Y, Pennypacker KR. Leukemia inhibitory factor-loaded nanoparticles with enhanced cytokine metabolic stability and anti-inflammatory activity. Pharm Res. 2018;35(1):6.
32. Lee S, Eun Y, Kim H, Cha HS, Koh EM, Lee J. Machine learning to predict early TNF inhibitor users in patients with ankylosing spondylitis. Sci Rep. 2020;10(1):20299.

Chapter 13
Cervical Spine Deformity in the Elderly

Young Min Lee and Dean Chou

Background

Cervical spine deformity (CSD) is known to negatively affect the healthcare quality of life in patients, and this effect may be particularly pronounced in elderly patients. Specifically, cervical spine deformity in the elderly represents an ever-growing problem of socioeconomic importance, especially in the context of the increasing proportion of the population in the United States that are older than 65 years of age [1]. The literature is sparse on the specific topic of CSD in the elderly, with the majority of publications in the literature focusing on thoracolumbar deformity and its effect on health-related quality of life (HRQOL) measures, but it is anticipated that this will become a topic of wide interest and activity as the population of the US ages. The elderly are particularly afflicted by disorders of CSD, as contributing factors to the development of CSD include prior thoracolumbar malalignment [2], history of prior cervical spine surgery, or consequences of inflammatory disorders, all of which are more likely to occur in the elderly population [3]. While the estimates of overall incidence and prevalence of CSD in the elderly population are lacking in the literature, Smith et al. reported in a multicenter prospective study of 470 patients with thoracolumbar deformity (TLD) with a mean age of 52 years and found that CSD had a prevalence of 52%, highlighting the need for evaluation for CSD in patients with TLD correction [4]. Although it is not as prevalent as TLD, symptomatic CSD can be quite debilitating, and its impact on health has been compared to that of stroke or blindness. It has been predicted that it will become a major area of focus for elderly spinal care in the United States.

Y. M. Lee (✉) · D. Chou
Department of Neurological Surgery, University of California San Francisco, CA, USA
e-mail: young.lee@ucsf.edu; dean.chou@ucsf.edu

K.-M. G. Fu et al. (eds.), *Treatment of Spine Disease in the Elderly*,
https://doi.org/10.1007/978-3-031-12612-3_13

Cervical Spinal Deformity Development in the Elderly

The most common type of CSD in adults is primarily sub-axial in the sagittal plane and manifests as a kyphotic deformity. Coronal plane deformities, such as scoliosis, are overall less common and especially so in the elderly, as they are usually caused by congenital anomalies and are more prevalent in younger patients. Typical pathologic CSD is considered to be kyphotic in nature, and it has been therefore theorized that cervical kyphosis usually increases with increasing age. However, there has been significant controversy regarding this finding, and some recent studies suggest that in patients with normal aging that are asymptomatic, cervical lordosis, not kyphosis, may actually increase [5, 6]. CSD in the sagittal plane is thought to originate from spondylosis in the facet joints. Shedid and Benzel state that with age, increasing facet hypertrophy from degenerative arthrosis can result in a progressively more kyphotic posture causing the development of symptomatic CSD [7]. This compensatory mechanism is thought to relieve pain by reducing the amount of load placed on the overgrown facet joints. With increasing degeneration as patients age, there is decreased range of motion of the cervical spine. This has been born out by Yukawa et al., who found that the C2-C7 range of motion in the third decade of life was 68 degrees compared to 45 degrees in the eight decade of life in asymptomatic healthy volunteers [7]. Most of this loss of range of motion occurred with extension, which is consistent with the theory of facet-initiated spondylosis and with the theory that degenerative changes are responsible for kyphosis initially, not vice-versa. However, in contrast to symptomatic age-related cervical kyphosis, asymptomatic patients may actually have increasing lordosis with increasing age. For example, a recent study by Kim et al. studied the radiographs of 104 patients with various types of thoracolumbar deformity who were asymptomatic from the perspective of their cervical spine. They found that with increasing age, cervical lordosis significantly increases in this asymptomatic group. This replicated the findings of prior studies in the general population (without spinal deformity or symptoms), which reported increasing rates of cervical lordosis with increasing age [5, 8, 9]. Interestingly, there was no correlation between radiographic cervical degeneration and cervical lordosis. In contrast to the cervical lordosis that develops with age in asymptomatic patients, causes of pathologic kyphotic CSD include advanced degenerative disease, prior trauma, inflammatory disorders (such as ankylosing spondylitis or rheumatoid arthritis), and cancer or can be iatrogenic after surgery. In the elderly population, however, the most common cause is iatrogenic development of CSD after prior laminectomy is post-laminectomy kyphosis [10]. It is estimated that the incidence of post-laminectomy kyphosis may be as high as 21% in patients undergoing a dorsal-only approach without posterior spinal instrumentation. This may be related to the preoperative kyphosis that has not been addressed during the index surgery or disruption of the posterior tension band that supports the cervical spine. Although there is not a clear association between laminectomy and development of post-laminectomy kyphosis in patients with normal preoperative cervical alignment, there is good evidence to suggest the presence of preoperative kyphosis puts patients at a significantly higher risk of kyphotic deformity after laminectomy [11, 12]. Kyphotic deformity is particularly common after laminectomy as the majority (64%) of cervical spine axial load bearing occurs through the posterior columns, including the articular processes and facet joints [13]. Loss of the integrity of this posterior column through disruption of the posterior tension band and/or the posterior facet complex can cause an initial loss of sagittal cervical alignment, shifting the weight-bearing axis anteriorly. This places the already weakened posterior cervical musculature at a mechanical disadvantage, eventually causing progression of kyphosis. For this reason, most authors recommend that the insertion of the semispinalis cervicis and capitis muscles into the C2 be preserved when performing a laminectomy, as these muscles have been shown to support neck extension [14]. As kyphosis progresses, patients may not be able to maintain upright head posture, affecting mobility and increasing the likelihood of falls. Secondary myelopathy may also occur as a complication, as the cervical spinal cord can "drape" over the kyphotic aspect of the vertebral bodies, causing increased tension and decreased blood flow to the spinal cord, leading to the development of myelopathy. To help prevent this complication, meticulous facet preservation and keeping the posterior tension band intact would be critical.

Evaluation for Surgery in Cervical Spine Deformity in the Elderly

Initial Evaluation

As with any patient being evaluated for surgery, a thorough history and physical examination is the basis of surgical decision-making. As elderly CSD is highly correlated with the presence of cervical myelopathy, there must be screening for symptoms of myelopathy that include the following: urinary changes, gait issues, hyperreflexia, pyramidal signs (Hoffman's sign, Romberg's), weakness, and loss of dexterity. Elderly patients may have a significant medical history, and a general medical evaluation into the presence of comorbidities, such as cardiovascular disease, respiratory disease, tobacco use, drug use, and prior infectious history, should be obtained. Evaluation of medical frailty will help risk-stratify patients for different surgical approaches or even exclude patients from CSD corrective surgery.

Patients should also be evaluated for their quality of life and disability. Studies have shown that cervical deformity exists in a significant percentage of the population, but these deformities are completely asymptomatic [15, 16]. Just because a patient has a cervical deformity does not necessarily mean it needs treatment. Issues such as pain, disability, ability to see the horizon, and activities of daily life should be taken into consideration.

Radiographic Evaluation

Radiographic evaluation should include 36-inch scoliosis radiographs, including an assessment of global sagittal and coronal alignment. The chin-brow angle should be captured, as well as the C2 to C2 cervical sagittal vertical axis (cSVA). In addition, computed tomography (CT) to assess the bony anatomy and magnetic resonance imaging (MRI) to assess spinal cord anatomy yield a more complete picture. The CT can detect presence of ankylosis, either of the disc spaces or the facets. If the anterior column and facets are fused, CSD correction may become much more difficult, often requiring a multistage surgical intervention, including posterior column release prior to anterior correction followed by posterior instrumentation. This can necessitate a closer assessment of patient frailty and goals of surgery. The flexibility of the CSD is also important to assess and can be performed via lateral flexion/extension cervical radiographs. A posterior-only approach may be an option, if the CSD is flexible with open anterior disc spaces and if the deformity corrects upon extension of the cervical spine.

The specific assessment of radiographic parameters (such as cervical lordosis, C2-C7 sagittal vertical axis, chin-brow vertical angle, T1 slope, T1 pelvic angle (TPA)) should be considered. Parameters to evaluate for include the following: (1) cervical kyphosis (C2-C7 Cobb angle greater than 10 degrees), (2) cervical scoliosis (coronal Cobb angle greater than 10 degrees), (3) C2-C7 sagittal-vertical axis (cSVA) > 4 cm, or (4) chin-brow vertical angle (CBVA) less than −10° or greater than 10° [17, 18].

Surgical Planning

Surgical planning in the elderly should be performed with a focus on the goals of surgery, specific to the individual patient but in generally to include correction of CSD with ability to maintain horizontal gaze, decompress the neural elements, and restore alignment of the cervical spine.

As described by Tan et al., a list of factors that are important for surgery when planning CD correction include the following: (1) presence of neural compression and any associated neurologic symptoms, (2) flexibility of the deformity, (3) presence of anterior or posterior ankylosis, (4) location of the deformity, (5) prior surgery, (6) presence of degenerative changes at other vertebral levels particularly at the proximal/distal end vertebral levels and the cervicothoracic junction, and (7) general medical status and presence of medical comorbidities.

The location of kyphotic deformity helps determine where correction should occur and what type of surgery will be necessary.

Location of kyphotic deformity	Surgical correction technique to consider
Focal deformity in cervical spine	Anterior corpectomy or osteotomy
Severe focal kyphotic deformity at cervicothoracic junction	C7 or T1/T2 PSO may be required
Severe CSD with concurrent severe thoracic kyphosis	Additional osteotomies in thoracic spine may be required

Many elderly patients undergoing evaluation for CSD correction will have a history of prior spine surgery. Figure 13.1 demonstrates sagittal CT scans of a patient who had a prior C4/C5 corpectomy and C3-C7 posterior spinal fusion who presented with distal junctional kyphosis and pseudarthrosis with kyphotic angulation at C7/T1. Figure 13.2 shows sagittal MRIs of the same patient showing flattening of

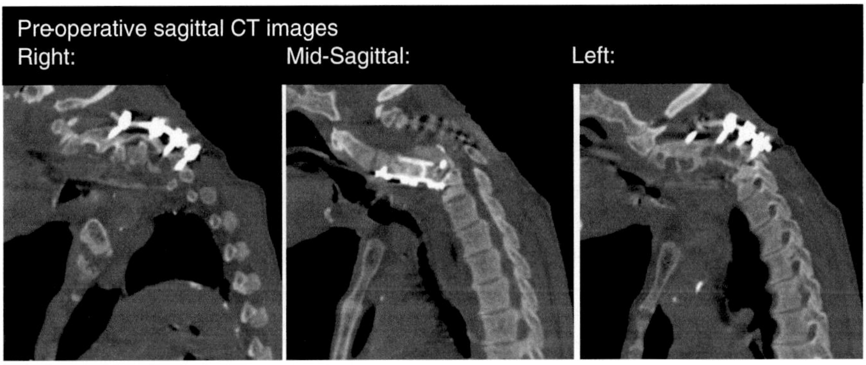

Fig. 13.1 Preoperative sagittal CT images demonstrate distal junctional kyphosis after a prior C4/C5 corpectomy with C3-C7 posterior spinal fusion. There is pseudarthrosis and a kyphotic angulation at C7-T1

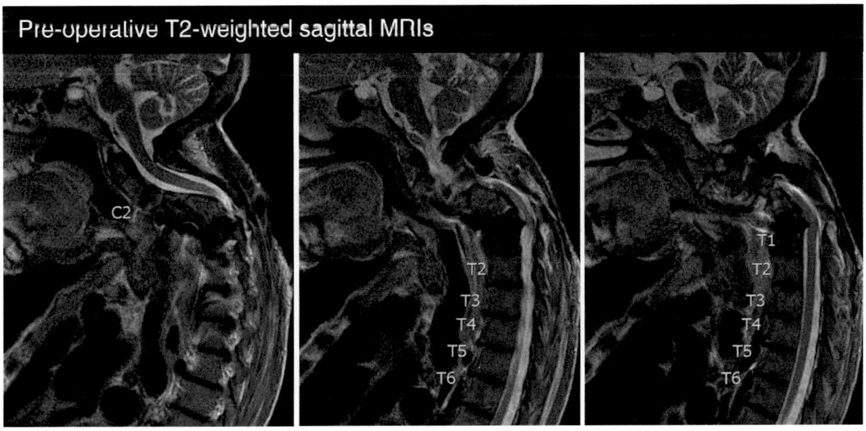

Fig. 13.2 Preoperative T2-weighted sagittal MRIs show kyphotic angulation at the distal junction of the prior C3-C7 posterior spine instrumentation with flattening of the cord at C7-T1 secondary to a dorsal osteophyte and a small dorsal epidural fluid collection

the cervical cord but no obvious cord compression or cord signal. It is critical to review prior operative reports to determine the presence of and type of implants in addition to any intraoperative findings that may have been discovered during prior surgeries. In addition, the evaluation of the prior surgical site(s) will yield high-value information that will help guide the specifics of CSD correction. Examples include the laterality of approach for anterior spine procedures, the necessity of otolaryngology consultation in cases of prior superior or recurrent laryngeal nerve damage, or plastic surgery consultation in cases of evidence of poor wound healing and wound coverage from prior surgeries.

Algorithmic Approach to Cervical Spine Deformity Correction

In general, CSD correction methods can be categorized into three broad categories as follows: (1) anterior only approaches, (2) posterior only approaches, and (3) combined anterior-posterior approaches. Within these broad categories, there exists several methods for cervical kyphosis correction:

1. Anterior cervical discectomy and fusion (ACDF): An ACDF allows sequential induction of lordosis via distraction over multiple segments and for further lordosis induction via sequential screw tightening, pulling the spine toward a lordotic cervical plate [19].
2. Anterior osteotomy: Anterior osteotomy techniques in the cervical spine performed through an anteriorly fused spine back to the level of the transverse foramen bilaterally is a powerful correction technique that can be applied throughout the cervical spine. Symmetric anterior osteotomies may be used for "chin-on-chest" deformities, while asymmetric anterior osteotomies may be used for "ear-on-shoulder" deformities [20].
3. Posterior osteotomy: Posterior osteotomy techniques in the cervical spine encompass techniques such as partial facet joint resection and complete facet joint resection. Partial and complete facet joint resections are performed across multiple levels for a cumulative lordotic effect and usually require mobility of the anterior column [21].
4. Three-column osteotomy: For ankylosed, fixed, and severe deformities, a three-column osteotomy is often required. Three-column osteotomies are typically done via a combined anterior-posterior approach (such as a vertebral body resection of pedicle subtraction osteotomy) or posterior-only approach [22]. Posterior-only approaches involve the opening-wedge osteotomy and the closing-wedge osteotomy. The opening-wedge osteotomy is performed at C7 involving a laminectomy, facetectomy, and pediculectomy with a fulcrum of rotation in the middle column. The closing-wedge osteotomy is similar to the opening-wedge osteotomy with the addition of an osteotomy in the vertebral body that is closed like a pedicle subtraction osteotomy [21]. In the example of our patient, Fig. 13.3 demonstrates the combination of a three-column pedicle-subtraction osteotomy with multiple posterior osteotomies for kyphosis correction.

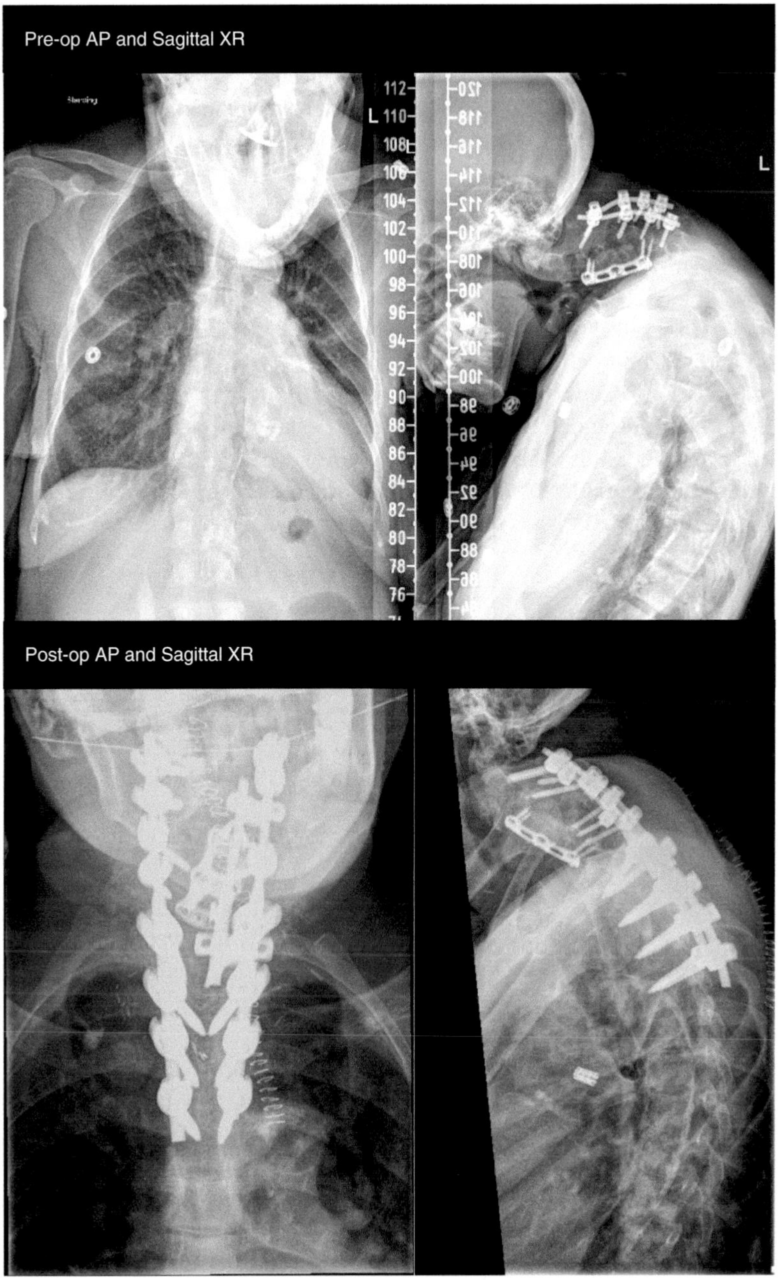

Fig. 13.3 The preoperative XR films and postoperative films are shown for a 65-year-old female patient who presented with dysphagia from "chin-on-chest" distal junctional kyphotic deformity with weakness of the hands and arms, 5 years after a prior C4-C5 corpectomy with C3-C7 posterior spinal fusion was performed at a different hospital. A posterior-only approach utilizing a T1 pedicle subtraction osteotomy was performed. The prior fusion was revised and expanded down to T5. Postoperative films demonstrate improvement of cervicothoracic deformity

The correct approach may not be obvious. There have been prior publications in the literature for algorithmic strategies for the correction of CSDs in the general population. One such algorithmic strategy, published by Hann et al. [23], is summarized in this section. CSDs are further divided into two main categories: (1) fixed (not flexible) and (2) nonfixed (flexible). Fixed deformities are then subclassified into those that are ankylosed and non-ankylosed.

Fixed Deformity Without Ankylosis

Patients with fixed deformity without ankylosis are recommended for anterior release and grafting with or without posterior fusion. An anterior approach alone may be possible because of the ability to extend the cervical spine after release of anterior soft tissue due to nonfused facet joints. Multiple segmental discectomies and distraction at each level with anterior wedge-shaped interbody grafts are generally preferable to long-segment corpectomy, which may be at higher risk of pseudarthrosis and result in more vertical distraction than angular correction.

Fixed Deformity with Anterior Ankylosis

Patients with fixed deformity with anterior ankylosis are recommended for anterior release or osteotomies and subsequent posterior correction. This combined approach allows for anterior lengthening, posterior shortening, and kyphosis correction.

Fixed Deformity with Posterior Ankylosis

Patients with fixed deformity with posterior ankylosis are typically treated with posterior osteotomy, followed by anterior release with interbody grafting and then followed by posterior instrumentation and fusion. Typically, these patients have posterior ankylosis in the setting of prior posterior fusion. Initial posterior osteotomies are aimed at releasing the posterior ankylosing fusion mass. Decompression can be performed at this time if necessary, and screws can be placed without rods. After this portion, the patient is turned supine, anterior osteotomies are performed at the ankylosed segments, and anterior discectomies and placement of interbody graft may be performed to correct kyphotic deformity. Subsequently, the patient is turned prone and posterior spine instrumentation, and deformity correction is completed.

Fixed Deformity with Circumferentially Fused Cervicothoracic Junction

Patients with a fixed deformity with circumferentially fused cervicothoracic junction typically require a three-column osteotomy or pedicle subtraction osteotomy (PSO) for correction. This type of autofusion may be secondary to diffuse idiopathic skeletal hyperostosis or ankylosing spondylitis. The PSO is performed across the cervicothoracic junction, and its advantages include that it does not require an intact anterior motion segment. However, the morbidity of the three-column osteotomy is more morbid, and this should be taken into consideration.

Flexible Deformity with Mild Kyphosis

Patients with flexible deformity with mild kyphosis can often benefit from an anterior cervical discectomy with fusion (ACDF). Typically, local kyphosis originating from cervical degeneration (not secondary to iatrogenic post-laminectomy kyphosis) from one segment can be treated via this method because of significant sequential distraction via ACDF [19]. Each segment can be significantly distracted anteriorly, resulting in kyphosis correction.

Flexible Deformity with Moderate Kyphosis

Patients with flexible deformity with moderate kyphosis spanning more than three levels and correctable with traction of postural change may benefit from a posterior only method of decompression and fusion. Mild to moderate post laminectomy kyphosis may be approached using this method. Although this method can decrease kyphosis, it is less effective in inducing lordosis than the anterior approach. Compared to the back-front-back method, it has less operative time, blood loss, and morbidity.

Flexible Deformity with Severe Kyphosis

Patients with flexible deformity with severe kyphosis should generally be treated with a combined 360-degree anterior and posterior approach. Typically, this involves an initial anterior approach with multilevel discectomy and interbody grafting without plating, followed by a turn to prone with posterior laminectomy, instrumentation, posterior osteotomies, and kyphosis correction.

Radiographic Success After Cervical Spine Deformity Correction in the Elderly

There is sparse literature on the radiographic success rates and predictors of radiographic failure after CSD in the elderly. Horn et al. reported on 89 patients who underwent CSD with an average age of 61.9 years and showed that 20% of patients had an overall poor outcome, where "poor outcome" was defined as either poor radiographic outcome or poor clinical outcome. The mean correction of the C2-C7 Cobb angle was from −7 degrees to 7 degrees ($p < 0.001$) and cSVA improved from 4.6 cm to 4.0 cm ($p = 0.008$). There was no significant difference in baseline C2-C7 Cobb angles and cSVA between those who suffered a poor outcome and those who did not, but at 1-year after surgery, there was a significant difference in cSVA (4.9 cm versus 3.9 cm, $p = 0.04$) between those who did and those who did not suffer poor outcome, respectively. Of those who had poor outcomes ($n = 18$), 73% of patients had persistently malaligned or worsened T1-slope cervical lordosis mismatch, and 8% had persistent or worsened severe cSVA. Osteoporosis, which is significantly correlated with increasing age, was identified as a predictor of poor outcome with an odds ratio of 5.9 [24].

Complications After Cervical Spine Deformity Correction in the Elderly

Increasing age has been identified as a significant, independent predictor of complications and morbidity after surgery. An analysis of a prospective registry by Boddapati et al. reported that predictors of postoperative respiratory compromise after anterior spine surgery included increasing age and history of chronic cardiac and/or chronic respiratory disease. Age over 70 has been identified as an independent predictor of a 30-day readmission after posterior cervical fusion in a large retrospective study of 3401 patients with an odds ratio of 1.61 compared to those younger than 70 years [25]. Katz et al. reported in a retrospective study of 15,600 patients undergoing both anterior cervical discectomy and fusion (ACDF) and anterior cervical corpectomy and fusion (ACCF) that increasing age predicted readmission, reoperation, and morbidity after surgery. Of note, the average ages of the groups undergoing ACDF and ACCF were 54.9 and 56.2 years, respectively [26]. Passias et al. reported on a comparison of perioperative complications between a multicenter prospective cervical deformity database and the Nationwide Inpatient Sample (NIS), finding that the NIS included significantly younger patients (age under 50 years). The younger patients had a significantly lower rate of neurologic, peripheral vascular, respiratory, gastrointestinal, and infectious complications but had higher device-related complications rates. This suggests that surgeon-maintained cervical deformity databases may have higher granularity and more precise reporting compared to nationwide databases, but nationwide databases may be better at capturing medical complications.

Although increasing age may be an important predictor of morbidity for preoperative and postoperative CSD, there is significant heterogeneity in the "frailty" definition in elderly patients. A more granular approach to identifying elderly patients that may benefit from CSD correction and those at high risk of serious complications requires an assessment of other comorbidities and health-related data that are independent of age alone. One such approach in surgical literature has been the development of the "frailty index (FI)," which is utilized to summarize and measure the health status of older individuals, to serve as a proxy measure for aging and vulnerability to poor outcomes. Miller et al. [27] reported on an initial study of 61 patients undergoing adult CSD correction, utilizing 40 patient-related variables to construct a CSD-related FI. They found that the incidence of major complications increased with greater frailty but did not have an association with surgical complications, discharge disposition, or length of stay. Another study, reported by Passias et al. [28], studied a modified version of the frailty index reported by Miller et al. This larger study of 121 adult CSD categorized into three groups as follows: (1) not frail, (2) frail, and (3) severely frail. They found that increased frailty was significantly associated with increased length of stay, neck pain, infection, mortality, and decreased HRQOL. Severely frail patients are at higher risk of mortality after CSD correction surgery, and this is likely related to preoperative comorbidities and health status. The vast majority of postoperative mortality after CSD correction occurs secondary to medical complications, such as myocardial infarction, pneumonia, cardiopulmonary failure, and sepsis [29]. Although outcomes after CSD surgery appear highly variable, and complications are likely largely secondary to complex deformity correction cases, it is clear that increasing age, significant comorbidities, and increased frailty contribute to a higher risk of poor outcomes after CSD correction surgery. There appears to be a relative dearth of literature on the specific management of elderly patients with CSD and their outcomes after surgery, and further studies are needed that specifically focus on the elderly. More importantly, it would be an incorrect assumption to assume that the elderly comprises a homogenous group. Rather, studies should focus on management strategies and risk mitigation in elderly patients stratified by evidence-derived factors to allow surgeons to better prescribe surgical versus alternative nonsurgical treatments.

Conclusion

Cervical spinal deformity may cause impairment of healthcare quality of life in elderly patients. Normal asymptomatic aging involves development of increased cervical lordosis or kyphosis, and many patients with cervical kyphosis are asymptomatic. However, once quality of life becomes impaired, intervention can be contemplated. Goals of surgery include correction of CSD to maintain horizontal gaze, decompress the neural elements, and restore alignment of the cervical spine. CSD and can involve several techniques, such as ACDF, anterior osteotomy, posterior osteotomy, and three-column osteotomy. Increased age, significant comorbidities, and increased frailty appear to have correlation with poor outcome for CSD correction.

References

1. Graffeo CS, et al. Odontoid fractures and the silver tsunami: evidence and practice in the very elderly. Neurosurgery. 2016;63:113–7.
2. Protopsaltis TS, et al. How the neck affects the back: changes in regional cervical sagittal alignment correlate to HRQOL improvement in adult thoracolumbar deformity patients at 2-year follow-up. J Neurosurg Spine. 2015;23:153–8.
3. Steinmetz MP, Stewart TJ, Kager CD, Benzel EC, Vaccaro AR. Cervical deformity correction. Neurosurgery. 2007;60:S1–90.
4. Smith JS, et al. Prevalence and type of cervical deformity among 470 adults with thoracolumbar deformity. Spine. 2014;39:E1001–9.
5. Gore DR, Sepic SB, Gardner GM. Roentgenographic findings of the cervical spine in asymptomatic people. Spine. 1986;11:521–4.
6. Ichihara D, et al. Longitudinal magnetic resonance imaging study on whiplash injury patients: minimum 10-year follow-up. J Orthop Sci. 2009;14:602–10.
7. Shedid D, Benzel EC. Cervical spondylosis anatomy: pathophysiology and biomechanics. Neurosurgery. 2007;60:S7–13.
8. Gore DR. Roentgenographic findings in the cervical spine in asymptomatic persons: a ten-year follow-up. Spine. 2001;26:2463–6.
9. Doual JM, Ferri J, Laude M. The influence of senescence on craniofacial and cervical morphology in humans. Surg Radiol Anat. 1997;19:175–83.
10. Albert TJ, Vacarro A. Postlaminectomy kyphosis. Spine. 1998;23:2738–45.
11. Mikawa Y, Shikata J, Yamamuro T. Spinal deformity and instability after multilevel cervical laminectomy. Spine. 1987;12:6–11.
12. Sim FH, Svien HJ, Bickel WH, Janes JM. Swan-neck deformity following extensive cervical laminectomy: a review of twenty-one cases. JBJS. 1974;56:564–80.
13. Pal GP, Sherk HH. The vertical stability of the cervical spine. Spine. 1988;13:447–9.
14. Nolan JPJ, Sherk HH. Biomechanical evaluation of the extensor musculature of the cervical spine. Spine. 1988;13:9–11.
15. Ao S, Liu Y, Wang Y, Zhang H, Leng H. Cervical kyphosis in asymptomatic populations: incidence, risk factors, and its relationship with health-related quality of life. J Orthop Surg. 2019;14:322.
16. Le Huec JC, Demezon H, Aunoble S. Sagittal parameters of global cervical balance using EOS imaging: normative values from a prospective cohort of asymptomatic volunteers. Eur Spine J. 2015;24:63–71.
17. Ames CP, et al. Reliability assessment of a novel cervical spine deformity classification system. J Neurosurg Spine. 2015;23:673–83.
18. Ames CP, et al. Cervical radiographical alignment: comprehensive assessment techniques and potential importance in cervical myelopathy. Spine. 2013;38:S149–60.
19. Guinn JMV, Pennicooke B, Rivera J, Mummaneni PV, Chou D. Anterior cervical discectomy with fusion and plating for correction of degenerative cervical kyphosis: 2-dimensional operative video. Oper Neurosurg (Hagerstown). 2021;20:E214.
20. Safaee MM, Tan LA, Riew KD. Anterior osteotomy for rigid cervical deformity correction. J Spine Surg. 2020;6:210–6.

21. Safaee MM, Tan LA, Ames CP. Posterior osteotomy techniques for rigid cervical deformity correction. J Spine Surg. 2020;6:274–9.
22. Lau D, Ames CP. Three column osteotomy for the treatment of rigid cervical deformity. Neurospine. 2020;17:525–33.
23. Hann S, et al. An algorithmic strategy for selecting a surgical approach in cervical deformity correction. Neurosurg Focus. 2014;36:E5.
24. Horn SR, et al. Predicting the combined occurrence of poor clinical and radiographic outcomes following cervical deformity corrective surgery. J Neurosurg Spine. 2019;32:182–90.
25. Choy W, Lam SK, Smith ZA, Dahdaleh NS. Predictors of 30-day hospital readmission after posterior cervical fusion in 3401 patients. Spine. 2018;43:356–63.
26. Katz AD, Mancini N, Karukonda T, Cote M, Moss IL. Comparative and predictor analysis of 30-day readmission, reoperation, and morbidity in patients undergoing multilevel ACDF versus single and multilevel ACCF using the ACS-NSQIP dataset. Spine. 2019;44:E1379.
27. Miller EK, et al. Assessment of a novel adult cervical deformity frailty index as a component of preoperative risk stratification. World Neurosurg. 2018;109:e800–6.
28. Passias PG, et al. Development of a modified cervical deformity frailty index: a streamlined clinical tool for preoperative risk stratification. Spine. 2019;44:169–76.
29. Smith JS, et al. Prospective multicenter assessment of all-cause mortality following surgery for adult cervical deformity. Neurosurgery. 2018;83:1277–85.

Chapter 14
Spinal Cord Injury in the Elderly Population

Jacob L. Goldberg, Sertac Kirnaz, and Michael S. Virk

Introduction

Spinal cord injury (SCI) is a significant cause of long-term neurological disability. In the United States, the incidence of SCI is estimated at approximately 12,000 new cases per year with a prevalence of 270,000 cases [1]. The estimated and inflation-adjusted direct and indirect costs annually for spinal cord injuries are $10B and $3.7B US dollars, respectively [2]. Acute care costs involving the initial hospitalization and rehabilitation reportedly costs $142,366 per patient [3]. In the first year alone, the average costs are $523,089, with subsequent annual cost totaling $79,759 [4].

SCI incidence follows a bimodal distribution, peaking in the young adult and elderly populations [5, 6]. The US population pyramid demonstrates a bulge between the ages of 52 and 64 years old, and approximately 16.5% of the population is over 65 years old, suggesting that the prevalence of elderly patients with SCI will increase. Moreover, the number of adults aged 65 years and older rapidly increases and is expected to double over the next several decades [7]. In young adults, SCI is predominantly the result of high velocity trauma. In contrast, 77% of SCI cases in the elderly result from the low velocity mechanism of traumatic falls followed by motor vehicle accidents [8]. Nonetheless the consequences of SCI in the elderly are severe. Among the geriatric population, the leading cause of unexpected death is related to traumatic injury, the most devastating of which are SCI [9]. Compared with young adults, the mortality rates among adults 65 years and older is significantly higher following SCI [10]. Further, older adults are also left

J. L. Goldberg (✉) · S. Kirnaz · M. S. Virk
Department of Neurological Surgery, Weill Cornell Medicine—New York Presbyterian Hospital, New York, NY, USA
e-mail: jag9177@nyp.org; sek2024@med.cornell.edu; miv2010@med.cornell.edu

K.-M. G. Fu et al. (eds.), *Treatment of Spine Disease in the Elderly*,
https://doi.org/10.1007/978-3-031-12612-3_14

with a greater degree of functional impairment despite similar rates of neurologic recovery [10]. Furlan et al. studied 396 patients with SCI and found the risk of death within 1 year of injury to proportionally increase with age at the time of injury [10].

Several factors converge to increase the risk and severity of SCI in the elderly. This population is particularly susceptible to falls. Age-related deterioration of vision, balance, and proprioception is the physiologic underpinning of impaired ambulation. Beyond these factors, polypharmacy regularly encountered in the elderly population can be sedating or contribute to postural hypotension, both of which increase fall prevalence. The sequela of falls is further compounded by anti-platelet and anticoagulation medications, which in turn contribute to hematomas. Genetic conditions, which manifest with higher prevalence and in more progressed states in older age such as ankylosing spondylitis and diffuse idiopathic skeletal hyperostosis, can alter spinal biomechanics. In these patients, traumatic injuries, including fractures, create long functional lever arms, which in turn increase the force transmitted across the vertebral column potentially leading to SCI, even following low velocity mechanisms. Similarly, as expected degenerative changes such as ligamentous hypertrophy, disc degeneration, and osteophyte formation accumulate, spinal stenosis increases with age. This increases the likelihood that relatively minor falls with neck hyperextension may result in SCI [11]. Indeed, cervical spondylotic myelopathy increases fall risk via gait impairment, which further threatens vertebral column integrity and spinal cord health. Finally, osteoporotic fractures, such as thoracolumbar burst fractures, increase with age jeopardizing the spinal cord at T12 and L1 in particular.

Elderly SCI is a clinical entity that will be commonly encountered by practicing spine surgeons. In this chapter, we review the common SCI's, evidence-based and consensus treatment recommendations, outcomes, and experimental treatments currently under investigation.

Central Cord Syndrome

The primary mechanism of elderly SCI is neck hyperextension during a fall resulting in cervical cord injury [12, 13]. Central cord syndrome (CCS) is the most common cause of incomplete spinal cord injury in the elderly [14]. CCS was initially described by Schneider et al. in the mid-1950s as "disproportionately more motor impairment of the upper than of the lower extremities, bladder dysfunction, usually urinary retention, and varying degrees of sensory loss below the level of the lesion[15]." Central cord syndrome in the absence of spinal cord compression results from a concussive force disrupting the functional activity of the centrally located spinal tracts. While the precise mechanism is not totally understood, one theory suggests that because the somatotopic organization of both the lateral corticospinal tracts and the dorsal columns consists of medial upper limb neuronal/axonal localization, the constellation of symptoms predominantly affects the upper extremities. After the primary traumatic injury occurs, the secondary injury develops as a result of inflammation and neuronal apoptosis [16]. While upper extremities are generally affected to a greater extent than lower extremities, the clinical manifestations of CCS range from mild upper extremity weakness with intact sensation to complete quadriparesis without sacral region involvement. Bladder, bowel, and/or sexual dysfunction can be observed in the most severe cases.

The diagnosis is often made on the basis of clinical symptoms. Often, there are no radiographic findings on plain X-rays or CT scans associated with acute cervical trauma, such as disco-ligamentous complex disruption, but canal stenosis and/or cord compression of uncertain chronicity are common [17, 18]. MRI can be helpful for evaluation of connective tissues and neural elements. The presence of prevertebral hematomas or edema and lesions of the posterior tension band raise concern for instability [19]. Intramedullary hyperintense signal on T2-weighted and STIR sequences is associated with spinal cord edema, or in some cases preexisting myelomalacia, and may include parenchymal hemorrhage [20]. A retrospective cohort in 2011 evaluating patients with acute traumatic central cord syndrome reported long-term ASIA motor scores could be correlated with MRI findings, including midsagittal diameter at the point of maximum compression, maximum canal compression, and length of parenchymal damage [21].

Thus, the primary mechanism of injury in elderly CCS involves a hyperextension injury of the cervical spine, particularly with superimposed spinal stenosis, osteophytosis, redundant ligamentum flavum, congenital stenosis, or rheumatoid arthritis [12, 13]. Fractures and/or dislocations are less frequently seen in elderly patients with CCS compared to a younger cohort due to the associated low velocity mechanism of injury [22]. In addition to trauma, other etiologies of CCS in the elderly include epidural infection and malignancy. The treatment of CCS, with or without ongoing cord compression, is discussed in subsequent sections (Fig. 14.1).

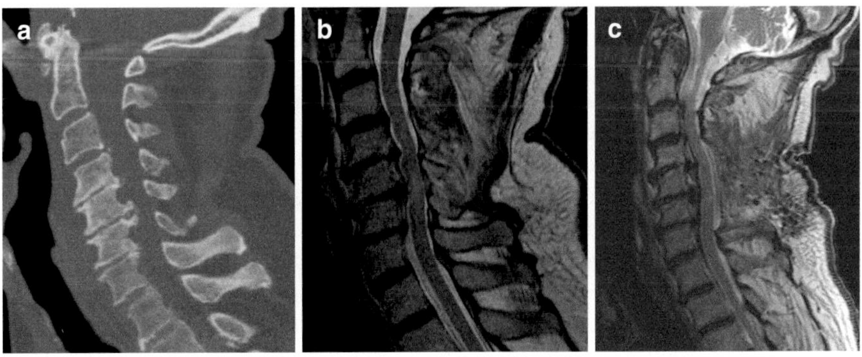

Fig. 14.1 Radiographic findings in a 91-year-old male patient presenting with dense central cord syndrome. (**a**) Sagittal CT cervical demonstrates C4-C5 and C5-C6 disc/osteophyte complexes, but no bony fracture or facet dislocation. (**b**) Sagittal MRI cervical spine demonstrates T2 cord signal at C4-C5 and diffusely at C5-C6 consistent with spinal cord edema. (**c**) Sagittal MRI 1 month following C4-C6 laminectomy without instrumentation. MRI revealing posterior decompression of cervical cord with consolidated intramedullary T2 cord signal

Spinal Trauma Associated with SCI: Odontoid Fracture, Penetrating Injury, and Fracture Dislocation

Odontoid Fractures

Odontoid fractures can occur with low velocity trauma and are the most common cervical spine fracture in adults 70 years and older [23]. The Anderson and D'Alonzo classification for odontoid fractures categorizes them the following way: type I, isolated fracture of the dens; type II, fracture along the base of the dens; and type III, extending through the vertebral body of C2 [24]. Patients with type I and III fractures are routinely managed conservatively with a rigid external collar 6–8 weeks and rates of fusion of 100% for type I and between 64% and 100% for type III [25]. Type II fractures are poorly healing with as many as 85% resulting in nonunion if managed conservatively [26]. Graffeo et al., in a single-center prospectively collected series of 111 elderly patients with type II odontoid fractures, found a significantly increased odds of poor outcomes associated with the presenting Glasgow Coma Scale and/or comorbid SCI [27]. Of note, only 3 of 111 patients with type 2 odontoid fractures presented with evidence of SCI.

In the elderly population, the risks, benefits, and treatment goals in patients with type II fractures require careful consideration. Molinari et al. published a surgical series, which demonstrated some of the decision-making complexities [28]. They evaluated elderly patients with type II odontoid fracture and treated those with >50% fracture displacement with C1-C2 posterior fusion (n = 25) and managed conservatively (for 12 weeks) the patients whose displacement was <50% (n = 33). The authors reported higher fracture healing in the operative (28%) compared with conservative management (6%) group. Sixty-seven percent in the nonoperative group had a nonmobile union. However, they also found higher rates of complication (24% vs. 6%) and mortality (20% vs. 12%) in the operative cohort. Of note, no patients in the nonoperative cohort and only two patients in the operative cohort presented with a neurologic deficit. No differences were observed between the groups on the basis of patient-reported pain outcomes, function, or satisfaction. The effect of treatment on neurologic outcome could not be ascertained. Though the generalizability of the study is limited by the fact that the operative group had worse fracture displacement, one conclusion suggests that fracture healing is not necessarily correlated with pain relief, function, or satisfaction but surgery did carry significant risks. In a separate report, Schroeder et al. published a meta-analysis evaluating the best available evidence and suggested that in well-selected geriatric patients, surgical management of type II fractures can be performed safely and with an associated decrease in short- and long-term mortality [29]. They reported that both short- and long-term mortality (odds ratios 0.43 and 0.47, respectively) were lower in patients who underwent surgery with no significant difference in mortality or complication rate related to surgical approach (anterior or posterior).

In practice, many type II odontoid fractures are managed with long-term rigid cervical collar immobilization. In a small but representative study, Molinari et al. published their experience describing 34 patients with type II fractures managed with collar alone [30]. At 15 months, 6% of patients demonstrated radiographic fusion while 70% had mobile non-union. Notably, patient-reported outcomes did not significantly differ on the basis of fracture healing or stability.

Penetrating Injury

SCI resulting from penetrating injury is rare in the elderly population [31]. Prognosis and outcomes are likely worse in the elderly population, due to the presence of comorbidities and overall health status. Unlike blunt trauma, which is more common in cervical spine, penetrating SCI usually occurs in thoracic spine, and the rate of neurological recovery is lower for penetrating SCI patients [32]. Roach et al. found that the rate of complete SCI was about 50% more for penetrating SCI patients then blunt SCI patients [32]. Morrow et al. further described the epidemiology of penetrating SCI reporting the results of a prospectively maintained spine trauma database [33]. Of 1130 patients presenting with traumatic spine fractures, 154 (13%) were secondary to penetrating injury. Sixty-three patients (41%) had concomitant spinal cord or cauda equina injury. Forty-four (70%) presented with ASIA A impairment with 10 (16%) improving by at least one grade. Nine patients in total underwent surgical intervention for either instability, ongoing compression with worsening exam, infectious concerns, or multiple reasons. Surgery was not correlated with an improvement in ASIA score. Although it is generally recommended to maintain elevated MAP goals in SCI patients among younger patients, Readdy et al. demonstrated that 71% penetrating SCI patient treated with vasopressors had cardiogenic complications [34]. Though evidence is unavailable due to the rarity of this condition in the elderly, the poor cardiac tolerance in a younger cohort cautions against the use of vasopressors in the elderly penetrating SCI patient.

Thoracolumbar Fracture/Dislocation Associated with SCI

Although cervical injuries are most prevalent in the setting of mechanical fall, other factors, such as decreased global range of motion, loss of disc elasticity, and overall stiffening of the spinal column, predispose to thoracic distraction injuries as well [35, 36]. For example, ankylosing spondylitis (AS) and diffuse idiopathic skeletal hyperostosis (DISH) predispose patients to multiple column vertebral fracture, which are often highly unstable with minor trauma (Fig. 14.2). Based on Finnish national patient register data, Alaranta et al. showed patients with AS are 11.4 times more likely to have SCI compared to general population [37]. Several other studies

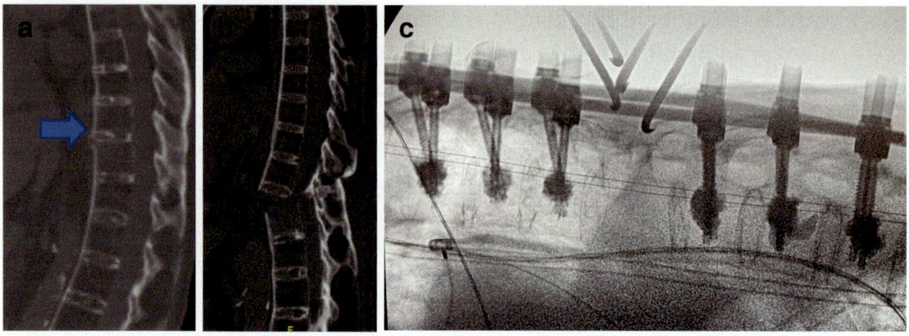

Fig. 14.2 (**a**) Sagittal CT demonstrating bridging bone throughout the thoracic spine consistent with ankylosing spondylitis. A fracture through the T10 superior endplate is marked with a blue arrow. (**b**) A subsequent CT taken after repositioning demonstrates loss of alignment. (**c**) Lateral fluoroscopy demonstrating posterior fusion 3 levels above and below the fracture level

also demonstrated that AS patients have a higher risk of complete SCI. Given the ability of these highly unstable fractures to auto-reduce, the finding of AS on imaging should prompt careful investigation for an unstable but well-aligned vertebral fracture (Fig. 14.3). Since AS patients suffer from long-standing pain, diagnosis of a cervical fracture or dislocation can be missed or delayed in this patient population. In a retrospective analysis by Anwar et al., fractures or dislocations were missed on initial cervical X-rays in 59.4% of patients with AS. With high clinical suspicion, MRI should be obtained [38]. Distraction fractures associated with AS carry an increased risk of morbidity and mortality, including SCI [39]. Multilevel pedicle screw fixation, generally three levels cranial and three levels caudal to the fracture, is routinely employed to prevent catastrophic neurologic injury [40] (Fig. 14.3).

Thoracolumbar burst fractures account for 15% of spinal injuries [41] and often occur between T12 and L3 [42] with ~50% occurring at either T12 or L1. Rates of associated neurological deficit vary widely and depend in part on mechanism of injury [41–44]. With nonoperative treatment (brace, recumbency, external casting, etc.), rates of partial neurological recovery range from 14% to 83%, while full neurological recovery is reported in <20% of cases [45]. Several retrospective and systemic reviewers have found stabilization within 3 days to be associated with shorter hospital stays, less morbidity, and better outcomes [45]. A prospective study by Cengiz et al. found surgery within 8 h to be associated with improvement in neurologic outcome (ASIA score) as well as shorter hospital and ICU stays and fewer complications [46].

Medical Management

Management of acute SCI patient is a critical and time-sensitive intervention. The general principles of advanced traumatic life support (ATLS) should be applied to any acute SCI patients [47]. If the patient is unconscious, the mechanism of injury

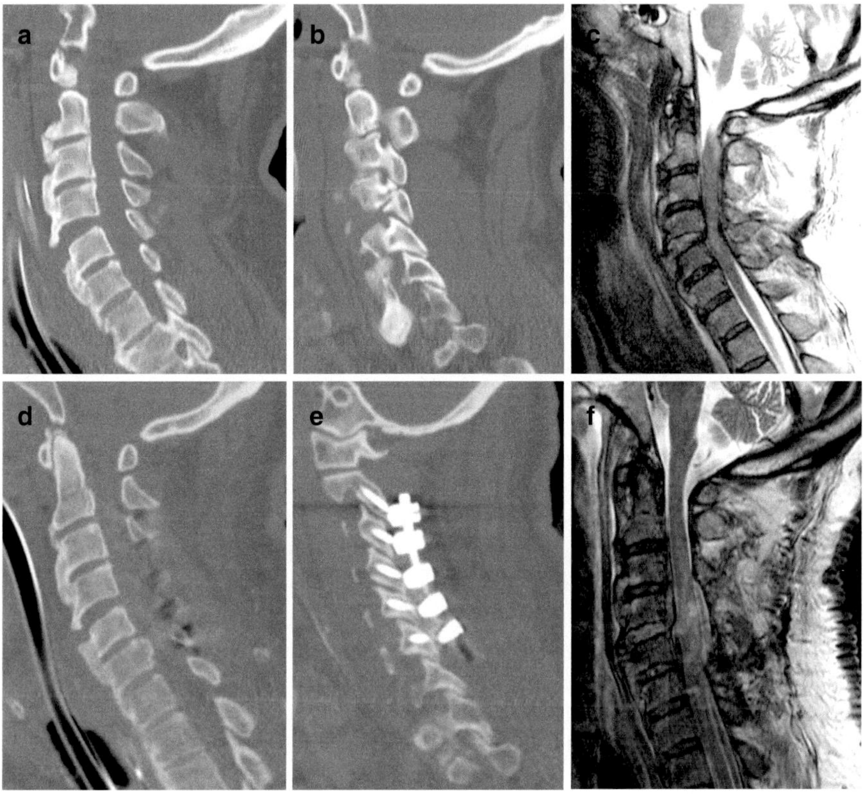

Fig. 14.3 76-year-old male with DISH after a fall downstairs while intoxicated resulting in central cord injury. (**a**) Sagittal CT demonstrating widening of the C4-C5 disc space and acute fracture through the overlying osteophyte, which (**b**) extends posteriorly into the lamina and facet. (**c**) Sagittal T2 MRI with intramedullary hyperintensity at C4-C5, C3-C6 severe stenosis with ventral epidural hematoma. (**d**) Postoperative sagittal CT demonstrating posterior decompression and (**e**) lateral mass instrumentation. (**f**) Postoperative sagittal T2 MRI with decompressed cord and evolution of cord edema

is suspicious, or the patient has a neurological deficit, immediate immobilization with a rigid cervical collar or a backboard is required prior to the transfer to a healthcare facility [48]. Collar and logroll should be maintained until proper imaging can be obtained. Optimization of tissue oxygenation and perfusion are the two most important preventive measures for possible long-term neurological disability due to secondary injury. Airway protection and ventilation should be considered especially for patients with high cervical injury. In case of a hypovolemic and neurogenic shock, IV fluids and infusion of pressors, including norepinephrine or dopamine, is indicated to maintain blood pressure, particularly since these patients are susceptible to systemic hypoperfusion. Therapeutic elevation of mean arterial pressure (MAP) to greater than 85 mm Hg during the first week post SCI is a nontargeted intervention being employed more commonly [49, 50]. On the other hand, while the use of high-dose steroids in the immediate SCI period is used by some practitioners in younger patient cohorts at early time points, it is not routinely used in the elderly as evidence in favor remains weak while the side effect profile is considerable.

Surgical Management

The surgical treatment goal in SCI is decompression of the spinal cord by directly removing mass occupying lesions from the spinal canal, opening the spinal canal around the compressed cord, realigning the vertebral column, and stabilizing unstable injuries [51]. In spite of minimizing the effects of the primary injury by rapid decompression, the resulting ischemia and reperfusion lead to further injury due to altered enzymatic activity, unregulated release of neurotransmitters, and apoptosis of neurons and their supporting cells [52]. Disappointingly, medical treatment aimed at halting and/or reversing this biochemically mediated injury remain elusive.

Several preclinical studies showed that early surgical decompression was helpful in terms of ameliorating secondary injury; however, early clinical studies failed to demonstrate this theory [53, 54]. In 1980s and 1990s, several studies failed to demonstrate the benefits of early surgical decompression over delayed decompression, and the timing of surgery remained a point of debate [55]. Moreover, in a multicenter prospective study in 1987, authors favored delaying surgery after observing deterioration in cervical SCI patients underwent decompression surgery within the first 5 days [56]. However, published studies have demonstrated positive results of early decompression (<24 h) in SCI patients. Fehlings et al. showed that patients undergoing decompression within 24 h were 2.8 times more likely to have at least a two-grade ASIA impairment scale improves at 6 months follow-up in a multicenter, prospective study on 313 patients with acute cervical SCI [57]. More recently, a meta-analysis by Lee et al. further demonstrated that ultra-early decompression (<8 h) is both safe and superior to late decompression in terms of neurological recovery [57]. Subsequent studies have shown that ultra-early decompression provide better long-term functional outcome and shorter length of hospital stays [58, 59]. Specifically, Jug et al. found statistically significant improvements in the motor component of the ASIA score in patients operated <8 h compared with 8–24 h after injury [58].

In the elderly population, treatment needs to account for the increased surgical risks in the context of a particular patient's medical comorbidities and baseline functional status. Most patients without radiographic abnormality experience neurologic improvement with medical management in rigid external immobilization. Although neurologic recovery is often seen with conservative management, recovery may be limited. It is also worth noting that a hard collar is associated with significant morbidity in the elderly, including dysphasia, aspiration, and falls.

In a study of 44 by Hagen et al., early surgery was associated with decreased length of stay and better motor recovery in patients with central cord associated with an acute traumatic disc herniation or cervical fracture compared with late surgery [8]. However, in patients with central cord without these acute traumatic radiographic abnormalities, neurologic function was no different in patients undergoing early compared with late surgery. Notably, surgery was well tolerated in both cohorts. Though the literature remains controversial over the years, many surgeons favor early surgical decompression in an acceptable risk surgical candidate [60]. A growing field of research is focusing on further investigating early decompression. In a recent retrospective study of 48 patients with cervical SCI, Burke et al. found a significant improvement in neurologic outcome among patients operated on within 12 h of presentation and those within 12–24 h of presentation with those in the ultra-early group faring the best [60].

Regarding hospital course, Lau et al. retrospectively studied 83 young and 23 elderly SCI patients and found significantly higher rates of cervical SCI in the elderly, similar length of ICU stays, and higher rates of complications and mortality (1.7× and 10.8×, respectively) [61].

Outcomes

After SCI, geriatric patients face a significantly increased rate of mortality [31]. For those with comorbid neurodegenerative disorders, outcomes are even worse [62]. Compared with young adults with SCI, elderly patients are more likely to end up with a permanent tracheostomy due to their decreased overall pulmonary function and out of concern for airway protection [63]. Improving these outcomes depends in part on anticipating and managing the commonly encountered acute and chronic complications [64, 65]. Depending partly on the mechanism and specific injury, elderly patients with SCI are at elevated risk for the following acute complications: neurogenic shock, autonomic dysfunction, stroke, myocardial infarction, dysphagia, respiratory impairment, and bowel and/or bladder dysfunction. The most commonly encountered complications related to prolonged immobility and included pressure ulcers, pain, osteoporosis, and deep venous thrombosis/pulmonary embolisms.

Spinal cord injury rehabilitation is especially important in the elderly, as they face higher rates of functional impairment after injury. Specialized programs have been demonstrated to lead to functional improvements associated with the activities of daily living similar to those observed in younger cohorts using independence assessments [66]. However, in aggregate the elderly SCI population faces significant hurdles after injury compared to younger populations [67]. DeVivo et al. illustrate this in their report of 886 SCI patients finding those older than 61 years of age (compared with those aged 16 to 30) are 22 times more likely to be discharged to a nursing home, 72 times more likely to remain in a nursing home 2 years after injury, and 7 times more likely to have hired attendants to assist them during the second year post injury [67]. Specialized elderly SCI programs ideally involve a multidisciplinary team, including physiatrists, geriatricians, physical and occupational therapists, nutritionists, and wound care specialists. Additional consultation from gastroenterologists and urologists are frequently required. Mental health professionals are also core members of this multidisciplinary team. Livneh et al. reported on 95 adults with SCI being treated in the outpatient setting finding that coping resources and strategies facilitated psychosocial adaptation to SCI [68].

Experimental Treatments

Several experimental medical interventions aimed at halting or reversing the secondary biochemical injury are being studied in trial settings and are not in routine clinical use. Polyunsaturated fatty acids experimentally protect the cord during acute injury and are being investigated for a possible treatment role in promoting cord restoration [69]. Other trials are investigating the role of minocycline in decreasing the amount of neuronal loss following injury [70]. Riluzole has shown early promise in decreasing the glutamate mediated loss of motor neurons after SCI and is now being evaluated in a multicenter phase III clinical trial [71].

Non-pharmacologic interventions such as therapeutic hypothermia after acute SCI are also being evaluated [72]. In their most recent position statement on the topic, the AANS/CNS Trauma Section noted encouraging evidence regarding the safety of modest therapeutic hypothermia but were unable to produce a recommendation for or against this intervention, citing the need for randomized trials [73].

Conclusion

The prevalence of spinal cord injury is highest among young adults and the elderly. As the overall population ages, spine surgeons will continue to see increasing numbers of elderly patients presenting with SCI. Several factors converge for elderly patients, including polypharmacy, degenerative processes, and certain disease states, which both increase the predisposition to falling and worsen the severity of these events. Treatment depends on the particular pattern of injury and patient-specific factors. Medical interventions designed to stop the biochemical secondary spinal cord damage are currently under investigation. Surgical treatment should be performed early when appropriate. SCI-focused rehabilitation comprised of a multidisciplinary team is an essential aspect of post SCI care.

Funding None.

Financial Disclosures The authors report no financial disclosures relevant to this submission with the exception of: JLG- none, SK – none. MSV: Depuy Synthes, Globus Medical, Brainlab Inc.

Conflicts of Interests The authors declare no conflicts of interest related to the information presented.

References

1. National Spinal Cord InjuryStatistical Center. Spinal cord injury facts and figures at a glance. J Spinal Cord Med. 2012;35:197–8.
2. Ma VY, Chan L, Carruthers KJ. Incidence, prevalence, costs, and impact on disability of common conditions requiring rehabilitation in the United States: stroke, spinal cord injury, traumatic brain injury, multiple sclerosis, osteoarthritis, rheumatoid arthritis, limb loss, and back pain. Arch Phys Med Rehabil. 2014;95:986–995.e1.
3. Mahabaleshwarkar R, Khanna R. National hospitalization burden associated with spinal cord injuries in the United States. Spinal Cord. 2014;52:139–44.
4. DeVivo M, Chen Y, Mennemeyer S, Deutsch A. Costs of care following spinal cord injury. Top Spinal Cord Inj Rehabil. 2011;16:1–9.
5. Wyndaele M, Wyndaele JJ. Incidence, prevalence and epidemiology of spinal cord injury: what learns a worldwide literature survey? Spinal Cord. 2006;44:523–9.
6. Pickett W, Simpson K, Walker J, Brison RJ. Traumatic spinal cord injury in Ontario, Canada. J Trauma. 2003;55:1070–6.
7. Miller KE, Zylstra RG, Standridge JB. The geriatric patient: a systematic approach to maintaining health. Am Fam Physician. 2000;61:1089–104.
8. Hagen EM, Aarli JA, Gronning M. The clinical significance of spinal cord injuries in patients older than 60 years of age. Acta Neurol Scand. 2005;112:42–7.
9. Sattin RW. Falls among older persons: a public health perspective. Annu Rev Public Health. 1992;13:489–508.
10. Furlan JC, Fehlings MG. The impact of age on mortality, impairment, and disability among adults with acute traumatic spinal cord injury. J Neurotrauma. 2009;26:1707–17.
11. Teresi LM, Lufkin RB, Reicher MA, Moffit BJ, Vinuela FV, Wilson GM, Bentson JR, Hanafee WN. Asymptomatic degenerative disk disease and spondylosis of the cervical spine: MR imaging. Radiology. 1987;164:83–8.
12. Penrod LE, Hegde SK, Ditunno JF. Age effect on prognosis for functional recovery in acute, traumatic central cord syndrome. Arch Phys Med Rehabil. 1990;71:963–8.
13. Ishida Y, Tominaga T. Predictors of neurologic recovery in acute central cervical cord injury with only upper extremity impairment. Spine. 2002;27:1652–8; discussion 1658
14. McKinley W, Santos K, Meade M, Brooke K. Incidence and outcomes of spinal cord injury clinical syndromes. J Spinal Cord Med. 2007;30:215–24.
15. Schneider RC, Cherry G, Pantek H. The syndrome of acute central cervical spinal cord injury; with special reference to the mechanisms involved in hyperextension injuries of cervical spine. J Neurosurg. 1954;11:546–77.
16. Nowak DD, Lee JK, Gelb DE, Poelstra KA, Ludwig SC. Central cord syndrome. J Am Acad Orthop Surg. 2009;17:756–65.
17. Henderson RL, Reid DC, Saboe LA. Multiple noncontiguous spine fractures. Spine. 1991;16:128–31.
18. Vaccaro AR, An HS, Lin S, Sun S, Balderston RA, Cotler JM. Noncontiguous injuries of the spine. J Spinal Disord. 1992;5:320–9.
19. Song J, Mizuno J, Inoue T, Nakagawa H. Clinical evaluation of traumatic central cord syndrome: emphasis on clinical significance of prevertebral hyperintensity, cord compression, and intramedullary high-signal intensity on magnetic resonance imaging. Surg Neurol. 2006;65:117–23.

20. Quencer RM, Bunge RP, Egnor M, Green BA, Puckett W, Naidich TP, Post MJ, Norenberg M. Acute traumatic central cord syndrome: MRI-pathological correlations. Neuroradiology. 1992;34:85–94.
21. Aarabi B, Alexander M, Mirvis SE, Shanmuganathan K, Chesler D, Maulucci C, Iguchi M, Aresco C, Blacklock T. Predictors of outcome in acute traumatic central cord syndrome due to spinal stenosis. J Neurosurg Spine. 2011;14:122–30.
22. Hashmi SZ, Marra A, Jenis LG, Patel AA. Current concepts: central cord syndrome. Clin Spine Surg. 2018;31:407–12.
23. Ryan MD, Henderson JJ. The epidemiology of fractures and fracture-dislocations of the cervical spine. Injury. 1992;23:38–40.
24. Anderson LD, D'Alonzo RT. Fractures of the odontoid process of the axis. J Bone Joint Surg Am. 1974;56:1663–74.
25. Julien TD, Frankel B, Traynelis VC, Ryken TC. Evidence-based analysis of odontoid fracture management. Neurosurg Focus. 2000;8:e1.
26. Sasso RC. C2 dens fractures: treatment options. J Spinal Disord. 2001;14:455–63.
27. Graffeo CS, Perry A, Puffer RC, Carlstrom LP, Chang W, Mallory GW, Clarke MJ. Deadly falls: operative versus nonoperative management of type II odontoid process fracture in octogenarians. J Neurosurg Spine. 2017;26:4–9.
28. Molinari WJ, Molinari RW, Khera OA, Gruhn WL. Functional outcomes, morbidity, mortality, and fracture healing in 58 consecutive patients with geriatric odontoid fracture treated with cervical collar or posterior fusion. Global Spine J. 2013;3:21–32.
29. Schroeder GD, Kepler CK, Kurd MF, Paul JT, Rubenstein RN, Harrop JS, Brodke DS, Chapman JR, Vaccaro AR. A systematic review of the treatment of geriatric type II odontoid fractures. Neurosurgery. 2015;77(Suppl 4):S6–14.
30. Molinari RW, Khera OA, Gruhn WL, McAssey RW. Rigid cervical collar treatment for geriatric type II odontoid fractures. Eur Spine J. 2012;21:855–62.
31. Fassett DR, Harrop JS, Maltenfort M, Jeyamohan SB, Ratliff JD, Anderson DG, Hilibrand AS, Albert TJ, Vaccaro AR, Sharan AD. Mortality rates in geriatric patients with spinal cord injuries. J Neurosurg Spine. 2007;7:277–81.
32. Roach MJ, Chen Y, Kelly ML. Comparing blunt and penetrating trauma in spinal cord injury: analysis of long-term functional and neurological outcomes. Top Spinal Cord Inj Rehabil. 2018;24:121–32.
33. Morrow KD, Podet AG, Spinelli CP, Lasseigne LM, Crutcher CL, Wilson JD, Tender GC, DiGiorgio AM. A case series of penetrating spinal trauma: comparisons to blunt trauma, surgical indications, and outcomes. Neurosurg Focus. 2019;46:E4.
34. Readdy WJ, Saigal R, Whetstone WD, et al. Failure of mean arterial pressure goals to improve outcomes following penetrating spinal cord injury. Neurosurgery. 2016;79:708–14.
35. Dvorak J, Froehlich D, Penning L, Baumgartner H, Panjabi MM. Functional radiographic diagnosis of the cervical spine: flexion/extension. Spine. 1988;13:748–55.
36. Jabbour P, Fehlings M, Vaccaro AR, Harrop JS. Traumatic spine injuries in the geriatric population. Neurosurg Focus. 2008;25:E16.
37. Alaranta H, Luoto S, Konttinen YT. Traumatic spinal cord injury as a complication to ankylosing spondylitis. An extended report. Clin Exp Rheumatol. 2002;20:66–8.
38. Jacobs WB, Fehlings MG. Ankylosing spondylitis and spinal cord injury: origin, incidence, management, and avoidance. Neurosurg Focus. 2008;24:E12.
39. Chaudhary SB, Hullinger H, Vives MJ. Management of acute spinal fractures in ankylosing spondylitis. ISRN Rheumatol. 2011;2011:150484.
40. Rustagi T, Drazin D, Oner C, York J, Schroeder GD, Vaccaro AR, Oskouian RJ, Chapman JR. Fractures in spinal ankylosing disorders: a narrative review of disease and injury types, treatment techniques, and outcomes. J Orthop Trauma. 2017;31(Suppl 4):S57–74.
41. Wilcox RK, Boerger TO, Allen DJ, Barton DC, Limb D, Dickson RA, Hall RM. A dynamic study of thoracolumbar burst fractures. J Bone Joint Surg Am. 2003;85:2184–9.

42. Holmes JF, Miller PQ, Panacek EA, Lin S, Horne NS, Mower WR. Epidemiology of thoracolumbar spine injury in blunt trauma. Acad Emerg Med. 2001;8:866–72.
43. Schouten R, Lewkonia P, Noonan VK, Dvorak MF, Fisher CG. Expectations of recovery and functional outcomes following thoracolumbar trauma: an evidence-based medicine process to determine what surgeons should be telling their patients. J Neurosurg Spine. 2015;22:101–11.
44. Bensch FV, Koivikko MP, Kiuru MJ, Koskinen SK. The incidence and distribution of burst fractures. Emerg Radiol. 2006;12:124–9.
45. Kato S, Murray J-C, Kwon BK, Schroeder GD, Vaccaro AR, Fehlings MG. Does surgical intervention or timing of surgery have an effect on neurological recovery in the setting of a thoracolumbar burst fracture? J Orthop Trauma. 2017;31(Suppl 4):S38–43.
46. Cengiz SL, Kalkan E, Bayir A, Ilik K, Basefer A. Timing of thoracolomber spine stabilization in trauma patients; impact on neurological outcome and clinical course. A real prospective (rct) randomized controlled study. Arch Orthop Trauma Surg. 2008;128:959–66.
47. Resnick DK. Updated guidelines for the management of acute cervical spine and spinal cord injury. Neurosurgery. 2013;72(Suppl 2):1.
48. Hachem LD, Ahuja CS, Fehlings MG. Assessment and management of acute spinal cord injury: from point of injury to rehabilitation. J Spinal Cord Med. 2017;40:665–75.
49. Karsy M, Hawryluk G. Modern medical management of spinal cord injury. Curr Neurol Neurosci Rep. 2019;19:65.
50. Saadeh YS, Smith BW, Joseph JR, Jaffer SY, Buckingham MJ, Oppenlander ME, Szerlip NJ, Park P. The impact of blood pressure management after spinal cord injury: a systematic review of the literature. Neurosurg Focus. 2017;43:E20.
51. Anderson KK, Tetreault L, Shamji MF, Singh A, Vukas RR, Harrop JS, Fehlings MG, Vaccaro AR, Hilibrand AS, Arnold PM. Optimal timing of surgical decompression for acute traumatic central cord syndrome: a systematic review of the literature. Neurosurgery. 2015;77(Suppl 4):S15–32.
52. Witiw CD, Fehlings MG. Acute spinal cord injury. J Spinal Disord Tech. 2015;28:202–10.
53. Batchelor PE, Wills TE, Skeers P, Battistuzzo CR, Macleod MR, Howells DW, Sena ES. Meta-analysis of pre-clinical studies of early decompression in acute spinal cord injury: a battle of time and pressure. PLoS One. 2013;8:e72659.
54. Wagner FC, Chehrazi B. Early decompression and neurological outcome in acute cervical spinal cord injuries. J Neurosurg. 1982;56:699–705.
55. Fehlings MG, Tator CH. An evidence-based review of decompressive surgery in acute spinal cord injury: rationale, indications, and timing based on experimental and clinical studies. J Neurosurg. 1999;91:1–11.
56. Marshall LF, Knowlton S, Garfin SR, Klauber MR, Eisenberg HM, Kopaniky D, Miner ME, Tabbador K, Clifton GL. Deterioration following spinal cord injury. A multicenter study. J Neurosurg. 1987;66:400–4.
57. Fehlings MG, Vaccaro A, Wilson JR, et al. Early versus delayed decompression for traumatic cervical spinal cord injury: results of the surgical timing in acute spinal cord injury study (STASCIS). PLoS One. 2012;7:e32037.
58. Jug M, Kejžar N, Vesel M, Al Mawed S, Dobravec M, Herman S, Bajrovic FF. Neurological recovery after traumatic cervical spinal cord injury is superior if surgical decompression and instrumented fusion are performed within 8 h versus 8–24 h after injury—a single Centre experience. J Neurotrauma. 2015;32(18):1385–92. https://doi.org/10.1089/neu.2014.3767.
59. Lee D-Y, Park Y-J, Kim H-J, Ahn H-S, Hwang S-C, Kim D-H. Early surgical decompression within 8 h for traumatic spinal cord injury: is it beneficial? A meta-analysis. Acta Orthop Traumatol Turc. 2018;52:101–8.
60. Burke JF, Yue JK, Ngwenya LB, et al. Ultra-early (<12 h) surgery correlates with higher rate of American Spinal Injury Association Impairment Scale Conversion After Cervical Spinal Cord Injury. Neurosurgery. 2019;85:199–203.
61. Lau D, Dalle Ore CL, Tarapore PE, et al. Value of aggressive surgical and intensive care unit in elderly patients with traumatic spinal cord injury. Neurosurg Focus. 2019;46:E3.

62. Babat LB, McLain RF, Bingaman W, Kalfas I, Young P, Rufo-Smith C. Spinal surgery in patients with Parkinson's disease: construct failure and progressive deformity. Spine. 2004;29:2006–12.
63. Harrop JS, Vaccaro A, Przybylski GJ. Acute respiratory compromise associated with flexed cervical traction after C2 fractures. Spine. 2001;26:E50–4.
64. Sezer N, Akkuş S, Uğurlu FG. Chronic complications of spinal cord injury. World J Orthop. 2015;6:24–33.
65. Hagen EM. Acute complications of spinal cord injuries. World J Orthop. 2015;6:17–23.
66. Kennedy P, Evans MJ, Berry C, Mullin J. Comparative analysis of goal achievement during rehabilitation for older and younger adults with spinal cord injury. Spinal Cord. 2003;41:44–52.
67. DeVivo MJ, Kartus PL, Rutt RD, Stover SL, Fine PR. The influence of age at time of spinal cord injury on rehabilitation outcome. Arch Neurol. 1990;47:687–91.
68. Livneh H, Martz E. Coping strategies and resources as predictors of psychosocial adaptation among people with spinal cord injury. Rehabil Psychol. 2014;59:329–39.
69. Yu WY, He DW. Current trends in spinal cord injury repair. Eur Rev Med Pharmacol Sci. 2015;19:3340–4.
70. Ahuja CS, Martin AR, Fehlings M. Recent advances in managing a spinal cord injury secondary to trauma. [version 1; peer review: 2 approved]. F1000Res. 2016;5:F1000 Faculty Rev-1017. https://doi.org/10.12688/f1000research.7586.1.
71. Fehlings MG, Nakashima H, Nagoshi N, Chow DSL, Grossman RG, Kopjar B. Rationale, design and critical end points for the Riluzole in acute spinal cord injury study (RISCIS): a randomized, double-blinded, placebo-controlled parallel multi-center trial. Spinal Cord. 2016;54:8–15.
72. Hansebout RR, Hansebout CR. Local cooling for traumatic spinal cord injury: outcomes in 20 patients and review of the literature. J Neurosurg Spine. 2014;20:550–61.
73. Creasey G, Steinberg GK. Study of systemic cooling in acute spinal cord injury. Neurosurgery. 2010;66:E1217.

Chapter 15
Cervical Spinal Oncology

Zach Pennington, Andrew Schilling, Andrew Hersh, and Daniel M. Sciubba

Abbreviations

AJCC	American Joint Commission on Cancer
ASA	American Society of Anesthesiologists
CCI	Charlson Comorbidity Index
ESCC	Epidural spinal cord compression
mFI-5	Modified Frailty Index—5-item
MIS	Minimally invasive surgery
MSTS	Musculoskeletal Tumor Society
R0	Resection with no evidence of tumor cells on microscopic examination
RFA	Radiofrequency ablation
SEER	Surveillance, Epidemiology, and End Results
SINS	Spinal Instability Neoplastic Score
SLITT	Spinal laser interstitial thermotherapy
WBB	Weinstein-Boriani-Biagini

IRB Approval: IRB approval was not required for the present book chapter.

Z. Pennington · A. Schilling · A. Hersh
Department of Neurosurgery, Johns Hopkins University School of Medicine, Baltimore, MD, USA
e-mail: aschill6@jhmi.edu; ahersh2@jhmi.edu

D. M. Sciubba (✉)
Department of Neurosurgery, Johns Hopkins University School of Medicine, Baltimore, MD, USA

Department of Neurosurgery, Donald and Barbara Zucker School of Medicine at Hofstra, Long Island Jewish Medical Center and North Shore University Hospital, Northwell Health, Manhasset, NY, USA
e-mail: dsciubb1@jhmi.edu

K.-M. G. Fu et al. (eds.), *Treatment of Spine Disease in the Elderly*,
https://doi.org/10.1007/978-3-031-12612-3_15

Introduction

Spinal oncology can be divided into four groups based upon two diagnostic axes—(1) whether the tumor is primary or metastatic and (2) whether the tumor arises from the vertebral column or from the spinal cord and meninges. Of these, metastases of the vertebral column are by far the most common lesion type, followed by primary lesions of the spinal cord and meninges [1]. Primary lesions of the vertebral column are far more uncommon – estimated to occur in 2–3 patients per million population per year [1, 2]. Metastases isolated to the spinal cord and meninges are exceedingly uncommon [3].

Among the elderly, which we operatively define here as those greater than 60 years of age, the most common lesion types are spinal column metastases (71–105 cases per 100,000 population per year), [4] primary tumors of the spinal cord and meninges (2–2.7 per 100,000 per year and 0.9–1.4 per 100,000 per year, respectively), [1] and primary vertebral column tumors (≈5 per million per year) [1]. The optimal management strategies of these lesion types will be the focus of this chapter.

Frailty in the Elderly Spine Oncology Patient

Frailty is a somewhat vague concept used to describe the increased vulnerability that comes with aging-associated decline in physical reserve and function [5]. Clinical surrogates that have been used for frailty include weight loss or cachexia, [6] muscle loss or sarcopenia, [7–9] physical endurance, hypoalbuminemia/malnutrition, [10] and nutritional risk [11]. Multiple frailty assessment instruments have also been developed, [12] of which the most common are the physical frailty phenotype, [13] the deficit accumulation index, [14] and the vulnerable elders survey [15]. Within the spine literature, the Modified Frailty Index-5 (mFI-5) [16–18] and the American Society of Anesthesiologists (ASA) classification have also been employed as frailty metrics [19].

Previous investigations into the impact of frailty on spine oncology outcomes has yielded mixed outcomes. Zakaria investigated the impact of sarcopenia—low skeletal muscle mass—in patients with spinal metastasis and found it to be an independent predictor of increased overall mortality for both surgical and radiosurgical patients [7, 8]. Similarly, Charest-Morin, using the mFI-5, found greater frailty to be an independent predictor of prolonged hospitalization in patients undergoing en bloc resection of a primary or metastatic vertebral column tumor [18]. By contrast, Bourassa-Moreau et al. [20] found that frailty, as measured by previously validated indices (e.g. the mFI-5), did not predict either mortality or complication in patients undergoing emergent surgery for spinal metastasis. Nevertheless, they did find that sarcopenia predicting poorer outcomes, suggesting that, in general, frailty, as defined by poorer physical reserve, portends poorer outcomes in spine tumor patients. Fig. 15.1 conceptually represents how age and physical degeneration may factor into the relative risk-benefit profile of spine tumor surgery.

An independent but related concern is the presence of medical comorbidities. In general, patient medical histories increase in complexity with age; diabetes mellitus, [21] hypertension, [22] chronic pulmonary disease, [23] and cancer [24] are all increasingly common in the aged population. These medical comorbidities have been previously analyzed using a number of metrics, of which those most commonly applied to the spinal surgery literature are the Charlson Comorbidity Index (CCI) and ASA class. Greater medical complexity as measured by a higher CCI score or ASA class has previously been tied to prolonged hospitalizations and higher 30-day mortality in patients operated for spinal tumors [25]. Using the National Surgical Quality Improvement Program (NSQIP) database, Lakomkin et al. [25] found that CCI was an even stronger predictor of poor outcomes than ASA class or patient frailty, as assessed by the mFI-5.

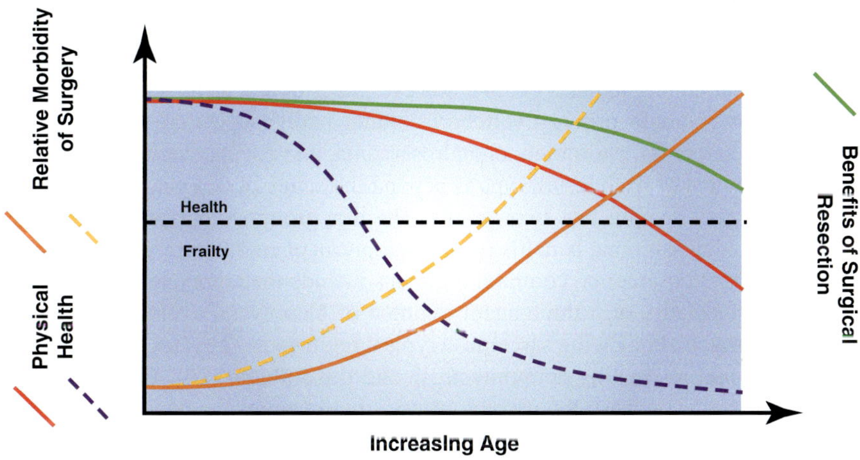

Fig. 15.1 Schematic representation of the relative costs and benefits of surgical intervention for spine tumors superimposed on a plot of physical health as a function of age. As the plot demonstrates, physical health worsens with increasing age. Under normal aging (red line), this process occurs gradually, whereas under certain conditions, patients experience a process of advanced aging (purple line). Those experiencing advanced aging cross the boundary between health and frailty at an earlier age than those aging at a normal rate. The incremental benefits of surgery (green)—commonly thought of in terms of overall or disease-specific survival—tend to decrease with age for most tumor pathologies, reaching a minimum at the point where the expected disease-specific survival equals or exceeds the actuarial survival for someone of the patient's age and general condition *without* active malignancy. Relative procedural morbidity also increases with age (orange line) as the pulmonary function and wound healing abilities of the patient decrease. Under the conditions of advanced aging (gold line), the relative morbidity may rise at an accelerated rate. Consequently, patients demonstrating advanced frailty may experience a relative reversal of the expected risks and benefits of surgery at an earlier age, as reflected by the intersection of the gold line with the green "benefit" line at a younger age relative to the orange line

Primary Spine Tumors

As stated above, primary spine tumors can be divided into those arising from the bones and those arising from the spinal cord, nerve roots, or meninges. The latter are far more common and surgery for these lesions is generally less morbid.

Tumors of the Vertebral Column

For the purposes of this discussion, we define primary tumors of the vertebral column as all malignancies arising from the bone of the mobile spine and sacrum. There are many benign lesions (e.g., chondroblastoma, enchondroma, giant cell tumor, osteoblastoma) that arise from the spinal column; however, these oftentimes do not require surgical management. Primary malignancies of the mobile spine and sacrum are exceedingly rare, occurring in only 2–3 patients per million population annually. Nevertheless, they are predominately seen in patients over the age of 50, with peak incidence in the sixth and seventh decade of life [1]. Disease burden is slightly higher among females (≈5:4); however, rates do not differ substantially.

The most common primary vertebral column malignancies are osteosarcoma (osteogenic sarcoma), chordoma, chondrosarcoma, and Ewing sarcoma. The optimal management of each lesion type is beyond the scope of this chapter; however, they can largely be split into two groups. The first group, comprised of osteosarcoma and Ewing sarcoma, benefits from neoadjuvant chemotherapy administration [26, 27]. For osteosarcoma, common regimens include methotrexate, doxorubicin, ifosfamide, cisplatin, or a three-agent regimen of bleomycin, cyclophosphamide, and dactinomycin. For Ewing sarcoma, a typical regimen is 12 cycles of vincristine, ifosfamide, and alternating actinomycin D and doxorubicin [26]. Chordoma and chondrosarcoma comprise the second group—those lesions for which chemotherapy has little to no efficacy.

Examination of population-level data, such as the Surveillance, Epidemiology, and End Results (SEER) database, suggest that all four lesion types benefit from surgical resection [28]. Specifically, en bloc resection with negative margins (R0 resection) has been demonstrated [29, 30] to offer superior survival in chordoma, [31–33] chondrosarcoma, [34–38] osteosarcoma, [39, 40] and Ewing sarcoma [41, 42]. Despite the apparent benefits in terms of local control and overall survival, surgery for primary osseous spinal malignancies is among the most morbid of neurosurgical procedures. Many elderly patients may be too ill to reasonably pursue surgical intervention and should instead be treated with a combination of radiotherapy for local control and pain relief, cementoplasty for spinal column stabilization, and chemotherapy for control of metastatic spread.

Patients, especially those who are advanced in age, benefit from multidisciplinary management and thorough evaluation of their preoperative health status. Those deemed healthy enough for surgery then undergo a process of oncologic staging (e.g., with positron emission tomography and/or computed tomography of the chest, abdomen, and pelvis) and surgical staging. The Enneking or Musculoskeletal Tumor Society (MSTS) system [43, 44] has been the staging system of choice for nearly 30 years. But recently, the American Joint Commission on Cancer (AJCC) published a TNM system for primary spine malignancies that incorporates elements of tumor morphology in addition to locoregional spread [45]. Many spinal oncologists still use the former system; however, it seems likely that in the near future the AJCC system may become standard due to shared features with the other TNM systems, which are widely employed in medical oncology [46].

Lesions that demonstrate no evidence of spread beyond local nodes may be reasonably approached for en bloc R0 resection. The Weinstein-Boriani-Biagini (WBB) [47] is a surgical staging system well-known to spinal oncologists that divides each spinal segment into concentric tissue layers, each comprised of 12 sectors arranged like a clockface (Fig. 15.2). The sectors involved dictate whether an anterior or posterior approach is preferrable. For lesions of the subaxial spine, an anterior approach is generally preferred for tumor delivery; a second posterior approach for stabilization may also be required. For lesions of the craniocervical junction, more invasive approaches are often necessary, including a staged posterior-anterior approach with a transmandibular anterior stage for lesions of the craniocervical junction or a transmanubrial approach for lesions of the cervicothoracic junction. Previous investigations have suggested that it may be used to accurately predict which lesions can be resected en bloc with wide or marginal margins in 88% of cases [48]. However, it must be noted that the vertebral arteries and nerve roots feeding the brachial plexus potentially complicate the resection of these lesions [49, 50]. In general, we favor preservation of the roots feeding the brachial plexus, given their vital role in daily function. Preservation of these nerves may lead to intralesional or marginal resection though. By contrast, we favor sacrifice of the vertebral artery to achieve en bloc R0 resection, if there is sufficient perfusion of the posterior circulation by the contralateral vertebral artery [51].

Though most primary sarcomas are conventionally thought of as radiation-resistant, modern radiation modalities, including focused photon therapy, proton therapy and hadron therapy (e.g. carbon ion therapy) have been shown to be effective [52]. Consequently, radiotherapy has become a key part of the treatment paradigm for most patients with primary bone tumors [2, 53–58]. Proton and hadron therapies may have advantages in terms of reduced radiation to adjacent healthy tissues. Lastly, some preliminary experiences have suggested that definitive, high-dose proton or hadron therapy may be useful for local control in those patients unable or unwilling to tolerate the morbidity of surgical management [59–61].

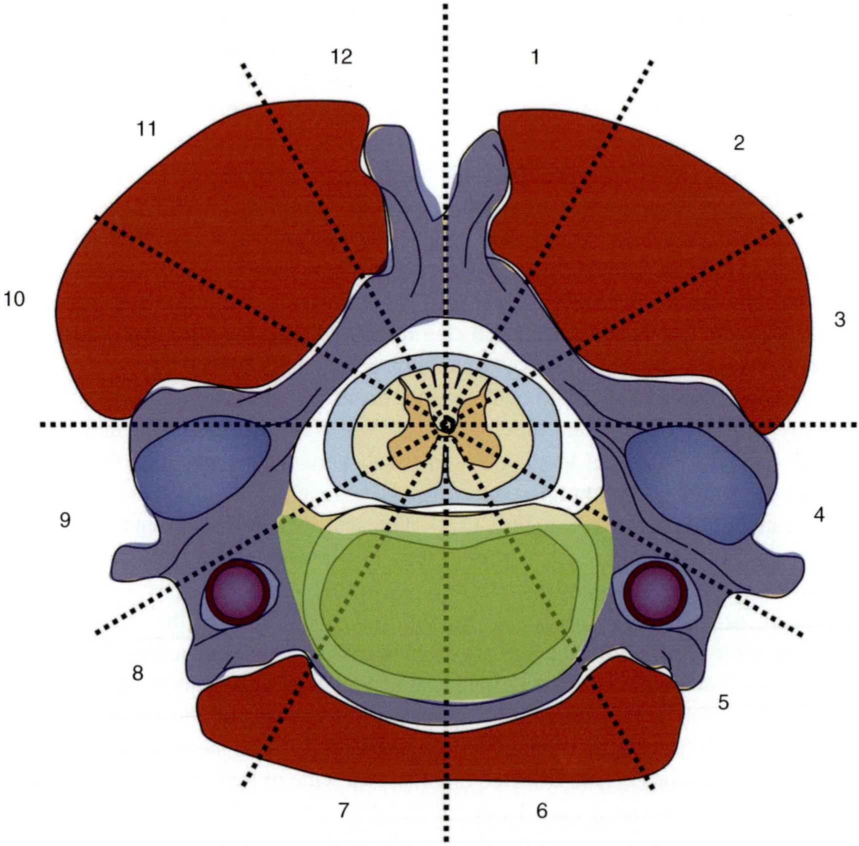

Fig. 15.2 Weinstein-Boriani-Biagini (WBB) system applied to the cervical spine. Concentric tissue layers are (A) the extraosseous soft tissues/muscle, (B) the superficial bone (intraosseous compartment—blue), (C) the deep bone (intraosseous compartment—green), (D) the epidural compartment, and (E) the intradural compartment

Tumors of the Spinal Cord and Meninges

Primary lesions of the spinal cord and meninges show peak incidence in the seventh decade of life; more than 40% of meningeal lesions and nearly 30% of spinal cord lesions are documented in patients over the age of 60 [1]. Like primary vertebral column tumors, lesions are more common among women (M:F $\approx$ 3:2 for meningeal lesions and 6:5 for spinal cord lesions) [1]. For both intramedullary and extramedullary lesions, cervical localization is less common than thoracic localization but accounts for a nontrivial proportion of cases [62].

Intradural Extramedullary Lesions

The most common histologies for intradural extramedullary tumors are schwannomas and meningiomas [63–66]. Surgical resection has conventionally been the treatment of choice for both pathologies [67, 68]. It is indicated for patients with neurological deficits secondary to neural element compression (e.g., spinal cord compression in meningiomas). Increased age is a known risk factor for postoperative venous thromboembolism, 30-day mortality, 30-day reoperation, 30-day unplanned readmission, and nonroutine discharge [69–71].

Meningiomas are uncommon in the cervical spine relative to the thoracic region, but 14–27% localize to the cervical spine [64]. Dorsal lesions can usually be addressed in patients that are considered poor substrates, such as elderly patients with extensive medical comorbidities, and definitive radiotherapy may be a reasonable alternative for spinal. A recent review of the SEER database demonstrated that this is only employed in ≈1% of patients though [72]. Such population-level data lacks the granularity to explain the reason for this treatment method. However, it can be speculated that patients generally receive surgery, as it is the best means of relieving preoperative neurological deficits. Gross total resection is possible in 82–99% of cases, though it may be difficult or impossible in calcified lesions [64]. The exact approach entertained is dependent upon the location of the lesion; dorsal lesions can be effectively treated with laminoplasty and Simpson grade I/II resection. However, anterior or anterolateral localization appears more common in cervical tumors [71, 73]. A dorsal or dorsolateral approach with sectioning of the dentate ligaments is generally effective for these lesions. However, for ventral lesions abutting the cervicothoracic cord, a transcervical approach with anterior cervical corpectomy and fusion may be entertained [73, 74]. In must be noted that such anterior approaches carry increased risk of dysphagia with age, especially among patients >60 years old [75, 76]. Complication rates are relatively low (0–3%) as is local recurrence (1–6%) [64]. Local control appears comparable for Simpson grade I and grade II resection, [77] though debate remains about this issue [78, 79].

Schwannomas, by contrast, are generally easily addressed from a posterior-only approach, and several large series have been published describing their management, including those of Conti et al., [80] Lenzi et al., [81] Seppälä et al., [82] and Safaee et al. [83, 84] Reported rates of gross total resection vary widely, ranging from 21% to 99% of cases; [80, 84] rates of gross total resection may be lower for cervical lesions [84]. All report relatively good outcomes, with neurological recovery seen in 56–73% of patients [80, 81] and significant improvements in functional status [80]. Based upon the result of Lenzi et al., [81] sensory deficits are both more common than motor deficits preoperatively and more likely to recover after surgical resection. However, many patients (up to 80%) are left with residual preoperative neurological deficit or a new postoperative neurological deficit [82]. It is essential that patients be warned of these likely complications prior to surgery. For patient unwilling to tolerate these deficits or who are unable to otherwise tolerate surgery, radiosurgery may also be an effective option for pain control and symptom stabilization [67, 68, 85–87].

Intradural Intramedullary (Intrinsic) Lesions

Increased age is similarly a predictor of worse outcomes amongst patients being treated for intrinsic/intramedullary spinal cord tumors. [88] The most common intrinsic lesions include ependymoma, astrocytoma, and hemangioblastoma [62, 65, 66, 89]. Unlike extramedullary lesions, surgery is generally the only option for the management of intrinsic lesions. In the case of ependymoma and hemangioblastoma, curative resection is often possible and improves progression-free survival [90–93]. Therefore, patients who are healthy enough to undergo surgical management should be treated with definitive resection, irrespective of age. By contrast, astrocytomas generally have ill-defined margins [92, 94]. Therefore, the patient and surgeon must have a more extensive discussion about the relative balance between the benefits spinal cord decompression and the new neurological deficits that are unavoidable with such surgeries. Cervical lesions are thought to have the highest rates of postoperative neurological worsening [92] and lowest likelihood of achieving optimal neurological outcomes [93]. Ill-defined tumor planes, [90] larger tumor size, [95] and increased age [93] are also associated with poorer neurological outcomes. Lastly, some prior series suggest that sensory symptoms are the most likely to improve following surgery [96]. Patients looking for improvements in motor or bowel/bladder function may therefore expect relatively less benefit than patients looking for sensory improvements. This warrants further investigation though.

Metastatic Lesions

The age profile of patients with metastatic spine tumors largely reflects the profile of all patients with oncologic disease, which is perhaps unsurprising, given that 40–70% of patients with newly diagnosed cancer will develop spine metastases [97]. However, only a small subset of patients with metastatic spine disease will have indications for surgical intervention [98]. The most common primary malignancies vary somewhat based upon the population under examination, but, in general, the most common primaries—lung, prostate, and breast—are the same as the most common primary malignancies in the general population [99]. Hepatocellular carcinoma and gastric adenocarcinoma are also common among East Asian populations, [4] consistent with the higher incidence of these cancers in Eastern Asia. Although cervical metastases are the least common, they are the easiest to address surgically.

Goals of Surgery

The primary goals of surgery for metastatic spine disease are to address underlying mechanical instability and to relieve compression on the neural elements. Assessment of mechanical instability relies on a combination of radiographic and clinical assessment. Biomechanical studies—finite element analyses and cadaveric experiments—have demonstrated that greater instability is associated with larger lesion size [100–103]. Additionally, finite analyses have suggested that decreases in axial loading capacity may be greatest for more cranially situated vertebrae [100]. Poor underlying bone quality, which is common in the elderly, also lowers vertebral body yield strength, [102] as does involvement of the posterolateral elements [104, 105].

The aggregate of these findings in turn led to the development of the Spinal Instability Neoplastic Score (SINS), a decision-making aid developed by the Spinal Oncology Study Group [106] that has been demonstrated to have high inter- and intra-rater reliability [107]. SINS scores lesions on a scale from 1 to 18 based upon underlying bone quality, extent of vertebral body involvement, the presence or absence of pain, posterolateral element involvement, location, and the presence of concurrent deformity. Lesions scoring >12 are deemed mechanically unstable enough to warrant surgical intervention, whereas those scoring ≤6 are deemed non-surgical. Intermediate scores (7–12) are classified as "potentially unstable"; however, more recent studies have suggested that scores of 10 or above generally benefit from surgical management [108, 109]. Additionally, a recent study by the Memorial Sloan Kettering group [110] suggested that blastic lesions, lesions causing mechanical pain, and lesions of the mobile or junctional spine segments were most likely to experience symptomatic benefit from intervention. Based upon this, it would appear that patient with cervical or cervicothoracic junctional lesions are more likely to experience benefit from surgery than those with lesions of the thoracic spine. Curiously, the results also suggest that patients with blastic lesions experience greater benefit, which is contrary to conventional thought. However, a 2020 finite element analysis suggested that the underlying loading characteristics of blastic lesions are poorer than those of lytic lesions [111]. Further investigations are necessary to evaluate this point.

Neurological deficits are the second major indication for surgical management of spinal metastases, and roughly 20,000 patients each year require intervention for metastatic epidural spinal cord compression (ESCC) [112]. With the publication of the findings of Patchell et al., [112] surgical decompression has been considered the gold standard as it provides superior functional outcomes to radiotherapy alone. Even with the advent of improved, focused radiation modalities (e.g., CyberKnife), surgical decompression remains the intervention of choice for those with tumor directly abutting the cord. Like mechanical instability, ESCC can also be assessed using a validated scoring system—the ESCC scale of Bilsky et al. [113]—that has previously been correlated with the severity of neurological impairment [114]. Lesions with direct tumor-cord contact (ESCC grade 2 and 3) should generally be treated with surgical decompression followed by radiotherapy, so-called separation surgery [115]. However, recent evidence suggests that radiotherapy alone may be reasonable for a select group of ESCC grade 2 patients presenting with either no neurological deficits or mild neurological deficits on presentation [116, 117]. Such decision should be made in consultation with a multidisciplinary care team and knowledge of the patient's treatment goals .However, it may be preferrable for some elderly patients with extensive medical comorbidities that would make them poor surgical candidates.

Who Is a Surgical Candidate?

Ensuring that a patient is a good surgical candidate is paramount for metastatic lesions, as the goal of surgery is symptom palliation, not cure. This is especially true for cervical metastases, which have the highest risk of multiple perioperative complications [118]. Conventionally, surgical candidacy for patients with spinal metastases has been based upon expected postoperative survival, with most spinal oncologists recommending surgery only for those patients with an expected survival of at least 3 months [98]. Pursuant to this, a number of survival predictors have been created, of which the best known are the Tomita [119] and Tokuhashi scales [120, 121]. Early scales were quite simplistic; however, more complex scores have been developed recently using multivariable analyses and machine learning. These newer scoring systems have proven more accurate and include the scoring systems of the Skeletal Oncology Research Group [122–124] and the New England Spinal Metastasis Score [125]. However, recently prospective work has suggested that even patients who do not meet these conventional survival guidelines may benefit from surgical intervention. Dea and the AOSpine Knowledge Forum Tumor [126] recently demonstrated that even patients with postoperative survival times less than 3 months may experience similar, clinically meaningful improvements in health-related quality-of-life outcomes. As a result, expected survival may not be an effective strategy for determining surgical candidacy. Rather, we favor an evaluation that balances the morbidity of surgery against the projected patient benefit in terms of neurological status and quality of life. Those with extensive comorbidities and concordantly high expected morbidity may be harmed more than helped by surgical intervention. By contrast, those with relatively few medical comorbidities may experience a net benefit from surgical treatment, even if they have poor expected survival.

Minimally Invasive Surgical Techniques and Alternatives for Frail Patients

As stated previously, the biggest concern with performing surgery for primary or metastatic lesions of the aged spine is whether the patient is too frail to tolerate the morbidity of surgery. As decreasing a patient's frailty is seldom an option, surgical optimization focuses on reducing procedural morbidity. The most popular means of doing so is through minimally invasive surgery (MIS). MIS techniques are defined by all surgical techniques that minimize soft tissue dissection and the disruption of normal anatomy en route to achieving the goals of surgery. MIS techniques are difficult to employ for primary vertebral body tumors, as en bloc resection with negative margins is the therapeutic gold standard [31, 32] and almost uniformly requires extensive soft tissue dissection. MIS approaches to primary lesions of the spinal cord and meninges, and metastatic vertebral column lesions have been described. For metastatic lesions, separation surgery is the most popular strategy [127, 128]. It makes use of percutaneous instrumentation and a small, posterior midline approach to resect the epidural tumor. The remaining tumor is then irradiated to achieve maximal control. In cases where anterior column reconstruction is required, a mini-open approach has been described, replacing the laminectomy with a transpedicular approach and piecemeal corpectomy [129]. In the cervical spine, however, a posterior approach may not be required, as the lower amount of prevertebral soft tissue means that an anterior cervical corpectomy and fusion via the Smith-Robinson approach is generally adequate [130]. However, for lesions of the craniocervical or cervicothoracic junction, a posterior approach may be necessary to access the tumor or to address underlying instability at these points of increased shear stress.

For primary lesions of the spinal cord and meninges, anterior approaches are generally contraindicated as they would require vertebral column resection to address the primary pathology. Posterior approaches are preferred, and minimally invasive approaches have been described, including endoscope-assisted, percutaneous resection of a cervical foraminal nerve sheath tumors, [131, 132] microscopic hemilaminectomy for resection of an intramedullary spinal cord tumors, [133] endoscope-assisted resection of intradural, intramedullary lesion, [134] and endoscope-assisted resection of intradural, extramedullary lesions [135, 136].

Nonsurgical Alternatives

Although MIS techniques have expanded the proportion of patients who can safely undergo surgical management of their tumors, there remains a nontrivial proportion of patients who are too ill to undergo surgery. For these patients, alternative interventions have been developed. Cementoplasty, which can be divided into vertebroplasty and kyphoplasty, is a percutaneous procedure aimed at stabilizing tumor-affected vertebra. Though uncommonly described in the cervical spine, [137] cementoplasty has been widely used for thoracolumbar lesion. Biomechanical analyses have shown cementoplasty significantly improves the axial loading properties of tumor-affected vertebrae [138]. Clinically, this likely translates to decreased rates of pathologic fracture. Downsides to cementoplasty are that it does not address neural element correction and provides minimal correction of de novo deformity secondary to pathologic fracture. Additionally, both vertebroplasty and kyphoplasty are associated with cement embolus formation and cement extravasation into the epidural space. Risk of cement-related embolic events may be reduced by using higher viscosity cements [139]. Disruption of the posterior vertebral body cortex increases the risk of epidural and venous leakage [140] and has been conventionally held as a contraindication to cementoplasty. However, case series have been published, demonstrating the relative safety of vertebroplasty or kyphoplasty with high viscosity cement in patients with pathologic fractures at high risk for cement leakage [141].

Cementoplasty does not address epidural disease or neural element compression. For this, other technologies have been described. Spinal laser interstitial thermotherapy (SLITT) places an ultraviolet laser probe transpedicularly into the tumor-affected vertebra. The laser heats the tumor up to 78 °C, causing rapid tumor cell death. The procedure is monitored using intraoperative magnetic resonance imaging, to ensure that the epidural space stays within preestablished safe limits [142]. It has been reported as safe even in patients with epidural tumor compressing the spinal cord [142, 143] and may be used as a neoadjuvant to stereotactic radiotherapy for local tumor control. Radiofrequency ablation (RFA) and cryoablation serve similar roles. Like SLITT, RFA uses a low-power (≤20 W per electrode) radiofrequency probe inserted transpedicularly under computed tomography or fluoroscopy guidance to induce coagulative necrosis of the tumor cells [144]. The epidural tumor can then collapse into the necrosed vertebral body lesion, decompressing the spinal cord. It has been shown to have high rates of pain relief and local control in small series [144–146]. Experience with cryoablation is far more limited in spine metastases [147]. It uses a transpedicularly inserted cryoablation probe to instill compressed argon gas into the lesion. The gas chills the tumor cells to ≤−130 °C, inducing coagulative necrosis. This results in indirect spinal cord decompression through a mechanism similar to that of SLITT and RFA. Though most published experiences describe a short post-procedural hospitalization (1–2 days), it may be amenable to outpatient implementation. All three techniques have low associated risk of wound complications, but careful temperature monitoring of the epidural space is necessary to prevent spinal cord injury [148].

Conclusion

Spinal oncology encompasses a breadth of pathologies with very different surgical interventions. Like degenerative disease, tumors are generally more common with age; lesion incidence peaks in the sixth or seventh decade of life for most lesion types. Cervical location is uncommon for most lesion types; however, metastatic and primary tumors of the cervical vertebral column, spinal cord, and meninges are seen at appreciable rates. In all cases, surgery is relatively morbid and care must be taken to ensure that the patient is healthy enough to tolerate surgery. Preoperative frailty scales may help to stratify patient risk and the adoption of minimally invasive surgical techniques and percutaneous treatments may reduce procedural morbidity.

Regardless of patient age though, preoperative consultation must focus on clearly identifying the goals of surgery and determining whether or not they align with the patient's treatment goals.

Funding None.

Devices None.

Previous Presentations None.

Disclosures Zach Pennington: None.

Andrew Schilling: None.

Andrew Hersh: None.

Daniel M. Sciubba: Consultant for Baxter, DePuy-Synthes, Globus Medical, K2M, Medtronic, NuVasive, Stryker. Unrelated grant support from Baxter Medical, North American Spine Society, and Stryker.

References

1. Sohn S, Kim J, Chung CK, Lee NR, Sohn MJ, Kim SH. A nation-wide epidemiological study of newly diagnosed primary spine tumor in the adult Korean population, 2009–2011. J Korean Neurosurg Soc. 2017;60:195–204.
2. Pennington Z, Ehresman J, McCarthy EF, Ahmed AK, Pittman PD, Lubelski D, Goodwin CR, Sciubba DM. Chordoma of the sacrum and mobile spine: a narrative review. Spine J. 2021;21(3):500–17. https://doi.org/10.1016/j.spinee.2020.10.009.
3. Goyal A, Yolcu Y, Kerezoudis P, Alvi MA, Krauss WE, Bydon M. Intramedullary spinal cord metastases: an institutional review of survival and outcomes. J Neuro-Oncol. 2019;142:347–54.
4. Sohn S, Kim J, Chung CK, Lee NR, Park E, Chang U-K, Sohn MJ, Kim SH. A nationwide epidemiological study of newly diagnosed spine metastasis in the adult Korean population. Spine J. 2016;16:937–45.
5. Xue Q-L. The frailty syndrome: definition and natural history. Clin Geriatr Med. 2011;27:1–15.
6. Tabouret E, Gravis G, Cauvin C, Loundou A, Adetchessi T, Fuentes S. Long-term survivors after surgical management of metastatic spinal cord compression. Eur Spine J. 2015;24:209–15.
7. Zakaria HM, Wilkinson BM, Pennington Z, et al. Sarcopenia as a prognostic factor for 90-day and overall mortality in patients undergoing spine surgery for metastatic tumors: a multicenter retrospective cohort study. Neurosurgery. 2020;87:1025–36.
8. Zakaria HM, Llaniguez JT, Telemi E, et al. Sarcopenia predicts overall survival in patients with lung, breast, prostate, or myeloma spine metastases undergoing stereotactic body radiation therapy (SBRT), independent of histology. Neurosurgery. 2020;86:705–16.
9. Gakhar H, Dhillon A, Blackwell J, Hussain K, Bommireddy R, Klezl Z, Williams J. Study investigating the role of skeletal muscle mass estimation in metastatic spinal cord compression. Eur Spine J. 2015;24:2150–5.

10. Hussain AK, Cheung ZB, Vig KS, Phan K, Lima MC, Kim JS, Di Capua J, Kaji DA, Arvind V, Cho SK. Hypoalbuminemia as an independent risk factor for perioperative complications following surgical decompression of spinal metastases. Glob Spine J. 2019;9:321–30.
11. Watanabe T, Kanayama M, Takahata M, Oda I, Suda K, Abe Y, Okumura J, Hojo Y, Iwasaki N. Perioperative complications of spine surgery in patients 80 years of age or older: a multicenter prospective cohort study. J Neurosurg Spine. 2020;32:622–30.
12. Buta BJ, Walston JD, Godino JG, Park M, Kalyani RR, Xue Q-L, Bandeen-Roche K, Varadhan R. Frailty assessment instruments: systematic characterization of the uses and contexts of highly-cited instruments. Ageing Res Rev. 2016;26:53–61.
13. Fried LP, Tangen CM, Walston J, et al. Frailty in older adults: evidence for a phenotype. J Gerontol A Biol Sci Med Sci. 2001;56:M146–57.
14. Mitnitski AB, Mogilner AJ, Rockwood K. Accumulation of deficits as a proxy measure of aging. Sci World J. 2001;1:323–36.
15. Saliba D, Elliott M, Rubenstein LZ, et al. The vulnerable elders survey: a tool for identifying vulnerable older people in the community. J Am Geriatr Soc. 2001;49:1691–9.
16. Wilson JRF, Badhiwala JH, Moghaddamjou A, Yee A, Wilson JR, Fehlings MG. Frailty is a better predictor than age of mortality and perioperative complications after surgery for degenerative cervical myelopathy: an analysis of 41,369 patients from the NSQIP database 2010–2018. J Clin Med. 2020;9:3491.
17. Yagi M, Michikawa T, Hosogane N, et al. The 5-item modified frailty index is predictive of severe adverse events in patients undergoing surgery for adult spinal deformity. Spine (Phila Pa 1976). 2019;44:E1083–91.
18. Charest-Morin R, Flexman AM, Srinivas S, et al. Perioperative adverse events following surgery for primary bone tumors of the spine and en bloc resection for metastases. J Neurosurg Spine. 2020;32:98–105.
19. Karhade AV, Vasudeva VS, Dasenbrock HH, Lu Y, Gormley WB, Groff MW, Chi JH, Smith TR. Thirty-day readmission and reoperation after surgery for spinal tumors: a National Surgical Quality Improvement Program analysis. Neurosurg Focus. 2016;41:E5.
20. Bourassa-Moreau É, Versteeg A, Moskven E, et al. Sarcopenia, but not frailty, predicts early mortality and adverse events after emergent surgery for metastatic disease of the spine. Spine J. 2020;20:22–31.
21. Mendola ND, Chen T-C, Gu Q, Eberhardt MS, Saydah S (2018) Prevalence of Total, diagnosed, and undiagnosed diabetes among adults: United States, 2013–2016. Hyattsville, MD.
22. Ostchega Y, Fryar CD, Nwankwo T, Nguyen DT (2020) Hypertension prevalence among adults aged 18 and over: United States, 2017–2018. Hyattsville, MD.
23. Tilert T, Paulose-Ram R, Howard D, Butler J, Lee S, Wang MQ. Prevalence and factors associated with self-reported chronic obstructive pulmonary disease among adults aged 40-79: the National Health and nutrition examination survey (NHANES) 2007-2012. EC Pulmonol Respir Med. 2018;7:650–62.
24. Siegel RL, Miller KD, Jemal A. Cancer statistics, 2020. CA Cancer J Clin. 2020;70:7–30.
25. Lakomkin N, Zuckerman SL, Stannard B, Montejo J, Sussman ES, Virojanapa J, Kuzmik G, Goz V, Hadjipanayis CG, Cheng JS. Preoperative risk stratification in spine tumor surgery. Spine (Phila Pa 1976). 2019;44:E782–7.
26. Ozturk AK, Gokaslan ZL, Wolinsky J-P. Surgical treatment of sarcomas of the spine. Curr Treat Options in Oncol. 2014;15:482–92.
27. Sciubba DM, Okuno SH, Dekutoski MB, Gokaslan ZL. Ewing and osteogenic sarcoma: evidence for multidisciplinary management. Spine (Phila pa 1976). 2009;34:S58.
28. Mukherjee D, Chaichana K, Parker S, Gokaslan Z, McGirt M. Association of surgical resection and survival in patients with malignant primary osseous spinal neoplasms from the surveillance, epidemiology, and end results (SEER) database. Eur Spine J. 2013;22:1375–82.
29. Schwab J, Gasbarrini A, Bandiera S, Boriani L, Amendola L, Picci P, Ferrari S, Boriani S. Osteosarcoma of the Mobile spine. Spine (Phila Pa 1976). 2012;37:E381–6.

30. Talac R, Yaszemski MJ, Currier BL, Fuchs B, Dekutoski MB, Kim CW, Sim FH. Relationship between surgical margins and local recurrence in sarcomas of the spine. Clin Orthop Relat Res. 2002;397:127–32.
31. Gokaslan ZL, Zadnik PL, Sciubba DM, et al. Mobile spine chordoma: results of 166 patients from the AOSpine knowledge forum tumor database. J Neurosurg Spine. 2016;24:644–51.
32. Varga PP, Szövérfi Z, Fisher CG, et al. Surgical treatment of sacral chordoma: prognostic variables for local recurrence and overall survival. Eur Spine J. 2015;24:1092–101.
33. Rotondo RL, Folkert W, Liebsch NJ, et al. High-dose proton-based radiation therapy in the management of spine chordomas: outcomes and clinicopathological prognostic factors. J Neurosurg Spine. 2015;23:788–97.
34. Bergh P, Gunterberg B, Meis-Kindblom JM, Kindblom L-G. Prognostic factors and outcome of pelvic, sacral, and spinal chondrosarcomas: a center-based study of 69 cases. Cancer. 2001;91:1201–12.
35. York JE, Berk RH, Fuller GN, Rao JS, Abi-Said D, Wildrick DM, Gokaslan ZL. Chondrosarcoma of the spine: 1954 to 1997. J Neurosurg Spine. 1999;90:73–8.
36. Yang X, Wu Z, Xiao J, Feng D, Huang Q, Zheng W, Chen H, Yuan W, Jia L. Chondrosarcomas of the cervical and cervicothoracic spine. J Spinal Disord Tech. 2012;25:1–9.
37. Boriani S, De Iure F, Bandiera S, Campanacci L, Biagini R, Di Fiore M, Bandello L, Picci P, Bacchini P. Chondrosarcoma of the Mobile spine: report on 22 cases. Spine (Phila Pa 1976). 2000;25:804–12.
38. Schoenfeld AJ, Hornicek FJ, Pedlow FX, Kobayashi W, Raskin KA, Springfield D, DeLaney TF, Nielsen GP, Mankin HJ, Schwab JH. Chondrosarcoma of the Mobile spine: a review of 21 cases treated at a single center. Spine (Phila Pa 1976). 2012;37:119–26.
39. Pombo B, Cristina Ferreira A, Cardoso P, Oliveira A. Clinical effectiveness of Enneking appropriate versus Enneking inappropriate procedure in patients with primary osteosarcoma of the spine: a systematic review with meta-analysis. Eur Spine J. 2020;29:238–47.
40. Dekutoski MB, Clarke MJ, Rose P, et al. Osteosarcoma of the spine: prognostic variables for local recurrence and overall survival, a multicenter ambispective study. J Neurosurg Spine. 2016;25:59–68.
41. Charest-Morin R, Dirks MS, Patel S, et al. Ewing sarcoma of the spine: prognostic variables for survival and local control in surgically treated patients. Spine (Phila Pa 1976). 2018;43:622–9.
42. Wan W, Lou Y, Hu Z, et al. Factors affecting survival outcomes of patients with non-metastatic Ewing's sarcoma family tumors in the spine: a retrospective analysis of 63 patients in a single center. J Neuro-Oncol. 2017;131:313–20.
43. Enneking WF, Spanier SS, Goodman MA. A system for the surgical staging of musculoskeletal sarcoma. Clin Orthop Relat Res. 1980;153:106–20.
44. Enneking WF. A system of staging musculoskeletal neoplasms. Clin Orthop Relat Res. 1986;204:9–4.
45. Tanaka K, Ozaki T. New TNM classification (AJCC eighth edition) of bone and soft tissue sarcomas: JCOG bone and soft tissue tumor study group. Jpn J Clin Oncol. 2019;49:103–7.
46. Rose PS, Holt GE, Kneisl JS. Changes to the American joint committee on cancer staging system for spine tumors—practice update. Ann Transl Med. 2019;7:215.
47. Boriani S, Weinstein JN, Biagini R. Primary bone tumors of the spine. Spine (Phila Pa 1976). 1997;22:1036–44.
48. Yamazaki T, McLoughlin GS, Patel SR, Rhines LD, Fourney DR. Feasibility and safety of en bloc resection for primary spine tumors: a systematic review by the spine oncology study group. Spine (Phila Pa 1976). 2009;34:S31–8.
49. Mattei TA, Mendel E. En bloc resection of primary malignant bone tumors of the cervical spine. Acta Neurochir. 2014;156:2159–64.
50. Kaloostian PE, Gokaslan ZL. Surgical management of primary tumors of the cervical spine: surgical considerations and avoidance of complications. Neurol Res. 2014;36:557–65.

51. Westbroek EM, Pennington Z, Ehresman J, Ahmed AK, Gailloud P, Sciubba DM. Vertebral artery sacrifice versus skeletonization in the setting of cervical spine tumor resection: case series. World Neurosurg. 2020;139:e601–7.
52. Konieczkowski DJ, DeLaney TF, Yamada YJ. Radiation strategies for spine chordoma: proton beam, carbon ions, and stereotactic body radiation therapy. Neurosurg Clin N Am. 2020;31:263–88.
53. Dial BL, Kerr DL, Lazarides AL, et al. The role of radiotherapy for chordoma patients managed with surgery. Spine (Phila Pa 1976). 2020;45:E742–51.
54. Pennicooke B, Laufer I, Sahgal A, Varga PP, Gokaslan ZL, Bilsky MH, Yamada YJ. Safety and local control of radiation therapy for chordoma of the spine and sacrum: a systematic review. Spine (Phila Pa 1976). 2016;41:S186–92.
55. Cuccia F, Fiore MR, Barcellini A, et al. Outcome and toxicity of carbon ion radiotherapy for axial bone and soft tissue sarcomas. Anticancer Res. 2020;40:2853–9.
56. Holliday EB, Mitra HS, Somerson JS, Rhines LD, Mahajan A, Brown PD, Grosshans DR. Postoperative proton therapy for chordomas and chondrosarcomas of the spine. Spine (Phila Pa 1976). 2015;40:544–9.
57. Kerr DL, Dial BL, Lazarides AL, Catanzano AA, Lane WO, Blazer DG, Brigman BE, Mendoza-Lattes S, Eward WC, Erickson ME. Epidemiologic and survival trends in adult primary bone tumors of the spine. Spine J. 2019;19:1941–9.
58. Indelicato DJ, Rotondo RL, Begosh-Mayne D, Scarborough MT, Gibbs CP, Morris CG, Mendenhall WM. A prospective outcomes study of proton therapy for chordomas and chondrosarcomas of the spine. Int J Radiat Oncol. 2016;95:297–303.
59. Matsumoto K, Imai R, Kamada T, Maruyama K, Tsuji H, Tsujii H, Shioyama Y, Honda H, Isu K. Impact of carbon ion radiotherapy for primary spinal sarcoma. Cancer. 2013;119:3496–503.
60. Jin CJ, Berry-Candelario J, Reiner AS, et al. Long-term outcomes of high-dose single-fraction radiosurgery for chordomas of the spine and sacrum. J Neurosurg Spine. 2020;32:79–88.
61. Indelicato DJ, Keole SR, Shahlaee AH, Morris CG, Gibbs CP, Scarborough MT, Pincus DW, Marcus RB. Spinal and paraspinal Ewing tumors. Int J Radiat Oncol. 2010;76:1463–71.
62. Hirano K, Imagama S, Sato K, et al. Primary spinal cord tumors: review of 678 surgically treated patients in Japan. A multicenter study. Eur Spine J. 2012;21:2019–26.
63. Kshettry VR, Hsieh JK, Ostrom QT, Kruchko C, Benzel EC, Barnholtz-Sloan JS. Descriptive epidemiology of spinal meningiomas in the United States. Spine (Phila Pa 1976). 2015;40:E886–9.
64. Gottfried ON, Gluf W, Quinones-Hinojosa A, Kan P, Schmidt MH. Spinal meningiomas: surgical management and outcome. Neurosurg Focus. 2003;14:1–7.
65. Suh Y-L, Koo H, Kim TS, et al. Tumors of the central nervous system in Korea: a multicenter study of 3221 cases. J Neuro-Oncol. 2002;56:251–9.
66. Schellinger KA, Propp JM, Villano JL, McCarthy BJ. Descriptive epidemiology of primary spinal cord tumors. J Neuro-Oncol. 2008;87:173–9.
67. Gerszten PC, Quader M, Novotny J, Flickinger JC. Radiosurgery for benign tumors of the spine: clinical experience and current trends. Technol Cancer Res Treat. 2012;11:133–9.
68. Meola A, Soltys S, Schmitt A, Gerszten PC, Chang SD. Stereotactic radiosurgery for benign spinal tumors. Neurosurg Clin N Am. 2020;31:231–5.
69. Phan K, Vig KS, Ho YT, Hussain AK, Di Capua J, Kim JS, White SJW, Lee NJ, Kothari P, Cho SK. Age is a risk factor for postoperative complications following excisional laminectomy for intradural extramedullary spinal tumors. Glob Spine J. 2019;9:126–32.
70. Ahn A, Phan K, Cheung ZB, White SJW, Kim JS, Cho SK-W. Predictors of discharge disposition following laminectomy for intradural extramedullary spinal tumors. World Neurosurg. 2019;123:e427–32.
71. Phan K, Cheung ZB, Vig KS, Hussain AK, Lima MC, Kim JS, Di Capua J, Cho SK. Age stratification of 30-day postoperative outcomes following excisional laminectomy for extradural cervical and thoracic tumors. Glob Spine J. 2018;8:490–7.

72. Yolcu YU, Goyal A, Alvi MA, Moinuddin F, Bydon M. Trends in the utilization of radiotherapy for spinal meningiomas: insights from the 2004–2015 National Cancer Database. Neurosurg Focus. 2019;46:E6.
73. Slin'ko EI, Al-Qashqish II. Intradural ventral and ventrolateral tumors of the spinal cord: surgical treatment and results. Neurosurg Focus. 2004;17:1–8.
74. Angevine PD, Kellner C, Haque RM, McCormick PC. Surgical management of ventral intradural spinal lesions. J Neurosurg Spine. 2011;15:28–37.
75. Wang T, Ma L, Yang D-L, Wang H, Bai Z-L, Zhang L-J, Ding W-Y. Factors predicting dysphagia after anterior cervical surgery. Medicine (Baltimore). 2017;96:e7916.
76. Chung W-F, Liu S-W, Huang L-C, Chang H-K, Wu J-C, Chen L-F, Chen Y-C, Huang W-C, Cheng H, Lo S-S. Serious dysphagia following anterior cervical discectomy and fusion: long-term incidence in a national cohort. J Neurosurg Sci. 2020;64:231–7.
77. Barber SM, Konakondla S, Nakhla J, Fridley JS, Xia J, Oyelese AA, Telfeian AE, Gokaslan ZL. Oncologic benefits of dural resection in spinal meningiomas: a meta-analysis of Simpson grades and recurrence rates. J Neurosurg Spine. 2020;32:441–51.
78. Voldřich R, Netuka D, Beneš V. Spinal meningiomas: is Simpson grade II resection radical enough? Acta Neurochir. 2020;162:1401–8.
79. Nakamura M, Tsuji O, Fujiyoshi K, Hosogane N, Watanabe K, Tsuji T, Ishii K, Toyama Y, Chiba K, Matsumoto M. Long-term surgical outcomes of spinal meningiomas. Spine (Phila Pa 1976). 2012;37:E617–23.
80. Conti P, Pansini G, Mouchaty H, Capuano C, Conti R. Spinal neurinomas: retrospective analysis and long-term outcome of 179 consecutively operated cases and review of the literature. Surg Neurol. 2004;61:34–43.
81. Lenzi J, Anichini G, Landi A, Piciocchi A, Passacantilli E, Pedace F, Delfini R, Santoro A. Spinal nerves schwannomas: experience on 367 cases—historic overview on how clinical, radiological, and surgical practices have changed over a course of 60 years. Neurol Res Int. 2017;2017:1–12.
82. Seppälä MT, Haltia MJJ, Sankila RJ, Jääskeläinen JE, Heiskanen O. Long-term outcome after removal of spinal schwannoma: a clinicopathological study of 187 cases. J Neurosurg. 1995;83:621–6.
83. Safaee M, Parsa AT, Barbaro NM, Chou D, Mummaneni PV, Weinstein PR, Tihan T, Ames CP. Association of tumor location, extent of resection, and neurofibromatosis status with clinical outcomes for 221 spinal nerve sheath tumors. Neurosurg Focus. 2015;39:E5.
84. Safaee MM, Lyon R, Barbaro NM, Chou D, Mummaneni PV, Weinstein PR, Chin CT, Tihan T, Ames CP. Neurological outcomes and surgical complications in 221 spinal nerve sheath tumors. J Neurosurg Spine. 2017;26:103–11
85. Kufeld M, Wowra B, Muacevic A, Zausinger S, Tonn J-C. Radiosurgery of spinal meningiomas and schwannomas. Technol Cancer Res Treat. 2012;11:27–34.
86. Sachdev S, Dodd RL, Chang SD, Soltys SG, Adler JR, Luxton G, Choi CYH, Tupper L, Gibbs IC. Stereotactic radiosurgery yields long-term control for benign intradural, extramedullary spinal tumors. Neurosurgery. 2011;69:533–9.
87. Hwang L, Okoye CC, Patel RB, et al. Stereotactic body radiotherapy for benign spinal tumors: meningiomas, schwannomas, and neurofibromas. J Radiosurgery SBRT. 2019;6:167–77.
88. Sharma M, Sonig A, Ambekar S, Nanda A. Discharge dispositions, complications, and costs of hospitalization in spinal cord tumor surgery: analysis of data from the United States Nationwide inpatient sample, 2003–2010. J Neurosurg Spine. 2014;20:125–41.
89. Man-Kai C. Spinal cord tumors in the People's republic of China. Neurosurgery. 1982;10:22–4.
90. Garcés-Ambrossi GL, McGirt MJ, Mehta VA, Sciubba DM, Witham TF, Bydon A, Wolinksy J-P, Jallo GI, Gokaslan ZL. Factors associated with progression-free survival and long-term neurological outcome after resection of intramedullary spinal cord tumors: analysis of 101 consecutive cases. J Neurosurg Spine. 2009;11:591–9.

91. Wostrack M, Ringel F, Eicker SO, et al. Spinal ependymoma in adults: a multicenter investigation of surgical outcome and progression-free survival. J Neurosurg Spine. 2018;28:654–62.
92. Karikari IO, Nimjee SM, Hodges TR, et al. Impact of tumor histology on Resectability and neurological outcome in primary intramedullary spinal cord tumors: a single-center experience with 102 patients. Neurosurgery. 2015;76:S4–S13.
93. Samuel N, Tetreault L, Santaguida C, Nater A, Moayeri N, Massicotte EM, Fehlings MG. Clinical and pathological outcomes after resection of intramedullary spinal cord tumors: a single-institution case series. Neurosurg Focus. 2016;41:E8.
94. Knafo S, Aghakhani N, David P, Parker F. Management of intramedullary spinal cord tumors: a single-center experience of 247 patients. Rev Neurol (Paris). 2020;177(5):508–14. https://doi.org/10.1016/j.neurol.2020.07.014.
95. Eroes CA, Zausinger S, Kreth F-W, Goldbrunner R, Tonn J-C. Intramedullary low grade astrocytoma and ependymoma. Surgical results and predicting factors for clinical outcome. Acta Neurochir. 2010;152:611–8.
96. Schebesch K-M, Mueller S, Wendl C, Brawanski A, Riemenschneider MJ, Proescholdt M. Recurrence rates and functional outcome after resection of intrinsic intramedullary tumors. Clin Neurol Neurosurg. 2015;134:60–6.
97. Pennington Z, Goodwin ML, Westbroek EM, Cottrill E, Ahmed AK, Sciubba DM. Lactate and cancer: spinal metastases and potential therapeutic targets (part 2). Ann Transl Med. 2019;7:221.
98. Pennington Z, Ehresman J, Cottrill E, Lubelski D, Lehner K, Feghali J, Ahmed AK, Schilling A, Sciubba DM. To operate, or not to operate? Narrative review of the role of survival predictors in patient selection for operative management of patients with metastatic spine disease. J Neurosurg Spine. 2020:1–15.
99. Siegel RL, Miller KD, Jemal A. Cancer statistics, 2019. CA Cancer J Clin. 2019;69:7–34.
100. Galbusera F, Qian Z, Casaroli G, Bassani T, Costa F, Schlager B, Wilke H-J. The role of the size and location of the tumors and of the vertebral anatomy in determining the structural stability of the metastatically involved spine: a finite element study. Transl Oncol. 2018;11:639–46.
101. Costa MC, Campello LBB, Ryan M, Rochester J, Viceconti M, Dall'Ara E (2020) Effect of size and location of simulated lytic lesions on the structural properties of human vertebral bodies, a micro-finite element study. Bone Reports 12:100257.
102. Whyne CM, Hu SS, Lotz JC. Parametric finite element analysis of vertebral bodies affected by tumors. J Biomech. 2001;34:1317–24.
103. Roth SE, Mousavi P, Finkelstein J, Chow E, Kreder H, Whyne CM. Metastatic burst fracture risk prediction using biomechanically based equations. Clin Orthop Relat Res. 2004;419:83–90.
104. Ebihara H, Ito M, Abumi K, Taneichi H, Kotani Y, Minami A, Kaneda K. A biomechanical analysis of metastatic vertebral collapse of the thoracic spine: a sheep model study. Spine (Phila Pa 1976). 2004;29:994–9.
105. Whyne CM, Hu SS, Lotz JC. Burst fracture in the metastatically involved spine: development, validation, and parametric analysis of a three-dimensional Poroelastic finite-element model. Spine (Phila Pa 1976). 2003;28:652–60.
106. Fisher CG, DiPaola CP, Ryken TC, et al. A novel classification system for spinal instability in neoplastic disease: an evidence-based approach and expert consensus form the spine oncology study group. Spine (Phila Pa 1976). 2010;35:E1221–9.
107. Pennington Z, Ahmed AK, Cottrill E, Westbroek EM, Goodwin ML, Sciubba DM. Intra- and interobserver reliability of the spinal instability neoplastic score system for instability in spine metastases: a systematic review and meta-analysis. Ann Transl Med. 2019;7:218.
108. Hussain I, Barzilai O, Reiner AS, DiStefano N, McLaughlin L, Ogilvie S, Bilsky M, Laufer I. Patient-reported outcomes after surgical stabilization of spinal tumors: symptom-based validation of the spinal instability neoplastic score (SINS) and surgery. Spine J. 2018;18:261–7.

109. Pennington Z, Ahmed AK, Westbroek EM, Cottrill E, Lubelski D, Goodwin ML, Sciubba DM. SINS score and stability: evaluating the need for stabilization within the uncertain category. World Neurosurg. 2019;128:e1034–47.
110. Hussain I, Barzilai O, Reiner AS, McLaughlin L, DiStefano NM, Ogilvie S, Versteeg AL, Fisher CG, Bilsky MH, Laufer I. Spinal instability neoplastic score component validation using patient-reported outcomes. J Neurosurg Spine. 2019;30:432–8.
111. Stadelmann MA, Schenk DE, Maquer G, Lenherr C, Buck FM, Bosshardt DD, Hoppe S, Theumann N, Alkalay RN, Zysset PK. Conventional finite element models estimate the strength of metastatic human vertebrae despite alterations of the bone's tissue and structure. Bone. 2020;141:115598.
112. Patchell RA, Tibbs PA, Regine WF, Payne R, Saris S, Kryscio RJ, Mohiuddin M, Young B. Direct decompressive surgical resection in the treatment of spinal cord compression caused by metastatic cancer: a randomised trial. Lancet. 2005;366:643–8.
113. Bilsky MH, Laufer I, Fourney DR, Groff M, Schmidt MH, Varga PP, Vrionis FD, Yamada Y, Gerszten PC, Kuklo TR. Reliability analysis of the epidural spinal cord compression scale. J Neurosurg Spine. 2010;13:324–8.
114. Maseda M, Uei H, Nakahashi M, Sawada H, Tokuhashi Y. Neurological outcome of treatment for patients with impending paralysis due to epidural spinal cord compression by metastatic spinal tumor. J Orthop Surg Res. 2019;14:291.
115. Laufer I, Iorgulescu JB, Chapman T, Lis E, Shi W, Zhang Z, Cox BW, Yamada Y, Bilsky MH. Local disease control for spinal metastases following "separation surgery" and adjuvant hypofractionated or high-dose single-fraction stereotactic radiosurgery: outcome analysis in 186 patients. J Neurosurg Spine. 2013;18:207–14.
116. Rothrock RJ, Li Y, Lis E, et al. Hypofractionated spinal stereotactic body radiation therapy for high-grade epidural disease. J Neurosurg Spine. 2020;33:680–7.
117. Redmond KJ, Lo SS, Soltys SG, et al. Consensus guidelines for postoperative stereotactic body radiation therapy for spinal metastases: results of an international survey. J Neurosurg Spine. 2017;26:299–306.
118. Hussain AK, Vig KS, Cheung ZB, Phan K, Lima MC, Kim JS, Kaji DA, Arvind V, Cho SK-W. The impact of metastatic spinal tumor location on 30-day perioperative mortality and morbidity after surgical decompression. Spine (Phila Pa 1976). 2018;43:E648–55.
119. Tomita K, Kawahara N, Kobayashi T, Yoshida A, Murakami H, Akamaru T. Surgical strategy for spinal metastases. Spine (Phila Pa 1976). 2001;26:298–306.
120. Tokuhashi Y, Matsuzaki H, Oda H, Oshima M, Ryu J. A revised scoring system for preoperative evaluation of metastatic spine tumor prognosis. Spine (Phila Pa 1976). 2005;30:2186–91.
121. Tokuhashi Y, Matsuzaki H, Toriyama S, Kawano H, Ohsaka S. Scoring system for the preoperative evaluation of metastatic spine tumor prognosis. Spine (Phila Pa 1976). 1990;15:1110–3.
122. Paulino Pereira NR, Janssen SJ, van Dijk E, Harris MB, Hornicek FJ, Ferrone ML, Schwab JH. Development of a prognostic survival algorithm for patients with metastatic spine disease. J Bone Joint Surg Am. 2016;98:1767–76.
123. Karhade AV, Thio QCBS, Ogink PT, et al. Development of machine learning algorithms for prediction of 30-day mortality after surgery for spinal metastasis. Neurosurgery. 2019;85:E83–91.
124. Karhade AV, Ahmed AK, Pennington Z, Chara A, Schilling A, Thio QCBS, Ogink PT, Sciubba DM, Schwab JH. External validation of the SORG 90-day and 1-year machine learning algorithms for survival in spinal metastatic disease. Spine J. 2020;20:14–21.
125. Schoenfeld AJ, Ferrone ML, Schwab JH, Blucher JA, Barton LB, Tobert DG, Chi JH, Shin JH, Kang JD, Harris MB. Prospective validation of a clinical prediction score for survival in patients with spinal metastases: the New England spinal metastasis score. Spine J. 2021;21(1):28–36. https://doi.org/10.1016/j.spinee.2020.02.009.

126. Dea N, Versteeg AL, Sahgal A, et al. Metastatic spine disease: should patients with short life expectancy be denied surgical care? An international retrospective cohort study. Neurosurgery. 2020;87:303–11.
127. Rothrock R, Pennington Z, Ehresman J, Bilsky MH, Barzilai O, Szerlip NJ, Sciubba DM. Hybrid therapy for spinal metastases. Neurosurg Clin N Am. 2020;31:191–200.
128. Barzilai O, Laufer I, Robin A, Xu R, Yamada Y, Bilsky MH. Hybrid therapy for metastatic epidural spinal cord compression: technique for separation surgery and spine radiosurgery. Oper Neurosurg. 2019;16:310–8.
129. Chou D, Lu DC. Mini-open transpedicular corpectomies with expandable cage reconstruction. J Neurosurg Spine. 2011;14:71–7.
130. Liu JK, Apfelbaum RI, Schmidt MH. Surgical management of cervical spinal metastasis: anterior reconstruction and stabilization techniques. Neurosurg Clin N Am. 2004;15:413–24.
131. Ying G-Y, Yao Y, Shen F, Wu Z-Y, Chen C-M, Zhu Y-J. Percutaneous endoscopic removal of cervical foraminal schwannoma via interlaminar approach: a case report. Oper Neurosurg. 2018;14:1–5.
132. Zhang J, Zhang X-H, Wang Z, et al. Transforaminal resection of cervical dumbbell schwannomas in patients with additional tumors. World Neurosurg. 2017;98:768–73.
133. Li J, Jiang X-H, Chen A-Q, Ying G-Y, Shen F, Zhu Y-J. Surgical management of a cervical intramedullary hemangioblastoma presenting with intracystic hemorrhage by hemi-semi-laminectomy via a posterior approach. J Int Med Res. 2019;47:3458–64.
134. Chern JJ, Gordon AS, Naftel RP, Tubbs RS, Oakes WJ, Wellons JC. Intradural spinal endoscopy in children. J Neurosurg Pediatr. 2011;8:107–11.
135. Parihar V, Yadav N, Yadav Y, Ratre S, Bajaj J, Kher Y. Endoscopic management of spinal intradural extramedullary tumors. J Neurol Surg A Cent Eur Neurosurg. 2016;78:219–26.
136. Barami K, Dagnew E. Endoscope-assisted posterior approach for the resection of ventral intradural spinal cord tumors: report of two cases. Minim Invasive Neurosurg. 2007;50:370–3.
137. Cazzato RL, de Marini P, Auloge P, Autreausseau PA, Koch G, Dalili D, Rao P, Garnon J, Gangi A. Percutaneous vertebroplasty of the cervical spine performed via a posterior trans-pedicular approach. Eur Radiol. 2020;31(2):591–8. https://doi.org/10.1007/s00330-020-07198-6.
138. Tschirhart CE, Roth SE, Whyne CM. Biomechanical assessment of stability in the metastatic spine following percutaneous vertebroplasty: effects of cement distribution patterns and volume. J Biomech. 2005;38:1582–90.
139. Chen WC, Tsai SHL, Goyal A, Fu T-S, Lin T-Y, Bydon M. Comparison between vertebroplasty with high or low viscosity cement augmentation or kyphoplasty in cement leakage rate for patients with vertebral compression fracture: a systematic review and network meta-analysis. Eur Spine J. 2021;30(9):2680–90. https://doi.org/10.1007/s00586-020-06636-9.
140. Tang B, Cui L, Chen X, Liu Y. Risk factors for cement leakage in percutaneous vertebroplasty for osteoporotic vertebral compression fractures. Spine (Phila Pa 1976). 2020. https://doi.org/10.1097/BRS.0000000000003773
141. Reyad RM, Ghobrial HZ, Hakim SM, Hashem RH, Elsaman A, Shaaban MH. Thick cement usage in percutaneous vertebroplasty for malignant vertebral fractures at high risk for cement leakage. Diagn Interv Imaging. 2017;98:721–8.
142. Tatsui CE, Stafford RJ, Li J, et al. Utilization of laser interstitial thermotherapy guided by real-time thermal MRI as an alternative to separation surgery in the management of spinal metastasis. J Neurosurg Spine. 2015;23:400–11.
143. Tatsui CE, Nascimento CNG, Suki D, et al. Image guidance based on MRI for spinal interstitial laser thermotherapy: technical aspects and accuracy. J Neurosurg Spine. 2017;26:605–12.
144. Mayer T, Cazzato RL, De Marini P, Auloge P, Dalili D, Koch G, Garnon J, Gangi A. Spinal metastases treated with bipolar radiofrequency ablation with increased (>70 °C) target temper-

ature: Pain management and local tumor control. Diagn Interv Imaging. 2020;102(1):27–34. https://doi.org/10.1016/j.diii.2020.04.012.
145. Bagla S, Sayed D, Smirniotopoulos J, Brower J, Neal Rutledge J, Dick B, Carlisle J, Lekht I, Georgy B. Multicenter prospective clinical series evaluating radiofrequency ablation in the treatment of painful spine metastases. Cardiovasc Intervent Radiol. 2016;39:1289–97.
146. Reyes M, Georgy M, Brook L, Ortiz O, Brook A, Agarwal V, Muto M, Manfre L, Marcia S, Georgy BA. Multicenter clinical and imaging evaluation of targeted radiofrequency ablation (t-RFA) and cement augmentation of neoplastic vertebral lesions. J Neurointerv Surg. 2018;10:176–82.
147. Gravel G, Tselikas L, Moulin B, et al. Early detection with MRI of incomplete treatment of spine metastases after percutaneous cryoablation. Eur Radiol. 2019;29:5655–63.
148. Westbroek EM, Goodwin ML, Hui F, Khan MA, Sciubba DM. Thermal injury to spinal cord, a rare complication of percutaneous microwave spine tumor ablation: case report. J Clin Neurosci. 2019;64:50–4.

Part III
Thoracolumbar Disease in the Elderly

Chapter 16
Management of Spondylolisthesis in the Elderly Population

Mohamad Bydon, Abdul Karim Ghaith, Yagiz Ugur Yolcu, and Kingsley Abode-Iyamah

Introduction

Spondylolisthesis, or the slippage of one vertebra over another, is a frequent condition encountered in the elderly population. History of this pathology dates back to the late eighteenth century, and the term itself was coined in 1854 by Kilian [1, 2]. Currently degenerative and isthmic spondylolisthesis are the two main types and have prevalence of 8.2% and 13.6%, respectively [3, 4]. The direction of the slippage is usually forward and called "anterolisthesis," while "retrolisthesis" or backward displacement of vertebrae may also be seen. Although any part of the vertebral column can be involved, spondylolisthesis is frequently seen in the lumbar spine with L4-L5 and L5-S1 levels being the most common location [5, 6]. The severity of the slippage has an important role in the clinical decision making and most commonly evaluated using Meyerding grading (grade 1–5 according to the percentage of slippage) [7].

In the elderly population, 30% of the patients were reported to have Meyerding grade I spondylolisthesis, and 12% has shown progression [8, 9]. Similar to the general population, the most commonly involved level for the elderly patients was also reported to be L4-L5 level [9]. In contrast, spondylolisthesis in cervical spine is rarely reported as an individual pathology and often mentioned in studies evaluating cervical myelopathy. In a study of 79 patients (age ≥ 65 years) undergoing

M. Bydon (✉) · A. K. Ghaith · Y. U. Yolcu
Mayo Clinic Neuro-Informatics Laboratory, Department of Neurologic Surgery, Mayo Clinic, Rochester, MN, USA

Department of Neurologic Surgery, Mayo Clinic, Rochester, MN, USA
e-mail: bydon.mohamad@mayo.edu; ghaith.abdulkarim@mayo.edu; yolcu.yagiz@mayo.edu

K. Abode-Iyamah
Department of Neurologic Surgery, Mayo Clinic, Jacksonville, FL, USA
e-mail: Abode-Iyamah.Kingsley@mayo.edu

K.-M. G. Fu et al. (eds.), *Treatment of Spine Disease in the Elderly*,
https://doi.org/10.1007/978-3-031-12612-3_16

surgery for cervical spondylotic myelopathy (CSM), all patients were found to have a certain degree of degenerative spondylolisthesis with the slippage varying from ~2.0 mm to 3.5 mm or more [10]. Tani et al. proposed that spondylolisthesis has a functional importance in patients presenting with cervical spondylotic myelopathy (CSM) and found a significant association between spondylolisthesis and conduction block in an electrophysiological study of 80 elderly patients undergoing surgery for CSM [11]. Spondylolisthesis is rarely encountered in thoracic spine, and mainly case reports and small case series have been reported to this date [12–14].

Diagnosis

Diagnosis of spondylolisthesis in elderly patients does not differ from the diagnosis in the general population. After a thorough history and physical examination, imaging modalities generally used to obtain a final diagnosis for spondylolisthesis. Historically, physical examination findings, such as palpable "step-off" in the back, have been frequently used as an indicator [15, 16]. However, most patients predominantly present with pain and are often evaluated before having a progressive disease with prominent signs in physical examination.

For imaging, standing lateral X-rays are usually preferred with the addition of flexion-extension X-rays in certain cases to identify any instability [17]. Magnetic resonance imaging (MRI) is an alternative, which can provide additional information with better visualization of the soft tissue and neural elements [18]. Due to the widespread availability of X-ray and higher cost of MRI, X-rays are more frequently utilized in the clinical practice. Moreover, MRI is thought to underestimate the degree of spondylolisthesis compared to X-ray as a result of the differences in positioning [19]. Recent studies have also demonstrated the discrepancies between the measurements from two imaging modalities with an intraclass correlation coefficient of 0.35, which is an indicator of a poor agreement [20]. Although it is not utilized as frequent as the X-ray, computerized tomography (CT) is also a useful modality in diagnosis of spondylolisthesis, especially in identifying potential pars interarticularis defects [21].

Nonsurgical Treatment

Physical Therapy

Flexion based physical therapy programs are thought to be more effective than extension-based programs, due to the theoretical advantage of opening the central canal and leading to better symptom relief. Although specific studies on elderly population have not been conducted, the study by Hicks et al. showed the mean age of the patients who failed physical therapy to be higher (46.5 years) than those who improved following physical therapy (38.2 years) [22].

Medications and Injections

Nonsteroidal anti-inflammatory drugs (NSAIDs) are utilized for the management of pain and were found to be effective in short-term symptomatic relief [23]. Yet, extra cautions should be taken with the choice of any medication in the elderly population and decision should be tailored according to comorbidities. Epidural corticosteroid injections (ESIs) constitute another option for short-term symptomatic relief. Kraiwattanapong et al. evaluated the short- and long-term outcomes of fluoroscopically guided lumbar transforaminal epidural steroid injection in a cohort of patients with degenerative spondylolisthesis [24]. Similar to the pain medication, ESIs were found to provide mainly pain relief and improvements in short-term outcomes [24]. Nerve blocks or radiofrequency ablation might also be utilized as alternative modalities when a nonsurgical treatment is preferred. Park et al. investigated the impact of radiofrequency neurotomy, nerve blocks, and instrumented fusion procedures on clinical outcomes in a study of 371 patients [25]. They found that 74% of the patients in surgery group had excellent or good outcomes compared to 71% in radiofrequency neurotomy group and 64% in nerve block group [25].

Conservative vs. Surgical Treatment

A few studies have compared the outcomes of conservative management to surgical management of the spondylolisthesis. Möller et al. presented a prospective randomized study of 111 patients with adult isthmic spondylolisthesis, comparing an exercise program to posterolateral fusion with regard to their impact on pain improvement and the functional outcome defined by Disability Rating Index, and found that the patients undergoing surgical management have shown greater degree of pain relief and functional improvement [26]. Similarly, 4-year outcomes from Spine Patient Outcomes Research Trial have suggested more favorable outcomes with surgical management for patients with degenerative spondylolisthesis [27].

Surgical Treatment

Indications for Surgical Treatment

Regardless of the nonsurgical approaches in treatment, patients might need to undergo surgery for correction of the underlying pathology to improve symptoms or prevent decline in neurological function. The common indications for surgical treatment are intractable back pain, failure with 3–6 months of conservative care, progressive neurological deficits such as severe radiculopathy, muscle weakness and loss of bowel/bladder control, sagittal imbalance, or severe interference with the activities of daily living affecting the quality of life of the patient. Variety of procedures ranging from simple decompression to fusion or dynamic stabilization might be preferred [28].

Overview of Surgical Alternatives for Lumbar Spondylolisthesis

Decompression alone is mostly recommended in patients with significant comorbidities and stable spondylolisthesis [29]. Posterior decompression procedures, such as laminectomy or laminotomy, are usually preferred for patients undergoing decompression alone [30]. In certain cases, involvement of multiple segments may require the surgeon expanding the laminectomy. However, more extensive decompression have the potential to destabilize the spinal segments, therefore necessitating a fusion procedure later [31]. Pedicle screws and rod instrumentation are frequently preferred options to achieve a higher rate of successful fusion with the process of pedicular screw insertion varying with the anatomical variations in the shape of the pedicles [32, 33]. Following the instrumentation, various graft materials are also utilized to augment the fusion process in the operated segment [34]. Local bone grafts, allograft, demineralized bone matrix (DBM), and bone morphogenetic protein (BMP) are among the commonly utilized grafts. While autografts and allografts have been a part of the standard approach, adjunctive BMP use (off-label) has shown promising results with regard to achieving bony union, and although the use is off-label, its utilization is trending up [35, 36]. Recently, dynamic stabilization using elastic materials has also emerged as a potential alternative to solid fusion of the vertebral column [37, 38].

As spondylolisthesis occurs frequently in the lumbar spine, approaches directed to primarily correct spondylolisthesis are usually performed for the patients presenting with lumbar spondylolisthesis (Fig. 16.1a–c). Posterior lumbar interbody fusion (PLIF) is a highly utilized option with rates of successful fusion rates approaching 98 to 100% in some series (Fig. 16.2a–c) [39, 40]. In the presence of conditions such as epidural fibrosis or conjoined nerve roots, alternative approaches could be pursued to avoid complications [41]. When an anterior approach is preferred, retroperitoneal approach is utilized to minimize complications, by avoiding manipulation of the bowel and other intra-abdominal contents (Fig. 16.3a–c) [42]. With this approach, it is important to be cognizant of the surrounding anatomy and landmarks to avoid injury to the vascular structures (i.e., aorta, iliac vessels) or the ureter. [42–44] In addition, limiting electrocautery use during the incision of the anterior longitudinal ligament is necessary to avoid the injury to the sympathetic plexus. On the other hand, transforaminal lumbar interbody fusion (TLIF) is usually performed with the help of minimally invasive surgery (MIS) techniques and showed favorable outcomes for the elderly population in recent studies (Fig. 16.4a–c) [45]. Recently, lateral lumbar interbody fusion techniques (anterior to psoas [ATP] and transpsoas) have been emerged as relatively newer approaches and are currently being utilized in the treatment of various pathologies as well as spondylolisthesis [46].

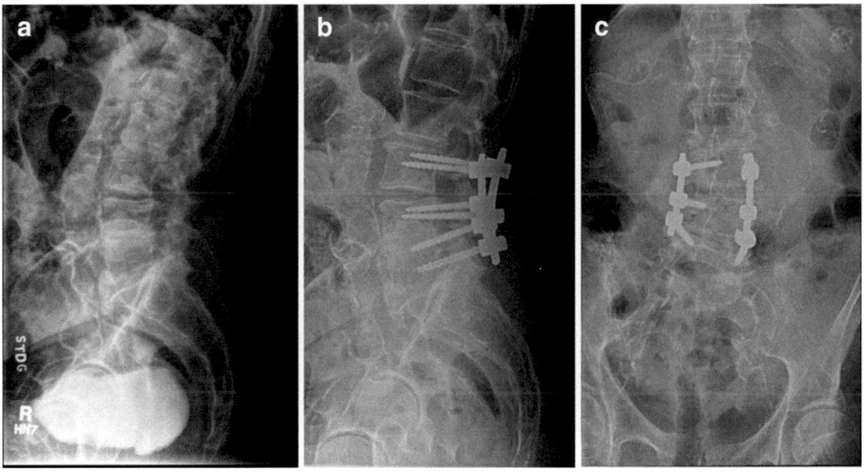

Fig. 16.1 A 69-year-old male patient with a past medical history of chronic back pain, presenting for general weakness in his limbs. Preoperative X-ray (**a**) shows advanced degenerative arthritis in the lower lumbar spine with multilevel degenerative disk disease with low-grade spondylolisthesis. The patient underwent posterior decompression and fusion of L3-L5. Postoperative lateral (**b**) and AP (**c**) X-rays show instrumentation and posterior fusion of L3-L5

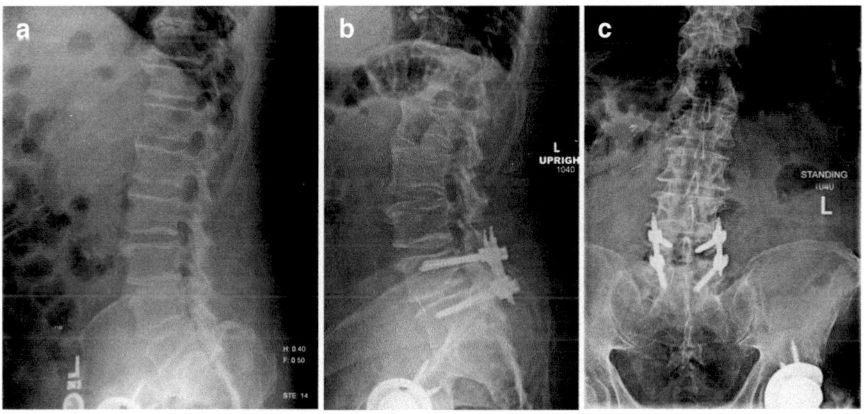

Fig. 16.2 A 72-year-old male patient presenting with a 2- to 3-month history of low back pain radiating down to the right lower extremity. Preoperative X-rays (**a**) showed minimal endplate spurring with lower lumbar facet arthropathy and low-grade spondylolisthesis. The patient underwent L4-L5 posterior interbody lumbar fusion with use of a PEEK cage. Postoperative X-rays (lateral (**b**) and AP (**c**)) showed stable appearing lumbar fusion L4-L5

Outcomes of Surgical Treatment

Although frequently performed with the addition of fusion, a few studies reported the outcomes of decompression alone for treatment of spondylolisthesis in the elderly population. Li et al. evaluated 18 patients (age range: 66–85 years)

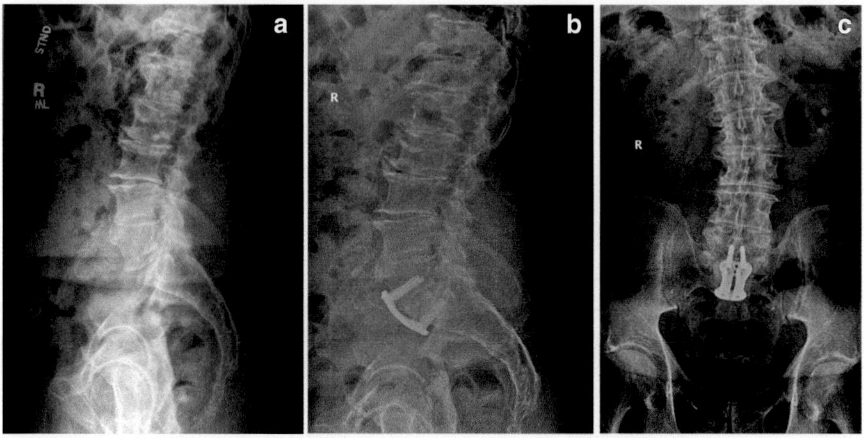

Fig. 16.3 A 69-year-old male presenting for right low back and lower extremity pain. Preoperative X-rays (**a**) showed degenerative disk disease at all of the lumbar interspaces with associated hypertrophic changes and facet arthropathy and low-grade retrolisthesis. Postoperative X-rays (lateral (**b**) and AP (**c**)) following ALIF showed stable L5-S1 fusion with reduction of the slippage

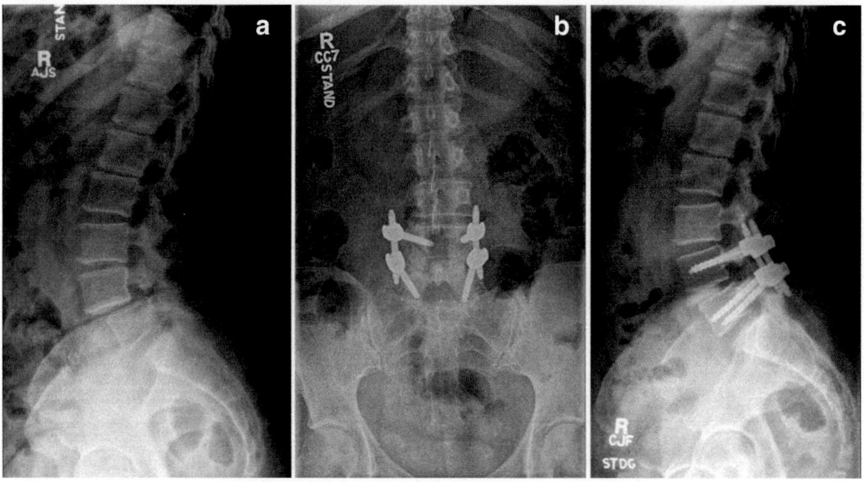

Fig. 16.4 A 71-year-old female patient presenting with pseudoclaudication and left leg pain. Preoperative X-ray (**a**) showed spondylolysis at L4 with grade II spondylolisthesis L4 on L5. Following MI-TLIF, postoperative X-rays (AP (**b**) and lateral (**c**)) showing L4-L5 fusion with posterior instrumentation and reduction of the slippage

undergoing percutaneous transforaminal endoscopic decompression (PTED) and found statistically significant improvements in ODI and VAS scores for back and leg pain at 1-month follow-up, which persisted at all subsequent follow-up points [46]. In addition, 83.3% of patients had good and excellent outcome according to modified MacNab criteria at the last follow-up [47]. Similarly, a recent study of 40 patients aged 60 years or older undergoing PTED showed improvements in VAS leg pain (from 7.5 ± 1.1 to 2.2 ± 1.1) and ODI (from 67.3 ± 9.3 to 20.7 ± 8.1) at 12-month follow-up [48].

Among studies evaluating the outcomes of fusion, Wu et al. evaluated the outcomes and value of the combined use of micro endoscopic discectomy (MED) and minimally invasive transforaminal lumbar interbody fusion (MI-TLIF) for the treatment of multilevel degenerative lumbar spinal stenosis with spondylolisthesis with a comparison to PLIF procedures [49]. The mean age of the study population was 63.4 years with the youngest patient being 53 years old. Authors concluded that the used combination of MED and MI-TLIF has the advantages of reduced blood loss, less damage to the paraspinal soft tissue, shorter length of incision, shorter bed rest time, improved outcomes, and shorter recovery times with similar short-term clinical outcomes to traditional PLIF [49].

A more recent study with a similar age range reported the clinical and radiographic outcomes of transpsoas lumbar interbody fusion for18 consecutive patients with grade I or II spondylolisthesis and neurogenic claudication [50]. None of the patients needed an additional decompression, and patients did not report any sensory loss or motor deficit. With regard to patient-reported outcomes (PROs) at 6-month follow-up, Oswestry Disability Index (ODI) improved by 26 points, and SF-12 mean physical and mental component scores improved by 11.9% and 9.6%, respectively [50].

With regard to individual fusion procedures, Takahashi et al. presented a study of 35 patients who are 70 years old or older undergoing one- or two-level TLIF for degenerative spondylolisthesis, evaluating the improvements in JOA, VAS, and ODI in 6-month, 12-month, 24-month, and further follow-ups [51]. Significant improvements were identified for each outcome at each follow-up point; however, when compared to a younger cohort of patients undergoing same surgery for the same diagnosis, it was found that improvements in mentioned outcomes are significantly better for younger patients [51].

A thorough analysis of different age groups among elderly population was conducted using the Quality Outcomes Database (QOD) lumbar spondylolisthesis registry [52]. Patients undergoing surgery for grade I spondylolisthesis were divided into four age groups as less than 60 (n = 239), 60 to 70 (n = 209), 71 to 80 (n = 128), and more than 80 (n = 32) years. With regard to outcomes, estimated blood loss, operative time, and discharge disposition were found to be different between four groups (p = 0.002, 0.0001 and 0.002, respectively). The length of hospital stay as well as readmission and reoperation rates were similar between the groups [52]. Among statistically significant outcomes, patients older than the age of 80 years had the lowest estimated blood loss (mean: 110 mL) and operative time (mean: 135 min). In contrast, patients older than the age of 80 years had the highest rate of nonroutine discharge (acute care facility in the context of the study) [52].

Complications

Great vessel injury can be one of the rare and devastating complications of the surgical treatment modalities, and the early recognition of the injury is essential, especially in the elderly population. The injury may present as uncontrolled hemorrhage in an acute setting and can be fatal. It can also be encountered as a late complication with arteriovenous fistula or pseudoaneurysm formation [53]. Durotomy is another complication encountered during surgical treatment of spondylolisthesis and might occur during the various stages of procedures, such as discectomy or laminectomy and medial facetectomy [54]. In addition, the excessive intraoperative retraction of the nerve roots in any surgical intervention may lead to neurologic injury [55].

The literature on complication rates following the surgical treatment of spondylolisthesis in elderly patients have shown contradicting findings. Some studies suggested that the advanced age was not associated with higher rates of complications when compared to younger patients after adjusting for type and grade of spondylolisthesis, while other studies showed an increase in the complication rate following posterior lumbar surgery in the elderly population [56–58].

Lieber et al. evaluated the postoperative complications following single-level lumbar fusion for degenerative spondylolisthesis among 224 patients, who are older than 80 years, and compared the complication rates to a younger (45–65 years) cohort of patients [58]. After adjusting for comorbidities, elderly patients were found to have significantly higher rates of complications only with regard to urinary tract infection (OR: 3.298, $p = 0.008$) and intraoperative/postoperative transfusions (OR: 2.186, $p < 0.001$), while the rates were similar for two groups with regard to the remaining list of medical and surgical complications [59]. In contrast, a recent study comparing complication rates following minimally invasive TLIF between elderly patients (mean age:75 years) and their younger counterparts (mean age:59 years) found similar rates for the two groups [60].

Conclusion

The management of spondylolisthesis in elderly population might be more challenging mainly due to increased comorbidities. Conservative and surgical approaches for the general population have also been adopted for the elderly patients and mainly resulted in improvements in short-term and long-term outcomes, respectively. However, there is controversy on whether the complication rates following surgical treatment are higher for the elderly patients, due to the conflicting results reported in the literature.

References

1. Kilian HF. Schilderungen neuer Beckenformen und ihres Verhaltens im Leben: der Praxis entnommen. Mannheim: Bassermann & Mathy; 1854. p. 131. Available from: https://play.google.com/store/books/details?id=BCFCAAAAcAAJ
2. Herbiniaux G Trait sur divers accouchments laborieux et sur les polypes de Ia matrice. Bruxelles, DeBoubers 1782
3. Wiltse LL, Winter RB. Terminology and measurement of spondylolisthesis. J Bone Joint Surg Am. 1983;65(6):768–72. Available from: https://www.ncbi.nlm.nih.gov/pubmed/6863359
4. Kalichman L, Kim DH, Li L, Guermazi A, Berkin V, Hunter DJ. Spondylolysis and spondylolisthesis: prevalence and association with low back pain in the adult community-based population. Spine. 2009;34(2):199–205. https://doi.org/10.1097/BRS.0b013e31818edcfd.
5. Lowe RW, Hayes TD, Kaye J, Bagg RJ, Luekens CA. Standing roentgenograms in spondylolisthesis. Clin Orthop Relat Res. 1976;117:80–4. Available from: https://www.ncbi.nlm.nih.gov/pubmed/1277688
6. Segebarth B, Kurd MF, Haug PH, Davis R. Routine upright imaging for evaluating degenerative Lumbar stenosis: incidence of degenerative Spondylolisthesis missed on supine MRI. J Spinal Disord Tech. 2015;28(10):394–7. https://doi.org/10.1097/BSD.0000000000000205.
7. Meyerding HW. Spondylolisthesis as an etiologic factor in backache. JAMA. 1938;111(22):1971–6. Available from: https://jamanetwork.com/journals/jama/article-abstract/283115?casa_token=EeTaaosvfakAAAAA:_2K7NI9y2TlICeFVcgg_BbSqs0g1Hw3wQgl9ZGRID3uXE4uh_k0iQahvkuamjZVWxEI7pK6JMg
8. Vogt MT, Rubin D, Valentin RS, Palermo L, Donaldson WF 3rd, Nevitt M, et al. Lumbar olisthesis and lower back symptoms in elderly white women. The Study of Osteoporotic Fractures. Spine. 1998;23(23):2640–7. https://doi.org/10.1097/00007632-199812010-00020.
9. Denard PJ, Holton KF, Miller J, Fink HA, Kado DM, Yoo JU, et al. Lumbar spondylolisthesis among elderly men: prevalence, correlates, and progression. Spine. 2010;35(10):1072–8. https://doi.org/10.1097/BRS.0b013e3181bd9e19.
10. Kawasaki M, Tani T, Ushida T, Ishida K. Anterolisthesis and retrolisthesis of the cervical spine in cervical spondylotic myelopathy in the elderly. J Orthop Sci. 2007;12(3):207–13. https://doi.org/10.1007/s00776-007-1122-5.
11. Tani T, Kawasaki M, Taniguchi S, Ushida T. Functional importance of degenerative spondylolisthesis in cervical spondylotic myelopathy in the elderly. Spine. 2003;28(11):1128–34. https://doi.org/10.1097/01.BRS.0000067263.73474.97.
12. Shimada Y, Kasukawa Y, Miyakoshi N, Hongo M, Ando S, Itoi E. Spondylolisthesis of the thoracic spine. Case report. J Neurosurg Spine. 2006;4(5):415–8. https://doi.org/10.3171/spi.2006.4.5.415.
13. Hsieh P-C, Lee S-T, Chen J-F. Lower thoracic degenerative spondylithesis with concomitant lumbar spondylosis. Clin Neurol Neurosurg. 2014;118:21–5. https://doi.org/10.1016/j.clineuro.2013.11.019.
14. Takagi Y, Yamada H, Ebara H, Hayashi H, Iwanaga T, Shimozaki K, et al. Thoracic spondylolisthesis and spinal cord compression in diffuse idiopathic skeletal hyperostosis: a case report. J Med Case Rep. 2017;11(1):90. https://doi.org/10.1186/s13256-017-1252-0.
15. Capener N. Spondylolisthesis. 1932. https://deepblue.lib.umich.edu/bitstream/handle/2027.42/37946/1800197505_ftp.pdf?sequence=1
16. Phalen GS, Dickson JA. Spondylolisthesis and tight hamstrings. JBJS. 1961;43(4):505. Available from: https://journals.lww.com/jbjsjournal/Abstract/1961/43040/Spondylolisthesis_and_Tight_Hamstrings.5.aspx
17. Hu SS, Tribus CB, Diab M, Ghanayem AJ. Spondylolisthesis and spondylolysis. Instr Course Lect. 2008;57:431–45. Available from: https://www.ncbi.nlm.nih.gov/pubmed/18399601

18. Maus TP. Imaging of the spine and nerve roots. Phys Med Rehabil Clin N Am. 2002;13(3):487–544, vi. https://doi.org/10.1016/s1047-9651(02)00009-8.
19. Bendo JA, Ong B. Importance of correlating static and dynamic imaging studies in diagnosing degenerative lumbar spondylolisthesis. Am J Orthop. 2001;30(3):247–50. Available from: https://www.ncbi.nlm.nih.gov/pubmed/11300136
20. Alvi MA, Sebai A, Yolcu Y, Wahood W, Elder BD, Kaufmann T, et al. Assessing the differences in measurement of degree of Spondylolisthesis between supine MRI and erect X-ray: An institutional analysis of 255 cases. Oper Neurosurg (Hagerstown). 2020;18(4):438–43. https://doi.org/10.1093/ons/opz180.
21. Kalichman L, Hunter DJ. Diagnosis and conservative management of degenerative lumbar spondylolisthesis. Eur Spine J. 2008;17(3):327–35. https://doi.org/10.1007/s00586-007-0543-3.
22. Hicks GE, Fritz JM, Delitto A, McGill SM. Preliminary development of a clinical prediction rule for determining which patients with low back pain will respond to a stabilization exercise program. Arch Phys Med Rehabil. 2005;86(9):1753–62. https://doi.org/10.1016/j.apmr.2005.03.033.
23. van Tulder MW, Scholten RJ, Koes BW, Deyo RA. Nonsteroidal anti-inflammatory drugs for low back pain: a systematic review within the framework of the Cochrane collaboration Back review group. Spine. 2000;25(19):2501–13. https://doi.org/10.1097/00007632-200010010-00013.
24. Kraiwattanapong C, Wechmongkolgorn S, Chatriyanuyok B, Woratanarat P, Udomsubpayakul U, Chanplakorn P, et al. Outcomes of fluoroscopically guided lumbar transforaminal epidural steroid injections in degenerative lumbar spondylolisthesis patients. Asian Spine J. 2014;8(2):119–28. https://doi.org/10.4184/asj.2014.8.2.119.
25. Park CK, Kim SB, Kim MK, Park BJ, Choi SG, Lim YJ, et al. Comparison of treatment methods in lumbar spinal stenosis for geriatric patient: nerve block versus radiofrequency neurotomy versus spinal surgery. Korean J Spine. 2014;11(3):97–102.
26. Möller H, Hedlund R. Surgery versus conservative management in adult isthmic spondylolisthesis--a prospective randomized study: part 1. Spine. 2000;25(13):1711–5. https://doi.org/10.1097/00007632-200007010-00016.
27. Weinstein JN, Lurie JD, Tosteson TD, Zhao W, Blood EA, Tosteson ANA, et al. Surgical compared with nonoperative treatment for lumbar degenerative spondylolisthesis: four-year results in the spine patient outcomes research trial (SPORT) randomized and observational cohorts. J Bone Joint Surg Am. 2009;91(6):1295. Available from: https://www.ncbi.nlm.nih.gov/pmc/articles/pmc2686131/
28. Lurie J, Tomkins-Lane C. Management of lumbar spinal stenosis. BMJ. 2016;352:h6234. https://doi.org/10.1136/bmj.h6234.
29. Rousing R, Jensen RK, Fruensgaard S, Strøm J, Brøgger HA, Degn JDM, et al. Danish national clinical guidelines for surgical and nonsurgical treatment of patients with lumbar spinal stenosis. Eur Spine J. 2019;28(6):1386–96. https://doi.org/10.1007/s00586-019-05987-2.
30. Sunderland G, Foster M, Dheerendra S, Pillay R. Patient-reported outcomes following Lumbar decompression surgery: a review of 2699 cases. Global Spine J. 2020:2192568219896541. https://doi.org/10.1177/2192568219896541.
31. Haddadi K, Qazvini HRG. Outcome after Surgery of Lumbar Spinal Stenosis: A Randomized Comparison of Bilateral Laminotomy, Trumpet Laminectomy, and Conventional Laminectomy. Front Surg. 2016;3:19. https://doi.org/10.3389/fsurg.2016.00019.
32. Nouh MR. Spinal fusion-hardware construct: basic concepts and imaging review. World J Radiol. 2012;4(5):193–207. https://doi.org/10.4329/wjr.v4.i5.193.
33. Basques BA, Espinoza Orías AA, Shifflett GD, Fice MP, Andersson GB, An HS, et al. The Kinematics and Spondylosis of the Lumbar Spine Vary Depending on the Levels of Motion Segments in Individuals With Low Back Pain. Spine. 2017;42:E767–74. https://doi.org/10.1097/brs.0000000000001967.
34. Gupta A, Kukkar N, Sharif K, Main BJ, Albers CE, El-Amin SF III. Bone graft substitutes for spine fusion: A brief review. World J Orthopedics. 2015;6:449. https://doi.org/10.5312/wjo.v6.i6.449.

35. Tannoury CA, An HS. Complications with the use of bone morphogenetic protein 2 (BMP-2) in spine surgery. Spine J. 2014;14:552–9. https://doi.org/10.1016/j.spinee.2013.08.060.
36. France JC, Schuster JM, Moran K, Dettori JR. Iliac crest bone graft in Lumbar fusion: the effectiveness and safety compared with local bone graft, and graft site morbidity comparing a Single-incision midline approach with a two-incision traditional approach. Global Spine J. 2015;5(3):195–206. https://doi.org/10.1055/s-0035-1552985.
37. Chang C-C, Kuo C-H, Chang H-K, Tu T-H, Fay L-Y, Wu J-C, et al. Minimally invasive dynamic screw stabilization using cortical bone trajectory. BMC Musculoskelet Disord. 2020;21(1):605. https://doi.org/10.1186/s12891-020-03629-z.
38. Greiner-Perth R, Sellhast N, Perler G, Dietrich D, Staub LP, Röder C. Dynamic posterior stabilization for degenerative lumbar spine disease: a large consecutive case series with long-term follow-up by additional postal survey. Eur Spine J. 2016;25(8):2563–70. https://doi.org/10.1007/s00586-016-4532-2.
39. Brantigan JW, Steffee AD, Lewis ML, Quinn LM, Persenaire JM. Lumbar interbody fusion using the Brantigan I/F cage for posterior lumbar interbody fusion and the variable pedicle screw placement system: two-year results from a Food and Drug Administration investigational device exemption clinical trial. Spine. 2000;25(11):1437–46. Available from: https://journals.lww.com/spinejournal/Fulltext/2000/06010/Lumbar_Interbody_Fusion_Using_the_Brantigan_I_F.17.aspx
40. Brantigan JW, Neidre A, Toohey JS. The Lumbar I/F cage for posterior lumbar interbody fusion with the variable screw placement system: 10-year results of a Food and Drug Administration clinical trial. Spine J. 2004;4:681–8. https://doi.org/10.1016/j.spinee.2004.05.253.
41. Chrastil J, Patel AA. Complications associated with posterior and transforaminal lumbar interbody fusion. J Am Acad Orthop Surg. 2012;20(5):283–91. https://doi.org/10.5435/JAAOS-20-05-283.
42. Manunga J, Alcala C, Smith J, Mirza A, Titus J, Skeik N, et al. Technical approach, outcomes, and exposure-related complications in patients undergoing anterior lumbar interbody fusion. J Vasc Surg. 2020; https://doi.org/10.1016/j.jvs.2020.06.129.
43. Isiklar ZU, Lindsey RW, Coburn M. Ureteral injury After anterior Lumbar interbody fusion. Spine. 1996;21:2379–82. https://doi.org/10.1097/00007632-199610150-00016.
44. Fantini GA, Pawar AY. Access related complications during anterior exposure of the lumbar spine. World J Orthop. 2013;4(1):19–23. https://doi.org/10.5312/wjo.v4.i1.19.
45. Joshi Nikhil N, Lim JW-A, Yeo W, Yue W-M. Elderly Patients Achieving Clinical and Radiological Outcomes Comparable with Those of Younger Patients Following Minimally Invasive Transforaminal Lumbar Interbody Fusion. Asian Spine J. 2017;11:230–42. https://doi.org/10.4184/asj.2017.11.2.230.
46. Rodgers WB, Lehmen JA, Gerber EJ, Rodgers JA. Grade 2 spondylolisthesis at L4-5 treated by XLIF: safety and midterm results in the "worst case scenario". ScientificWorldJournal. 2012;2012:356712. https://doi.org/10.1100/2012/356712.
47. Li X-F, Jin L-Y, Lv Z-D, Su X-J, Wang K, Shen H-X, et al. Efficacy of percutaneous transforaminal endoscopic decompression treatment for degenerative lumbar spondylolisthesis with spinal stenosis in elderly patients. Exp Ther Med. 2020;19(2):1417–24. https://doi.org/10.3892/etm.2019.8337.
48. Cheng X-K, Cheng Y-P, Liu Z-Y, Bian F-C, Yang F-K, Yang N, et al. Percutaneous transforaminal endoscopic decompression for lumbar spinal stenosis with degenerative spondylolisthesis in the elderly. Clin Neurol Neurosurg. 2020;194:105918. https://doi.org/10.1016/j.clineuro.2020.105918.
49. Wu H, Yu W-D, Jiang R, Gao Z-L. Treatment of multilevel degenerative lumbar spinal stenosis with spondylolisthesis using a combination of microendoscopic discectomy and minimally invasive transforaminal lumbar interbody fusion. Exp Ther Med. 2013;5(2):567–71. https://doi.org/10.3892/etm.2012.812.
50. Campbell PG, Nunley PD, Cavanaugh D, Kerr E, Utter PA, Frank K, et al. Short-term outcomes of lateral lumbar interbody fusion without decompression for the treatment of symp-

tomatic degenerative spondylolisthesis at L4-5. Neurosurg Focus. 2018;44(1):E6. https://doi.org/10.3171/2017.10.FOCUS17566.

51. Takahashi T, Hanakita J, Minami M, Kitahama Y, Kuraishi K, Watanabe M, et al. Clinical outcomes and adverse events following transforaminal interbody fusion for lumbar degenerative spondylolisthesis in elderly patients. Neurol Med Chir. 2011;51(12):829–35. https://doi.org/10.2176/nmc.51.829.
52. Karsy M, Chan AK, Mummaneni PV, Virk MS, Bydon M, Glassman SD, et al. Outcomes and Complications with age in Spondylolisthesis: An evaluation of the Elderly from the quality outcomes database. Spine. 2020;45(14):1000–8. https://doi.org/10.1097/BRS.0000000000003441.
53. Bae HJ, Cho TG, Kim CH, Lee HK, Moon JG, Choi JI. Aortic injury during transforaminal lumbar interbody fusion. Korean J Spine. 2017;14(3):118–20. https://doi.org/10.14245/kjs.2017.14.3.118.
54. Klingler J-H, Volz F, Krüger MT, Kogias E, Rölz R, Scholz C, et al. Accidental durotomy in minimally invasive transforaminal Lumbar interbody fusion: frequency, risk factors, and management. ScientificWorldJournal. 2015;2015:532628. https://doi.org/10.1155/2015/532628.
55. Lykissas MG, Aichmair A, Hughes AP, Sama AA, Lebl DR, Taher F, et al. Nerve injury after lateral lumbar interbody fusion: a review of 919 treated levels with identification of risk factors. Spine J. 2014;14:749–58. https://doi.org/10.1016/j.spinee.2013.06.066.
56. Sansur CA, Reames DL, Smith JS, Kojo Hamilton D, Berven SH, Broadstone PA, et al. Morbidity and mortality in the surgical treatment of 10,242 adults with spondylolisthesis: Presented at the 2009 Joint Spine Section Meeting. J Neurosurg Spine. 2010;13(5):589–93. Available from: https://thejns.org/spine/view/journals/j-neurosurg-spine/13/5/article-p589.xml
57. Raffo CS, Lauerman WC. Predicting morbidity and mortality of lumbar spine arthrodesis in patients in their ninth decade. Spine. 2006;31:99–103. https://doi.org/10.1097/01.brs.0000192678.25586.e5.
58. Carreon LY, Puno RM, Dimar JR, Glassman SD, Johnson JR. Perioperative complications of posterior lumbar decompression and arthrodesis in older adults. J Bone Joint Surg Am. 2003;85:2089–92. https://doi.org/10.2106/00004623-200311000-00004.
59. Lieber BA, Chiang V, Prabhu AV, Agarwal N, Henry JK, Lin D, et al. Postoperative complications for elderly patients after single-level lumbar fusions for spondylolisthesis. World Neurosurg. 2016;91:149–53. https://doi.org/10.1016/j.wneu.2016.03.052.
60. Goh GS-H, Tay YWA, Liow MHL, Gatot C, Ling ZM, Fong PL, et al. Elderly Patients undergoing minimally invasive transforaminal Lumbar interbody fusion may have similar clinical outcomes, Perioperative Complications, and fusion rates as their younger counterparts. Clin Orthop Relat Res. 2020;478:822–32. https://doi.org/10.1097/corr.0000000000001054.

Chapter 17
Sagittal Plane Deformity Considerations in the Elderly

Michael J. Strong, Timothy J. Yee, Robert Y. North, and Paul Park

Adult spinal deformity (ASD) is a heterogeneous disorder affecting the entire musculoskeletal system of the spine, predominately in the lumbar and/or thoracolumbar region [1–3]. Multiple etiologies have been identified for ASD, including de novo degenerative, iatrogenic "flatback" post fusion surgery, and progressive degeneration after spinal surgery. In general, ASD is considered a spectrum disorder that is usually multifactorial [1, 2, 4]. It is estimated that roughly a quarter of the US population will be over the age of 65 years by 2060 [5]. Since ASD is prevalent in individuals aged 60 years and older, ranging from 32% to 68% [6], the number of patients requiring surgical treatment will continue to grow.

Pathophysiology

The spine is designed to achieve an efficient, upright posture through its unique curvature. In particular, lumbar lordosis is vital to bipedalism, preserving the center of gravity over a narrow area over the feet [7]. The pelvis transfers weight from the spine and trunk to the lower limbs through the hips. Through this interplay, the pelvis is a key structure in spine stability as well as maintaining alignment and has been referred to as the pelvic vertebra [8, 9].

Sagittal malalignment can result in pain and disability. This occurs because with positive sagittal imbalance, natural compensatory mechanisms are triggered [10]. These include hyperlordosis of the cervical spine, reduction of thoracic kyphosis, lumbar retrolisthesis, hyperextension of the lumbar segments, pelvic retroversion,

M. J. Strong · T. J. Yee · R. Y. North · P. Park (✉)
Department of Neurosurgery, University of Michigan, Ann Arbor, MI, USA
e-mail: mistrong@med.umich.edu; tjyee@med.umich.edu; RNorth@mdanderson.org; ppark@med.umich.edu

K.-M. G. Fu et al. (eds.), *Treatment of Spine Disease in the Elderly*, https://doi.org/10.1007/978-3-031-12612-3_17

hip extension, knee flexion, and ankle extension [7, 11–14]. These compensatory maneuvers can require tremendous energy expenditure with resultant pain and disability leading to deterioration of quality of life.

Radiographic Parameters

Evaluating patients with ASD requires a careful assessment of the entire spine. Traditionally, spinal alignment has been measured through standing anteroposterior and lateral scoliosis (36-inch) radiographs. More recently, EOS imaging (EOS, Paris, France) is an alternative modality that allows whole-body skeletal imaging with low-radiation dosage. Based on these imaging studies, a variety of radiographic parameters are recorded to analyze regional as well as global spinal balance. The primary focus of this chapter will be on sagittal spinopelvic alignment (Fig. 17.1).

Pelvic Parameters

Three parameters are utilized to assess the pelvis, including pelvic incidence (PI), pelvic tilt (PT), and sacral slope (SS) (Fig. 17.1). These variables are related according to the equation PI = PT + SS.

Pelvic Incidence

Pelvic incidence is the angle between a line drawn from the midpoint of the bi-femoral heads to the midpoint of the sacral endplate and a line drawn perpendicular to the mid-S1 endplate. Since the sacroiliac joint has limited mobility and pelvic morphology is variable, PI is unique to each individual. Furthermore, the PI is typically fixed after adolescence. It has been reported that the mean for asymptomatic adults aged 20–70 years was 54.7° with a range of 33° to 82° [15].

Pelvic Tilt

Pelvic tilt is the angle between a line drawn from the midpoint of the sacral endplate to the midpoint of the femoral heads and a vertical line drawn through the bi-femoral heads. PT is a measure of pelvic rotation around the femoral heads and is therefore not fixed. If the pelvis is retroverted, PT increases, and if the pelvis is anteverted, PT decreases. In addition, if the sacral endplate is positioned behind the femoral heads, PT is positive, and if it is in front of the femoral heads, PT is negative. The mean value for asymptomatic adults aged 20–70 years has been reported to be 13.2° with a range of −4.5° to 27° [15].

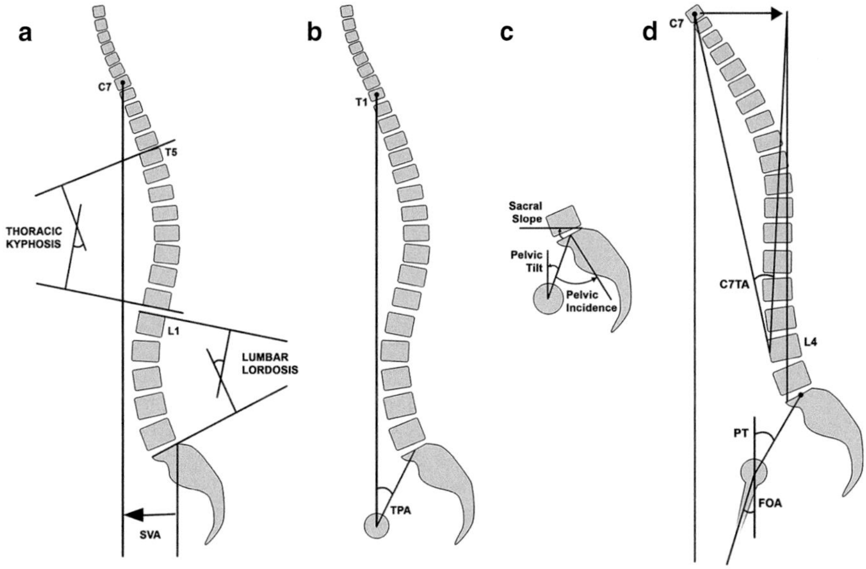

Fig. 17.1 Schematic of spinopelvic radiographic parameters. (**a**) Sagittal vertical axis (SVA) is measured as the horizontal distance from the superior posterior point of the S1 endplate to the C7 centroid vertical plumb line. Thoracic kyphosis (TK) and lumbar lordosis (LL) are measured typically using the Cobb method. TK is the angle between either the upper endplate of T1, T4, or T5 and the lower endplate of T12. LL is the angle between the upper endplate of L1 and the upper endplate of S1. (**b**) The T1 pelvic angle (TPA) is measured as the angle between a line drawn from the center of the T1 vertebral body to the midpoint of the femoral heads and a line drawn from this point to the midpoint of the sacral endplate. (**c**) Pelvic parameters include pelvic incidence (PI), pelvic tilt (PT), and sacral slope (SS), which are related as follows: PI = PT + SS. Pelvic incidence is the angle between a line drawn from the midpoint of the bi-femoral heads to the midpoint of the sacral endplate and a line drawn perpendicular to the mid-S1 endplate. Pelvic tilt is the angle between a line drawn from the midpoint of the sacral endplate to the midpoint of the femoral heads and a vertical line drawn through the bi-femoral heads. Sacral slope is the angle between a line drawn tangent to the upper sacral endplate and the horizontal. (**d**) The full balance integrated (FBI) method is based on the sum of three measured angles, represented as C7TA + FOA + PTCA. The first angle, C7-translation angle (C7TA), is the angle between the midpoint of the C7 inferior endplate and a line projected from the C7 plumb line to the S1 plateau with the L4 vertebra as a reference point. The second angle, angle of femur obliquity (FOA), is the angle of the femoral axis relative to vertical. The last angle, angle of tilt compensation (PTCA), takes into account pelvic tilt. If PT is less than 25°, add 5° to the equation, and if greater than 25°, add 10°

Sacral Slope

Sacral slope is the angle between a line drawn tangent to the upper sacral endplate and the horizontal. A vertical oriented pelvis has a low SS, while a pelvis in a more horizontal orientation has a higher SS. The mean value for asymptomatic adults aged 20–70 years has been reported to be 41.2° with range of 17° to 63° [15].

These pelvic parameters are related geometrically through the equation, PI = PT + SS. Patients with a low PI will typically have small pelvic diameters with a vertical orientation. In this configuration, both the SS and PT will be low, given the limited ability of the pelvis to tilt due to the positioning of the sacral plate directly over the femoral head axis. On the other hand, patients with a high PI typically have large pelvic diameters in a more horizontal orientation. The femoral head axis is oriented anterior to the sacral plate in this configuration, leading to a higher SS and PT. The ability to retrovert the pelvis will be higher in these patients with high PI.

Regional Spine Alignment

Thoracic kyphosis and lumbar lordosis (LL) are typically calculated using the Cobb method [16] (Fig. 17.1). The Cobb method measures the angle between the two-end vertebra of a regional spine curve. The thoracic kyphosis angle is measured as the angle between the T1 upper endplate and the T12 lower endplate. However, oftentimes, due to the difficulty visualizing the upper thoracic spine on lateral X-rays, an acceptable measurement for thoracic kyphosis is from T4 or T5 to the T12 lower endplate or even T4 to T9 [17–21]. LL is the angle between the upper endplate of L1 and the upper endplate of S1.

Relationship of Lumbar Lordosis to Pelvic Incidence

Lumbar lordosis tends to be matched closely to PI in asymptomatic individuals who are able to maintain an economic upright posture. This relationship between PI and LL is the rationale for calculating the difference in these two variables (PI-LL) to help guide deformity corrective surgery and has been extensively studied [7, 22]. This parameter, PI-LL, measures the mismatch between the pelvis and the lumbar lordosis. Early studies suggested that a mismatch of less than 10° was as an ideal sagittal alignment goal [22]. More recent studies have shown that certain factors such as increasing age can impact the target PI-LL mismatch goals [13, 23, 24].

Roussouly Spine Types

Recently, the classically accepted definition that the thoracic spine is kyphotic and the lumbar spine is lordotic has been questioned. Roussouly et al. have proposed that there are four spine types with varying inflection points, which is where the transition from lordosis to kyphosis occurs [25]. This inflection point is related to PI, where higher PIs result in the inflection point moving more superiorly even into the thoracic spine. Therefore, in patients with high PI, the lordotic region would encompass the lower thoracic spine [14]. In other words, the inflection point for lumbar lordosis is not always located at T12-L1. Roussouly et al. have also proposed dividing the lumbar curve into upper and lower curvatures. It has been shown that the lower curve from L4-S1 is more clinically relevant, as the majority of the lumbar lordosis is achieved at this location [25]. Therefore, appropriate treatment of this lower curve is often essential in restoring sagittal balance.

Global Spinal Alignment

A variety of parameters have been used to assess global spinal alignment, the most popular being the measurement of the C7-S1 sagittal vertical axis (SVA) (Fig. 17.1). Alternative radiographic parameters for global alignment include the T1 pelvic angle and the full balance integrated (FBI) method, among others (Fig. 17.1).

SVA is measured as the horizontal distance from the superior posterior point of the S1 endplate to the C7 centroid vertical plumb line. By convention, a C7 plumb line anterior to the posterosuperior margin of the S1 endplate results in a positive SVA. Historically, a value greater than 5 cm was considered abnormal [26, 27]. While SVA is used ubiquitously, one vital caveat to consider is that SVA is dynamic and can be affected by patient posture and pelvic version. SVA is not representative of the center of gravity and may not provide a comprehensive measure of a patient's balance as it does not take into account pelvic compensation [28]. In response to these concerns raised about the SVA, the T1 pelvic angle was developed [29].

The T1 pelvic angle (TPA) is measured as the angle between a line drawn from the center of the T1 vertebral body to the midpoint of the femoral heads and a line drawn from this point to the midpoint of the sacral endplate. In contrast to SVA, the TPA takes into account pelvic version [29, 30]. Both SVA and TPA are also referred to as truncal inclination. A major advantage of the T1 pelvic angle over the SVA is that the former is less affected by postural compensation [29].

The full balance integrated (FBI) method has been suggested to be a more comprehensive approach toward assessing spinal alignment. FBI is based on the sum of three measured angles, which provides the value of sagittal angle correction needed to restore optimal balance to the patient [31]. The first angle, C7-translation angle (C7TA), is the angle between the midpoint of the C7 inferior endplate and a line projected from the C7 plumb line to the S1 plateau with the L4 vertebra as a reference point. The second angle, angle of femur obliquity (FOA), is the angle of the femoral axis relative to vertical. The last angle, angle of tilt compensation (PTCA), takes into account pelvic tilt. If PT is less than 25°, add 5° to the equation, and if greater than 25°, add 10°. Therefore, the equation is as follows: FBI angle of correction = C7TA + FOA + PTCA [31].

Radiographic Parameters and Patient-Reported Outcomes

Numerous studies have highlighted the correlation between spinopelvic alignment and clinical outcomes [27, 32–36]. In 2002, Schwab et al. analyzed radiographic parameters in a small cohort of patients with scoliosis and determined that upper endplate obliquities of L3 and L4, lateral spondylolisthesis, lumbar lordosis, and thoracolumbar kyphosis were significantly correlated with patient-reported pain scores [33]. Subsequent investigations identified SVA, PT, and PI-LL as key spinopelvic parameters, as they appeared to be associated most strongly with disability. In one large study of ASD, SVA $\geq$ 47 mm, PT $\geq$ 22°, and PI-LL $\geq$ 11° significantly correlated with severe disability as defined as Oswestry Disability Index (ODI) more than 40 [36]. In another multicenter prospective comparative study, surgical correction of spinopelvic malalignment resulted in significantly better health-related quality of life (HRQoL) scores than nonoperative treatment, despite having worse sagittal deformity and HRQoL scores in the surgery group at baseline [37].

Given the importance of specific radiographic parameters, Schwab et al. initially introduced a simple classification system, which included curve type, lordosis modifier, and subluxation modifier [38]. This classification system, while reliable and predictive of HRQoL scores, did not incorporate pelvic parameters. Therefore, in 2012, the Schwab classification system was revised to the Scoliosis Research Society (SRS)-Schwab classification and included curve type, PI-LL modifier, global alignment modifier, and pelvic tilt modifier [39]. While reliable in guiding surgical planning and correlative with HRQoL scores [40], the use of the sagittal modifiers can be cumbersome. Kieser et al. have proposed using a single sagittal modifier to simplify the model [41]. Although the authors demonstrate this simplified SRS-Schwab classification model correlates with both HRQoL scores and surgical indication, further validation studies are warranted before this modified classification system is accepted into clinical practice.

Age-Adjusted Radiographic Parameters

Age-related changes to spinal alignment have been well described and include loss of lumbar lordosis and progressive thoracic kyphosis [42, 43]. Not surprisingly, a progressively forward stooping posture with increasing SVA has been correlated with age [44–46]. The increased SVA is multifactorial, likely due to the loss of lumbar lordosis, which pushes the C7 plumb line further anteriorly.

Given the expected alignment changes with aging, recent studies have questioned whether less stringent spinopelvic parameters are needed in the elderly

Table 17.1 Spinopelvic radiographic parameters by age group

	PT (°)	PI-LL (°)	SVA (mm)
Ideal	<20	10	< 50
<35 years	11.1	−11.3	−29.1
35–44 years	15.5	−6.2	−4.0
45–54 years	18.9	−1.7	16.5
55–64 years	22.1	3.3	37.0
65–74 years	25.2	7.5	55.6
≥74 years	28.8	13.7	79.9

Data adapted from Schwab et al. [22], Lafage et al. [23], and Ames et al. [50]
PT pelvic tilt, *PI-LL* difference between pelvic incidence and lumbar lordosis, *SVA* sagittal vertical axis

population to achieve symptomatic improvement [23]. In one investigation, new radiographic thresholds were determined based on age-specific ODI US norms, extrapolated from US norms SF-36 Physical Component Score [23]. These spinopelvic parameters approximated the optimal thresholds according to age group and demonstrated these values increased with age, ranging from SVA of −29.1 mm, PT of 11.1°, and PI-LL of −11.3° in patients under 35 years of age to SVA of 79.9 mm, PT of 28.8°, and PI-LL of 13.7° in patients 74 years or older [23] (Table 17.1).

Other investigations have also shown that obtaining optimal spinopelvic parameters is not essential to achieving symptomatic improvement in the elderly. In one such study of older patients with deformity undergoing surgery, there were no significant differences in visual analog scale back and leg pain scores or ODI scores between patients classified as aligned versus malaligned postoperatively [24]. This was present despite the significant differences in postoperative spinopelvic parameters, including SVA (13.9 mm vs. 64.8 mm), PT (21.1° vs. 29°), and PI-LL (2.8° vs. 19.6°) for the aligned and malaligned groups, respectively [24].

Although increasing age and its associated physiologic changes likely alter the optimal radiographic alignment target, other factors may explain the lack of clinical difference in malaligned older patients versus younger patients. Specifically, other studies investigating the impact of age on clinical and radiographic outcomes following lumbar spinal fusion have demonstrated similar observations [47–49]. Differences in patient expectation have been suggested to explain the lack of differences in clinical outcomes. Younger patients typically have a higher baseline activity level and more to lose if they do not regain their normal function compared to elderly patients. Therefore, expectations for improvement following surgery may be lower in elderly patients [47].

Surgical Correction of Adult Spinal Deformity in the Elderly

In evaluating elderly deformity patients for corrective surgery, it is important to assess the presenting spinopelvic alignment as well as compensatory mechanisms in order to determine the appropriate amount of surgical correction needed to restore optimal spinal balance [37, 42]. Historically, the alignment goals in the elderly were based on ideal spinopelvic radiographic parameters, which include SVA less than 50 mm, PT less than 20°, and PI-LL within 10° [22, 50]. Notably, early on, some even advocated overcorrection of ASD patients to mitigate the loss of alignment correction in the elderly due to the progressive degenerative changes [51, 52]. More recently, it has been postulated that loss of some degree of sagittal balance with aging is physiologic, and so modification of the "ideal" radiographic parameters is needed. Thus, elderly patients may not have to be held to the same rigorous alignment parameters as younger patients. In addition, the concept of sagittal balance is a dynamic phenomenon with multiple influences, such as neuro-sensorial modulation, soft tissue response to gravity, and bony alignment [23]. Surgical correction can only directly address bony alignment. As such, it may be better to strive for good sagittal balance, even if there is compensation [11].

Although radiographic alignment is an important treatment goal, other important factors should be considered when developing a surgical treatment. An individualized patient-specific surgical approach is most appropriate, taking into account not just the radiographic alignment but also comorbidities (e.g., osteoporosis), advanced imaging (e.g., MRI findings), and presenting symptoms. Deformity surgery in general carries high risk and this risk is elevated in the elderly. For example, Smith et al. conducted a study investigating the complication rate in a cohort of ASD patients with a mean age of 60.7 years who underwent three-column osteotomy for deformity correction. Seventy-eight percent of patients experienced at least one complication from the time of surgery through their 2-year follow-up visit [53]. In addition, the elderly population has a higher prevalence of chronic comorbidities that need to be taken into account when considering surgical intervention [47].

Surgical treatment of ASD in the elderly can encompass multiple techniques. Figures 17.2, 17.3, 17.4, and 17.5 present four cases that each highlight important aspects in deformity correction in the elderly. Figure 17.2 illustrates a hybrid circumferential approach for deformity correction with the use of multilevel interbody fusion. Figure 17.3 highlights the use of cement augmentation to mitigate instrumentation failure in cases of poor bone quality. Figure 17.4 shows an example of three-column osteotomy in a patient with a fixed defect. Finally, Fig. 17.5 details an example of radiculopathy due to the fractional curve.

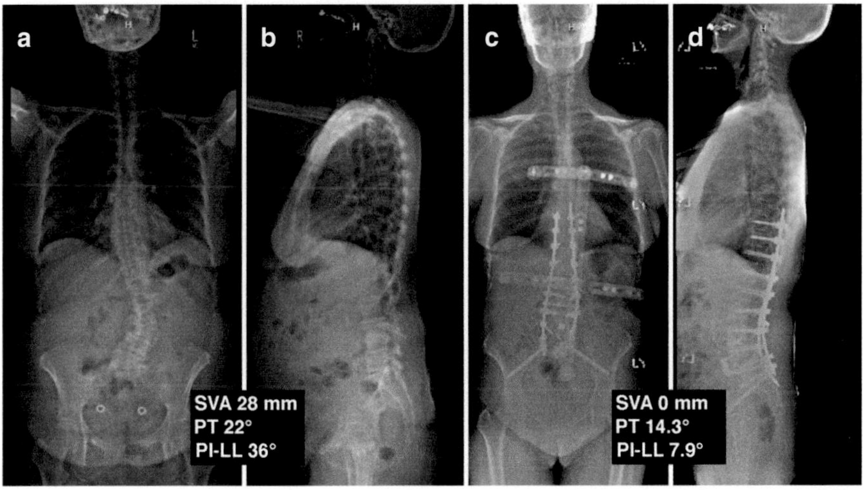

Fig. 17.2 A 63-year-old woman with back and leg pain and adult spinal deformity (SVA = 28 mm, PT = 22°, PI-LL = 36°) (**a** and **b**) underwent L2-L3 and L3-L4 lateral lumbar interbody fusion, L5-S1 oblique lumbar interbody fusion, L4-L5 transforaminal lumbar interbody fusion, and T10-ilium fusion. Postoperative imaging demonstrated marked improvement in sagittal alignment (SVA = 0 mm, PT = 14.3°, and PI-LL = 7.9°) (**c** and **d**). This case highlights a hybrid approach, using a primarily lateral approach for interbody fusion followed by second-stage posterior surgery to obtain correction

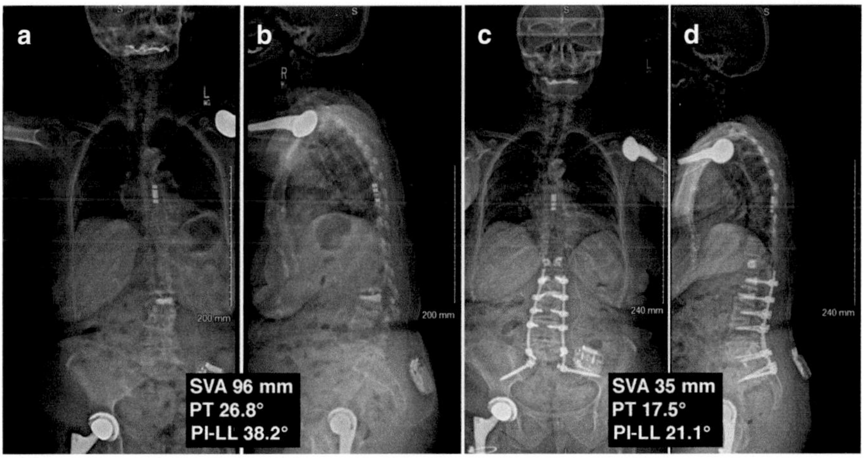

Fig. 17.3 A 71-year-old woman with history of osteoporosis s/p L2 kyphoplasty presented with severe back and leg pain and inability to ambulate (SVA = 96 mm, PT = 26.8°, and PI-LL = 38.2°) (**a** and **b**). She underwent T12 vertebroplasty, L2–L4 laminectomies and facet osteotomies, and L1-ilium fusion with cement-augmented screws. Postoperative imaging demonstrated improved sagittal parameters (SVA = 35 mm, PT = 17.5°, and PI-LL = 21.1°) (**c** and **d**). This case highlights the use of cement augmentation to prevent instrumentation failure as it facilitates with screw purchase

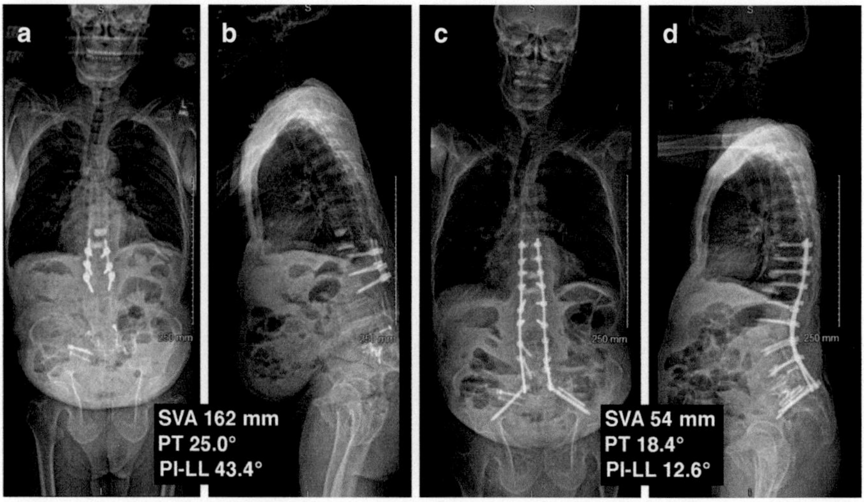

Fig. 17.4 A 68-year-old man with history of right SI fusion, L3-S1 fusion, L1-L3 fusion, and T11 and T12 vertebroplasty presented with disabling back and right leg pain (SVA = 162 mm, PT = 25.0°, and PI-LL = 43.4°) (**a** and **b**). He underwent T10-T12 laminectomies, L3 PSO, and T9-ilium fusion with cement-augmented screws. Postoperative imaging demonstrated marked improvement in sagittal alignment (SVA = 54 mm, PT = 18.4°, and PI-LL = 12.6°) (**c** and **d**). This case highlights the need for three-column osteotomy for a fixed defect

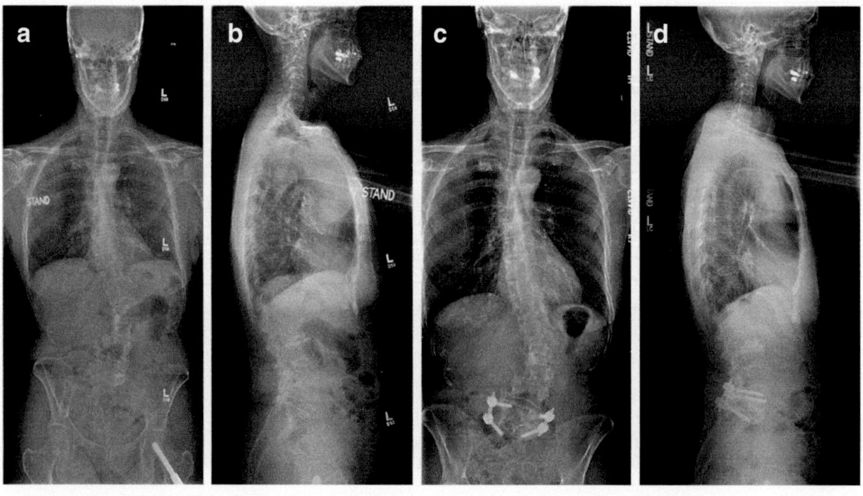

Fig. 17.5 A 69-year-old woman with history of chronic low back pain presented with recent onset of left leg pain and was found to have a fractional curve causing nerve root entrapment (**a** and **b**). The patient underwent left L5-S1 minimally invasive transforaminal lumbar interbody fusion. Postoperative imaging demonstrates appropriate implant and screw placement (**c** and **d**). This case shows that a deformity correction is not always required. Treating the symptom can result in a smaller operation with good outcomes

Conclusion

Special consideration is needed for elderly patients with ASD. The prevalence of ASD will only increase, and a better understanding of the pathophysiology and biomechanics of this progressive disease is warranted. Key spinopelvic radiographic parameters, including the SVA, TPA, PT, and PI-LL mismatch, are used to assess the degree of malalignment. Recently, there has been an emphasis on age-adjusted radiographic alignment targets. In addition, factors beyond radiographic alignment need to be considered, including comorbidities, presenting symptoms, and degree of neurologic compression. Balancing benefit versus risk may result in consideration of a compensated sagittal balance rather than an optimal sagittal balance in these patients.

References

1. Smith JS, Shaffrey CI, Bess S, Shamji MF, Brodke D, Lenke LG, et al. Recent and emerging advances in spinal deformity. Neurosurgery. 2017;80(3s):S70–s85. https://doi.org/10.1093/neuros/nyw048.
2. Aebi M. The adult scoliosis. Eur Spine J. 2005;14(10):925–48. https://doi.org/10.1007/s00586-005-1053-9.
3. Diebo BG, Shah NV, Boachie-Adjei O, Zhu F, Rothenfluh DA, Paulino CB, et al. Adult spinal deformity. Lancet. 2019;394(10193):160–72. https://doi.org/10.1016/s0140-6736(19)31125-0.
4. Ailon T, Smith JS, Shaffrey CI, Lenke LG, Brodke D, Harrop JS, et al. Degenerative spinal deformity. Neurosurgery. 2015;77(Suppl 4):S75–91. https://doi.org/10.1227/neu.0000000000000938.
5. Lutz W, Sanderson W, Scherbov S. The coming acceleration of global population ageing. Nature. 2008;451(7179):716–9. https://doi.org/10.1038/nature06516.
6. Schwab F, Dubey A, Gamez L, El Fegoun AB, Hwang K, Pagala M, et al. Adult scoliosis: prevalence, SF-36, and nutritional parameters in an elderly volunteer population. Spine (Phila Pa 1976). 2005;30(9):1082–5. https://doi.org/10.1097/01.brs.0000160842.43482.cd.
7. Diebo BG, Varghese JJ, Lafage R, Schwab FJ, Lafage V. Sagittal alignment of the spine: what do you need to know? Clin Neurol Neurosurg. 2015;139:295–301. https://doi.org/10.1016/j.clineuro.2015.10.024.
8. Duval-Beaupère G, Schmidt C, Cosson P. A Barycentremetric study of the sagittal shape of spine and pelvis: the conditions required for an economic standing position. Ann Biomed Eng. 1992;20(4):451–62. https://doi.org/10.1007/bf02368136.
9. Legaye J, Duval-Beaupère G, Hecquet J, Marty C. Pelvic incidence: a fundamental pelvic parameter for three-dimensional regulation of spinal sagittal curves. Eur Spine J. 1998;7(2):99–103. https://doi.org/10.1007/s005860050038.
10. Lafage V, Schwab F, Skalli W, Hawkinson N, Gagey PM, Ondra S, et al. Standing balance and sagittal plane spinal deformity: analysis of spinopelvic and gravity line parameters. Spine (Phila Pa 1976). 2008;33(14):1572–8. https://doi.org/10.1097/BRS.0b013e31817886a2.
11. Le Huec JC, Thompson W, Mohsinaly Y, Barrey C, Faundez A. Sagittal balance of the spine. Eur Spine J. 2019;28(9):1889–905. https://doi.org/10.1007/s00586-019-06083-1.
12. Obeid I, Hauger O, Aunoble S, Bourghli A, Pellet N, Vital JM. Global analysis of sagittal spinal alignment in major deformities: correlation between lack of lumbar lordosis and flexion of the knee. Eur Spine J. 2011;20(Suppl 5):681–5. https://doi.org/10.1007/s00586-011-1936-x.

13. Diebo BG, Ferrero E, Lafage R, Challier V, Liabaud B, Liu S, et al. Recruitment of compensatory mechanisms in sagittal spinal malalignment is age and regional deformity dependent: a full-standing axis analysis of key radiographical parameters. Spine (Phila Pa 1976). 2015;40(9):642–9. https://doi.org/10.1097/brs.0000000000000844.
14. Cheung JPY. The importance of sagittal balance in adult scoliosis surgery. Ann Transl Med. 2020;8(2):35. https://doi.org/10.21037/atm.2019.10.19.
15. Vialle R, Levassor N, Rillardon L, Templier A, Skalli W, Guigui P. Radiographic analysis of the sagittal alignment and balance of the spine in asymptomatic subjects. J Bone Joint Surg Am. 2005;87(2):260–7. https://doi.org/10.2106/jbjs.D.02043.
16. Cobb J. Outline for the study of scoliosis. Instr Course Lect. 1947;5:261–75.
17. Goh S, Price RI, Leedman PJ, Singer KP. A comparison of three methods for measuring thoracic kyphosis: implications for clinical studies. Rheumatology (Oxford). 2000;39(3):310–5. https://doi.org/10.1093/rheumatology/39.3.310.
18. Briggs AM, Wrigley TV, Tully EA, Adams PE, Greig AM, Bennell KL. Radiographic measures of thoracic kyphosis in osteoporosis: Cobb and vertebral centroid angles. Skelet Radiol. 2007;36(8):761–7. https://doi.org/10.1007/s00256-007-0284-8.
19. Singer KP, Jones TJ, Breidahl PD. A comparison of radiographic and computer-assisted measurements of thoracic and thoracolumbar sagittal curvature. Skelet Radiol. 1990;19(1):21–6. https://doi.org/10.1007/bf00197923.
20. Goh S, Price RI, Leedman PJ, Singer KP. The relative influence of vertebral body and intervertebral disc shape on thoracic kyphosis. Clin Biomech. 1999;14(7):439–48. https://doi.org/10.1016/S0268-0033(98)00105-3.
21. Ohrt-Nissen S, Cheung JPY, Hallager DW, Gehrchen M, Kwan K, Dahl B, et al. Reproducibility of thoracic kyphosis measurements in patients with adolescent idiopathic scoliosis. Scoliosis Spinal Disord. 2017;12:4. https://doi.org/10.1186/s13013-017-0112-4.
22. Schwab F, Patel A, Ungar B, Farcy JP, Lafage V. Adult spinal deformity-postoperative standing imbalance: how much can you tolerate? An overview of key parameters in assessing alignment and planning corrective surgery. Spine (Phila Pa 1976). 2010;35(25):2224–31. https://doi.org/10.1097/BRS.0b013e3181ee6bd4.
23. Lafage R, Schwab F, Challier V, Henry JK, Gum J, Smith J, et al. Defining spino-pelvic alignment thresholds: should operative goals in adult spinal deformity surgery account for age? Spine (Phila Pa 1976). 2016;41(1):62–8. https://doi.org/10.1097/brs.0000000000001171.
24. Park P, Fu KM, Mummaneni PV, Uribe JS, Wang MY, Tran S, et al. The impact of age on surgical goals for spinopelvic alignment in minimally invasive surgery for adult spinal deformity. J Neurosurg Spine. 2018;29(5):560–4. https://doi.org/10.3171/2018.4.SPINE171153.
25. Roussouly P, Gollogly S, Berthonnaud E, Dimnet J. Classification of the normal variation in the sagittal alignment of the human lumbar spine and pelvis in the standing position. Spine (Phila Pa 1976). 2005;30(3):346–53. https://doi.org/10.1097/01.brs.0000152379.54463.65.
26. Booth KC, Bridwell KH, Lenke LG, Baldus CR, Blanke KM. Complications and predictive factors for the successful treatment of flatback deformity (fixed sagittal imbalance). Spine (Phila Pa 1976). 1999;24(16):1712–20. https://doi.org/10.1097/00007632-199908150-00013.
27. Glassman SD, Berven S, Bridwell K, Horton W, Dimar JR. Correlation of radiographic parameters and clinical symptoms in adult scoliosis. Spine (Phila Pa 1976). 2005;30(6):682–8. https://doi.org/10.1097/01.brs.0000155425.04536.f7.
28. Roussouly P, Gollogly S, Noseda O, Berthonnaud E, Dimnet J. The vertical projection of the sum of the ground reactive forces of a standing patient is not the same as the C7 plumb line: a radiographic study of the sagittal alignment of 153 asymptomatic volunteers. Spine (Phila Pa 1976). 2006;31(11):E320–5. https://doi.org/10.1097/01.brs.0000218263.58642.ff.
29. Protopsaltis T, Schwab F, Bronsard N, Smith JS, Klineberg E, Mundis G, et al. TheT1 pelvic angle, a novel radiographic measure of global sagittal deformity, accounts for both spinal inclination and pelvic tilt and correlates with health-related quality of life. J Bone Joint Surg Am. 2014;96(19):1631–40. https://doi.org/10.2106/jbjs.M.01459.

30. Ryan DJ, Protopsaltis TS, Ames CP, Hostin R, Klineberg E, Mundis GM, et al. T1 pelvic angle (TPA) effectively evaluates sagittal deformity and assesses radiographical surgical outcomes longitudinally. Spine (Phila Pa 1976). 2014;39(15):1203–10. https://doi.org/10.1097/BRS.0000000000000382.
31. Le Huec JC, Leijssen P, Duarte M, Aunoble S. Thoracolumbar imbalance analysis for osteotomy planification using a new method: FBI technique. Eur Spine J. 2011;20(Suppl 5):669–80. https://doi.org/10.1007/s00586-011-1935-y.
32. Jackson RP, McManus AC. Radiographic analysis of sagittal plane alignment and balance in standing volunteers and patients with low back pain matched for age, sex, and size. A prospective controlled clinical study. Spine (Phila Pa 1976). 1994;19(14):1611–8. https://doi.org/10.1097/00007632-199407001-00010.
33. Schwab FJ, Smith VA, Biserni M, Gamez L, Farcy JP, Pagala M. Adult scoliosis: a quantitative radiographic and clinical analysis. Spine (Phila Pa 1976). 2002;27(4):387–92. https://doi.org/10.1097/00007632-200202150-00012.
34. Lafage V, Schwab F, Patel A, Hawkinson N, Farcy JP. Pelvic tilt and truncal inclination: two key radiographic parameters in the setting of adults with spinal deformity. Spine (Phila Pa 1976). 2009;34(17):E599–606. https://doi.org/10.1097/BRS.0b013e3181aad219.
35. Schwab F, Lafage V, Patel A, Farcy JP. Sagittal plane considerations and the pelvis in the adult patient. Spine (Phila Pa 1976). 2009;34(17):1828–33. https://doi.org/10.1097/BRS.0b013e3181a13c08.
36. Schwab FJ, Blondel B, Bess S, Hostin R, Shaffrey CI, Smith JS, et al. Radiographical spinopelvic parameters and disability in the setting of adult spinal deformity: a prospective multicenter analysis. Spine (Phila Pa 1976). 2013;38(13):E803–12. https://doi.org/10.1097/BRS.0b013e318292b7b9.
37. Smith JS, Lafage V, Shaffrey CI, Schwab F, Lafage R, Hostin R, et al. Outcomes of operative and nonoperative treatment for adult spinal deformity: a prospective, multicenter, propensity-matched cohort assessment with minimum 2-year follow-up. Neurosurgery. 2016;78(6):851–61. https://doi.org/10.1227/neu.0000000000001116.
38. Schwab F, Farcy JP, Bridwell K, Berven S, Glassman S, Harrast J, et al. A clinical impact classification of scoliosis in the adult. Spine (Phila Pa 1976). 2006;31(18):2109–14. https://doi.org/10.1097/01.brs.0000231725.38943.ab.
39. Schwab F, Ungar B, Blondel B, Buchowski J, Coe J, Deinlein D, et al. Scoliosis Research Society-Schwab adult spinal deformity classification: a validation study. Spine (Phila Pa 1976). 2012;37(12):1077–82. https://doi.org/10.1097/BRS.0b013e31823e15e2.
40. Smith JS, Klineberg E, Schwab F, Shaffrey CI, Moal B, Ames CP, et al. Change in classification grade by the SRS-Schwab adult spinal deformity classification predicts impact on health-related quality of life measures: prospective analysis of operative and nonoperative treatment. Spine (Phila Pa 1976). 2013;38(19):1663–71. https://doi.org/10.1097/BRS.0b013e31829ec563.
41. Kieser DC, Boissiere L, Cawley DT, Larrieu D, Yilgor C, Takemoto M, et al. Validation of a simplified SRS-Schwab classification using a sagittal modifier. Spine Deformity. 2019;7(3):467–71. https://doi.org/10.1016/j.jspd.2018.09.008.
42. Le Huec JC, Charosky S, Barrey C, Rigal J, Aunoble S. Sagittal imbalance cascade for simple degenerative spine and consequences: algorithm of decision for appropriate treatment. Eur Spine J. 2011;20(Suppl 5):699–703. https://doi.org/10.1007/s00586-011-1938-8.
43. Schwab F, Lafage V, Boyce R, Skalli W, Farcy JP. Gravity line analysis in adult volunteers: age-related correlation with spinal parameters, pelvic parameters, and foot position. Spine (Phila Pa 1976). 2006;31(25):E959–67. https://doi.org/10.1097/01.brs.0000248126.96737.0f.
44. Gelb DE, Lenke LG, Bridwell KH, Blanke K, McEnery KW. An analysis of sagittal spinal alignment in 100 asymptomatic middle and older aged volunteers. Spine (Phila Pa 1976). 1995;20(12):1351–8.
45. Hammerberg EM, Wood KB. Sagittal profile of the elderly. J Spinal Disord Tech. 2003;16(1):44–50. https://doi.org/10.1097/00024720-200302000-00008.

46. Asai Y, Tsutsui S, Oka H, Yoshimura N, Hashizume H, Yamada H, et al. Sagittal spino-pelvic alignment in adults: the Wakayama spine study. PLoS One. 2017;12(6):e0178697. https://doi.org/10.1371/journal.pone.0178697.
47. Khan JM, Basques BA, Harada GK, Louie PK, Chen I, Vetter C, et al. Does increasing age impact clinical and radiographic outcomes following lumbar spinal fusion? Spine J. 2020;20(4):563–71. https://doi.org/10.1016/j.spinee.2019.11.003.
48. Becker P, Bretschneider W, Tuschel A, Ogon M. Life quality after instrumented lumbar fusion in the elderly. Spine (Phila Pa 1976). 2010;35(15):1478–81. https://doi.org/10.1097/BRS.0b013e3181c62294.
49. Takahashi T, Hanakita J, Minami M, Kitahama Y, Kuraishi K, Watanabe M, et al. Clinical outcomes and adverse events following transforaminal interbody fusion for lumbar degenerative spondylolisthesis in elderly patients. Neurol Med Chir (Tokyo). 2011;51(12):829–35. https://doi.org/10.2176/nmc.51.829.
50. Ames CP, Smith JS, Scheer JK, Bess S, Bederman SS, Deviren V, et al. Impact of spinopelvic alignment on decision making in deformity surgery in adults: a review. J Neurosurg Spine. 2012;16(6):547–64. https://doi.org/10.3171/2012.2.Spine11320.
51. Cho KJ, Kim KT, Kim WJ, Lee SH, Jung JH, Kim YT, et al. Pedicle subtraction osteotomy in elderly patients with degenerative sagittal imbalance. Spine (Phila Pa 1976). 2013;38(24):E1561–6. https://doi.org/10.1097/BRS.0b013e3182a63c29.
52. Lafage R, Schwab F, Glassman S, Bess S, Harris B, Sheer J, et al. Age-adjusted alignment goals have the potential to reduce PJK. Spine (Phila Pa 1976). 2017;42(17):1275–82. https://doi.org/10.1097/brs.0000000000002146.
53. Smith JS, Shaffrey CI, Klineberg E, Lafage V, Schwab F, Lafage R, et al. Complication rates associated with 3-column osteotomy in 82 adult spinal deformity patients: retrospective review of a prospectively collected multicenter consecutive series with 2-year follow-up. J Neurosurg Spine. 2017;27(4):444–57. https://doi.org/10.3171/2016.10.Spine16849.

Chapter 18
Revision Surgery in the Elderly

Barry Cheaney II and Khoi D. Than

Introduction

There has been a dramatic increase in spinal surgery rates over the past few decades, and with improving health care and life expectancy, there is a rising need for spine care in the elderly population [1–3]. With this, revision spine surgery rates are expected to rise. The elderly patient is unique in that they often have several major comorbidities in addition to the natural aging process of the body. Several changes to the bone and intervertebral discs occur with aging, leading to altered mechanics and damage accumulation [4]. Changes in alignment (loss of lumbar lordosis, increase in thoracic kyphosis, and scoliosis) and bone mineral density of the vertebrae can lead to a stiffer and weaker spine [4]. A loss of disc height naturally occurs with aging and places nonphysiological loads on adjacent segments and facet joints [5]. These factors predispose the elderly population to several degenerative conditions of the thoracolumbar spine and contribute to the challenges faced during revision surgery.

Revision spine surgery requires a thorough evaluation of the patient's symptomatic and surgical history, and special considerations must be taken with elderly patients that the operating surgeon must address. These special considerations go beyond the chief complaint and include proper management of comorbidities, knowledge of how those comorbidities may affect intraoperative decisions, surgical clearance from multidisciplinary teams, as well as remaining up to date on current

B. Cheaney II
Department of Neurological Surgery, Oregon Health & Science University, Portland, OR, USA
e-mail: Cheaney@ohsu.edu

K. D. Than (✉)
Department of Neurosurgery, Duke University, Durham, NC, USA
e-mail: Khoi.than@duke.edu

K.-M. G. Fu et al. (eds.), *Treatment of Spine Disease in the Elderly*,
https://doi.org/10.1007/978-3-031-12612-3_18

Surgical Revision Considerations

The changes to the aged spine predispose the elderly population to postoperative complications. In addition to medical optimization of this patient population, modified surgical techniques may decrease the occurrence of these complications [7, 22, 23]. The following sections include common complications of spine surgery in the elderly and options for when revision surgery is necessary.

Infection

Surgical site infection is an important complication after spine surgery (Fig. 18.1) [24, 25]. Compared to younger populations, elderly patients are more vulnerable to adverse health and functional effects of postoperative infections [26]. McGarry et al. [27] reported that surgical site infections was associated with greater than fivefold mortality rate and twofold prolonged duration of hospitalization in elderly patients than that of younger patients. Indications for surgery in patients with suspected or confirmed infection include progression of infection despite antibiotic therapy, epidural abscesses causing pain and/or neurologic symptoms, and progressive collapse of the vertebral bodies or disks, leading to spinal deformity [1]. Treatment usually involves the surgical debridement of infected and necrotic tissues and intravenous antibiotic therapy for 4 to 9 weeks [28]. For patients with instrumentation, removal of implants and direct or staged reimplantation should be considered, especially in cases with high risk of treatment failure [25]. Titanium instrumentation is a good option as titanium exhibits less bacterial glycocalyx adherence than stainless steel [29].

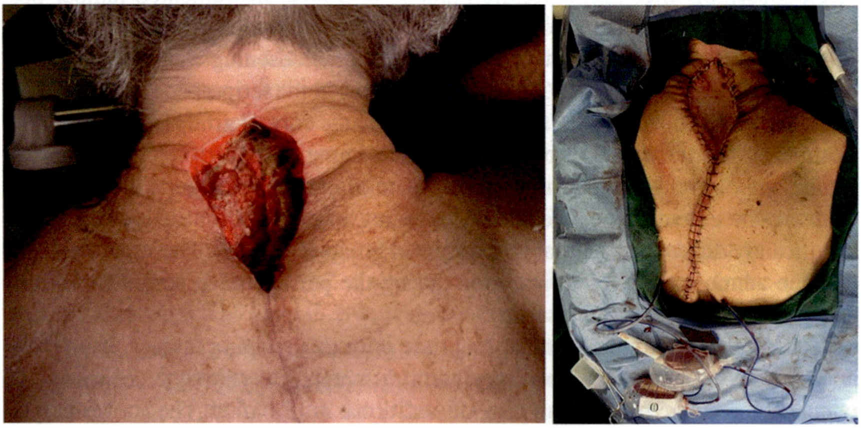

Fig. 18.1 Wound dehiscence and infection in an 80-year-old woman who underwent extension of thoracolumbar fusion to C2. The wound was repaired with rotational flap coverage by plastic surgery

Proximal Junctional Kyphosis

Proximal junctional kyphosis (PJK) is defined as a proximal junctional angle (PJA) greater than 10 degrees postoperatively, and at least 10 degrees greater than the corresponding preoperative measurement, with bony compromise or instrumentation failure at the upper instrumented vertebrae (UIV) or adjacent rostral vertebrae (UIV +1). When PJK results in fractures and/or symptoms requiring reoperation, proximal junctional failure (PJF) is diagnosed (Fig. 18.2) [30]. This junctional disorder can lead to cord compression, which may warrant emergent surgery [31]. The incidence of PJK has been reported in up to 40% following adult spinal deformity correction and long-instrumented fusion, [23, 32, 33] and complications due to PJK or additional remote level vertebral fracture following adult spinal deformity surgery is a major concern for elderly patients with low bone mineral density [34]. A number of groups have studied the protective and risks factors of developing PJK, and due to controversial data, Liu et al. [33] conducted a meta-analysis. The pooled results suggested that age >55 years old, fusion to the sacrum, preoperative thoracic kyphosis angle (T5–T12) >40°, low bone mineral density, and preoperative SVA >5 cm are risk factors for PJK. Preventative techniques to consider during the index operation and during revision surgery when extension of fusion is necessary include the use of laminar hooks, [22, 23] ligament reinforcement, and vertebroplasty/kyphoplasty at the UIV and UIV + 1 [23]. Ghobrial et al. [32] studied the incidence of PJK/PJF in patients treated with prophylactic polymethylmethacrylate (PMMA) cement augmentation at the UIV and UIV + 1 versus a control group (no vertebroplasty). The incidence of PJK was 36% in the control group and 23.7% in the vertebroplasty group (p = 0.020, OR = 0.548, 95% CI = 0.211–1.424). The authors concluded that the use of prophylactic vertebral cement augmentation at the UIV

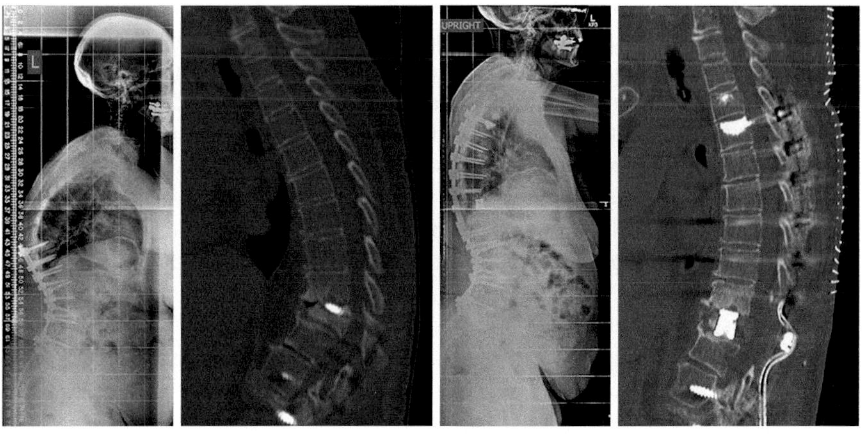

Fig. 18.2 A 73-year-old woman status post previous T10-S1 fusion presented with back and right leg pain, and was found to have proximal junctional kyphosis. She was treated via a T10 vertebral column resection, extension of fusion to T4, and T3 and T4 vertebroplasties

and UIV + 1 segment at the time of deformity correction appears to be preventative in the development of PJK/PJF.

The length of pedicle screws may have effects on the incidence of PJK. Park et al. [35] investigated the risk of UIV fractures associated with UIV screw fixation (unicortical vs. bicortical) and PMMA augmentation after adult spinal deformity surgery. All thoracolumbar fusions spanned 4 levels or more. Of the 52 included patients, 15 underwent unicortical screw fixation at the UIV, 16 patients underwent bicortical screw fixation with PMMA augmentation at the UIV, and 21 patients underwent bicortical screw fixation at the UIV without PMMA augmentation. UIV fracture rates were 0%, 31.3%, and 42.9%, respectively. UIV bicortical screw fixation increased the risk for UIV fracture (OR 5.39; $p = 0.02$). The authors concluded that bicortical screw fixation at the UIV should be avoided in long thoracolumbar fusion surgery to avoid PJF, with a preference for unicortical screws.

Pedicle Screws

Loosening of pedicle screws is a major complication of posterior spine surgery [36]. As pedicle screw performance is highly dependent on bone quality, [37] osteoporotic patients are predisposed to higher implant failure rates [17, 38]. Augmentation of the pedicle screw with bone cement, such as PMMA, calcium-based cements, or hydroxyapatite, is one technique to enhance fixation purchase [36, 37, 39]. Indications for augmentation for pedicle screws include osteoporosis and revision surgery in the elderly [37]. Sawakami et al. [40] evaluated the clinical efficacy of PMMA augmentation in reinforcing pedicle screws in osteoporotic spines. Of the 38 patients with osteoporotic vertebral fractures that underwent posterior fusion using pedicle screws, 17 had pedicle screw augmentation with PMMA. The augmentation group had significantly decreased incidence of pedicle screw lucency (determined as present on both anteroposterior and lateral radiographs when the radiolucency was 1 mm or wider at the bone-screw interface) compared to the control (29.4% vs. 71.4%), significantly decreased correction loss (3 degrees vs. 7.2 degrees), and significantly higher bony fusion rate [determined as present on lateral radiographs when bone formation (consolidation) was disclosed surrounding the collapsed vertebra or the movement was <2 degrees in the flexion-extension radiographs] (94.1% vs. 76.1%). The use of pedicle screw augmentation has been supported by other study groups as a safe and practical technique that increases the strength and stiffness of fixation (Fig. 18.3) [37, 39, 41, 42].

Revision spine surgery often requires extension of fusion with rods and pedicle screws or replacement of internal fixation. The type of screw used can have differing radiologic and clinical effects, especially in the elderly, often osteoporotic, patient. Wu et al. [43] compared the rate of screw loosening and clinical outcomes of expandable pedicle screws (EPS) with those of conventional pedicle screws (CPS) in patients treated for spinal stenosis combined with osteoporosis. One hundred and

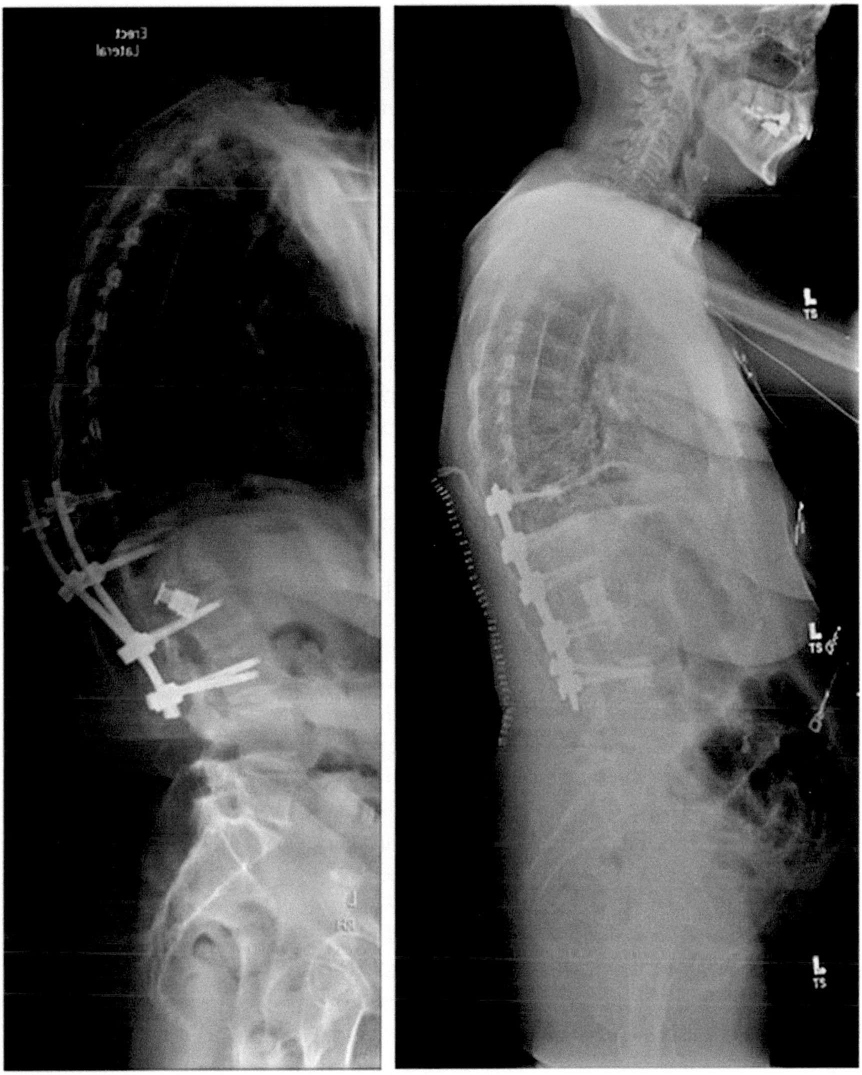

Fig. 18.3 A 66-year-old woman underwent T11-L3 fusion with L1 corpectomy for plasmacytoma. She returned with evidence for cage migration and hardware loosening. She underwent reexploration for extension of fusion to T10, replacement of instrumentation with fenestrated screws for cement augmentation, and minimally invasive lateral approach for redo T12-L2 interbody fusion

fifty-seven consecutive patients with spinal stenosis received either EPS fixation (n = 80) or CPS fixation (n = 77) to obtain lumbosacral stabilization. In the EPS group, 20 screws became loose (4.1%) in 6 patients (7.5%), and two screws (0.4%) had broken. In the CPS group, 48 screws became loose (12.9%) in 15 patients

(19.5%), but no screws were broken. The fusion rate in the EPS group (92.5%) was significantly higher than that of the CPS group (80.5%). The authors conclude that EPS can decrease the risk of screw loosening and achieve better fixation strength and clinical results in osteoporotic lumbar spine fusion.

Anterior Versus Posterior Approach

A separate consideration to revision spine surgeries is approach. In patients with a prior posterolateral approach, unintended neural structural injury or CSF leakage during the dissection of scarred neural tissue may occur with a repeat posterior procedure [44, 45]. Additionally, a repeat posterior procedure entails re-dissection of back muscles, resulting in further weakening of spinal supportive structures, hindering proper healing [46–48]. An anterior approach for the revision procedure minimizes these risks because an unscarred tissue plane is used to approach the spine [45, 49] and extensive epidural scarring due to a repeat posterior procedure is avoided [50]. Lee and colleagues [2] studied the efficacy of anterior lumbar interbody fusion (ALIF) with percutaneous screw fixation for revision surgery in lumbar spine and reported positive outcomes. The mean visual analog scale score for back and leg pain decreased, respectively, from 7.8 to 2.3 and 8.0 to 2.3 ($p < 0.001$). The mean Oswestry Disability Index score improved from 70 to 25% ($p < 0.001$). Radiological evidence of fusion (defined as the absence of radiographic motion of more than 5 degrees on the dynamic radiographs, absence of radiolucencies around a large area of the cages, and absence of implant failure) was noted in 52 of 54 patients. The mean preoperative segmental lordosis, whole lumbar lordosis, and sacral tilt were 15.2, 35.5, and 28.3 degrees, respectively; these values were significantly increased to 20.4, 40.7, and 31.4 degrees, respectively, after revision surgery from an anterior approach ($p < 0.001$). The increase in sacral tilt was positively correlated with improvement in back pain ($p = 0.028$) and functional status ($p = 0.025$). This study demonstrated that ALIF and percutaneous screw fixation can be an effective surgical option in revision surgery of the lumbosacral spine, as clinical and functional outcomes were significantly improved in the majority of the patients with instability, degenerative disc disease, recurrent herniation, and pseudarthrosis. Another group studied the outcomes of ALIF procedure for the treatment of failed back surgery syndrome (degenerative disc disease, postsurgical spondylolisthesis, or pseudarthrosis) and found similar findings. Back pain, leg pain, and functional status improved significantly, by 76% ($P < 0.01$), 80% ($P < 0.01$), and 67% ($P < 0.01$), respectively [45]. The anterior approach has proven to be a safe and viable alternative to repeat posterior approaches in select patient populations [2, 45, 51].

Sacral Insufficiency

Sacral insufficiency fractures are a common source of back pain in the elderly and are associated with significant morbidity [52–54]. Sacral insufficiency fractures are typically a result of an increased amount of stress on osteoporotic bone in elderly patients; however, these fractures may occur as a result of short- and long-fusion constructs to the sacrum [52, 55, 56]. Meredith and colleagues [54] reviewed 24 patients that developed sacral fractures caudal to instrumented spinal fusions. Eight of these patients were successfully treated conservatively. The authors identified anterolisthesis of the fracture greater than 2 mm and kyphotic angulation to be significantly associated with failure of conservative treatment. Those who failed nonoperative treatment underwent posterior extension of the fusion construct to S2 and the iliac wings with sacroiliac joint fusion, and in 10 cases, a combined anterior and posterior approach was used that consisted of either revision ALIF or trans-sacral posterior lumbar interbody fusion.

Buell et al. [52] reported their experience of nine patients who developed sacral insufficiency fracture after lumbosacral fusion. Six of these patients had osteopenia/osteoporosis and presenting symptoms, including back/leg pain or lower extremity weakness. All patients underwent lumbopelvic fixation via a posterior-only approach, resulting in successful healing; however, two patients underwent revision for rod fractures at 1 and 2 years postoperatively. Spine surgeons should have a high index of suspicion to diagnose sacral insufficiency fracture after lumbosacral arthrodesis. Sacral insufficiency is often unrecognized on plain radiographs; CT, MRI, and nuclear scintigraphy can be used to establish the diagnosis [54]. Conservative management is appropriate for select patients; [57] however, indications for surgical revision include pain refractory to nonoperative management, neurological deficits, fracture nonunion with anterolisthesis or kyphotic angulation, L5-S1 pseudarthrosis, and spinopelvic malalignment. High-risk patients may benefit from prophylactic lumbopelvic fixation at the time of index lumbosacral arthrodesis [52].

Conclusion

As life expectancy continues to increase, more and more elderly patients are pursuing spine surgery. Unfortunately, complications do arise that require revision surgeries. The elderly patient presents with unique characteristics, making revision surgery challenging. The spine surgeon must understand these challenges and adjust their approach to treating these patients.

References

1. Bederman SS, Le VH, Pahlavan S. An approach to lumbar revision spine surgery in adults. J Am Acad Orthop Surg. 2016;24(7):433–42.
2. Lee SH, Kang BU, Jeon SH, Park JD, Maeng DH, Choi YG, et al. Revision surgery of the lumbar spine: anterior lumbar interbody fusion followed by percutaneous pedicle screw fixation. J Neurosurg Spine. 2006;5(3):228–33.
3. Puvanesarajah V, Shen FH, Cancienne JM, Novicoff WM, Jain A, Shimer AL, et al. Risk factors for revision surgery following primary adult spinal deformity surgery in patients 65 years and older. J Neurosurg Spine. 2016;25(4):486–93.
4. Cloyd JM, Acosta FL Jr, Ames CP. Complications and outcomes of lumbar spine surgery in elderly people: a review of the literature. J Am Geriatr Soc. 2008;56(7):1318–27.
5. Cavanaugh JM, Lu Y, Chen C, Kallakuri S. Pain generation in lumbar and cervical facet joints. J Bone Joint Surg Am. 2006;88(Suppl 2):63–7.
6. Poorman GW, Zhou PL, Vasquez-Montes D, Horn S, Bortz C, Segreto F, et al. Differences in primary and revision deformity surgeries: following 1,063 primary thoracolumbar adult spinal deformity fusions over time. J Spine Surg. 2018;4(2):203–10.
7. Zileli M, Dursun E. How to improve outcomes of spine surgery in geriatric patients. World Neurosurg. 2020;140:519–26.
8. Worley N, Marascalchi B, Jalai CM, Yang S, Diebo B, Vira S, et al. Predictors of inpatient morbidity and mortality in adult spinal deformity surgery. Eur Spine J. 2016;25(3):819–27.
9. Cancienne JM, Werner BC, Chen DQ, Hassanzadeh H, Shimer AL. Perioperative hemoglobin A1c as a predictor of deep infection following single-level lumbar decompression in patients with diabetes. Spine J. 2017;17(8):1100–5.
10. Guzman JZ, Iatridis JC, Skovrlj B, Cutler HS, Hecht AC, Qureshi SA, et al. Outcomes and complications of diabetes mellitus on patients undergoing degenerative lumbar spine surgery. Spine. 2014;39(19):1596–604.
11. Hikata T, Iwanami A, Hosogane N, Watanabe K, Ishii K, Nakamura M, et al. High preoperative hemoglobin A1c is a risk factor for surgical site infection after posterior thoracic and lumbar spinal instrumentation surgery. J Orthop Sci. 2014;19(2):223–8.
12. Hwang JU, Son DW, Kang KT, Lee SH, Lee JS, Song GS, et al. Importance of hemoglobin A1c levels for the detection of post-surgical infection following single-level lumbar posterior fusion in patients with diabetes. Korean J Neurotrauma. 2019;15(2):150–8.
13. Peng W, Liang Y, Lu T, Li M, Li DS, Du KH, et al. Multivariate analysis of incision infection after posterior lumbar surgery in diabetic patients: a single-center retrospective analysis. Medicine. 2019;98(23):e15935.
14. Kezerle L, Shalev L, Barski L. Treating the elderly diabetic patient: special considerations. Diabetes Metab Syndr Obes. 2014;7:391–400.
15. Kim CH, Chung CK, Shin S, Choi BR, Kim MJ, Park BJ, et al. The relationship between diabetes and the reoperation rate after lumbar spinal surgery: a nationwide cohort study. Spine J. 2015;15(5):866–74.
16. O'Lynnger TM, Zuckerman SL, Morone PJ, Dewan MC, Vasquez-Castellanos RA, Cheng JS. Trends for spine surgery for the elderly: implications for access to healthcare in North America. Neurosurgery. 2015;77(Suppl 4):S136–41.
17. Carlson BC, Robinson WA, Wanderman NR, Sebastian AS, Nassr A, Freedman BA, et al. A review and clinical perspective of the impact of osteoporosis on the spine. Geriatr Orthop Surg Rehabil. 2019;10:2151459319861591.
18. Fischer CR, Hanson G, Eller M, Lehman RA. A systematic review of treatment strategies for degenerative lumbar spine fusion surgery in patients with osteoporosis. Geriatr Orthop Surg Rehabil. 2016;7(4):188–96.

19. Pickhardt PJ, Pooler BD, Lauder T, del Rio AM, Bruce RJ, Binkley N. Opportunistic screening for osteoporosis using abdominal computed tomography scans obtained for other indications. Ann Intern Med. 2013;158(8):588–95.
20. Ohtori S, Inoue G, Orita S, Yamauchi K, Eguchi Y, Ochiai N, et al. Teriparatide accelerates lumbar posterolateral fusion in women with postmenopausal osteoporosis: prospective study. Spine. 2012;37(23):E1464–8.
21. Ohtori S, Inoue G, Orita S, Yamauchi K, Eguchi Y, Ochiai N, et al. Comparison of teriparatide and bisphosphonate treatment to reduce pedicle screw loosening after lumbar spinal fusion surgery in postmenopausal women with osteoporosis from a bone quality perspective. Spine. 2013;38(8):E487–92.
22. Helgeson MD, Shah SA, Newton PO, Clements DH 3rd, Betz RR, Marks MC, et al. Evaluation of proximal junctional kyphosis in adolescent idiopathic scoliosis following pedicle screw, hook, or hybrid instrumentation. Spine. 2010;35(2):177–81.
23. Zhao J, Chen K, Zhai X, Chen K, Li M, Lu Y. Incidence and risk factors of proximal junctional kyphosis after internal fixation for adult spinal deformity: a systematic evaluation and meta-analysis. Neurosurg Rev. 2021;44(2):855–66.
24. Atesok K, Papavassiliou E, Heffernan MJ, Tunmire D, Sitnikov I, Tanaka N, et al. Current strategies in prevention of postoperative infections in spine surgery. Global Spine J. 2020;10(2):183–94.
25. Maruo K, Berven SH. Outcome and treatment of postoperative spine surgical site infections: predictors of treatment success and failure. J Orthop Sci. 2014;19(3):398–404.
26. Liang Z, Rong K, Gu W, Yu X, Fang R, Deng Y, et al. Surgical site infection following elective orthopaedic surgeries in geriatric patients: incidence and associated risk factors. Int Wound J. 2019;16(3):773–80.
27. McGarry SA, Engemann JJ, Schmader K, Sexton DJ, Kaye KS. Surgical-site infection due to Staphylococcus aureus among elderly patients: mortality, duration of hospitalization, and cost. Infect Control Hosp Epidemiol. 2004;25(6):461–7.
28. Bas T, Bas P, Blasco A, Bas JL. Chronic infections of the spine. Eur J Orthop Surg Traumatol. 2013;23(Suppl 1):S35–40.
29. Sheehan E, McKenna J, Mulhall KJ, Marks P, McCormack D. Adhesion of staphylococcus to orthopaedic metals, an in vivo study. J Orthop Res. 2004;22(1):39–43.
30. Glattes RC, Bridwell KH, Lenke LG, Kim YJ, Rinella A, Edwards C 2nd. Proximal junctional kyphosis in adult spinal deformity following long instrumented posterior spinal fusion: incidence, outcomes, and risk factor analysis. Spine. 2005;30(14):1643–9.
31. Arlet V, Aebi M. Junctional spinal disorders in operated adult spinal deformities: present understanding and future perspectives. Eur Spine J. 2013;22(Suppl 2):S276–95.
32. Ghobrial GM, Eichberg DG, Kolcun JPG, Madhavan K, Lebwohl NH, Green BA, et al. Prophylactic vertebral cement augmentation at the uppermost instrumented vertebra and rostral adjacent vertebra for the prevention of proximal junctional kyphosis and failure following long-segment fusion for adult spinal deformity. Spine J. 2017;17(10):1499–505.
33. Liu FY, Wang T, Yang SD, Wang H, Yang DL, Ding WY. Incidence and risk factors for proximal junctional kyphosis: a meta-analysis. Eur Spine J. 2016;25(8):2376–83.
34. Uei H, Tokuhashi Y, Maseda M, Nakahashi M, Sawada H, Matsumoto K, et al. Exploratory analysis of predictors of revision surgery for proximal junctional kyphosis or additional postoperative vertebral fracture following adult spinal deformity surgery in elderly patients: a retrospective cohort study. J Orthop Surg Res. 2018;13(1):252.
35. Park YS, Hyun SJ, Choi HY, Kim KJ, Jahng TA. Association between bicortical screw fixation at upper instrumented vertebra and risk for upper instrumented vertebra fracture. J Neurosurg Spine. 2017;26(5):638–44.

36. Weiser L, Huber G, Sellenschloh K, Viezens L, Püschel K, Morlock MM, et al. Insufficient stability of pedicle screws in osteoporotic vertebrae: biomechanical correlation of bone mineral density and pedicle screw fixation strength. Eur Spine J. 2017;26(11):2891–7.
37. Hoppe S, Keel MJ. Pedicle screw augmentation in osteoporotic spine: indications, limitations and technical aspects. Eur J Trauma Emerg Surg. 2017;43(1):3–8.
38. Bjerke BT, Zarrabian M, Aleem IS, Fogelson JL, Currier BL, Freedman BA, et al. Incidence of osteoporosis-related complications following posterior lumbar fusion. Global Spine J. 2018;8(6):563–9.
39. Chang MC, Liu CL, Chen TH. Polymethylmethacrylate augmentation of pedicle screw for osteoporotic spinal surgery: a novel technique. Spine. 2008;33(10):E317–24.
40. Sawakami K, Yamazaki A, Ishikawa S, Ito T, Watanabe K, Endo N. Polymethylmethacrylate augmentation of pedicle screws increases the initial fixation in osteoporotic spine patients. J Spinal Disord Tech. 2012;25(2):E28–35.
41. Chang MC, Kao HC, Ying SH, Liu CL. Polymethylmethacrylate augmentation of cannulated pedicle screws for fixation in osteoporotic spines and comparison of its clinical results and biomechanical characteristics with the needle injection method. J Spinal Disord Tech. 2013;26(6):305–15.
42. Piñera AR, Duran C, Lopez B, Saez I, Correia E, Alvarez L. Instrumented lumbar arthrodesis in elderly patients: prospective study using cannulated cemented pedicle screw instrumentation. Eur Spine J. 2011;20(Suppl 3):408–14.
43. Wu ZX, Gong FT, Liu L, Ma ZS, Zhang Y, Zhao X, et al. A comparative study on screw loosening in osteoporotic lumbar spine fusion between expandable and conventional pedicle screws. Arch Orthop Trauma Surg. 2012;132(4):471–6.
44. Brodke DS, Dick JC, Kunz DN, McCabe R, Zdeblick TA. Posterior lumbar interbody fusion. A biomechanical comparison, including a new threaded cage. Spine. 1997;22(1):26–31.
45. Duggal N, Mendiondo I, Pares HR, Jhawar BS, Das K, Kenny KJ, et al. Anterior lumbar interbody fusion for treatment of failed back surgery syndrome: an outcome analysis. Neurosurgery. 2004;54(3):636–43; discussion 43–4
46. Kim DY, Lee SH, Chung SK, Lee HY. Comparison of multifidus muscle atrophy and trunk extension muscle strength: percutaneous versus open pedicle screw fixation. Spine. 2005;30(1):123–9.
47. Rantanen J, Hurme M, Falck B, Alaranta H, Nykvist F, Lehto M, et al. The lumbar multifidus muscle five years after surgery for a lumbar intervertebral disc herniation. Spine. 1993;18(5):568–74.
48. Sihvonen T, Herno A, Paljärvi L, Airaksinen O, Partanen J, Tapaninaho A. Local denervation atrophy of paraspinal muscles in postoperative failed back syndrome. Spine. 1993;18(5):575–81.
49. Choi JY, Choi YW, Sung KH. Anterior lumbar interbody fusion in patients with a previous discectomy: minimum 2-year follow-up. J Spinal Disord Tech. 2005;18(4):347–52.
50. Skaf G, Bouclaous C, Alaraj A, Chamoun R. Clinical outcome of surgical treatment of failed back surgery syndrome. Surg Neurol. 2005;64(6):483–8, discussion 8–9
51. Kuslich SD, Ulstrom CL, Griffith SL, Ahern JW, Dowdle JD. The Bagby and Kuslich method of lumbar interbody fusion. History, techniques, and 2-year follow-up results of a United States prospective, multicenter trial. Spine. 1998;23(11):1267–78; discussion 79
52. Buell TJ, Yener U, Wang TR, Buchholz AL, Yen CP, Shaffrey ME, et al. Sacral insufficiency fractures after lumbosacral arthrodesis: salvage lumbopelvic fixation and a proposed management algorithm. Journal of neurosurgery. Spine. 2020:1–12.
53. Mahmood B, Pasternack J, Razi A, Saleh A. Safety and efficacy of percutaneous sacroplasty for treatment of sacral insufficiency fractures: a systematic review. J Spine Surg. 2019;5(3):365–71.
54. Meredith DS, Taher F, Cammisa FP Jr, Girardi FP. Incidence, diagnosis, and management of sacral fractures following multilevel spinal arthrodesis. Spine J. 2013;13(11):1464–9.

55. Kolz JM, Mitchell SA, Elder BD, Sebastian AS, Huddleston PM, Freedman BA. Sacral insufficiency fracture following short-segment lumbosacral fusion: case series and review of the literature: Global Spine J. 2020:2192568220950332.
56. Salzmann SN, Ortiz Miller C, Carrino JA, Yang J, Shue J, Sama AA, et al. BMI and gender increase risk of sacral fractures after multilevel instrumented spinal fusion compared with bone mineral density and pelvic parameters. Spine J. 2019;19(2):238–45.
57. Khan MH, Smith PN, Kang JD. Sacral insufficiency fractures following multilevel instrumented spinal fusion: case report. Spine. 2005;30(16):E484–8.

Chapter 19
Thoracolumbar Trauma in the Elderly

Nathan B. Han, Charles A. Sansur, and Kenneth M. Crandall

Introduction

Thoracolumbar fractures occur in around 5–6.9% of blunt trauma with an associated rate of neurological injury in approximately 26% of those patients [1, 2]. The high percentage of neurological injury related to the fracture can leave patients with devastating consequences. The most common mechanism of thoracolumbar injury in the general population is motor vehicle accidents followed by falls; however, in the elderly population, falls are the leading mechanism of thoracolumbar trauma. A retrospective analysis by Winkler et al. showed that the elderly cohort (age >70) with thoracolumbar trauma had a lower incidence of severe GCS category (GCS 3–8) compared to middle-aged cohort (5% elderly vs. 7.4% middle-aged) and lower injury severity score (13.3 elderly vs. 15.3 middle-aged). In addition, there are other unique aspects of the elderly patient population that need to be considered when managing and treating their thoracolumbar fractures. This chapter will discuss the unique biomechanical differences and factors to consider in the elderly, classifications of thoracolumbar trauma, conservative and operative management, and complications pertinent to elderly population.

Supplementary Information The online version contains supplementary material available at [https://doi.org/10.1007/978-3-031-12612-3_19].

N. B. Han · C. A. Sansur (✉) · K. M. Crandall
Department of Neurosurgery, University of Maryland School of Medicine, Baltimore, MD, USA
e-mail: nhan@som.umaryland.edu; csansur@som.umaryland.edu; kcrandall@som.umaryland.edu

K.-M. G. Fu et al. (eds.), *Treatment of Spine Disease in the Elderly*, https://doi.org/10.1007/978-3-031-12612-3_19

Unique Factors in Thoracolumbar Trauma of the Elderly

Osteoporosis

Osteoporosis constitutes bone of low density leading to increased risk of fracture and, in the case of vertebral osteoporosis, can lead to kyphosis and neurological deficits. It is defined by the World Health Organization as bone mineral density at the hip or lumbar spine less than or equal to 2.5 standard deviations below that of the young adult reference. In the United States, there are more than 9.9 million people with osteoporosis with annual estimate of 750,000 osteoporotic vertebral fractures [3]. The prevalence of osteoporosis increases with age and is greater in females [4].

In the setting of thoracolumbar trauma, osteoporotic patients present unique challenges. First, in the diagnosis of osteoporotic fractures with concomitant degenerative pathologies, it may be more difficult to identify acute osteoporotic fractures using plain radiographs, necessitating MRI to assess for vertebral body edema suggestive of an acute or subacute fracture. Second, there is increased chance of non-union in fractures of osteoporotic bones leading to failed conservative treatments and necessity of surgical intervention. Approximately 15–35% of patients with osteoporotic fractures do not heal completely [3]. Third, in cases requiring instrumentation for fusion, osteoporosis increases the risk of screw pullout rate and consequent need for revision surgery. These factors must be considered when diagnosing and treating elderly patients at risk of osteoporosis.

Ankylosing Spondylitis (AS)

Ankylosing spondylitis is a seronegative spondyloarthropathy, in which 90–95% of patients are positive for major histocompatibility complex class I molecule HLA-B27. It is defined by the Modified New York criteria with radiographic bilateral sacroiliitis greater than grade 2 or unilateral grade 3–4 with one of the clinical symptoms, including inflammatory back pain, limitation of lumbar spine motion in sagittal and coronal planes, and limitation of chest expansion. The pathology of AS involves inflammation of ligaments leading to ectopic bone formation and the uncoupling of bone formation and resorption with increased osteoclastic activity leading to weakening of bones. It is important to note that patients with AS have increased incidence of spinal epidural hematoma, due to bleeding from epidural venous plexus and diploë of the pathologic bone [5]. When patients with AS manifest paralysis, one must have a high index of suspicion for epidural hematoma, as the etiology for paralysis cannot be solely attributed to instability. As such, MRI should be performed in these patients to rule out the presence of epidural hematoma.

Diffuse Idiopathic Skeletal Hyperostosis (DISH)

DISH is a spinal ankylosing disorder of unclear etiology where there is spontaneous osseous fusion of the spinal ligaments, which is clinically diagnosed when anterior bridging osteophytes of the ankylosed anterior longitudinal ligament is seen on four consecutive levels [6]. Ossification is most commonly seen in the thoracic spine (T7–11) with right side prominence as pulsations of the descending aorta prevents bony formation along the left side of the thoracic spine [7]. There is a wide range of reported prevalence (3.5–42%), but the prevalence does increase with age (mean 68.2 years, male predominant), making this condition relatively common in the elderly population [8, 9]. The pertinent importance of DISH in thoracolumbar trauma is that the ossified levels of the spine act as an autologous fused segment creating higher stress at adjacent vertebral levels and fractures can lead to increased secondary displacement, delayed/nonunion, and neurological deterioration. Review by Westerveld et al. observed that the distribution of mechanism of injury in DISH patients were as follows: extension 51.5%, rotation 34.9%, compression 14%, and flexion 0% [8].

Classification of Thoracolumbar Injuries

Although there is no universally accepted thoracolumbar injury classification system, two commonly used methods are Thoracolumbar Injury Severity Score (TLISS) and Thoracolumbar Injury Classification and Severity Score (TLICS), which developed from TLISS [10]. While TLISS focused only on injury mechanism rather than morphology, TLICS replaced the mechanism of injury with a morphologic description of the injury. Specifically, TLICS addresses the following information for the injury: fracture pattern/morphology, integrity of posterior ligamentous complex, and neurological status of the patient. Scores of 0–4 are assigned in each category and total score of 3 or less deems nonoperative treatment, 4 is indeterminate, and 5 or greater recommends surgical intervention. The intra-/interobserver reliability ranged from moderate to substantial reproducibility (kappa score of 0.45–0.74). Retrospective application of TLICS in comparison to clinical decision made for surgical vs. nonsurgical intervention of thoracolumbar injuries show 96% matched in surgical decision-making and 99% of nonsurgical decision-making. The limitations of this classification include injuries with burst fractures, where the score may be less than 3. For example, patients with burst fractures may be at risk of developing progressive kyphotic deformity with retropulsion of the fractured elements, leading to canal compromise and neurological decline. As such, classification systems like the TLICS should be used as a guide in management, but not as a definitive algorithmic decision-making tool [11].

Another drawback of TLICS classification system is that it requires evaluation of the posterior ligamentous complex requiring MRI imaging, which does not have great interobserver reliability (kappa 0.11–0.45). The AO thoracolumbar classification adds patient-specific modifiers in addition to morphologic classification to further guide treatment with modifier M1 used with uncertain posterior element status and M2 for patients with underlying conditions affecting bone status, such as osteoporosis, DISH, and AS. Overall interobserver reliability for AO classification among 100 spine surgeons had kappa of 0.56 [12].

In elderly patients with osteoporotic fractures from low velocity trauma, the TLICS method does not specifically incorporate the osteoporotic nature and prognosis of such fractures. Sugita et al. developed a classification of osteoporotic vertebral fractures with five different classifications based on morphology of the vertebral body with observation that certain morphology of fractures (swelled, pinched, projecting anterior body) had poor prognosis with higher incidence of vertebral body collapse. Schnake et al. also developed a morphologic osteoporotic fracture classification (OF) with five different subgroups with distinction of posterior wall involvement and vertebral frame and structure. This classification had a substantial interrater kappa value of 0.63 [13, 14].

Conservative Management

In thoracolumbar trauma of the elderly with isolated vertebral fracture without neurological deficit and instability, conservative management involving pain management, early mobilization, and orthosis are initial treatment options. For patients with osteoporotic fractures, medications such as calcitonin and bisphosphonates are used to provide pain relief in addition to increasing bone density in the long run. Pamidronate demonstrated significant pain relief in acute osteoporotic fractures in a randomized control trial [15]. Lifestyle modifications, such as diet changes with adequate calcium and vitamin D intake, regular muscle strengthening and weight bearing exercise, and tobacco cessation, are beneficial for patients with osteoporotic fractures or at risk of osteoporosis.

Thoracolumbosacral orthotic (TLSO) bracing is commonly used in neurologically intact patients with stable fractures. Many non-load-bearing element fractures, such as spinous process or transverse process fractures, are stable fractures that can be managed with analgesics, with or without an orthotic brace. Anterior wedge compression fractures can also be treated with a brace. In this setting, the brace prevents forward flexion and diminishes load-bearing forces on the anterior compartment of the fractured body. When deciding to use orthotic bracing, one must be careful to ensure stability of fracture in standing position with the brace, so that there is no occult instability that would not be identified on a supine CT scan. Compression fractures with greater than 30° of kyphosis, 50% vertebral height loss, involvement of three contiguous levels, and flexion distraction fractures should be managed surgically. Some advocate bracing for 8–12 weeks with intermittent standing radiographs every 4–6 weeks to evaluate fracture healing and assess for progressive kyphotic deformity [16].

Operative Management

In elderly patients having thoracolumbar vertebral fractures with initial conservative treatment without clinical improvement or with radiographic worsening of fracture, vertebral augmentation is commonly performed as a next step in management. Vertebroplasty involves percutaneous injection of high-power cement through pedicles into the fractured vertebral body. It is indicated in traumatic fractures refractory to conservative therapy of more than 3–4 weeks [17]. Balloon kyphoplasty introduces an inflatable balloon in the fractured vertebral body and aims to correct the kyphotic deformity prior to cement injection, which is administered at low pressure [18]. Balloon kyphoplasty has similar indications to vertebroplasty in addition to traumatic vertebral fracture less than 7–10 days with kyphotic angle >15°. Absolute contraindication to the above procedures includes improvement in clinical symptom with conservative treatment, asymptomatic vertebral fracture, systemic/local infection, cement allergy, coagulopathy, and myelopathy originating at fracture level [19].

Meta-analysis of studies examining vertebroplasty or kyphoplasty versus control/sham procedures showed that both percutaneous kyphoplasty and vertebroplasty have similar long-term pain relief and functional outcome benefit compared to control groups; however, kyphoplasty tended to be more expensive and had longer operational time compared to vertebroplasty [20, 21]. Minamide et al. studied the efficacy of kyphoplasty in early (<4 weeks) vs. late (>4 weeks) in 51 patients and noted that kyphoplasty provides initial improvement in spine alignment at time of surgery, but in long term, the alignment returns to the value near initial time of surgery. Thus, their data suggests that earlier treatment group, which had better initial kyphotic angle compared to the late group, ultimately had significant improvement in long-term alignment compared to late treatment group with reduced rate of subsequent fractures [22].

For unstable fractures that require surgical instrumentation in elderly patients, factors such as elderly co-morbidities, spinal ankylosing disorders, and osteoporotic bone quality should be considered. Common standard treatment for unstable thoracolumbar fractures involves dorsal fusion above and below the fracture level, using pedicle screws with or without vertebroplasty/kyphoplasty. Figure 19.1 demonstrates a standing scoliosis film and MRI of a 67-year-old female with prior T4-T11 and L4-S1 fusion with new T12 compression fracture with retropulsion of T12 vertebral body causing cord compression. Due to the unstable nature of injury, the patient was taken to the operating room with extension of construct to include L1-L3 pedicles with realignment of fracture using in situ rod benders. T12 and

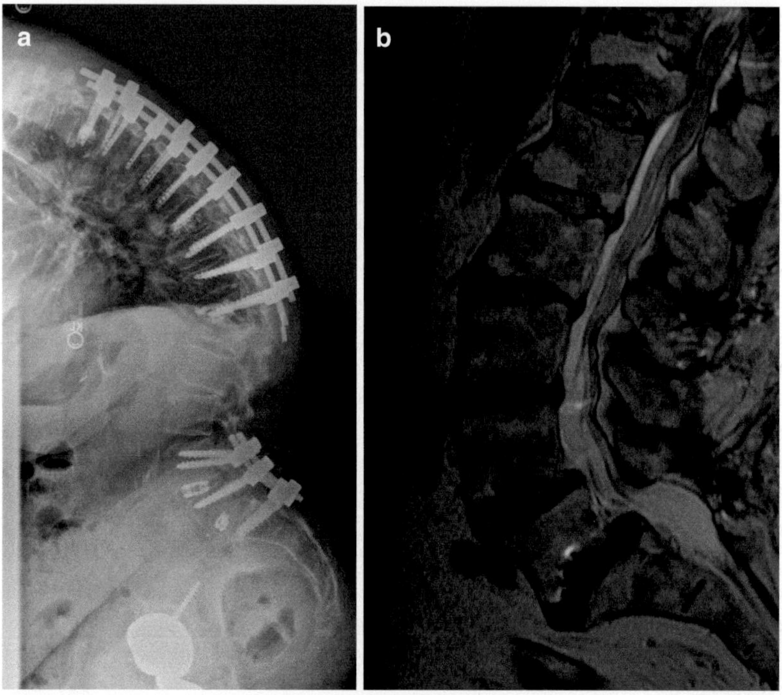

Fig. 19.1 (**a**) Standing scoliosis film of 67 year old female with prior T4-T11 and L4-S1 fusion with new T12 compression fracture. (**b**) MRI lumbar without contrast demonstrating T12 compression fracture with retropulsion of T12 vertebral body causing moderate to severe spinal canal stenosis

partial L1 and T11 laminectomies were performed for decompression, and bilateral pelvic screws were placed for additional stability and connected to construct. Intraoperative ultrasound was used to verify satisfactory decompression of the spinal cord. Eight-month follow-up imaging demonstrates continued resolution of deformity and corrected sagittal imbalance (Fig. 19.2).

In patients with osteoporosis, there are higher rates of complications, including screw loosening and pullout [23]. As such, different methods have been used to overcome the poor bone quality of such patients. Cement augmented pedicle screws are commonly performed with cannulated pedicle screws filled with polymethyl methacrylate cement. It is important to note that the FDA approves the use of cemented pedicle screws for patients with weakened bone secondary to malignancy. When cement is used in patients with osteoporosis or osteopenia, it is at the discretion of the surgeon and should be considered as off-label use. Figure 19.3 demonstrates pre- and post-cement administration into cannulated pedicle screws (see "Cement Augmented Pedicle Screw" video for steps of the procedure). Single-center retrospective observational study by Girardo et al. studied 636 screw placement of standard pedicle, cannulated, and PMMA augmented screws in 91

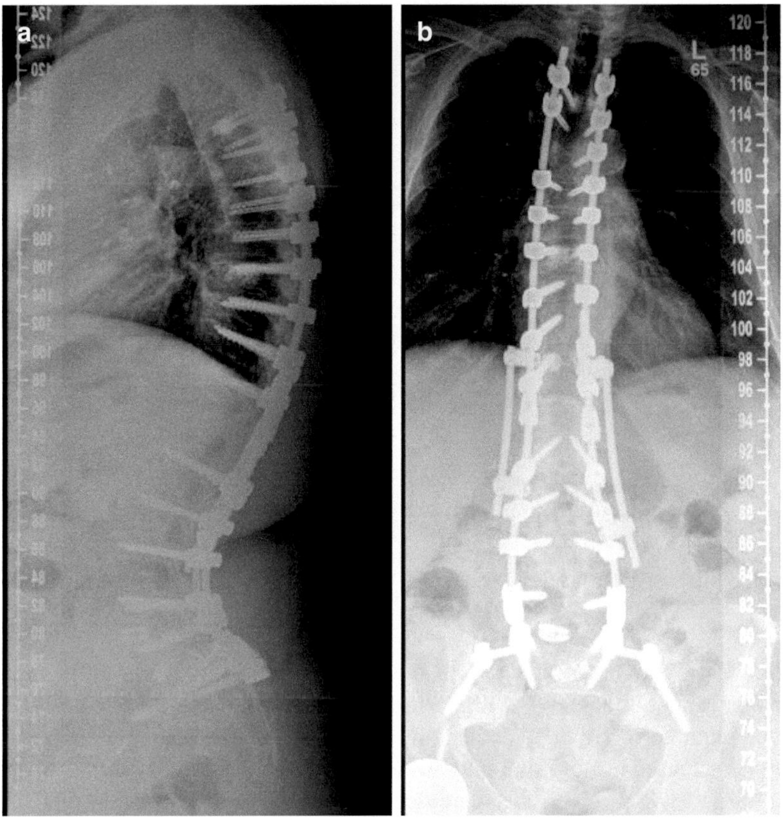

Fig. 19.2 Five months post-operative (**a**) sagittal and (**b**) coronal standing scoliosis film demonstrating extension of fusion construct connecting T11-L3 with bilateral pelvic fixation. Restoration of sagittal balance was achieved

osteoporotic patients age >65 with thoracolumbar fractures requiring fusion instrumentation. Post-op and follow-up X-rays were obtained and were evaluated for bisegmental Cobb angle, fractured vertebral angle, and pedicle screw loosening. In this study, augmented screws had no screw loosening (standard 1, cannulated 4) and significantly less worsening of segmental Cobb angle and fractured vertebra kyphosis angle compared to other screw types [24].

In elderly patients with DISH or AS presenting with thoracolumbar fracture, careful attention should be given, as there is higher risk of instability with secondary displacement and delayed/nonunion of fracture. A posterior approach for surgical management is usually performed in order to provide opportunity for decompression, recreate preexisting alignment, and confer stability to injured segment. Care must be taken when positioning patients, as the mere act of positioning can create additional extension-distraction forces, leading to further injury and/or deformity. Werner et al. suggests incorporating three levels of fixation above and below the

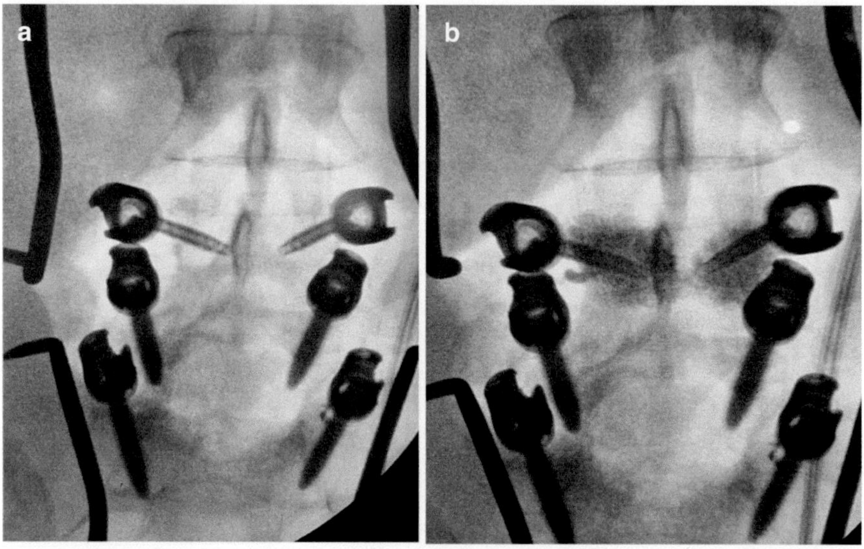

Fig. 19.3 Bilateral L4 cannulated screws (**a**) pre-cement augmentation and (**b**) post-cement augmentation

fracture to provide stress reduction on the instrumentation at each level. If complete reduction cannot be achieved with posterior procedure alone, an anterior procedure may be required to provide adequate reduction and anterior column support [25]. There is increased use of minimally invasive posterior instrumentation for patients with AS and DISH, given the increased benefit of shorter operative time, lower blood loss, and less operative soft tissue trauma; however, in cases with neurologic deficits, there should be a high index of suspicion for epidural hematoma and an open decompression may be needed [26].

Complications

Elderly patients have greater medical comorbidities, and hence have greater postoperative medical complications. Winkler et al. performed a retrospective analysis of 22,835 thoracolumbar trauma patients age >55 and observed that the elderly cohort (age >70) had a higher rate of cardiac arrest (0.1% vs. 0.2%), myocardial infarction (0.6% vs. 1.2%), and urinary tract infection (1.7% vs. 2.8%). Other complications, which did not have significant difference between the two groups, include pneumonia (7%), ARDS (3.6%), deep venous thrombosis (3%), surgical site infection (1.5%), and unplanned return to operating room (0.2%). Inpatient mortality rate, however, was lower in the elderly group with 5% in elderly and 9.3% in middle-aged group with significant lower odds ratio for mortality in elderly undergoing vertebroplasty/kyphoplasty (OR 0.14) [2].

Complications seen after percutaneous kyphoplasty or vertebroplasty include symptomatic cement leakage, cement embolism, pulmonary embolism, osteomyelitis, adjacent vertebral fracture, spinal cord compression, and radiculopathy. Overall complication rates of above procedures are less than 2%, with neurological decline seen in 0.6% of vertebroplasty and 0.03% of kyphoplasty patients. Pulmonary embolism can occur at rates of 0.6% for vertebroplasty and 0.01% for kyphoplasty [27].

Conclusion

Thoracolumbar trauma in the elderly is becoming more relevant in our society as a result of the increasing lifespan. As such, knowledge of unique elderly characteristics relevant in thoracolumbar trauma should be more widespread in order to provide more appropriate surgical and medical care of this population. Traits such as osteoporosis and ankylosing spinal disorders have substantial impact on the biomechanics of the elderly spine. As such, extra attention is needed in this patient population to reduce the risk of peri and postoperative complications.

References

1. Katsuura Y, Osborn JM, Cason GW. The epidemiology of thoracolumbar trauma: a meta-analysis. J Orthop. 2016;13(4):383–8.
2. Winkler EA, Yue JK, Birk H, Robinson CK, Manley GT, Dhall SS, et al. Perioperative morbidity and mortality after lumbar trauma in the elderly. Neurosurg Focus. 2015;39(4):E2.
3. Rajasekaran S, Kanna RM, Schnake KJ, Vaccaro AR, Schroeder GD, Sadiqi S, et al. Osteoporotic thoracolumbar fractures-how are they different?—classification and treatment algorithm. J Orthop Trauma. 2017;31(Suppl 4):S49–56.
4. Looker AC, Johnston CC, Wahner HW, Dunn WL, Calvo MS, Harris TB, et al. Prevalence of low femoral bone density in older U.S. women from NHANES III. J Bone Miner Res. 1995;10(5):796–802.
5. Jacobs WB, Fehlings MG. Ankylosing spondylitis and spinal cord injury: origin, incidence, management, and avoidance. Neurosurg Focus. 2008;24(1):E12.
6. Resnick D, Shaul SR, Robins JM. Diffuse idiopathic skeletal hyperostosis (Dish): Forestier's disease with extraspinal manifestations. Radiology. 1975;115(3):513–24.
7. Rustagi T, Drazin D, Oner C, York J, Schroeder GD, Vaccaro AR, et al. Fractures in spinal ankylosing disorders: a narrative review of disease and injury types, treatment techniques, and outcomes. J Orthop Trauma. 2017;31(Suppl 4):S57–74.
8. Westerveld LA, Verlaan JJ, Oner FC. Spinal fractures in patients with ankylosing spinal disorders: a systematic review of the literature on treatment, neurological status and complications. Eur Spine J. 2009;18(2):145–56.
9. Okano I, Tachibana T, Nishi M, Midorikawa Y, Hoshino Y, Sawada T, et al. Conservative treatment for stable low-energy thoracolumbar vertebral fractures in nonfused segments among elderly patients with diffuse idiopathic skeletal hyperostosis: a matched case-control study. Medicine (Baltimore). 2019;98(24):e16032.

10. Lee JY, Vaccaro AR, Lim MR, Oner FC, Hulbert RJ, Hedlund R, et al. Thoracolumbar injury classification and severity score: a new paradigm for the treatment of thoracolumbar spine trauma. J Orthop Sci. 2005;10(6):671–5.
11. Jiménez-Almonte JH, King JD, Luo TD, Cassidy RC, Aneja A. Classifications in brief: thoracolumbar injury classification and injury severity score system. Clin Orthop Relat Res. 2018;476(6):1352–8.
12. Divi SN, Schroeder GD, Oner FC, Kandziora F, Schnake KJ, Dvorak MF, et al. Aospine-spine trauma classification system: the value of modifiers: a narrative review with commentary on evolving descriptive principles. Global Spine J. 2019;9(1 Suppl):77S–88S.
13. Schnake KJ, Blattert TR, Hahn P, Franck A, Hartmann F, Ullrich B, et al. Classification of osteoporotic thoracolumbar spine fractures: recommendations of the spine section of the German Society for Orthopaedics and Trauma (DGOU). Global Spine J. 2018;8(2 Suppl):46S–9S.
14. Sugita M, Watanabe N, Mikami Y, Hase H, Kubo T. Classification of vertebral compression fractures in the osteoporotic spine. J Spinal Disord Tech. 2005;18(4):376–81.
15. Armingeat T, Brondino R, Pham T, Legré V, Lafforgue P. Intravenous pamidronate for pain relief in recent osteoporotic vertebral compression fracture: a randomized double-blind controlled study. Osteoporos Int. 2006;17(11):1659–65.
16. Chang V, Holly LT. Bracing for thoracolumbar fractures. Neurosurg Focus. 2014;37(1):E3.
17. Baerlocher MO, Saad WE, Dariushnia S, Barr JD, McGraw JK, Nikolic B, et al. Quality improvement guidelines for percutaneous vertebroplasty. J Vasc Interv Radiol. 2014;25(2):165–70.
18. Aparisi F. Vertebroplasty and kyphoplasty in vertebral osteoporotic fractures. Semin Musculoskelet Radiol. 2016;20(4):382–91.
19. Yimin Y, Zhiwei R, Wei M, Jha R. Current status of percutaneous vertebroplasty and percutaneous kyphoplasty—a review. Med Sci Monit. 2013;19:826–36.
20. Wang H, Sribastav SS, Ye F, Yang C, Wang J, Liu H, et al. Comparison of percutaneous vertebroplasty and balloon kyphoplasty for the treatment of single level vertebral compression fractures: a meta-analysis of the literature. Pain Physician. 2015;18(3):209–22.
21. Yuan W-H, Hsu H-C, Lai K-L. Vertebroplasty and balloon kyphoplasty versus conservative treatment for osteoporotic vertebral compression fractures: a meta-analysis. Medicine (Baltimore). 2016;95(31):e4491.
22. Minamide A, Maeda T, Yamada H, Murakami K, Okada M, Enyo Y, et al. Early versus delayed kyphoplasty for thoracolumbar osteoporotic vertebral fractures: the effect of timing on clinical and radiographic outcomes and subsequent compression fractures. Clin Neurol Neurosurg. 2018;173:176–81.
23. Chotigavanich C, Sanpakit S, Wantthanaapisith T, Thanapipatsiri S, Chotigavanich C. The surgical treatment of the osteoporotic vertebral compression fracture in the elderly patients with the spinal instrumentation. J Med Assoc Thail. 2009;92(Suppl 5):S109–15.
24. Girardo M, Rava A, Fusini F, Gargiulo G, Coniglio A, Cinnella P. Different pedicle osteosynthesis for thoracolumbar vertebral fractures in elderly patients. Eur Spine J. 2018;27(Suppl 2):198–205.
25. Werner BC, Samartzis D, Shen FH. Spinal fractures in patients with ankylosing spondylitis: etiology, diagnosis, and management. J Am Acad Orthop Surg. 2016;24(4):241–9.
26. Krüger A, Frink M, Oberkircher L, El-Zayat BF, Ruchholtz S, Lechler P. Percutaneous dorsal instrumentation for thoracolumbar extension-distraction fractures in patients with ankylosing spinal disorders: a case series. Spine J. 2014;14(12):2897–904.
27. Hulme PA, Krebs J, Ferguson SJ, Berlemann U. Vertebroplasty and kyphoplasty: a systematic review of 69 clinical studies. Spine (Phila Pa 1976). 2006;31(17):1983–2001.

Chapter 20
Osteomyelitis

Jacob S. Blitstein, Ashraf E. El Naga, Sanjay S. Dhall, and Anthony M. DiGiorgio

Case Presentation

A 65-year-old male patient presented with 3 weeks of back pain and abdominal pain. His medical history includes end-stage renal disease (ESRD) on hemodialysis along with hypertension, coronary artery disease, and hepatitis C. He denied any fevers, arthralgias, myalgias, nausea, or vomiting. He denied any numbness, weakness, or radicular pain. His vital signs were normal on presentation, and he was afebrile. His physical exam was notable for a right chest wall indwelling dialysis catheter and bilateral below-knee amputations secondary to peripheral artery disease. On physical examination, he was ill appearing but had no notable neurologic deficits. His laboratory workup was notable for a white cell count of 6.3, CRP of

J. S. Blitstein
Touro University College of Osteopathic Medicine, Vallejo, CA, USA
e-mail: Jacob.blitstein@tu.edu

A. E. El Naga
Department of Orthopaedic Surgery, University of California, San Francisco, UCSF/ZSFGH Orthopaedic Trauma Institute, San Francisco, CA, USA
e-mail: Ashraf.elnaga@ucsfe.du

S. S. Dhall
University of California, San Francisco, Zuckerberg San Francisco General Hospital, San Francisco, CA, USA
e-mail: Sanjay.dhall@ucsf.edu

A. M. DiGiorgio (✉)
Department of Neurological Surgery, University of California, San Francisco, San Francisco, CA, USA
e-mail: Anthony.digiorgio@ucsf.edu

K.-M. G. Fu et al. (eds.), *Treatment of Spine Disease in the Elderly*,
https://doi.org/10.1007/978-3-031-12612-3_20

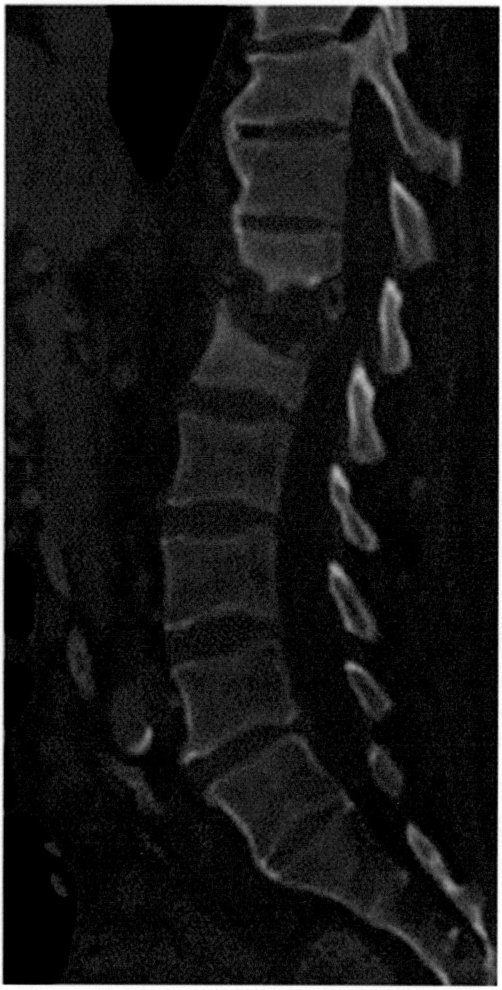

Fig. 20.1 Sagittal non-contrast CT scan of the lumbar spine showing bony destruction of the L1-L2 vertebral bodies with a focal kyphotic deformity

71 mg/dL (normal <8.1) and ESR of 130. A CT scan of the abdomen revealed a psoas abscess and bony destruction of the L1-L2 vertebral bodies (Fig. 20.1). A biopsy of the psoas abscess grew out *Staphylococcus epidermidis*, and a culture-guided antibiotic therapy was initiated. MRI scan did not reveal compression of neural elements (Fig. 20.2). Shortly after completing a 12-week IV antibiotic course, he represented with worsening abdominal pain, and a CT scan revealed worsening collapse of the L1-L2 vertebral bodies and a fracture through the L1 spinous process and laminae (Fig. 20.3). The patient underwent a lateral L1-L2 corpectomy with insertion of an expandable titanium cage and posterior instrumentation from T10 to L4 in a staged approach (Fig. 20.4). He tolerated the procedure well and achieved solid arthrodesis.

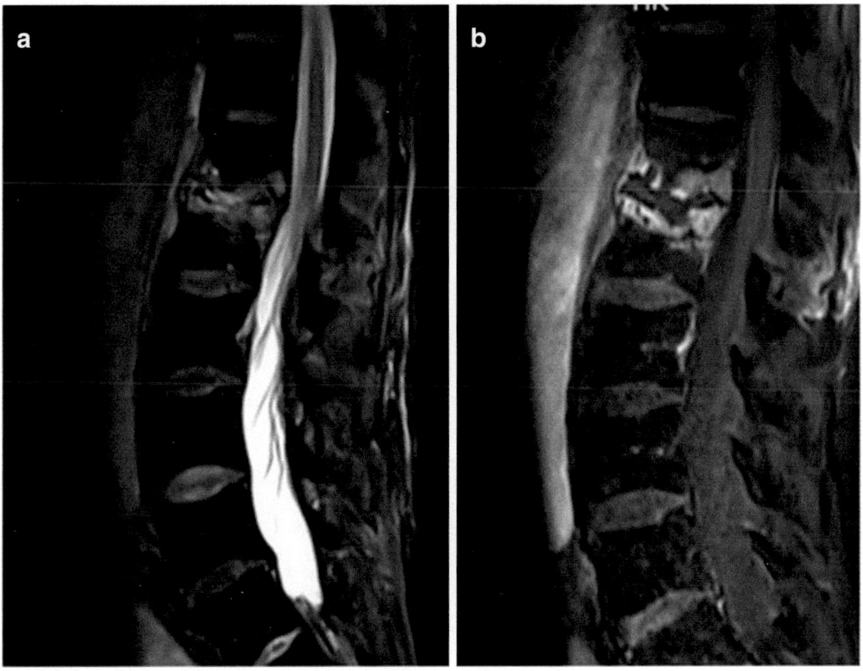

Fig. 20.2 Sagittal T2 (**a**) and contrast (**b**) MRI showing contrast-enhancing osteodiscitis but no compression of neural elements

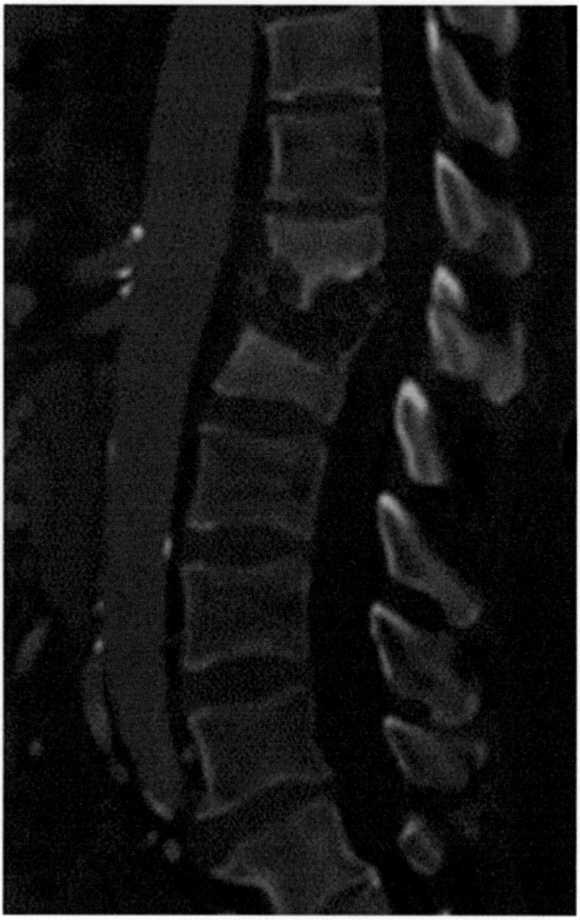

Fig. 20.3 Sagittal non-contrast CT showing a new spinous process fracture at L1

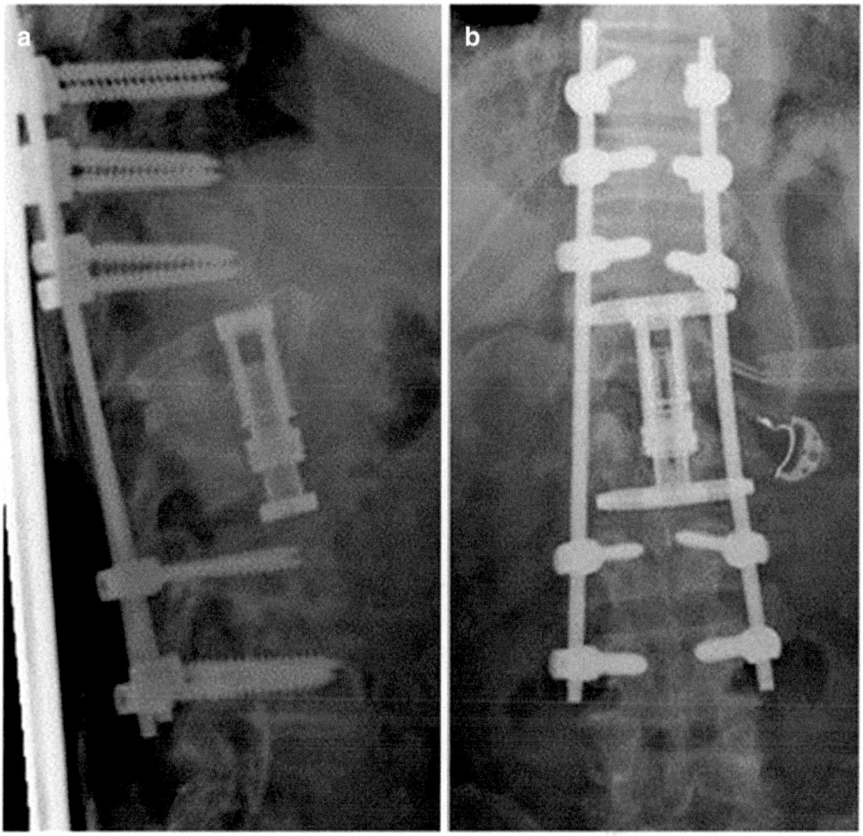

Fig. 20.4 Postoperative lateral (**a**) and AP (**b**) x-rays of the thoracolumbar spine showing the titanium expandable corpectomy cage at L1-L2 and posterior fixation with pedicle screws from T10-L4

Epidemiology

Demographics

Vertebral osteomyelitis (VO) is a disease affecting both young and old patients. Most commonly, VO occurs in adult males in their sixth and seventh decades of life [1]. VO exhibits a male predominance [1] and incidence increases with age [2, 3]. In older patients, VO is associated with the use of intravenous access ports, iatrogenic inoculation, and hematogenous spread from urinary tract infections. In contrast, VO is typically related to intravenous (IV) drug use in younger patients [4]. VO typically occurs in patients with underlying medical conditions, with most patients reporting more than one comorbidity, such as diabetes (29.3% of VO patients), liver cirrhosis (9.2%), and malignancy (8.7%) [5]. It has also been associated with immunosuppression, such as with corticosteroid use or chemotherapy [6]. These comorbidities are likely contributing factors to the increasing VO incidence in older patients, as they are more likely to have underlying medical conditions or compromised immune systems and are living longer with these chronic conditions.

Incidence

VO represents between 3% and 5% of all osteomyelitis cases with an incidence rate of 4–24 per million annually in the world [7–9]. The incidence of VO has been increasing, both in the USA and globally, over the past two decades. This increase can be attributed to a growing elderly population with a higher prevalence of chronic diseases in addition to increases in IV drug use in the younger age group. However, it has been suggested that increased recognition, given improved diagnostic capability, can also be contributing to this rise [7, 9–12]. The incidence of VO associated with venous access devices (such as for hemodialysis or long-term chemotherapy use) is also increasing, as patients are living longer with the diseases necessitating their use [5, 13].

Etiology

VO infection can occur due to bacterial (pyogenic), granulomatous, fungal, or parasitic pathogens. See Table 20.1 for an overview of the relative frequencies of causative pathogens. Gram-positive organisms are by far the most common pathogens in pyogenic VO (PVO), typically *Staphylococcus aureus* and *Streptococcus* species. Granulomatous infection includes those of fungal, mycobacterial, tubercular, or brucellar origin, while the parasitic form, which is rare, is most commonly caused by *Echinococcal* infections [19].

Most PVO infections involve a single organism, with polymicrobial infections are reported in 9% of cases [20]. While most cases of hematogenous VO (HVO) are due to methicillin-sensitive *Staphylococcus aureus* (MSSA) (33.5%), an increasing trend of VO due to methicillin-resistant *Staphylococcus aureus* (MRSA) has been seen, especially in cases associated with IV drug use [9, 10]. MRSA is also more commonly associated with chronic renal disease patients [21] and can be hospital acquired from accessing vascular ports. Though rare, the most common Gram-negative organisms in HVO include *Enterobacteriaceae*, *Klebsiella* sp., *Proteus mirabilis*, *Escherichia coli*, and *Pseudomonas* sp. [3, 9, 20].

Coagulase-negative staphylococci (CoNS) and *Propionibacterium* are commonly isolated in cases of VO that occur after spinal surgery, especially in the

Table 20.1 The relative frequencies of causative pathogens in vertebral osteomyelitis

Gram + bacteria	Frequency	Gram – bacteria	Frequency	Granulomatous	Frequency	Parasitic	Frequency
MSSA	+++++	*E. coli*	+++	TB	+	Echinococcus	~
MSRA	++++	*Pseudomonas aeruginosa*	++	*Brucella*	–		
Streptococcus	+++	*Klebsiella*	+				
S. epidermidis	++	*Proteus mirabilis*	+				
Enterococcus	~	*Candida/Aspergillus*	+				
Propionibacterium sp.	~						

[13–18]

setting of prior spinal instrumentation [22]. *Staphylococcus epidermidis* is a bacterial species that is frequently isolated as a VO infectious agent in patients with previous spinal surgery, in the elderly, and in the immunocompromised [7, 23, 24]. CoNS and *Propionibacterium* are low virulence organisms that can be introduced to the bloodstream following low-grade oral trauma events, such as toothbrushing, but have also been reported following instrumentation. These have recently been found to cause an increasing proportion of microbiologically confirmed cases of PVO [6, 9, 12]. VO due to Gram-negative organisms is less common but has seen an increasing prevalence associated with IV drug users [1].

Tuberculosis of the spine, also known as Pott's disease, is only seen in 1% of all tuberculosis infections globally [25]. With global TB rates declining, the overall prevalence of Pott's disease also continues to decline. Of the ten million people who fell ill with TB in 2019, eight countries accounted for two-thirds (India, Indonesia, China, the Philippines, Pakistan, Nigeria, Bangladesh, and South Africa). Only 2.5% of all TB infections occur in Europe and 2.9% in the Americas [26]. TVO commonly affects the thoracic spine [27]. In contrast to PVO, TVO typically presents with more than two infected vertebrae with approximately 25% of TVO cases having multifocal, noncontiguous skip lesions [28]. Brucella species can also cause a granulomatous form of VO in endemic regions, such as the Mediterranean, the Middle East, and South America [9, 29]. Exposure is often due to exposure to infected livestock. Brucellar VO has a predilection for the lumbar spine, and multilevel involvement is rare [30].

Fungal VO (FVO) is a much less common etiology of VO. Most FVO cases are associated with immunosuppression or IVDU, but FVO has also been associated with spinal surgeries [9, 31]. *Candidiasis, aspergillosis, coccidioidomycosis,* and *cryptococcosis are the most frequent fungi identified in FVO,* though *histoplasmosis* and *blastomycosis* have also been associated in endemic regions [31, 32]. FVO most commonly affects the lumbar spine. While very rare, parasitic infections from *Echinococcal species can cause VO* in endemic areas of temperate zone countries in southern South America, coastal Mediterranean countries, south and central parts of Russia, central Asia, and China [33].

Location

While the lumbar spine is the most common location, VO can involve any part of the spine. It usually involves ≥2 contiguous vertebral bodies and the intervening disc spaces [17]. Occasionally, infection can involve noncontiguous vertebrae with normal intervening vertebrae or can present as disease of a singular vertebrae, usually with a collapse vertebra body that resembles a spinal compression fracture [17]. The infection can also involve the epidural space, posterior elements, and surrounding soft tissue.

Pathophysiology and Pathogenesis

While the majority of VO cases are caused due to a hematogenous route (HVO), VO can also occur from direct inoculation (12–26% of cases) or from contiguous spread from adjacent tissue (3%) [17, 34]. Common primary sites of infection in HVO include the urinary tract, GI tract, respiratory system, the oral cavity, skin, subcutaneous tissues, endocarditis, bursitis, and septic arthritis as well as infected extravertebral implanted device or vascular access sites [17, 25]. VO caused by direct inoculation is primarily iatrogenic from surgery, spinal instrumentation, lumbar punctures, or epidural procedures [9]. While less common, trauma can also lead to VO [32].

HVO begins when bacteria enter the metaphyseal vascular arcades and spreads into the disc periphery or metaphysis of vertebral bodies [18, 25]. Once in the intervertebral disc space, proteolytic enzymes released by bacterial cause progressive destruction [25]. The migration of acute inflammatory cells to the site of local infection leads to the occurrence of edema, vascular congestion, and small vessel thrombosis [35]. Extension of infection into surrounding soft tissues can compromise the vascular supply of the bone and can lead to bone necrosis. Polymorphic leukocytes, macrophages, and osteoclasts then release inflammatory cytokines and proteolytic enzymes, which break down areas of necrotic bone, infected tissues, as well as normal surrounding tissue [36]. Intact regions of remaining periosteum fragments permit the formation of new bone, called an involucrum, which surrounds the necrotic sequestrum. This new bone continues to increase in density and size for weeks to months [37, 38].

Surgical attention is typically needed when there is extensive vertebral destruction, progressive spread of uncontrolled infection or in the presence of neurologic deficits. Extensive vertebral destruction can lead to loss of spinal stability or progressive deformity [25]. Acute neurological deficits secondary to VO are a surgical emergency. This can be from retropulsed bone or disc material into the spinal canal or from direct spread of the infection, causing an epidural abscess [32, 39, 40].

Clinical Presentation

VO has a wide spectrum of clinical presentations, ranging from patients with an acute illness, with more typical signs and symptoms, to a more subacute clinical presentation without bacteremia and less characteristic inflammatory pattern [12]. This disparity in presentation contributes to diagnostic difficulties and delays in diagnoses.

The most common occurring symptom of VO is axial back or neck pain (67–100%), followed by fever and neurologic deficit (weakness, sensory changes, or radicular pain). Absence of fever does not rule out VO, however [20]. The average duration of back pain is greater than 2 weeks, and can be up to a few months, and typically followed by generalized weakness with fever being the last symptom [14, 18, 19]. A systemic review by Mylona et al. reported that the mean time from onset of symptoms to diagnosis ranged from 11 to 59 days, reflecting the broad spectrum of clinical presentations seen in VO [20].

When present, neurological symptoms can range from mild deficits, such as sensory loss, paresthesias, or radiculopathy, to severe neurological compromise with subsequent weakness. The extent of the neurological sequelae seen depends on the site of infection and the aggressiveness of microorganism involved. Patients may present with dysphagia and torticollis due to cervical involvement or with dysautonomic symptoms due to thoracic involvement [25, 41]. Infections of the lumbosacral spine can produce single or multiple nerve root deficits [1, 42]. Rapid-onset paraplegia or quadriplegia is typically to be due to spinal epidural abscesses (SEA) [42]. The "classic triad" of SEA (back pain, fever, and neurologic deficit) is not a sensitive predictor of SEA or VO [1].

A readily identified primary infection can alert the clinician to the possibility of VO, such as a UTI or skin/soft tissue infection. Other sources of infection that have been reported with associated symptoms include the respiratory tract, often due to sinusitis; the oral cavity, due to low-grade tooth or gum trauma; and the GI tract [20]. The increasing incidence of cases caused by low-virulence bacteria, especially in the elderly with comorbidities, had led to an increasing number of cases presenting subacutely with a slower progression of VO signs and symptoms [43].

Diagnosis/Workup

The ubiquity of back pain as a chief complaint in the emergency setting often contributes to the frequent diagnostic delay seen in VO cases, with patients often reporting symptoms for months [4, 17, 44], and a significant portion of cases are initially missed on presentation [9]. A detailed history and physical with a high-level of suspicion will reduce the likelihood this diagnosis is missed. If VO is suspected, further investigation with laboratory and imaging testing should be completed in a timely manner to avoid delays and complications [1].

The Infectious Disease Society of America's (IDSA) "clinical guidelines for diagnosis and treatment of native vertebral osteomyelitis" recommends that a diagnosis of VO should be considered in patients with new or worsening back or neck pain and fever, elevated ESP or CRP, bacteremia, or endocarditis [41]. Patients will often present with an inflammatory pattern of axial pain (as opposed to mechanical, which improves with rest) and constitutional signs/symptoms, such as anorexia, lethargy, weight loss, nausea, or vomiting. The pain is often focal with paravertebral point tenderness. Important risk factors associated with VO include a history of IV drug use, diabetes mellitus, recent spinal surgery or injection, immunosuppression (congenital or acquired), and chronic kidney or liver disease [41]. Evaluation for concomitant infective endocarditis should also be considered in all VO patients [5, 21, 45].

Current recommendations for laboratory testing are to obtain a complete blood count, sedimentation rate, c-reactive protein, basic metabolic panel, and blood cultures in all patients with a suspicion of VO. BMP lab values allow clinicians to assess for coincident conditions, such as uncontrolled hyperglycemia and uremia, which have been associated with a significantly higher incidence of VO and SEA [1]. ESR and CRP levels are both considered highly sensitive markers for VO but are nonspecific [14, 25].

In contrast to the ESR and CRP trends, leukocytosis or neutrophilia (with >80% neutrophils) does not have a high sensitivity for VO diagnosis [46]. Although most patients present with a moderate elevation of 11.0–17.0 WBC k/μL, the presence of leukocytosis in VO patients is widely variable with no correlation found between degree of elevation and disease severity [1, 46].

Spinal imaging should be performed in any patient with suspected VO and be done so emergently, if there are any neurologic deficits [1]. CT scan is highly sensitive for erosive bony pathology and often able to detect paraspinal and epidural involvement [47]. MRI should be performed in all patients to quantify the extent of infection, provide a baseline, and rule out any epidural component [48]. Gadolinium should be used if there are no contraindications, such as an allergy or kidney disease.

Etiologic confirmation prior to treatment is important for selection of an appropriate antibiotic. Preventing delays to effective treatment delay contributes to reduced morbidity and mortality [16, 49, 50]. Obtaining a blood culture is recommended to help guide initial diagnostic or treatment decisions and may be used in conjunction with a direct tissue culture, or independently, to confirm the infective agent causing VO [1, 3].

A diagnosis of VO or discitis on imaging should prompt urgent image-guided biopsy within 24 h while holding antibiotics until after biopsy if the patient is hemodynamically stable. If patient is hemodynamically unstable, antibiotics are recommended immediately [1]. In hemodynamically stable patients in whom antibiotics have not been initiated, it is suggested to wait until blood culture results are returned to help guide effective treatment choice. Close neurological monitoring advised while awaiting results of the initial blood cultures. Neurological compromise and/or SEA, with or without hemodynamic instability, is an indication for starting empiric antibiotics without waiting for culture results [45].

Biopsy is used to confirm microbial etiology, which can help guide treatment decisions [1, 14]. Image-guided percutaneous biopsies are favored over open biopsy when etiology is unknown; however, open biopsy may be considered with recent spinal surgeries [20, 51].

Treatment

Most cases of VO can be managed by conservative measures, without the need for surgical management. The typical antibiotic regimen is IV vancomycin and ceftriaxone [1, 22].

In order to assess response to antimicrobial treatment, imaging, CRP, and ESR monitoring can be used in addition to assessment of overall clinical picture [52]. CRP levels were found to be the best independent predictor for early switch from IV to oral antibiotics, especially in cases of postoperative infections [53, 54]. Both MRIs and PET scans can be used to monitor disease progression [55].

Surgical management is indicated for compression of neural structures, leading to a neurologic deficit, instability, progressive deformity, or failure of medical therapy [4, 18]. Patients at a high risk for failure of medical treatment include those with diabetes, multifocal infection, and epidural abscesses [56].

With the bony destruction of the infection, instrumentation is often needed when surgery is indicated [57]. While it was long thought that placing instrumentation in an infected field would lead to persistent infection, more recent literature has shown this to not necessarily be the case [15, 58–61]. Surgical treatment options include anterior, posterior, or combined approaches. The location of pathology and neural compression is a key consideration in choice of approach. If an epidural abscess is present, an approach allowing access to the canal should be selected. Since VO favors the vertebral bodies, correction of deformity typically requires reconstruction of the anterior column with posterior instrumentation as well [62].

Reconstruction of the anterior thoracolumbar vertebral body can be done via anterior, posterior, or lateral-based approaches, while the anterior column in the cervical spine is reconstructed through the standard anterior approach to the cervical spine. Posteriorly based approaches such as a costotransversectomy-type approach is commonly considered in the thoracic spine. In such approaches, the adjacent costovertebral joint is removed so as to access the anterior vertebral body obliquely for corpectomy and anterior cage reconstruction. This typically involves sacrificing a thoracic nerve root, especially when performing multilevel reconstruction. As such, such a posterolateral approach is not considered in distal to L1, where nerve sacrifice would have significant functional implications. In the lumbar spine, a lateral or retroperitoneal approach is often considered and performed. In this case, the vertebral body is accessed lateral to the great vessels with several approaches described in relation to the traversing psoas muscle. The lateral retro pleural approach can also be employed for thoracic pathology, up to approximately T5, where the axilla obstructs exposure.

With any approach to anterior vertebral body reconstruction, posterior instrumentation is often considered, especially with any multilevel corpectomy. The addition of posterior instrumentation will improve fusion rates, especially in the cervical spine [63]. Epidural abscesses, if they can be accessed through a laminectomy alone, are often managed with a posterior only approach [50].

With many surgical variations available, a patient-centered approach is recommended based on each patient's pathology and risk factors. Spinal bracing may be an alternative to spinal surgery in appropriate candidates, in whom there are no neurologic deficits, especially if comorbidities preclude surgical intervention. However, one cohort study that compared rigid spinal bracing with percutaneous posterior screw-rod instrumentation found that "significantly faster recovery, lower pain scores and improved quality of life" was associated with the surgical treatment group [64].

Outcomes and Complications

Prognosis depends primarily on early diagnosis and treatment in order to avoid neurological sequelae and other complications. Park et al. reported that major sequelae risk factors include ≥3 weeks to diagnosis, neurologic deficits, and cervical or thoracic involvement. While overall mortality is low, poor functional outcomes are much more common, with 27% of patients reporting complications with a severe effect on quality of life [18, 20]. When compared to degenerative processes, surgical outcomes for VO include less neurological improvement and higher rates of complication [61].

Conclusion

VO is a notable cause of back pain that can lead to serious neurological deficits and pronounced spine instability or deformity if not identified and treated appropriately. The increasing incidence of VO highlights the need for clinicians to have enough knowledge necessary to avoid delays in diagnosis [12]. Advanced imaging and culture studies are both key components of establishing a diagnosis. In patients without neurologic deficits or evidence of instability, culture-guided antibiotics are the first line of treatment along with addressing any comorbid conditions. Surgery is indicated for spinal instability, progressive deformity, neurologic compression, and failed medical management. Instrumentation is often necessary and often performed in conjunction with anterior vertebral body reconstruction through any of a number of well-established surgical approaches.

References

1. Chenoweth CE, Bassin BS, Mack MR, Oppenlander ME, Patel RD, Quint DJ, Seagull FJ. Vertebral osteomyelitis, discitis, and spinal epidural abscess in adults. Michigan Medicine University of Michigan; 2018. http://www.ncbi.nlm.nih.gov/books/NBK547443/.
2. Grammatico L, Baron S, Rusch E, Lepage B, Surer N, Desenclos JC, Besnier JM. Epidemiology of vertebral osteomyelitis (VO) in France: analysis of hospital-discharge data 2002-2003. Epidemiol Infect. 2008;136(5):653–60. https://doi.org/10.1017/S0950268807008850.

3. Nickerson EK, Sinha R. Vertebral osteomyelitis in adults: an update. Br Med Bull. 2016;117(1):121–38. https://doi.org/10.1093/bmb/ldw003.
4. Gasbarrini AL, Bertoldi E, Mazzetti M, Fini L, Terzi S, Gonella F, Mirabile L, Barbanti Bròdano G, Furno A, Gasbarrini A, Boriani S. Clinical features, diagnostic and therapeutic approaches to haematogenous vertebral osteomyelitis. Eur Rev Med Pharmacol Sci. 2005;9(1):53–66.
5. Park K-H, Kim DY, Lee Y-M, Lee MS, Kang K-C, Lee J-H, Park SY, Moon C, Chong YP, Kim S-H, Lee S-O, Choi S-H, Kim YS, Woo JH, Ryu B-H, Bae I-G, Cho O-H. Selection of an appropriate empiric antibiotic regimen in hematogenous vertebral osteomyelitis. PLoS One. 2019;14(2):e0211888. https://doi.org/10.1371/journal.pone.0211888.
6. Carragee EJ. Pyogenic vertebral osteomyelitis. J Bone Joint Surg Am. 1997;79(6):874–80. https://doi.org/10.2106/00004623-199706000-00011.
7. Issa K, Diebo BG, Faloon M, Naziri Q, Pourtaheri S, Paulino CB, Emami A. The epidemiology of vertebral osteomyelitis in the United States from 1998 to 2013. Clin Spine Surg. 2018;31(2):E102–8. https://doi.org/10.1097/BSD.0000000000000597.
8. Kremers HM, Nwojo ME, Ransom JE, Wood-Wentz CM, Melton LJ, Huddleston PM. Trends in the epidemiology of osteomyelitis: a population-based study, 1969 to 2009. J Bone Joint Surg. 2015;97(10):837–45. https://doi.org/10.2106/JBJS.N.01350.
9. Saeed K, Esposito S, Ascione T, Bassetti M, Bonnet E, Carnelutti A, Chan M, Lye DC, Cortes N, Dryden M, Fernando S, Gottlieb T, Gould I, Hijazi K, Madonia S, Pagliano P, Pottinger PS, Segreti J, Spera AM, International Society of Antimicrobial Chemotherapy (ISAC) Bone and Skin & Soft Tissue Infections Working Group. Hot topics on vertebral osteomyelitis from the International Society of Antimicrobial Chemotherapy. Int J Antimicrob Agents. 2019;54(2):125–33. https://doi.org/10.1016/j.ijantimicag.2019.06.013.
10. DiGiorgio AM, Stein R, Morrow KD, Robichaux JM, Crutcher CL, Tender GC. The increasing frequency of intravenous drug abuse-associated spinal epidural abscesses: a case series. Neurosurg Focus. 2019;46(1):E4. https://doi.org/10.3171/2018.10.FOCUS18449.
11. Kehrer M, Pedersen C, Jensen TG, Lassen AT. Increasing incidence of pyogenic spondylodiscitis: a 14-year population-based study. J Infect. 2014;68(4):313–20. https://doi.org/10.1016/j.jinf.2013.11.011.
12. Lora-Tamayo J, Euba G, Narváez JA, Murillo O, Verdaguer R, Sobrino B, Narváez J, Nolla JM, Ariza J. Changing trends in the epidemiology of pyogenic vertebral osteomyelitis: the impact of cases with no microbiologic diagnosis. Semin Arthritis Rheum. 2011;41(2):247–55. https://doi.org/10.1016/j.semarthrit.2011.04.002.
13. Pigrau C, Rodríguez-Pardo D, Fernández-Hidalgo N, Moretó L, Pellise F, Larrosa M-N, Puig M, Almirante B. Health care associated hematogenous pyogenic vertebral osteomyelitis: a severe and potentially preventable infectious disease. Medicine. 2015;94(3):e365. https://doi.org/10.1097/MD.0000000000000365.
14. Bhavan KP, Marschall J, Olsen MA, Fraser VJ, Wright NM, Warren DK. The epidemiology of hematogenous vertebral osteomyelitis: a cohort study in a tertiary care hospital. BMC Infect Dis. 2010;10:158. https://doi.org/10.1186/1471-2334-10-158.
15. Carragee E, Iezza A. Does acute placement of instrumentation in the treatment of vertebral osteomyelitis predispose to recurrent infection: long-term follow-up in immune-suppressed patients. Spine. 2008;33(19):2089–93. https://doi.org/10.1097/BRS.0b013e3181839b9c.
16. Colmenero JD, Ruiz-Mesa JD, Sanjuan-Jimenez R, Sobrino B, Morata P. Establishing the diagnosis of tuberculous vertebral osteomyelitis. Eur Spine J. 2013;22(Suppl 4):579–86. https://doi.org/10.1007/s00586-012-2348-2.
17. McHenry MC, Easley KA, Locker GA. Vertebral osteomyelitis: long-term outcome for 253 patients from 7 Cleveland-area hospitals. Clin Infect Dis. 2002;34(10):1342–50. https://doi.org/10.1086/340102.
18. Nolla JM, Ariza J, Gómez-Vaquero C, Fiter J, Bermejo J, Valverde J, Escofet DR, Gudiol F. Spontaneous pyogenic vertebral osteomyelitis in nondrug users. Semin Arthritis Rheum. 2002;31(4):271–8. https://doi.org/10.1053/sarh.2002.29492.

19. Courjon J, Lemaignen A, Ghout I, Therby A, Belmatoug N, Dinh A, Gras G, Bernard L, DTS (Duration of Treatment for Spondylodiscitis) Study Group. Pyogenic vertebral osteomyelitis of the elderly: characteristics and outcomes. PLoS One. 2017;12(12):e0188470. https://doi.org/10.1371/journal.pone.0188470.
20. Mylona E, Samarkos M, Kakalou E, Fanourgiakis P, Skoutelis A. Pyogenic vertebral osteomyelitis: a systematic review of clinical characteristics. Semin Arthritis Rheum. 2009;39(1):10–7. https://doi.org/10.1016/j.semarthrit.2008.03.002.
21. Kim DY, Kim UJ, Yu Y, Kim S-E, Kang S-J, Jun K-I, Kang CK, Song K-H, Choe PG, Kim ES, Kim HB, Jang H-C, Jung SI, Oh M, Park K-H, Kim NJ. Microbial etiology of pyogenic vertebral osteomyelitis according to patient characteristics. Open Forum Infect Dis. 2020;7(6):ofaa176. https://doi.org/10.1093/ofid/ofaa176.
22. Zimmerli W. Clinical practice. Vertebral osteomyelitis. N Engl J Med. 2010;362(11):1022–9. https://doi.org/10.1056/NEJMcp0910753.
23. Le Moal G, Juhel L, Grollier G, Godet C, Azais I, Roblot F. Vertebral osteomyelitis due to Fusobacterium species: report of three cases and review of the literature. J Infect. 2005;51(2):E5–9. https://doi.org/10.1016/j.jinf.2004.06.012.
24. Love C, Patel M, Lonner BS, Tomas MB, Palestro CJ. Diagnosing spinal osteomyelitis: a comparison of bone and Ga-67 scintigraphy and magnetic resonance imaging. Clin Nucl Med. 2000;25(12):963–77. https://doi.org/10.1097/00003072-200012000-00002.
25. Mavrogenis AF, Megaloikonomos PD, Igoumenou VG, Panagopoulos GN, Giannitsioti E, Papadopoulos A, Papagelopoulos PJ. Spondylodiscitis revisited. EFORT Open Rev. 2017;2(11):447–61. https://doi.org/10.1302/2058-5241.2.160062.
26. WHO Global Tuberculosis Report 2020. https://www.who.int/teams/global-tuberculosis-programme/tb-reports/global-tuberculosis-report-2020.
27. Park DW, Sohn JW, Kim E-H, Cho D-I, Lee J-H, Kim K-T, Ha K-Y, Jeon C-H, Shim D-M, Lee J-S, Lee J-B, Chun BC, Kim MJ. Outcome and management of spinal tuberculosis according to the severity of disease: a retrospective study of 137 adult patients at Korean teaching hospitals. Spine. 2007;32(4):E130–5. https://doi.org/10.1097/01.brs.0000255216.54085.21.
28. Griffith JF, Kumta SM, Leung PC, Cheng JCY, Chow LTC, Metreweli C. Imaging of musculoskeletal tuberculosis: a new look at an old disease. Clin Orthop Relat Res. 2002;398:32–9. https://doi.org/10.1097/00003086-200205000-00006.
29. Lucero NE, Ayala SM, Escobar GI, Jacob NR. Brucella isolated in humans and animals in Latin America from 1968 to 2006. Epidemiol Infect. 2008;136(4):496–503. https://doi.org/10.1017/S0950268807008795.
30. Colmenero JD, Jiménez-Mejías ME, Sánchez-Lora FJ, Reguera JM, Palomino-Nicás J, Martos F, García de las Heras J, Pachón J. Pyogenic, tuberculous, and brucellar vertebral osteomyelitis: a descriptive and comparative study of 219 cases. Ann Rheum Dis. 1997;56(12):709–15. https://doi.org/10.1136/ard.56.12.709.
31. Gamaletsou MN, Rammaert B, Bueno MA, Moriyama B, Sipsas NV, Kontoyiannis DP, Roilides E, Zeller V, Prinapori R, Taj-Aldeen SJ, Brause B, Lortholary O, Walsh TJ. Aspergillus osteomyelitis: epidemiology, clinical manifestations, management, and outcome. J Infect. 2014;68(5):478–93. https://doi.org/10.1016/j.jinf.2013.12.008.
32. Lehovsky J. Pyogenic vertebral osteomyelitis/disc infection. Baillieres Best Pract Res Clin Rheumatol. 1999;13(1):59–75. https://doi.org/10.1053/berh.1999.0006.
33. Charles RW, Govender S, Naidoo KS. Echinococcal infection of the spine with neural involvement. Spine. 1988;13(1):47–9. https://doi.org/10.1097/00007632-198801000-00011.
34. Govender S. Spinal infections. J Bone Joint Surg Br. 2005;87(11):1454–8. https://doi.org/10.1302/0301-620X.87B11.16294.
35. Loughran AJ, Gaddy D, Beenken KE, Meeker DG, Morello R, Zhao H, Byrum SD, Tackett AJ, Cassat JE, Smeltzer MS. Impact of sarA and phenol-soluble modulins on the pathogenesis of osteomyelitis in diverse clinical isolates of Staphylococcus aureus. Infect Immun. 2016;84(9):2586–94. https://doi.org/10.1128/IAI.00152-16.

36. Vigorita VJ, Ghelman B, Mintz D. Orthopaedic pathology. 2nd ed. Lippincott Williams and Wilkins; 2008.
37. Kavanagh N, Ryan EJ, Widaa A, Sexton G, Fennell J, O'Rourke S, Cahill KC, Kearney CJ, O'Brien FJ, Kerrigan SW. Staphylococcal osteomyelitis: disease progression, treatment challenges, and future directions. Clin Microbiol Rev. 2018;31(2) https://doi.org/10.1128/CMR.00084-17.
38. Waldvogel FA, Medoff G, Swartz MN. Osteomyelitis: a review of clinical features, therapeutic considerations and unusual aspects. N Engl J Med. 1970;282(4):198–206. https://doi.org/10.1056/NEJM197001222820406.
39. Eismont FJ, Bohlman HH, Soni PL, Goldberg VM, Freehafer AA. Pyogenic and fungal vertebral osteomyelitis with paralysis. J Bone Joint Surg Am. 1983;65(1):19–29.
40. Moritani T, Kim J, Capizzano AA, Kirby P, Kademian J, Sato Y. Pyogenic and non-pyogenic spinal infections: emphasis on diffusion-weighted imaging for the detection of abscesses and pus collections. Br J Radiol. 2014;87(1041):20140011. https://doi.org/10.1259/bjr.20140011.
41. Berbari EF, Kanj SS, Kowalski TJ, Darouiche RO, Widmer AF, Schmitt SK, Hendershot EF, Holtom PD, Huddleston PM, Petermann GW, Osmon DR, Infectious Diseases Society of America, null. 2015 Infectious Diseases Society of America (IDSA) clinical practice guidelines for the diagnosis and treatment of native vertebral osteomyelitis in adults. Clin Infect Dis. 2015;61(6):e26–46. https://doi.org/10.1093/cid/civ482.
42. Shanahan MD, Ackroyd CE. Pyogenic infection of the sacro-iliac joint. A report of 11 cases. J Bone Joint Surg. 1985;67(4):605–8. https://doi.org/10.1302/0301-620X.67B4.4030859.
43. Murillo O, Roset A, Sobrino B, Lora-Tamayo J, Verdaguer R, Jiménez-Mejias E, Nolla JM, Colmenero JD, Ariza J. Streptococcal vertebral osteomyelitis: multiple faces of the same disease. Clin Microbiol Infect. 2014;20(1):O33–8. https://doi.org/10.1111/1469-0691.12302.
44. Gouliouris T, Aliyu SH, Brown NM. Spondylodiscitis: update on diagnosis and management. J Antimicrob Chemother. 2010;65(Suppl 3):iii11–24. https://doi.org/10.1093/jac/dkq303.
45. Pigrau C, Almirante B, Flores X, Falco V, Rodríguez D, Gasser I, Villanueva C, Pahissa A. Spontaneous pyogenic vertebral osteomyelitis and endocarditis: incidence, risk factors, and outcome. Am J Med. 2005;118(11):1287. https://doi.org/10.1016/j.amjmed.2005.02.027.
46. Hopkinson N, Stevenson J, Benjamin S. A case ascertainment study of septic discitis: clinical, microbiological and radiological features. QJM. 2001;94(9):465–70. https://doi.org/10.1093/qjmed/94.9.465.
47. Burke DR, Brant-Zawadzki M. CT of pyogenic spine infection. Neuroradiology. 1985;27(2):131–7. https://doi.org/10.1007/BF00343784.
48. Colip CG, Lotfi M, Buch K, Holalkere N, Setty BN. Emergent spinal MRI in IVDU patients presenting with back pain: do we need an MRI in every case? Emerg Radiol. 2018;25(3):247–56. https://doi.org/10.1007/s10140-017-1572-9.
49. D'Agostino C, Scorzolini L, Massetti AP, Carnevalini M, d'Ettorre G, Venditti M, Vullo V, Orsi GB. A seven-year prospective study on spondylodiscitis: epidemiological and microbiological features. Infection. 2010;38(2):102–7. https://doi.org/10.1007/s15010-009-9340-8.
50. Skaf GS, Kanafani ZA, Araj GF, Kanj SS. Non-pyogenic infections of the spine. Int J Antimicrob Agents. 2010;36(2):99–105. https://doi.org/10.1016/j.ijantimicag.2010.03.023.
51. Duarte RM, Vaccaro AR. Spinal infection: state of the art and management algorithm. Eur Spine J. 2013;22(12):2787–99. https://doi.org/10.1007/s00586-013-2850-1.
52. Khan MH, Smith PN, Rao N, Donaldson WF. Serum C-reactive protein levels correlate with clinical response in patients treated with antibiotics for wound infections after spinal surgery. Spine J. 2006;6(3):311–5. https://doi.org/10.1016/j.spinee.2005.07.006.
53. Babouee Flury B, Elzi L, Kolbe M, Frei R, Weisser M, Schären S, Widmer AF, Battegay M. Is switching to an oral antibiotic regimen safe after 2 weeks of intravenous treatment for primary bacterial vertebral osteomyelitis? BMC Infect Dis. 2014;14:226. https://doi.org/10.1186/1471-2334-14-226.

54. Grados F, Lescure FX, Senneville E, Flipo RM, Schmit JL, Fardellone P. Suggestions for managing pyogenic (non-tuberculous) discitis in adults. Joint Bone Spine. 2007;74(2):133–9. https://doi.org/10.1016/j.jbspin.2006.11.002.
55. Leone A, Dell'Atti C, Magarelli N, Colelli P, Balanika A, Casale R, Bonomo L. Imaging of spondylodiscitis. Eur Rev Med Pharmacol Sci. 2012;16(Suppl 2):8–19.
56. de Graeff JJ, Paulino Pereira NR, van Wulfften Palthe OD, Nelson SB, Schwab JH. Prognostic factors for failure of antibiotic treatment in patients with osteomyelitis of the spine. Spine. 2017;42(17):1339–46. https://doi.org/10.1097/BRS.0000000000002084.
57. Park K-H, Cho O-H, Lee JH, Park JS, Ryu KN, Park SY, Lee Y-M, Chong YP, Kim S-H, Lee S-O, Choi S-H, Bae I-G, Kim YS, Woo JH, Lee MS. Optimal duration of antibiotic therapy in patients with hematogenous vertebral osteomyelitis at low risk and high risk of recurrence. Clin Infect Dis. 2016;62(10):1262–9. https://doi.org/10.1093/cid/ciw098.
58. Heary RF, Agarwal N, Agarwal P, Goldstein IM. Surgical treatment with thoracic pedicle screw fixation of vertebral osteomyelitis with long-term follow-up. Oper Neurosurg. 2019;17(5):443–51. https://doi.org/10.1093/ons/opy398.
59. Lu DC, Wang V, Chou D. The use of allograft or autograft and expandable titanium cages for the treatment of vertebral osteomyelitis. Neurosurgery. 2009;64(1):122–30. https://doi.org/10.1227/01.NEU.0000336332.11957.0B.
60. Mondorf Y, Gaab MR, Oertel JMK. PEEK cage cervical ventral fusion in spondylodiscitis. Acta Neurochir. 2009;151(11):1537–41. https://doi.org/10.1007/s00701-009-0486-z.
61. Wadhwa R, Mummaneni PV, Lau D, Le H, Chou D, Dhall SS. Perioperative morbidity and mortality comparison in circumferential cervical fusion for osteomyelitis versus cervical spondylotic myelopathy. Neurosurg Focus. 2014;37(2):E7. https://doi.org/10.3171/2014.5.FOCUS14140.
62. D'Aliberti G, Talamonti G, Villa F, Debernardi A. The anterior stand-alone approach (ASAA) during the acute phase of spondylodiscitis: results in 40 consecutively treated patients. Eur Spine J. 2012;21(Suppl 1):S75–82. https://doi.org/10.1007/s00586-012-2238-7.
63. Mummaneni PV, Dhall SS, Rodts GE, Haid RW. Circumferential fusion for cervical kyphotic deformity: clinical article. J Neurosurg Spine. 2008;9(6):515–21. https://doi.org/10.3171/SPI.2008.10.08226.
64. Nasto LA, Colangelo D, Mazzotta V, Di Meco E, Neri V, Nasto RA, Fantoni M, Pola E. Is posterior percutaneous screw-rod instrumentation a safe and effective alternative approach to TLSO rigid bracing for single-level pyogenic spondylodiscitis? Results of a retrospective cohort analysis. Spine J. 2014;14(7):1139–46. https://doi.org/10.1016/j.spinee.2013.07.479.

Chapter 21
Thoracolumbar Spinal Oncology in the Geriatric Population

Jacob L. Goldberg, Ori Barzilai, Dennis Timothy Lockney, Anubhav G. Amin, and Mark H. Bilsky

Introduction

Symptomatic spinal cord compression due to metastatic cancer is common, affecting up to 20% of cancer patients, and often requires surgical intervention [1–4]. In symptomatic patients, surgery can improve pain, neurological status, and quality of life [5, 6]. The incidence of spinal metastases is expected to increase as advances in targeted therapies improve overall survival; however, targeted therapies are disproportionately effective against nonskeletal disease [7]. Coincident with the rise in incidence of spine metastatic disease is the projected rise in the elderly population [8]. This presents unique challenges in decision-making as the elderly face heightened perioperative risks. Taken together, the importance of surgery in this setting and the increased risk profile faced by the elderly often present a dilemma with regard to best treatment.

While studies have demonstrated the safety of surgery in elderly population for a variety of primary cancer types, spine surgery poses unique challenges in this age

J. L. Goldberg
Department of Neurosurgery, New York Presbyterian Hospital/Weill Cornell and Memorial Sloan Kettering Cancer Center, New York, NY, USA

Department of Neurosurgery, Memorial Sloan Kettering Cancer Center, New York, NY, USA
e-mail: jag9177@nyp.org

O. Barzilai · A. G. Amin
Department of Neurosurgery, Memorial Sloan Kettering Cancer Center, New York, NY, USA
e-mail: barzilao@mskcc.org

D. T. Lockney · M. H. Bilsky (✉)
Departmeny of Neurosurgery, University of California at San Francisco, San Francisco, CA, USA
e-mail: Dennis.lockney@ucsf.edu; bilskym@mskcc.org

K.-M. G. Fu et al. (eds.), *Treatment of Spine Disease in the Elderly*,
https://doi.org/10.1007/978-3-031-12612-3_21

group. At baseline, elderly patients are at increased risk of perioperative complication due to decreased physiologic reserve, poor tolerance of blood loss, lower rates of mobility, and often worse nutritional status [9–11]. In fact, patients aged 65 years and older are at increased risk of perioperative complication and rehospitalization after elective lumbar spine surgery, and this risk grows further, correlating with surgical invasiveness and medical comorbidities, among octogenarians [12, 13]. Octogenarians undergoing elective degenerative spinal fusion face rates as high as 71% and 8% of perioperative complication and mortality, respectively [14–17]. Of concern, the risk of spine surgery in the elderly is highest in cases of instrumented fusion which is often essential in addressing spine tumors. Deyo et al. found an increased risk associated with fusion compared to non-instrumented lumbar surgery with respect to rates of complication, blood transfusion, and nursing home placement [18]. Additionally, with operations requiring significant narcotic pain medication, the elderly face an increased risk of poorly managed postoperative pain and/or delirium [19, 20]. This may prompt concerns for safety with ambulation leading to increased immobilization and its associated consequences.

Despite all of these, recent technological advancements including the integration of minimally invasive surgical techniques; increased utilization of advanced photon-beam radiation therapy, i.e., stereotactic radiosurgery (SRS); stringent medical preoperative assessment; and postoperative medical co-management by geriatric medicine have made surgery in the elderly more tolerable. As a result of significant and evolving changes in treatment strategies, a cohesive team approach with multiple different subspecialists helps ensure patients receive optimal treatment. The NOMS (Neurologic, Oncologic, Mechanical stability, and Systemic disease/medical comorbidity) framework uses a multifaceted assessment to optimize patient outcomes [1]. NOMS was designed to synthesize essential clinical components to guide surgical decision-making. While systemic disease/medical comorbidity has always played an important role in NOMS, it takes on added emphasis in surgical decision-making as it relates to elderly oncology patients.

In this chapter, we present the application of the NOMS framework to the elderly patient population. We discuss complications and modifiable risk factors and predictive tools and indices and present the available literature evaluating minimally invasive techniques. Last, we present an example of a successful minimally invasive as well as open surgery for spinal metastases reviewing the key pre-, intra-, and postoperative considerations. Primary bony thoracolumbar tumors are exceedingly rare in the elderly and beyond the scope of this chapter.

Historical Data

Outcome data on surgical treatment of spinal metastases in the elderly are limited. Generally, cancer (requiring significant surgery) in octogenarians has historically been difficult to treat, given the high incidence of medical comorbidities and lack of quality, long-term survival data following complex operations [21–24]. A series of recent studies have evaluated the safety and efficacy of surgery for other primary malignancies in this age group, which have shown acceptable outcomes for patients diagnosed with colorectal [25, 26], breast [27, 28], lung [29–31], endometrial [28], renal [28, 32, 33], and bladder [32, 34] cancers. Specifically for spinal metastases, Amelot et al. published a large prospective multicenter study evaluating age at the time of surgery for spinal metastases in 1266 patients at 22 centers internationally [22]. Several interesting findings emerged. Patients 80 years and older compared with those younger than 70 years presented with worse neurologic status, required urgent surgery at presentation, and trended toward having more involved spinal levels. A significant difference was observed in the rate of complications between patients older than 80 (33%) and those younger than 70 (17%). This difference was mostly explained on the basis of postoperative wound complications. Quality of life improvements were noted in all age groups.

Evaluation of an Elderly Patient with Spinal Metastases

The NOMS framework standardizes surgical decision-making for spine metastases by integrating neurologic function, degree of spinal cord compression, sensitivity to conventional external beam radiotherapy (cERT), and extent of disease as well as medical comorbidities to achieve optimal patient outcomes [35]. This model accounts for the fact that while the treatment goals of palliation, pain control, preservation of neurologic function, maintenance of stability, and local tumor control remain unchanged, advances in radiotherapy and medical oncology have shifted paradigms changing the surgical objectives.

The neurologic and oncologic considerations in NOMS are intertwined and considered in tandem. Historically, the neurologic emphasis was placed on the severity of the presence of myelopathy or functional radiculopathy, but this determination is now largely made on the basis of radiographic parameters. The standardized assessment of epidural spinal cord compression (ESCC) is reliably evaluated using a 6-point scoring system (also known as the "Bilsky score") [36]. In this validated grading scheme, grades 0–1c range from bone only involvement to increasing degrees of canal encroachment without spinal cord compression. Grade 2 and 3, which are considered high-grade compression, represent cord compression with and without surrounding cerebral spinal fluid, respectively. The oncologic component considers the tumor's sensitivity to conventional external beam radiation (cEBRT), or spine stereotactic radiosurgery which is determined by tumor type/histology [37]. cEBRT is often delivered as 20–40 Gy in 2–3 Gy per fraction. Whereas the hematologic malignancies and breast and prostate carcinoma are moderately to highly sensitive to cEBRT, response rates in the remaining solid tumor malignancies are as low as 30% at 3-month follow-up. With the exception of hematologic malignancies and breast and prostate carcinoma, the remaining solid tumors are considered resistant to conventional external beam radiation with response rates as low as 30% at 3 months [38, 39]. In cases of severe cord compression by radiosensitive tumor histology, cEBRT alone still offers good results with radiographic cord decompression and maintenance or recovery of neurologic function.

The use and efficacy of stereotactic body radiotherapy (SBRT) in the postoperative setting have changed goals and invasiveness of surgery for spinal metastases. SBRT allows for the highly conformal delivery of high Gy per fraction ablative radiation doses to be precisely delivered to tumor tissue while sparing the spinal cord, resulting in durable local control for even the conventionally radioresistant tumors [40]. This was paradigm shifting as it allows for tumors causing low-grade compression to be treated with SBRT regardless of histology. Patients with high-grade compression and/or myelopathic signs require surgical decompression to relieve pressure on the cord and create a margin for delivery of SBRT to stay within accepted cord radiation tolerances. Treating with SBRT in the setting of high-grade compression carries the risk of either overexposure of the cord causing radiation-induced myelopathy or underdosing the tumor predisposing to epidural progression [41]. Use of SBRT in the postoperative setting changed the role of surgery. Previously, aggressive surgery was needed to achieve gross total resection as the local control rate with postoperative cEBRT is poor. With aggressive surgery and postoperative cEBRT, published rates of local control at 1 year were around 30% [42]. With the availability of postoperative SBRT, the goal of surgery changed from gross total resection to simple cord decompression and creating a thin (2 mm) margin (separation surgery) around the cord to allow for conformal, ablative stereotactic radiosurgery. Laufer et al. reported the results of separation surgery followed by SBRT with an overall rate of failure of 16% in a cohort among whom half had already experienced a local RT failure and 77% had radioresistant histology [43]. Though patients often require instrumented stabilization, minimally invasive short segment constructs which minimize tissue damage can be employed due to the stability conferred by cement-augmented screw fixation.

The determination of mechanical instability is made on the basis of the spinal instability neoplastic score (SINS) [44]. This classification assesses six components of tumor-related instability including location of lesion, presence and characteristics of associated pain, bone quality, spinal alignment, degree of vertebral body collapse, and involvement of the posterior spinal elements. Summative scores of 0–6 are considered stable, 13 or greater unstable, and 7–12 potentially unstable.

The last and most important factor in NOMS is the assessment of extent of disease and coexistent medical comorbidities. When assessing non-elderly patients, this determination is often best made by the treating medical oncologist. Assessment of overall survival can be aided by several predictive models. In a retrospective study of 165 patients with metastatic spinal disease, the Skeletal Oncology Research Group (SORG) nomogram was found to most accurately predict survival at 30 and 90 days, while the original Tokuhashi score was most predictive of survival at 1 year [45–47]. Of note, these scoring systems were not specifically designed to model the elderly population.

Minimally Invasive Spine Surgery

With advances in intraoperative navigation, instrumentation, and surgical techniques, minimally invasive surgery (MIS) is gaining traction in all areas of spine surgery. In the degenerative and deformity literature, MIS techniques have been correlated with less blood loss, shorter length of stay, early ambulation, and reduction in postoperative narcotic requirements and infections [48–51]. Some of these benefits, particularly those associated with percutaneous pedicle screws and/or fenestrated pedicle screws with cement augmentation, have been observed in cohorts of general spinal tumor patients [52, 53]. To date in the metastatic spinal literature, no difference in performance status, neurological status, or patient reported outcomes have been found between MIS and open technique. However, MIS techniques have been correlated with less blood loss and shorter length of stay [54]. Needless to say, further study to evaluating outcomes based upon MIS or open technique is underway.

Frailty

To aid in assessing the suitability of elderly spinal metastatic patients for surgery, the concept of frailty has emerged. Frailty is a way to assess geriatric patients for their fitness to undergo surgery. Frailty scores seek to objectively quantify and contextualize comorbidities, nutritional status, physiologic ability to tolerate surgery, and functional status. In a prospective study of 594 elderly patients presenting for elective surgery (all types), frailty scores were assigned to patients on the basis of their baseline weakness, weight loss, physical activity, and walking speed, and independently predicted postoperative complications, length of stay, and discharge to a rehabilitation facility (after previously living at home) [55]. Several modified frailty indices have been published to predict physiologic reserve in patients undergoing spinal deformity surgery [56–58]. Further, the metastatic spine tumor frailty index (MSTFI) has been developed to capture physiologic reserve in the unique population of elderly patients with spine metastases [59]. The MSTFI model is constructed using nine parameters: anemia, chronic lung disease, coagulopathy, electrolyte disorder, pulmonary circulation disorders, renal failure, malnutrition, nonelective admission, and anterior/combined surgical approach. Based upon these metrics, patient frailty was determined. In this population of over 4500 metastatic spinal tumor patients, the complication rate and in-patient mortality were 19% and 3%, respectively. However, compared with non-frail patients, even the mildly frail were found to be at significantly higher risk of developing a major in-hospital complication and staying in-patient for a longer duration postoperatively.

Geriatric Co-management

Interdisciplinary management, including medical and radiation oncologists, for patients with spinal metastases has long been recognized as foundational in the delivery of high-quality care [60]. The addition of a geriatric specialist when the patient is elderly may continue to improve both pre- and postoperative treatment. Festen et al. evaluated the implementation of an onco-geriatric multidisciplinary tumor board team [61]. By comparing the recommendations of the usual tumor board against those made by the onco-geriatric team for 197 geriatric oncology patients, Festen reported differing recommendations in 25% of cases with the onco-geriatric team favoring less intensive or palliative treatment. In the general surgical oncologic literature, Shahrokni et al. highlighted a role for geriatricians emphasizing preoperative optimization with prehabilitation, co-management with the surgical team postoperatively, and optimizing use of transitional care models [62]. While studies of geriatric patients with spinal metastases managed in this model are forthcoming, promising trends were observed in the elderly lumbar spinal surgery population. Adogwa et al. evaluated 125 elderly patients undergoing elective lumbar fusion for degenerative scoliosis and found reduced rates of postoperative complications, shorter length of stay, and improved perioperative functional status [63]. Taken together, these data suggest a role for geriatric specialist involvement at all stages of intervention.

Illustrative Case

A 76-year-old male with no previous cancer history presented with back pain and severe gait instability. His back pain was mechanical and biological in nature. Physical exam was most notable for myelopathy in his lower extremities. Workup revealed a T8 osseous metastasis causing ESCC3 (high grade) cord compression (Fig. 21.1). He underwent an emergent T7–9 posterior instrumented fusion with cement augmentation of the fenestrated pedicle screws, and a dorsolateral decompression (Fig. 21.2). Postoperatively, a CT myelogram was obtained for radiation planning which revealed reconstitution of the thecal sac (Fig. 21.3). The patient returned to his neurological baseline ambulating on his own without an assistive device. The pathology was consistent with a poorly differentiated adenocarcinoma of unknown primary origin. He subsequently underwent SBRT of 30 Gy in three fractions. In this case, the surgical goals are to relieve the symptomatic high-grade cord compression, create a safe margin around the spinal cord to allow for the delivery of SBRT, and obtain tissue for diagnosis.

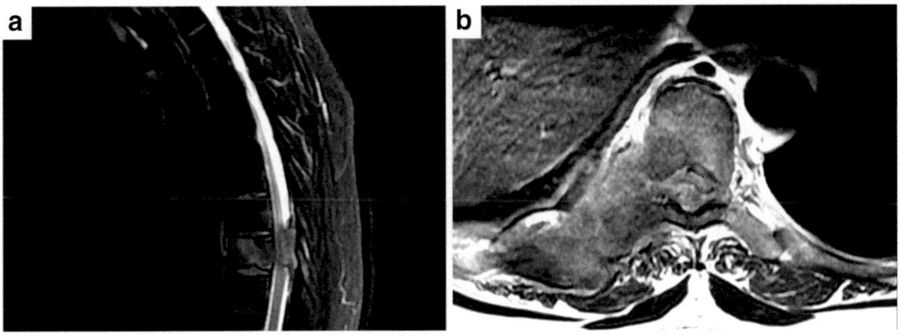

Fig. 21.1 Preoperative MRI. (**a**). Sagittal T2 MRI with an osseous metastasis at T8. (**b**) Axial T2 MRI at T8 demonstrating complete loss of CSF surrounding the spinal cord with high-grade cord compression (ESCC3)

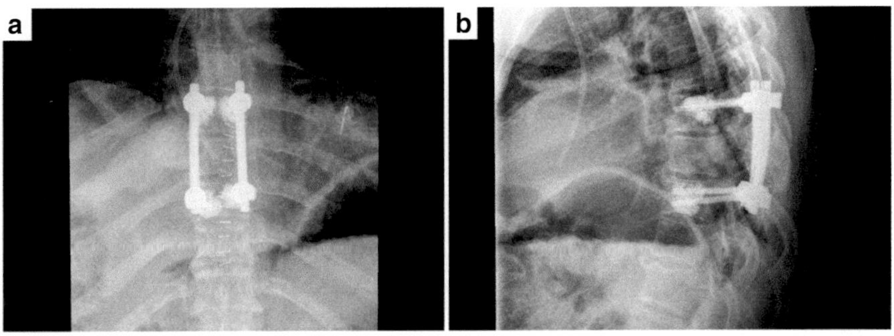

Fig. 21.2 Postoperative x-rays demonstrating T7–9 posterior instrumented fusion with cement-augmented pedicle screws. (**a**) AP. (**b**) Lateral

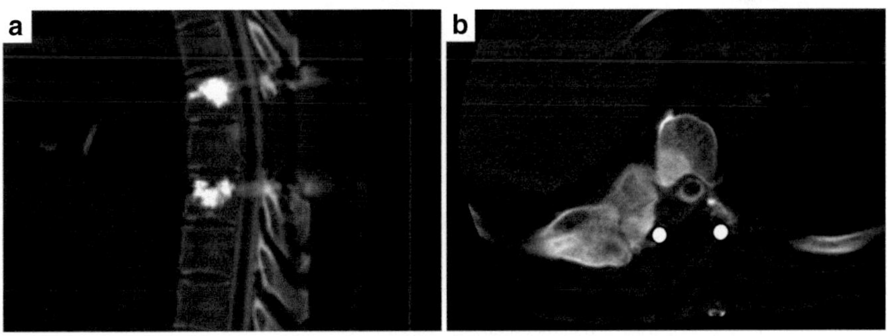

Fig. 21.3 Postoperative CT myelogram demonstrating contrast filling through the thecal sac at the level of previous high-grade spinal cord compression. (**a**) Sagittal. (**b**) Axial

Conclusion

Advances in our understanding of oncologic processes resulting in new targeted biologic and immunologic therapies are resulting in increased survival across many cancer types. While these treatments have improved systemic responses against cancer, they show poorer efficacy against skeletal metastases leading to an increased number of spinal metastases. As the incidence of spinal metastases increases, there is a coincident rise in the proportion of the population who are elderly. Elderly patients are in a high-risk group and generally have poor tolerance for invasive surgery. Fortunately, advances in the delivery of radiotherapy are resulting in less aggressive surgical goals. The evidence remains limited but does suggest that separation surgery in the geriatric population can be done safely and effectively. Mitigation of the perioperative risks in this population requires multidisciplinary involvement including a geriatric specialist.

References

1. Laufer I, Rubin DG, Lis E, Cox BW, Stubblefield MD, Yamada Y, Bilsky MH. The NOMS framework: approach to the treatment of spinal metastatic tumors. Oncologist. 2013;18:744–51.
2. Patchell RA, Tibbs PA, Regine WF, Payne R, Saris S, Kryscio RJ, Mohiuddin M, Young B. Direct decompressive surgical resection in the treatment of spinal cord compression caused by metastatic cancer: a randomised trial. Lancet. 2005;366:643–8.
3. Byrne TN. Spinal cord compression from epidural metastases. N Engl J Med. 1992;327:614–9.
4. Greenlee RT, Murray T, Bolden S, Wingo PA. Cancer statistics, 2000. CA Cancer J Clin. 2000;50:7–33.
5. Choi D, Fox Z, Albert T, et al. Prediction of quality of life and survival after surgery for symptomatic spinal metastases: a multicenter cohort study to determine suitability for surgical treatment. Neurosurgery. 2015;77:698–708; discussion 708.
6. Fehlings MG, Nater A, Tetreault L, et al. Survival and clinical outcomes in surgically treated patients with metastatic epidural spinal cord compression: results of the prospective multicenter AOSpine study. J Clin Oncol. 2016;34:268–76.
7. Hernandez RK, Adhia A, Wade SW, O'Connor E, Arellano J, Francis K, Alvrtsyan H, Million RP, Liede A. Prevalence of bone metastases and bone-targeting agent use among solid tumor patients in the United States. Clin Epidemiol. 2015;7:335–45.
8. Fehlings MG, Tetreault L, Nater A, Choma T, Harrop J, Mroz T, Santaguida C, Smith JS. The aging of the global population: the changing epidemiology of disease and spinal disorders. Neurosurgery. 2015;77(Suppl 4):S1–5.
9. Wu W-C, Schifftner TL, Henderson WG, Eaton CB, Poses RM, Uttley G, Sharma SC, Vezeridis M, Khuri SF, Friedmann PD. Preoperative hematocrit levels and postoperative outcomes in older patients undergoing noncardiac surgery. JAMA. 2007;297:2481–8.
10. Dunne JR, Malone D, Tracy JK, Gannon C, Napolitano LM. Perioperative anemia: an independent risk factor for infection, mortality, and resource utilization in surgery. J Surg Res. 2002;102:237–44.
11. Schwab F, Dubey A, Gamez L, El Fegoun AB, Hwang K, Pagala M, Farcy JP. Adult scoliosis: prevalence, SF-36, and nutritional parameters in an elderly volunteer population. Spine. 2005;30:1082–5.

12. Deyo RA, Mirza SK, Martin BI, Kreuter W, Goodman DC, Jarvik JG. Trends, major medical complications, and charges associated with surgery for lumbar spinal stenosis in older adults. JAMA. 2010;303:1259–65.
13. Kobayashi K, Imagama S, Ando K, et al. Complications associated with spine surgery in patients aged 80 years or older: Japan Association of Spine Surgeons with Ambition (JASA) multicenter study. Global Spine J. 2017;7:636–41.
14. Watanabe T, Kanayama M, Takahata M, Oda I, Suda K, Abe Y, Okumura J, Hojo Y, Iwasaki N. Perioperative complications of spine surgery in patients 80 years of age or older: a multicenter prospective cohort study. J Neurosurg Spine. 2019:1–9.
15. Saleh A, Thirukumaran C, Mesfin A, Molinari RW. Complications and readmission after lumbar spine surgery in elderly patients: an analysis of 2,320 patients. Spine J. 2017;17:1106–12.
16. Cloyd JM, Acosta FL, Ames CP. Complications and outcomes of lumbar spine surgery in elderly people: a review of the literature. J Am Geriatr Soc. 2008;56:1318–27.
17. Rajpal S, Lee Nelson E, Villavicencio AT, Telang J, Kantha R, Beasley K, Burneikiene S. Medical complications and mortality in octogenarians undergoing elective spinal fusion surgeries. Acta Neurochir. 2018;160:171–9.
18. Deyo RA, Ciol MA, Cherkin DC, Loeser JD, Bigos SJ. Lumbar spinal fusion. A cohort study of complications, reoperations, and resource use in the Medicare population. Spine. 1993;18:1463–70.
19. Halaszynski T. Influences of the aging process on acute perioperative pain management in elderly and cognitively impaired patients. Ochsner J. 2013;13:228–47.
20. Fong HK, Sands LP, Leung JM. The role of postoperative analgesia in delirium and cognitive decline in elderly patients: a systematic review. Anesth Analg. 2006;102:1255–66.
21. Aebi M. Spinal metastasis in the elderly. Eur Spine J. 2003;12(Suppl 2):S202–13.
22. Amelot A, Balabaud L, Choi D, et al. Surgery for metastatic spine tumors in the elderly. Advanced age is not a contraindication to surgery! Spine J. 2017;17:759–67.
23. Rades D, Evers JN, Bajrovic A, Veninga T, Schild SE. Re-irradiation of spinal cord compression due to metastasis in elderly patients. Anticancer Res. 2014;34:2555–8.
24. Given B, Given CW. Older adults and cancer treatment. Cancer. 2008;113:3505–11.
25. Wan Kim Y. Surgical treatment for colorectal cancer in octogenarians and nonagenarians. J BUON. 2017;22:578–85.
26. Weerink LBM, Gant CM, van Leeuwen BL, de Bock GH, Kouwenhoven EA, Faneyte IF. Long-term survival in octogenarians after surgical treatment for colorectal cancer: prevention of postoperative complications is key. Ann Surg Oncol. 2018;25:3874–82.
27. Glaser R, Marinopoulos S, Dimitrakakis C. Breast cancer treatment in women over the age of 80: a tailored approach. Maturitas. 2018;110:29–32.
28. Damhuis RAM, Meurs CJC, Meijer WS. Postoperative mortality after cancer surgery in octogenarians and nonagenarians: results from a series of 5,390 patients. World J Surg Oncol. 2005;3:71.
29. Tanita T, Hoshikawa Y, Tabata T, Noda M, Handa M, Kubo H, Chida M, Suzuki S, Ono S, Fujimura S. Functional evaluations for pulmonary resection for lung cancer in octogenarians. Investigation from postoperative complications. Jpn J Thorac Cardiovasc Surg. 1999;47:253–61.
30. Pagni S, Federico JA, Ponn RB. Pulmonary resection for lung cancer in octogenarians. Ann Thorac Surg. 1997;63:785–9.
31. Dominguez-Ventura A, Allen MS, Cassivi SD, Nichols FC, Deschamps C, Pairolero PC. Lung cancer in octogenarians: factors affecting morbidity and mortality after pulmonary resection. Ann Thorac Surg. 2006;82:1175–9.
32. Liguori G, Trombetta C, Pomara G, Amodeo A, Bucci S, Garaffa G, Francesca F, Belgrano E. Major invasive surgery for urologic cancer in octogenarians with comorbid medical conditions. Eur Urol. 2007;51:1600–4; discussion 1605.

33. Miller C, Raza SJ, Davaro F, May A, Siddiqui S, Hamilton ZA. Trends in the treatment of clinical T1 renal cell carcinoma for octogenarians: analysis of the National Cancer Database. J Geriatr Oncol. 2018;10:285–91.
34. De Groote R, Gandaglia G, Geurts N, et al. Robot-assisted radical cystectomy for bladder cancer in octogenarians. J Endourol. 2016;30:792–8.
35. Barzilai O, Laufer I, Yamada Y, Higginson DS, Schmitt AM, Lis E, Bilsky MH. Integrating evidence-based medicine for treatment of spinal metastases into a decision framework: neurologic, oncologic, mechanicals stability, and systemic disease. J Clin Oncol. 2017;35:2419–27.
36. Bilsky MH, Laufer I, Fourney DR, Groff M, Schmidt MH, Varga PP, Vrionis FD, Yamada Y, Gerszten PC, Kuklo TR. Reliability analysis of the epidural spinal cord compression scale. J Neurosurg Spine. 2010;13:324–8.
37. Gerszten PC, Mendel E, Yamada Y. Radiotherapy and radiosurgery for metastatic spine disease: what are the options, indications, and outcomes? Spine. 2009;34:S78–92.
38. Mizumoto M, Harada H, Asakura H, et al. Radiotherapy for patients with metastases to the spinal column: a review of 603 patients at Shizuoka Cancer Center Hospital. Int J Radiat Oncol Biol Phys. 2011;79:208–13.
39. Maranzano E, Latini P. Effectiveness of radiation therapy without surgery in metastatic spinal cord compression: final results from a prospective trial. Int J Radiat Oncol Biol Phys. 1995;32:959–67.
40. Yamada Y, Katsoulakis E, Laufer I, et al. The impact of histology and delivered dose on local control of spinal metastases treated with stereotactic radiosurgery. Neurosurg Focus. 2017;42:E6.
41. Lovelock DM, Zhang Z, Jackson A, Keam J, Bekelman J, Bilsky M, Lis E, Yamada Y. Correlation of local failure with measures of dose insufficiency in the high-dose single-fraction treatment of bony metastases. Int J Radiat Oncol Biol Phys. 2010;77:1282–7.
42. Klekamp J, Samii H. Surgical results for spinal metastases. Acta Neurochir. 1998;140:957–67.
43. Laufer I, Iorgulescu JB, Chapman T, Lis E, Shi W, Zhang Z, Cox BW, Yamada Y, Bilsky MH. Local disease control for spinal metastases following "separation surgery" and adjuvant hypofractionated or high-dose single-fraction stereotactic radiosurgery: outcome analysis in 186 patients. J Neurosurg Spine. 2013;18:207–14.
44. Fisher CG, DiPaola CP, Ryken TC, et al. A novel classification system for spinal instability in neoplastic disease: an evidence-based approach and expert consensus from the Spine Oncology Study Group. Spine. 2010;35:E1221–9.
45. Ahmed AK, Goodwin CR, Heravi A, Kim R, Abu-Bonsrah N, Sankey E, Kerekes D, De la Garza Ramos R, Schwab J, Sciubba DM. Predicting survival for metastatic spine disease: a comparison of nine scoring systems. Spine J. 2018;18:1804–14.
46. Paulino Pereira NR, Mclaughlin L, Janssen SJ, van Dijk CN, Bramer JAM, Laufer I, Bilsky MH, Schwab JH. The SORG nomogram accurately predicts 3- and 12-months survival for operable spine metastatic disease: external validation. J Surg Oncol. 2017;115:1019–27.
47. Tokuhashi Y, Matsuzaki H, Toriyama S, Kawano H, Ohsaka S. Scoring system for the preoperative evaluation of metastatic spine tumor prognosis. Spine. 1990;15:1110–3.
48. O'Toole JE, Eichholz KM, Fessler RG. Surgical site infection rates after minimally invasive spinal surgery. J Neurosurg Spine. 2009;11:471–6.
49. Than KD, Mummaneni PV, Bridges KJ, et al. Complication rates associated with open versus percutaneous pedicle screw instrumentation among patients undergoing minimally invasive interbody fusion for adult spinal deformity. Neurosurg Focus. 2017;43:E7.
50. Nerland US, Jakola AS, Solheim O, et al. Minimally invasive decompression versus open laminectomy for central stenosis of the lumbar spine: pragmatic comparative effectiveness study. BMJ. 2015;350:h1603.
51. Imada AO, Huynh TR, Drazin D. Minimally invasive versus open laminectomy/discectomy, transforaminal lumbar, and posterior lumbar interbody fusions: a systematic review. Cureus. 2017;9:e1488.

52. Versteeg AL, Verlaan J-J, de Baat P, Jiya TU, Stadhouder A, Diekerhof CH, van Solinge GB, Oner FC. Complications after percutaneous pedicle screw fixation for the treatment of unstable spinal metastases. Ann Surg Oncol. 2016;23:2343–9.
53. Barzilai O, McLaughlin L, Amato M-K, Reiner AS, Ogilvie SQ, Lis E, Yamada Y, Bilsky MH, Laufer I. Minimal access surgery for spinal metastases: prospective evaluation of a treatment algorithm using patient-reported outcomes. World Neurosurg. 2018;120:e889–901.
54. Hansen-Algenstaedt N, Kwan MK, Algenstaedt P, Chiu CK, Viezens L, Chan TS, Lee CK, Wellbrock J, Chan CYW, Schaefer C. Comparison between minimally invasive surgery and conventional open surgery for patients with spinal metastasis: a prospective propensity score-matched study. Spine. 2017;42:789–97.
55. Makary MA, Segev DL, Pronovost PJ, et al. Frailty as a predictor of surgical outcomes in older patients. J Am Coll Surg. 2010;210:901–8.
56. Miller EK, Ailon T, Neuman BJ, et al. Assessment of a novel adult cervical deformity frailty index as a component of preoperative risk stratification. World Neurosurg. 2018;109:e800–6.
57. Yagi M, Michikawa T, Hosogane N, et al. Treatment for frailty does not improve complication rates in corrective surgery for adult spinal deformity. Spine. 2019;44:723–31.
58. Ali R, Schwalb JM, Nerenz DR, Antoine HJ, Rubinfeld I. Use of the modified frailty index to predict 30-day morbidity and mortality from spine surgery. J Neurosurg Spine. 2016;25:537–41.
59. De la Garza Ramos R, Goodwin CR, Jain A, Abu-Bonsrah N, Fisher CG, Bettegowda C, Sciubba DM. Development of a metastatic spinal tumor frailty index (MSTFI) using a nationwide database and its association with inpatient morbidity, mortality, and length of stay after spine surgery. World Neurosurg. 2016;95:548–55.e4.
60. Newman WC, Patel A, Goldberg JL, Bilsky MH. The importance of multidisciplinary care for spine metastases: initial tumor management. Neurooncol Pract. 2020;7:i25–32.
61. Festen S, Kok M, Hopstaken JS, van der Wal-Huisman H, van der Leest A, Reyners AKL, de Bock GH, de Graeff P, van Leeuwen BL. How to incorporate geriatric assessment in clinical decision-making for older patients with cancer. An implementation study. J Geriatr Oncol. 2019;10:951–9.
62. Shahrokni A, Alexander K. The age of talking about age alone is over. Ann Surg Oncol. 2019;26:12–4.
63. Adogwa O, Elsamadicy AA, Vuong VD, Moreno J, Cheng J, Karikari IO, Bagley CA. Geriatric comanagement reduces perioperative complications and shortens duration of hospital stay after lumbar spine surgery: a prospective single-institution experience. J Neurosurg Spine. 2017;27:670–5.

Part IV
Surgical Technical Advances

Chapter 22
Surgical Technical Advances: Interbody Arthrodesis

Andrew K. Chan, Alexander Haddad, and Praveen V. Mummaneni

Introduction

With the increasing age of the general population, there has been a rise in the incidence of degenerative lumbar disease, including stenosis, spondylolisthesis, and scoliosis, as well as other lumbar pathologies, such as spinal tumors and fractures. These disorders disproportionately impact elderly patients over the age of 65 and are associated with increased disability and reductions in health-related quality of life measures [1]. The significant morbidity of spinal pathologies in the elderly and their increasing incidence have brought about an increased focus on surgical treatment modalities, including spinal fusion [2]. Spinal fusion can be accomplished through the use of posterior instrumentation with or without the use of interbody supplementation. First described by Briggs and Milligan in 1944, lumbar interbody fusion is used to treat a wide range of spinal pathologies, including degenerative disease, neoplasm, deformity, and trauma [3]. In contrast to posterior or posterolateral-based arthrodesis alone, approaches leveraging interbody devices involve the removal of the intervertebral disc, with insertion of a graft or implant that promotes anterior column arthrodesis between the upper and lower vertebrae [4, 5]. Arthrodesis of the anterior column via interbody approaches has a number of posited advantages compared to posterior-based approaches alone, including increased fusion rates as well as a greater ability to restore disc height, increase

A. K. Chan (✉) · A. Haddad
Department of Neurological Surgery, University of California, San Francisco, San Francisco, CA, USA
e-mail: andrew.chan@ucsf.edu; Alexander.Haddad@ucsf.edu

P. V. Mummaneni
UCSF Neurosurgery, San Francisco, CA, USA
e-mail: praveen.mummaneni@ucsf.edu

K.-M. G. Fu et al. (eds.), *Treatment of Spine Disease in the Elderly*,
https://doi.org/10.1007/978-3-031-12612-3_22

segmental lordosis, and—depending on surgical technique employed—correct spinal radiographic alignment parameters, although this remains an active area of investigation with conflicting reports in the literature [6–8]. Nevertheless, interbody fusions are commonly utilized, with rapidly evolving technologies.

A number of approaches exist to gain access to the intervertebral disc space and facilitate the performance of an interbody fusion. The five most commonly utilized approaches in the lumbar spine include posterior lumbar interbody fusion (PLIF), transforaminal lumbar interbody fusion (TLIF), anterior lumbar interbody fusion (ALIF), and lateral lumbar interbody fusion (LLIF) via a trans-psoas or pre-psoas approach, with each named with respect to their respective access route [4]. The PLIF and ALIF represent older, more traditional approaches, while TLIF and LLIF have only been utilized more recently. Approach selection and utilization is highly variable and surgeon/patient specific; there remains a paucity of high-quality evidence supporting one approach over another [5]. Similarly, the implant type used for interbody arthrodesis can vary. The most commonly used implants include polyetheretherketone (PEEK) and titanium, with a trend toward higher fusion rates in titanium cages [5, 9]. However, the use of newer technologies, such as expandable cages, mixed PEEK/titanium cages, and 3D printing, is also gaining popularity and continues to be studied [10].

The investment into further developing and evolving interbody fusion technologies highlights the promise of these surgeries in the treatment of a wide range of spinal pathologies. The diversity in approaches and techniques provides surgeons with a variety of options to choose from when selecting the ideal surgery for a specific patient. Indeed, patient characteristics are of utmost consideration when planning how to best perform an interbody fusion. This is especially true for elderly patients, who have unique patient characteristics that can impact the success of an interbody fusion and perioperative complications. In this chapter, we discuss the performance of interbody fusion in elderly patients and important considerations in this growing and vital patient population.

Spinal Fusion Surgery in Elderly Patients: Key Considerations

In 2000, approximately 606 million people were over the age of 60; this is expected to triple by 2050 to over two billion [11]. In fact, the population of patients over the age of 60 is projected to grow at 3.5 times the speed of the overall world population [11]. The rapidly expanding older patient population, coupled with a higher incidence of degenerative spinal disease in the elderly, highlights the need for surgeons to more completely understand the clinical characteristics of geriatric patients. This is especially true when considering clinical and radiographic nuances that might impact the ability for a patient to completely fuse following an interbody arthrodesis. Identifying and understanding clinical characteristics that impact the efficacy and success of interbody fusions is vital to preoperative planning, patient counseling, and improvements in patient symptomatology and quality of life.

A primary comorbidity that should be considered in elderly patients is osteoporosis. Defined as a bone mineral density (BMD) T-score of less than −2.5, osteoporosis is estimated to have affected 10.3 million adults over the age of 50 years in

2010, with another 43.4 million older adults having a low bone mineral density [12]. The pathophysiology of osteoporosis involves an imbalance between osteoclast and osteoblast activity, overall favoring increased bone reabsorption [13]. This increased reabsorption then leads to reduced BMD. Biomechanical studies have demonstrated reduced fixation strength of posterior instrumentation in osteoporotic vertebrae when compared to normal vertebrae [14–16]. The clinical consequence of low bone mineral density on spine surgery is well documented; complications include compression fractures, graft subsidence, proximal junctional kyphosis, and/or non-union [14]. Mechanisms of failure associated with reduced BMD can also vary depending on the type of fusion. In interbody fusions, osteoporosis is associated with an increased incidence of graft subsidence, iatrogenic fracture, and screw loosening [16–19]. Osteoporosis is also subsequently linked with worse clinical outcomes in select populations, including associations with increased revision surgeries, highlighting the impact it can have on patients and hospital resources [16, 18, 20]. Interestingly, osteoporosis is likely underdiagnosed in patients undergoing spine surgery; recent studies have demonstrated an increased incidence of low BMD when using Hounsfield units from preoperative computed tomography (CT) scans as a diagnostic tool [21, 22]. As a result, osteoporosis should be considered in every elderly patient undergoing spinal surgery, with preoperative optimization through treatments such as calcium, vitamin D, and bisphosphonates when appropriate [23]. A number of surgical techniques, such as increased screw size or cement augmentation of screws, have also been investigated for the treatment of patients with osteoporosis and can be utilized in patients who are appropriately identified [14].

Similarly, other comorbidities that frequently accrue with advanced age, such as insulin-dependent diabetes mellitus [24–28], obesity [29, 30], and reduced nutritional status [31], have been associated with increased complication rates and worse clinical outcomes, highlighting the importance of considering these as well. In fact, a rat model of insulin-dependent diabetes mellitus has demonstrated reduced rates of fusion. Similar trends have also been seen in human patients, further emphasizing the importance of identifying insulin-dependent diabetes mellitus in patients preoperatively [24, 32]. Medical preoperative optimization of these patients is crucial to reduce the impact of these comorbidities on outcomes following surgery. Despite the high incidence of comorbidities in elderly patients, multiple studies have demonstrated that this population can benefit from the appropriate surgical intervention with regard to clinical symptomology and health-related quality of life measures [33, 34]. In addition, studies have shown that surgical treatments for spinal pathologies in elderly patients is cost-effective [35].

Interbody Fusion in Geriatric Patients: A Review of the Literature

As previously discussed, a number of approaches exist to gain access to the intervertebral disc space providing surgeons with a variety of options to choose from based on their preference, the patient's anatomy, and the target disc space. Each approach has unique advantages and disadvantages making them more or less suited for particular clinical and radiographic situations. Traditionally, decision-making surrounding the utilization of specific approaches has been subject to individual surgeon preference without clear guidance on approach selection. Fortunately, a recent algorithm to aid surgeons in deciding on approach selection has been developed.

The minimally invasive interbody selection algorithm (MIISA) was developed through the consensus agreement of expert minimally invasive spine deformity surgeons across the United States [36]. The algorithm was generated by reviewing 223 MIS spine deformity surgeries, including approach selection and target disc space, and finalized through the agreement of contributing surgeons. Approaches that were included in the algorithm included ALIF, TLIF, and LLIF. Performance of a transpsoas LLIF with placement of a hyperlordotic cage and release of the anterior longitudinal ligament (ALL) was also included in the algorithm (anterior column realignment, ACR). The goal of the algorithm was to provide surgeons with guidance surrounding which approaches are most commonly used at specific levels within the lumbar spine as well as the degree of sagittal correction that can be achieved with each type of approach. When developing the algorithm, Mummaneni et al. found that the LLIF was often used for levels from L1 to L4, with TLIF at L4–5, and ALIF at L5–S1. They also found that, in general, the ALIF, LLIF, and TLIF were decreasingly able to induce segmental lordosis, in that order. This led to the finalized algorithm in Fig. 22.1.

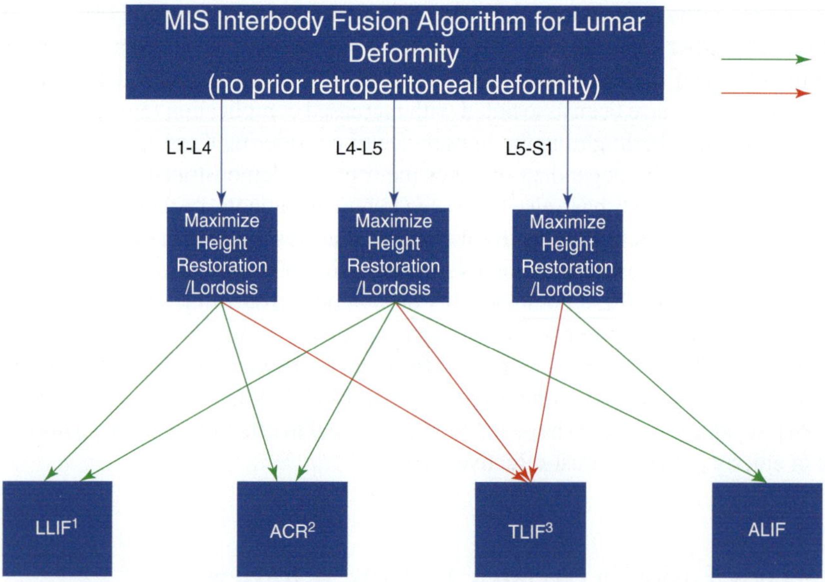

LLIF[1]: Prepsoas or transpsoas lateral interbody fusion; use when up to 5° of segmental lordosis is desired. Lordosis between L1-L4 is inconsistent while height restoration is consistent.
ACR[2]: Use when ≥10° of segmental lordosis is desired.
TLIF[3]: Allows for direct decompression of foraminal/lateral recess stenosis.

Fig. 22.1 Schematic demonstrating the MIS Lumbar Interbody Fusion Algorithm [36]

In the following section, we will discuss the use of individual approaches specifically in elderly patients, with a focus on perioperative, mechanical, and long-term quality of life outcomes when available in the literature.

ALIF

ALIFs are a commonly used to approach the intervertebral disc space with increasing popularity among surgeons [10]. The advantages associated with ALIFs surround the full access to disc space afforded by the anterior approach, which allows for ALL resection, complete discectomy, and the placement of a tall and lordotic interbody graft that is associated with high rates of fusion and the restoration of lumbar lordosis [4, 37]. Disadvantages include the need for an access surgeon, limited access to the L2/3 and L3/4 disc spaces, and a higher risk of vascular injury relative to other approaches [4]. In male patients, an ALIF approach has also been associated with the development of postoperative retrograde ejaculation, with a reported incidence of 0.9–7.4% [38–42]. The impact of age on outcomes following ALIF has been briefly explored in the literature. A 2017 study by Phan et al., including 137 patients who underwent ALIF by a single surgeon, showed a trend toward an increased risk of postoperative hematoma in older patients (relative to patients less than or equal to 49 years old); increasing age was also independently associated with an increased risk of delayed subsidence on multivariable analysis. This study was followed by Safaee et al. who, utilizing a cohort of 938 patients who underwent an ALIF at a single institution, identified increasing age, obesity, number of levels fused, and a preoperative surgical indication of degenerative disease/spondylolisthesis as independently associated with increased postoperative complications on multivariable analysis. However, they were not able to define an age threshold for complications. The increasing incidence of complications seen with increasing age is likely due to the comorbidities associated with elderly patients. Interestingly, Safaee et al. did include the Charlson Comorbidity Index (CCI), a measure of patient comorbidity burden, and diabetes as variables in their study, but neither was found to be significantly associated with complications on multivariable analysis. This may indicate that comorbidities in elderly patients outside of the CCI or diabetes are contributing to their increased rate of complications, such as osteoporosis. In addition, previous studies have correlated the modified frailty index (mFI) with increasing complications following ALIF, suggesting perhaps that disparate variables between the mFI and CCI, such as functional status, play an increased role in predicting complications in these patients [43]. Nevertheless, ALIFs are a reasonable surgical approach with significant benefits in elderly patients. Additional, larger prospective studies further investigating their use in geriatric patients are warranted. An example ALIF case is demonstrated in Fig. 22.2.

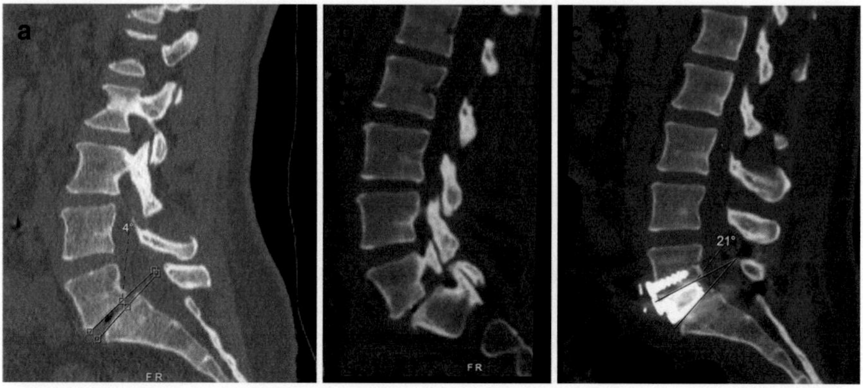

Fig. 22.2 This case illustrates use of an L5–S1 ALIF for isthmic spondylolisthesis. (**a**) Preoperative sagittal computed tomography (CT) image demonstrating L5–S1 spondylolisthesis and degenerative disc disease with loss of height and segmental lordosis. (**b**) Preoperative parasagittal CT image demonstrating a fracture of the pars interarticularis. (**c**) Postoperative CT image demonstrating a marked increase in disc height and segmental lordosis (from 4° to 21°), following L5–S1 ALIF

LLIF (Trans-psoas)

Originally described in 2006 [44], the trans-psoas LLIF achieves access to the disc space through a lateral retroperitoneal approach [4]. Trans-psoas LLIFs are especially well suited for achieving access to the T12/L1 to L4/L5 levels. In addition, LLIFs are particularly useful for achieving increased segmental lordosis [36]. When performed in the setting of ACR, with placement of a hyperlordotic cage and ALL release, trans-psoas LLIFs can significantly correct lordotic deformity and demonstrate a favorable complication profile to traditional deformity correction techniques [45]. However, disadvantages of the trans-psoas LLIF include limited access to the L5/S1 level as a result of the iliac crest as well as the potential for injury to the lumbar plexus and iliac vessels [4]. Multiple studies have evaluated the perioperative and long-term clinical outcomes associated with trans-psoas LLIFs in elderly patients. In a study of 55 patients over the age of 70 who underwent trans-psoas LLIF, Agarwal et al. showed a significant reduction in the mean 1-year postoperative Oswestry Disability Index (ODI) score when compared to the mean preoperative ODI, demonstrating the efficacy of the intervention in these patients. However, a preoperative T-score of <-1.0 conferred a significantly higher risk of graft subsidence; this further emphasizes reduced BMD as an important consideration in these patients as even a T-score above the definition of osteoporosis had a negative impact on patient outcomes [46]. These findings are further supported by Wang et al. who, in a cohort of 286 patients who underwent an trans-psoas LLIF, demonstrated similar improvements in ODI and visual analog scale (VAS) back and leg pain scores between geriatric and non-geriatric patients at 1 and 2 years postoperatively [47].

Finally, Saadeh et al. demonstrated no difference in 90-day complications between elderly and non-elderly patients who underwent 3D-guided trans-psoas LLIFs, although multilevel fusion was associated with increased complications. These studies demonstrate the relative safety and efficacy of trans-psoas LLIFs in elderly patients, supporting the continued use of this technique in geriatric patients. An example trans-psoas LLIF case is demonstrated in Fig. 22.3.

LLIF (Pre-psoas)

First described by Mayer, the pre-psoas approach LLIF facilitates access to the intervertebral disc space by utilizing a corridor ventral to the psoas, between the psoas and the peritoneum. This technique is similar to the trans-psoas LLIF, but proponents suggest it minimizes risk of injury to the lumbar plexus. However, there remain the risks of vascular injury and postoperative sympathetic dysfunction. The pre-psoas LLIF is also not recommended for patients with severe spondylolisthesis and central canal stenosis [4]. There is a general paucity of data surrounding the use of pre-psoas LLIFs in elderly patients. In a study of 63 patients who underwent a pre-psoas LLIF, Chengzhen et al. demonstrated a significant reduction in numeric rating scale (NRS) and ODI scores in both elderly and non-elderly patients with no difference between groups. Similarly, they found no differences in complications between the two groups, highlighting the efficacy and safety of pre-psoas LLIFs in elderly patients [48]. However, while promising, additional studies with greater sample sizes are warranted to further validate these findings and more completely evaluate the use of pre-psoas LLIFs in elderly patients.

PLIF

The PLIF was one of the original approaches for a lumbar interbody fusion. Some of the primary advantages associated with PLIFs are that many surgeons are comfortable performing it, and it allows for a posterior and anterior fusion through one incision in the back. However, it is also associated with a number of disadvantages, including injury to the paraspinal muscles, inadequate ability to restore lumbar lordosis, and the potential for retraction injury of the nerve roots; these contribute to the reduced utilization of the technique in modern neurosurgical practice [4]. A study in 2006 by Okuda et al., including 101 patients with >3 years of follow-up, found that both elderly and non-elderly patients clinically benefited when comparing their pre- and postoperative Japanese Orthopaedic Association (JOA) scores, with no difference between the groups. However, cage subsidence/graft bone collapse and delayed union (delayed arthrodesis more than 1 year, but less than 2 years

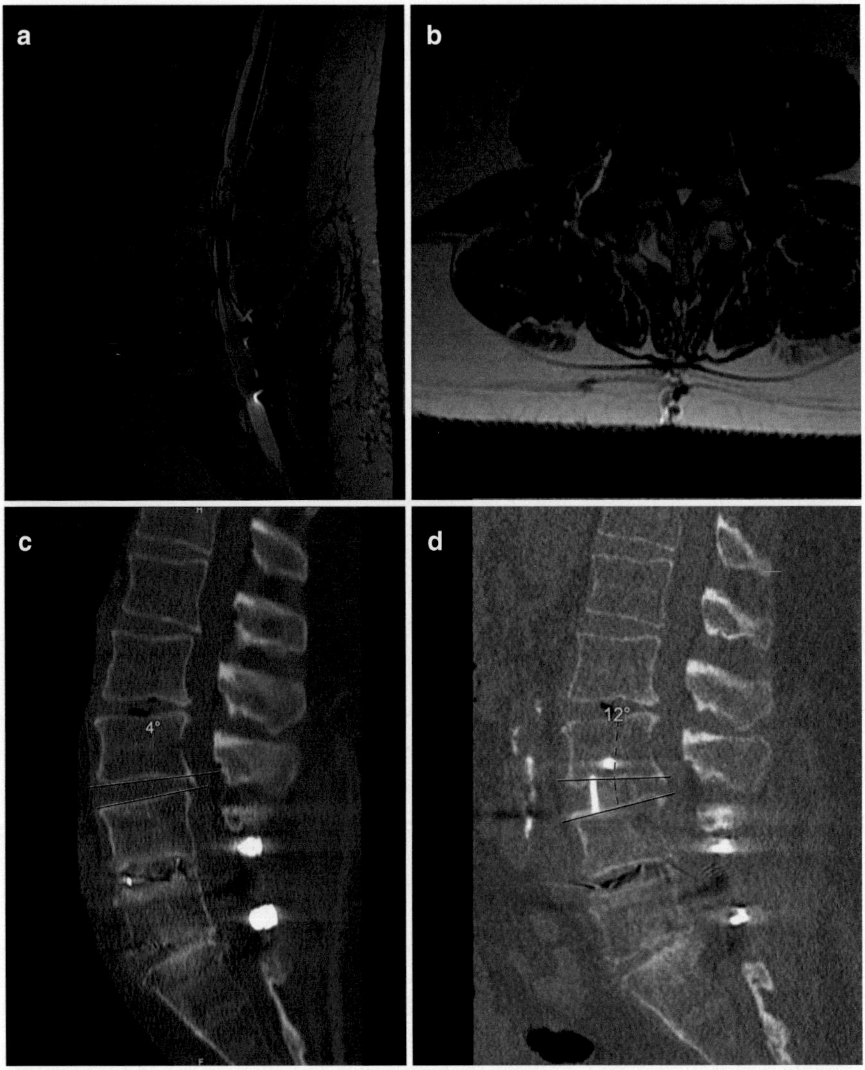

Fig. 22.3 This case illustrates use of an L3–4 LLIF for treatment of adjacent segment disease in a patient with prior history of a L4–S1 posterior spinal instrumented fusion. (**a**) Preoperative T2-weighted sagittal magnetic resonance imaging (MRI) reveals stenosis at L3–4. (**b**) A corresponding preoperative T2-weighted axial MRI image through the L3–4 disc space reveals central, lateral recess, and foraminal stenosis. (**c**) Preoperative sagittal CT image demonstrating loss of disc height and segmental lordosis at L3–4. (**d**) Postoperative sagittal CT image demonstrating increased disc height and a modest increase in segmental lordosis (from 4° to 12°) following L3–4 LLIF

postoperatively) were more common in the elderly population. This may have been due to a higher incidence of low BMD in elderly patients, though this was not specifically explored in the investigation. A subsequent study by Hayashi et al. demonstrated similar findings, with similar clinical outcomes between elderly and non-elderly patients, but a higher rate of bony non-union in elderly patients. Interestingly, they found no difference in osteoporotic vertebral fractures between the groups but saw a worsening of JOA improvement in elderly patients with osteoporotic vertebral fractures, again highlighting the importance of this comorbidity in older patients [49]. However, the presence of superior alternatives—which mitigate the risk associated with a midline approach and neural retraction—limits the application of PLIF to the elderly.

TLIF

The TLIF is one of the most commonly utilized approaches for lumbar interbody fusions. Like PLIFs, TLIFs are conducted from the posterior aspect of the spine. However, unlike PLIFs, TLIFs have a reduced risk of complications, including nerve root injury by utilizing a transforaminal, posterolateral-based approach. This avoids the neural retraction required of the PLIF. TLIFs can also be particularly useful if a patient requires direct decompression of a nerve root in addition to fusion, as a facetectomy is performed in order to facilitate a TLIF. TLIFs have reduced ability to induce lordosis, however, limiting their utility in the some adult spinal deformity cases. The TLIF is acceptable for thoracic and lumbar levels including L5/S1. However, it has a higher pseudarthrosis rate at L5–S1 compared to ALIF. A number of studies have evaluated the use of TLIFs in elderly patients. In a study of 210 patients who underwent an open TLIF, Chung et al. demonstrated similar clinical benefit between elderly and non-elderly patients, but with higher rates of non-union and complications, including durotomy, postoperative delirium, adult spinal deformity, and instrumentation failure in elderly patients. This may be due to the increased invasiveness associated with open TLIF surgery as subsequent studies investigating minimally invasive (MIS) TLIF approaches have demonstrated favorable outcomes with small, if any, differences between elderly and non-elderly patients [50–52]. Because of this, MIS-TLIF may be preferred to open TLIF in the elderly. However, studies are limited by relatively low sample sizes, highlighting the need for larger studies investigating MIS TLIF techniques in elderly patients. Nevertheless, the TLIF remains a promising technique, especially as it allows for single-stage, same-position posterior segmental instrumentation to be placed during one operation and using the same incision. An example TLIF case is demonstrated in Fig. 22.4.

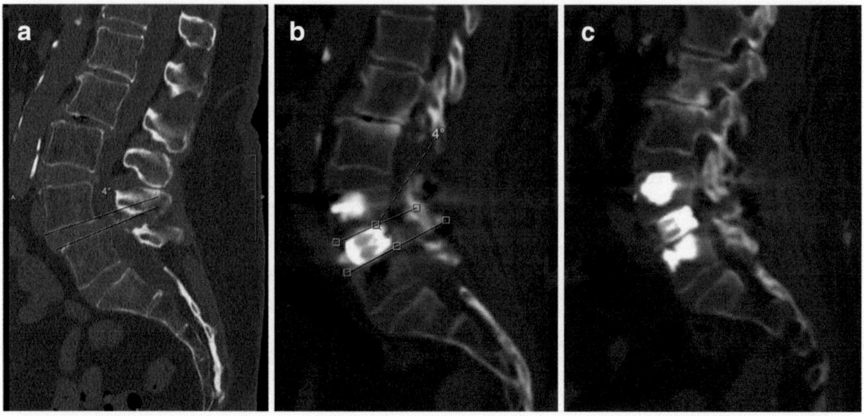

Fig. 22.4 This case illustrates use of an L4–5 TLIF for degenerative spondylolisthesis in an elderly patient with osteoporosis. (**a**) Preoperative sagittal CT image demonstrating Meyerding grade 1 spondylolisthesis at L4–5. (**b**) Postoperative sagittal CT image demonstrating L4–5 TLIF with a modest increase in disc height without change in segmental lordosis (4° both pre- and post-operatively). (**c**) Postoperative parasagittal CT image demonstrating cement augmentation of pedicle screw fixation, which was pursued given the patient's osteoporosis

Future Directions

Interbody arthrodesis plays an important role in the treatment of many spinal pathologies and will become increasingly utilized as the prevalence of these pathologies continues to grow with the aging population. Aging causes a general decline in physiologic reserve, organ function, and regenerative capacity [53]. As a result of this decline, and their higher incidence of medical comorbidities, such as diabetes, obesity, nutritional deficits, and osteoporosis, elderly patients represent a unique high-risk patient population that deserves careful consideration. Nevertheless, surgical intervention, when appropriate, can significantly improve the lives of elderly patients [54]. Thus, a better understanding of risk factors and outcomes in these patients will aid surgeons in preoperative planning, patient counseling, optimization of eligible patients, and conservative management of those who are deemed "too high-risk." In addition, surgeons should understand the interplay between specific surgical approaches, elderly patients, and outcomes.

As previously discussed, each approach to the intervertebral disc space has unique advantages and disadvantages with varying amounts of literature in elderly patients. One commonality across approaches was the low number of high-quality literature describing the approach and outcomes in elderly populations. Larger studies with long-term follow-up, and collected in a prospective manner, investigating each individual approach in elderly patients are required to more completely understand associated outcomes and complications. These studies should include clinical, radiographic, and quality of life outcomes. Generating large enough patient cohorts may require the use of multicenter collaborations [55, 56]. Further investigation into cage development and selection in elderly patients should also be performed. Similarly, there is also a paucity of research on the impact of graft materials and subsequent arthrodesis in elderly patients [57]. Cages with improved bioactivity and ability to stimulate bone growth and fusion will likely play an increased role in the care of elderly patients in the future, especially given their increased risk for osteoporosis.

Finally, a greater emphasis should be placed on understanding the biology behind how the aging process impacts spine surgery outcomes. Traditional risk stratification scores, such as the revised cardiac index, have shown little predictive ability in spine surgery, highlighting the need for a better understanding of the underlying physiology in these patients [58]. Different scoring methodologies, such as frailty measures, may play an increased role in the preoperative risk stratification of elderly patients in the future and warrant additional consideration. Given the clear relationship between certain comorbidities, such as osteoporosis, diabetes, and obesity, and complications, additional investigation into the screening and preoperative optimization of these variables should be performed for the elderly. Melding preoperative scoring systems and information on patient comorbidities with systemic biomarkers, such as c-reactive protein, with the ability to provide insight into a patient's biological age or inflammatory state may also allow for improved risk stratification when utilized as a holistic view on a patient's physiology [59, 60]. Nevertheless, there remains an important role of interbody arthrodesis for elderly patients, and outcomes will continue to improve as better technologies are developed.

Disclosures Dr. Chan reports receiving research support from Orthofix Medical, Inc. Dr. Mummaneni reports being a consultant to DePuy Synthes, Globus, and Stryker; having direct stock ownership in Spinicity/ISD; receiving support of clinical research effort from the NREF; receiving royalties from DePuy Synthes, Thieme, and Springer; receiving honoraria from Spineart; and receiving a grant from AO Spine.

References

1. Waldrop R, Cheng J, Devin C, McGirt M, Fehlings M, Berven S. The burden of spinal disorders in the elderly. Neurosurgery. 2015;77(4):S46–50. https://doi.org/10.1227/NEU.0000000000000950.
2. Siemionow K, An H, Masuda K, Andersson G, Cs-Szabo G. The effects of age, sex, ethnicity, and spinal level on the rate of intervertebral disc degeneration: a review of 1712 intervertebral discs. Spine (Phila Pa 1976). 2011;36(17):1333–9. https://doi.org/10.1097/BRS.0b013e3181f2a177.
3. Briggs H, Milligan PR. Chip fusion of the low back following exploration of the spinal canal. J Bone Jt Surg Am. 1944;26:125–30.
4. Mobbs RJ, Phan K, Malham G, Seex K, Rao PJ. Lumbar interbody fusion: techniques, indications and comparison of interbody fusion options including PLIF, TLIF, MI-TLIF, OLIF/ATP, LLIF and ALIF. J Spine Surg (Hong Kong). 2015;1(1):2–18. https://doi.org/10.3978/j.issn.2414-469X.2015.10.05.
5. Verma R, Virk S, Qureshi S. Interbody fusions in the lumbar spine: a review. HSS J. 2020;16(2):162–7. https://doi.org/10.1007/s11420-019-09737-4.

6. Fujimori T, Le H, Schairer WW, Berven SH, Qamirani E, Hu SS. Does transforaminal lumbar interbody fusion have advantages over posterolateral lumbar fusion for degenerative spondylolisthesis? Glob Spine J. 2014;5(2):102–9. https://doi.org/10.1055/s-0034-1396432.
7. Mummaneni PV, Haid RW, Rodts GE. Lumbar interbody fusion: state-of-the-art technical advances. J Neurosurg. 2004;101:24–30. https://doi.org/10.3171/spi.2004.1.1.0024.
8. Campbell RC, Mobbs RJ, Lu VM, Xu J, Rao PJ, Phan K. Posterolateral fusion versus interbody fusion for degenerative spondylolisthesis: systematic review and meta-analysis. Glob Spine J. 2017;7(5):482–90. https://doi.org/10.1177/2192568217701103.
9. Seaman S, Kerezoudis P, Bydon M, Torner JC, Hitchon PW. Titanium vs. polyetheretherketone (PEEK) interbody fusion: meta-analysis and review of the literature. J Clin Neurosci. 2017;44:23–9. https://doi.org/10.1016/j.jocn.2017.06.062.
10. Phan K, Mobbs RJ. Evolution of design of interbody cages for anterior lumbar interbody fusion. Orthop Surg. 2016;8(3):270–7. https://doi.org/10.1111/os.12259.
11. McNicoll G. World population ageing 1950-2050. Popul Dev Rev. 2002;28(4):814–6. https://go-gale-com.ucsf.idm.oclc.org/ps/i.do?p=AONE&sw=w&issn=00987921&v=2.1&it=r&id=GALE%7CA96904156&sid=googleScholar&linkaccess=fulltext. Accessed 24 Nov 2020.
12. Wright NC, Looker AC, Saag KG, et al. The recent prevalence of osteoporosis and low bone mass in the United States based on bone mineral density at the femoral neck or lumbar spine. J Bone Miner Res. 2014;29(11):2520–6. https://doi.org/10.1002/jbmr.2269.
13. Drake MT, Clarke BL, Lewiecki EM. The pathophysiology and treatment of osteoporosis. Clin Ther. 2015;37(8):1837–50. https://doi.org/10.1016/j.clinthera.2015.06.006.
14. Goldstein CL, Brodke DS, Choma TJ. Surgical management of spinal conditions in the elderly osteoporotic spine. Neurosurgery. 2015;77(4):S98–S107. https://doi.org/10.1227/NEU.0000000000000948.
15. Paxinos O, Tsitsopoulos PP, Zindrick MR, et al. Evaluation of pullout strength and failure mechanism of posterior instrumentation in normal and osteopenic thoracic vertebrae: laboratory investigation. J Neurosurg Spine. 2010;13(4):469–76. https://doi.org/10.3171/2010.4.SPINE09764.
16. Carlson BC, Robinson WA, Wanderman NR, et al. A review and clinical perspective of the impact of osteoporosis on the spine. Geriatr Orthop Surg Rehabil. 2019;10:2151459319861591. https://doi.org/10.1177/2151459319861591.
17. Cho JH, Hwang CJ, Kim H, Joo YS, Lee DH, Lee CS. Effect of osteoporosis on the clinical and radiological outcomes following one-level posterior lumbar interbody fusion. J Orthop Sci. 2018;23(6):870–7. https://doi.org/10.1016/j.jos.2018.06.009.
18. Tempel ZJ, Gandhoke GS, Okonkwo DO, Kanter AS. Impaired bone mineral density as a predictor of graft subsidence following minimally invasive transpsoas lateral lumbar interbody fusion. Eur Spine J. 2015;24:414–9. https://doi.org/10.1007/s00586-015-3844-y.
19. Formby PM, Kang DG, Helgeson MD, Wagner SC. Clinical and radiographic outcomes of transforaminal lumbar interbody fusion in patients with osteoporosis. Glob Spine J. 2016;6(7):660–4. https://doi.org/10.1055/s-0036-1578804.
20. Bjerke BT, Zarrabian M, Aleem IS, et al. Incidence of osteoporosis-related complications following posterior lumbar fusion. Glob Spine J. 2018;8(6):563–9. https://doi.org/10.1177/2192568217743727.
21. Wagner SC, Formby PM, Helgeson MD, Kang DG. Diagnosing the undiagnosed osteoporosis in patients undergoing lumbar fusion. Spine (Phila Pa 1976). 2016;41(21):E1279–83. https://doi.org/10.1097/BRS.0000000000001612.
22. Zou D, Jiang S, Zhou S, et al. Prevalence of osteoporosis in patients undergoing lumbar fusion for lumbar degenerative diseases. Spine (Phila Pa 1976). 2020;45(7):E406–10. https://doi.org/10.1097/BRS.0000000000003284.
23. Lubelski D, Choma TJ, Steinmetz MP, Harrop JS, Mroz TE. Perioperative medical management of spine surgery patients with osteoporosis. Neurosurgery. 2015;77(4):S92–7. https://doi.org/10.1227/NEU.0000000000000939.

24. Moazzeni K, Kazemi KA, Khanmohammad R, Eslamian M, Rostami M, Faghih-Jouibari M. Comparison of surgical outcome between diabetic versus nondiabetic patients after lumbar fusion. Int J Spine Surg. 2018;12(4):528–32. https://doi.org/10.14444/5064.
25. Golinvaux NS, Varthi AG, Bohl DD, Basques BA, Grauer JN. Complication rates following elective lumbar fusion in patients with diabetes: insulin dependence makes the difference. Spine (Phila Pa 1976). 2014;39(21):1809–16. https://doi.org/10.1097/BRS.0000000000000506.
26. Takahashi S, Suzuki A, Toyoda H, et al. Characteristics of diabetes associated with poor improvements in clinical outcomes after lumbar spine surgery. Spine (Phila Pa 1976). 2013;38(6):516–22. https://doi.org/10.1097/BRS.0b013e318273583a.
27. Epstein N. Predominantly negative impact of diabetes on spinal surgery: a review and recommendation for better preoperative screening. Surg Neurol Int. 2017;8(1):107. https://doi.org/10.4103/sni.sni_101_17.
28. Arinzon Z, Adunsky A, Fidelman Z, Gepstein R. Outcomes of decompression surgery for lumbar spinal stenosis in elderly diabetic patients. Eur Spine J. 2004;13(1):32–7. https://doi.org/10.1007/s00586-003-0643-7.
29. Puvanesarajah V, Werner BC, Cancienne JM, et al. Morbid obesity and lumbar fusion in patients older than 65 years. Spine (Phila Pa 1976). 2017;42(2):122–7. https://doi.org/10.1097/BRS.0000000000001692.
30. McGuire KJ, Khaleel MA, Rihn JA, Lurie JD, Zhao W, Weinstein JN. The effect of high obesity on outcomes of treatment for lumbar spinal conditions: subgroup analysis of the Spine Patient Outcomes Research Trial. Spine (Phila Pa 1976). 2014;39(23):1975–80. https://doi.org/10.1097/BRS.0000000000000577.
31. Phan K, Kim JS, Xu J, et al. Nutritional insufficiency as a predictor for adverse outcomes in adult spinal deformity surgery. Glob Spine J. 2018;8(2):164–71. https://doi.org/10.1177/2192568217708777.
32. NaPier Z, Kanim LEA, Nelson TJ, et al. The effect of insulin dependent diabetes on bone metabolism and growth after spinal fusion. Spine J. 2020;20(5):800–8. https://doi.org/10.1016/j.spinee.2019.11.011.
33. Shamji MF, Mroz T, Hsu W, Chutkan N. Management of degenerative lumbar spinal stenosis in the elderly. Neurosurgery. 2015;77(4):S68–74. https://doi.org/10.1227/NEU.0000000000000943.
34. Shamji MF, Goldstein CL, Wang M, Uribe JS, Fehlings MG. Minimally invasive spinal surgery in the elderly. Neurosurgery. 2015;77(4):S108–15. https://doi.org/10.1227/NEU.0000000000000941.
35. Devin CJ, Chotai S, Parker SL, Tetreault L, Fehlings MG, McGirt MJ. A cost-utility analysis of lumbar decompression with and without fusion for degenerative spine disease in the elderly. Neurosurgery. 2015;77(4):S116–24. https://doi.org/10.1227/NEU.0000000000000949.
36. Mummaneni PV, Shaffrey CI, Eastlack R, et al. The minimally invasive interbody selection algorithm (MIISA) for spinal deformity. Neurosurgery. 2019;66(Suppl_1). https://doi.org/10.1093/neuros/nyz310_338.
37. Phan K, Thayaparan GK, Mobbs RJ. Anterior lumbar interbody fusion versus transforaminal lumbar interbody fusion—systematic review and meta-analysis. Br J Neurosurg. 2015;29(5):705–11. https://doi.org/10.3109/02688697.2015.1036838.
38. Comer GC, Smith MW, Hurwitz EL, Mitsunaga KA, Kessler R, Carragee EJ. Retrograde ejaculation after anterior lumbar interbody fusion with and without bone morphogenetic protein-2 augmentation: a 10-year cohort controlled study. Spine J. 2012;12(10):881–90. https://doi.org/10.1016/j.spinee.2012.09.040.
39. Lindley EM, McBeth ZL, Henry SE, et al. Retrograde ejaculation after anterior lumbar spine surgery. Spine (Phila Pa 1976). 2012;37(20):1785–9. https://doi.org/10.1097/BRS.0b013e31825752bc.
40. Burkus JK, Dryer RF, Peloza JH. Retrograde ejaculation following single-level anterior lumbar surgery with or without recombinant human bone morphogenetic protein-2 in 5 random-

ized controlled trials; Clinical article. J Neurosurg Spine. 2013;18(2):112–21. https://doi.org/10.3171/2012.10.SPINE11908.
41. Malham GM, Parker RM, Ellis NJ, Blecher CM, Chow FY, Claydon MH. Anterior lumbar interbody fusion using recombinant human bone morphogenetic protein-2: a prospective study of complications. J Neurosurg Spine. 2014;21(6):851–60. https://doi.org/10.3171/2014.8.SPINE13524.
42. Mobbs RJ, Phan K, Daly D, Rao PJ, Lennox A. Approach-related complications of anterior lumbar interbody fusion: results of a combined spine and vascular surgical team. Glob Spine J. 2015;6(2):147–54. https://doi.org/10.1055/s-0035-1557141.
43. Phan K, Kim JS, Lee NJ, et al. Frailty is associated with morbidity in adults undergoing elective anterior lumbar interbody fusion (ALIF) surgery. Spine J. 2017;17(4):538–44. https://doi.org/10.1016/j.spinee.2016.10.023.
44. Ozgur BM, Aryan HE, Pimenta L, Taylor WR. Extreme lateral interbody fusion (XLIF): a novel surgical technique for anterior lumbar interbody fusion. Spine J. 2006;6(4):435–43. https://doi.org/10.1016/j.spinee.2005.08.012.
45. Godzik J, Pereira BA, Hemphill C, et al. Minimally invasive anterior longitudinal ligament release for anterior column realignment. Glob Spine J. 2020;10(2_suppl):101S–10S. https://doi.org/10.1177/2192568219880178.
46. Agarwal N, Faramand A, Alan N, et al. Lateral lumbar interbody fusion in the elderly: a 10-year experience: presented at the 2018 AANS/CNS Joint Section on Disorders of the Spine and Peripheral Nerves. J Neurosurg Spine. 2018;29(5):525–9. https://doi.org/10.3171/2018.3.SPINE171147.
47. Wang TY, Shammas R, Gottfried ON, Pimenta L, Brown C, Isaacs RE. A comparison of geriatric and nongeriatric patient outcomes following extreme lateral interbody fusion (XLIF). Spine J. 2016;16(10):S362. https://doi.org/10.1016/j.spinee.2016.07.485.
48. Jin C, Jaiswal MS, Jeun SS, Ryu KS, Hur JW, Kim JS. Outcomes of oblique lateral interbody fusion for degenerative lumbar disease in patients under or over 65years of age. J Orthop Surg Res. 2018;13(1) https://doi.org/10.1186/s13018-018-0740-2.
49. Hayashi K, Matsumura A, Konishi S, Kato M, Namikawa T, Nakamura H. Clinical outcomes of posterior lumbar interbody fusion for patients 80 years of age and older with lumbar degenerative disease: minimum 2 years' follow-up. Glob Spine J. 2016;6(7):665–72. https://doi.org/10.1055/s-0036-1578806.
50. Goh GSH, Tay YWA, Liow MHL, et al. Elderly patients undergoing minimally invasive transforaminal lumbar interbody fusion may have similar clinical outcomes, perioperative complications, and fusion rates as their younger counterparts. Clin Orthop Relat Res. 2020;478(4):822–32. https://doi.org/10.1097/CORR.0000000000001054.
51. Dong YL, Jung TG, Lee SH. Single-level instrumented mini-open transforaminal lumbar interbody fusion in elderly patients. J Neurosurg Spine. 2008;9(2):137–44. https://doi.org/10.3171/SPI/2008/9/8/137.
52. Nikhil JN, Wei-An LJ, Yeo W, Yue WM. Elderly patients achieving clinical and radiological outcomes comparable with those of younger patients following minimally invasive transforaminal lumbar interbody fusion. Asian Spine J. 2017;11(2):230–42. https://doi.org/10.4184/asj.2017.11.2.230.
53. Clegg A, Young J, Iliffe S, Rikkert MO, Rockwood K. Frailty in elderly people. Lancet. 2013;381:752–62. https://doi.org/10.1016/S0140-6736(12)62167-9.
54. Ibrahim JM, Singh P, Beckerman D, et al. Outcomes and quality of life improvement after multilevel spinal fusion in elderly patients. Glob Spine J. 2020;10(2):153–9. https://doi.org/10.1177/2192568219849393.
55. Mummaneni PV, Bydon M, Alvi MA, et al. Predictive model for long-term patient satisfaction after surgery for grade I degenerative lumbar spondylolisthesis: insights from the Quality Outcomes Database. Neurosurg Focus. 2019;46(5). https://doi.org/10.3171/2019.2.FOCUS18734.

56. Chan AK, Bisson EF, Bydon M, et al. Laminectomy alone versus fusion for grade 1 lumbar spondylolisthesis in 426 patients from the prospective Quality Outcomes Database. J Neurosurg Spine. 2019;30(2):234–41. https://doi.org/10.3171/2018.8.SPINE17913.
57. Ajiboye RM, Hamamoto JT, Eckardt MA, Wang JC. Clinical and radiographic outcomes of concentrated bone marrow aspirate with allograft and demineralized bone matrix for posterolateral and interbody lumbar fusion in elderly patients. Eur Spine J. 2015;24(11):2567–72. https://doi.org/10.1007/s00586-015-4117-5.
58. Carabini LM, Zeeni C, Moreland NC, et al. Predicting major adverse cardiac events in spine fusion patients: is the revised cardiac risk index sufficient? Spine (Phila Pa 1976). 2014;39(17):1441–8. https://doi.org/10.1097/BRS.0000000000000405.
59. Gaudillière B, Fragiadakis GK, Bruggner RV, et al. Clinical recovery from surgery correlates with single-cell immune signatures. Sci Transl Med. 2014;6(255):255ra131. https://doi.org/10.1126/scitranslmed.3009701.
60. Zhang L-J, Li N, Li Y, Zeng X-T, Liu M-Y. Cardiac biomarkers predicting MACE in patients undergoing noncardiac surgery: a meta-analysis. Front Physiol. 2019;9:1923. https://doi.org/10.3389/fphys.2018.01923.

Chapter 23
Pedicle Screw Fixation

Connor D. Berlin, Parantap Patel, and Avery Buchholz

Indications for pedicle screw placement:

- Existing spinal instability: trauma, tumors, and infection
- Potential spinal instability: spondylolisthesis, wide destabilizing decompression, stabilization after osteotomy, and pseudoarthrosis
- Scoliosis correction

Contraindications:

- Pedicle instability or fracture
- Inadequate pedicle size or morphology
- Severe osteopenia (relative contraindication)

History

The first application of sagittally oriented screws through the vertebral pedicle is widely attributed to Roy-Camille in the 1970s [1].This technique for spinal fixation was successfully utilized for the treatment of vertebral fractures, tumors, malunions, spondylolisthesis, and low-back pain disorders. Further studies by Louis (1986) using this pedicle screw fixation technique demonstrated high fusion rates in single-stage posterior and combined approaches in a review of 455 patients [2].With the advent of the pedicle screw also came the concurrent need for development of techniques for connecting multiple pedicles screws at varying vertebral levels.

C. D. Berlin · P. Patel · A. Buchholz (✉)
Department of Neurosurgery, University of Virginia Health, Charlottesville, VA, USA
e-mail: cdb5zm@hscmail.mcc.virginia.edu; PP7HY@hscmail.mcc.virginia.edu; alb8jp@hscmail.mcc.virginia.edu

K.-M. G. Fu et al. (eds.), *Treatment of Spine Disease in the Elderly*,
https://doi.org/10.1007/978-3-031-12612-3_23

Roy-Camille, Magerl, and Steffee are all credited with developing different methods for connecting adjacent screws, utilizing either metal plates or external fixation techniques [1, 3, 4].

Biomechanics

When pedicle screws are combined with plates or rods to form a rigid fixation construct, force is applied to the spine by a fixed moment arm cantilever [5].The stable fixation technique allows biomechanical stressors to be distributed across all three vertebral columns which resists motion in all three planes [6]. This has laid the foundation for modern spinal fixation. This technique has also allowed for the incorporation of fewer normal spinal segments to stabilize an abnormal segment. Thus, pedicle screws have increased our modern capability for correcting spinal deformity, decreased the need for external orthoses to stabilize the spine, and allowed for extensive nerve and cord decompression without threat of destabilizing the spine [7]. Although not universal, the use of pedicle screws has consistently demonstrated superior fusion rates compared to noninstrumented fusion [7].

Failure of these constructs can occur with axial loading, with the tips of the pedicle screw becoming more cranial angled while the screw head/rod construct translates caudally. Toeing-in the tip of the pedicle screw within the vertebral body may help to prevent such translocation [8]. However, it is more common for failure to occur at the screw-bone junction [5]. If a screw does pull out, break, or toggle in location, it is usually due to inappropriate biomechanical application. In the elderly, considerations of osteoporosis and techniques to prevent pullout, break, and toggling are discussed in a separate section below.

Screw Characteristics

Pedicle screws have a cancellous thread, with outer diameters ranging from 4.0 to 8.5 mm or greater and typically lengths from 30 to 55 mm in 5 mm increments. The screw types can further be subdivided into self-tapping and non-tapping (in which case a separate tap is used to create threads with the pedicle for the screw threads to lock into) [5].

In general, the concept of pedicle screws is the same as those of all machined screws. The key to the screw strength is the inner (core) diameter. The cube of the core diameter is proportional to the torsional strength of the screw, or the force required to resist screw bending or breakage [9]. The outer thread diameter, on the other hand, affords the screw much of its pullout resistance, which is directly proportional to the volume of bone between threads. Thus, pullout resistance can be modified by thread pitch (the distance between adjacent threads—cortical screws tend to have a smaller pitch and cancellous screws a larger pitch), thread lead (the distance a screw advances with each turn—in general threads that interface with cortical bone have a smaller lead than threads that interface with cancellous bone as a smaller lead affords greater mechanical advantage required for cortical bone),thread design ("V" profile produces shear and compression forces, versus compression forces only from a buttress design), and thread length (with some systems having a smooth, thick screw neck to prevent fractures near the head of the screw where it is most likely to fail) [9]. The additional advent of polyaxial screw heads has made intraoperative connection to rods much easier, although these systems are still vulnerable to failure at the polyaxial head-neck interface [10].

Pedicle Screw Insertion

Pedicle Anatomy

The pedicle is the anatomic bridge between the posterior spinal elements and the vertebral body. It is composed of hard cortical bone on the outside and an internal cancellous core. In general, the pedicle is thicker in the sagittal axis (pedicle height) than it is in the transverse axis [9]. Therefore, for considerations of screw placement, transverse pedicle screw thickness is an important consideration. In a study measuring pedicle diameters with CT, Bernard and Seibert demonstrated that 20% of pedicles were less than 7 mm at L2, 15.6% at L3, and 1.9% at L4, with no pedicles less than 7 mm at L5 and S1 [5, 11]. Nonetheless, the use of preoperative CT is recommended to confirm pedicle size and plan screw selection as there are instances of pedicle diameters being much less (i.e., 3–4 mm) at some of the thoracic and higher lumbar levels.

Additionally, surgeons should note the degree of pedicle angulation. The transverse pedicle angle decreases with caudal progression of the spine up until the lumbar spine, after which the angle increases [5]. The sagittal angle of the pedicle is relatively steep throughout the thoracolumbar spine, but less so at the lower lumbar spine.

It is important to recognize that the dural sac and intrathecal nerve roots are just adjacent to the medial pedicle in the transverse plane. In the sagittal plane, immediately below the pedicle is the neural foramen, with the nerve root positioned ventrally and cranially within. Thus, any medial or caudal violation of the pedicle can result in significant injury to neural structures.

Cervical Spine Although there are challenges to pedicle screw fixation in the cervical spine, some surgeons opt for this method compared to traditional lateral mass screws when technical experience and anatomy are favorable. Pedicle screw fixation in the cervical spine is biomechanically superior when compared to lateral mass screws [12]. Nevertheless, surgeons must be aware of dangers pedicle screws pose in the cervical spine, specifically the adjacent vertebral artery laterally or cervical nerve root inferiorly. The correct entry point is below the facet joint, halfway between the medial and lateral margins of the lateral mass [13]. Laminotomies are optional to better visualize the margins of the pedicle [13] (Fig. 23.1a). Preoperative planning is crucial, especially in cases of degenerative or rheumatoid changes to the posterior elements (as is often the case with elderly patients), a known risk factor for malpositioning of screws [14]. Medial-lateral inclination ranges from 30° to 60° between the midsagittal plane and the longitudinal axis of the screw, but is usually around 45° [13, 15] (Fig. 23.1b). Cranial-caudal angulation is typically perpendicular to the posterior elements' axis, or parallel to the cranial endplate for C5, C6, and C7 pedicles and slightly cephalad for C3 and C4 pedicles [13, 15] (Fig. 23.1c). In addition to high-resolution computed-tomography of the cervical spine, some surgeons routinely perform four-vessel magnetic resonance angiography preoperatively to assess for aberrant vertebral artery morphologies [16].

Thoracic Spine In the thoracic spine, care must be taken to avoid medial breaches, which can result in spinal cord injury, and lateral breaches, which can result in significant vascular, lymphatic, pleural, or esophageal injuries. Particular care must be taken at the mid-thoracic levels, T3 through T9, which have the narrowest pedicles and the smallest distance between the spinal cord and the medial aspect of each pedicle [17]. Entry points can be subdivided into four groups: T1–T3, T4–T6, T7–T9, and T10–T12 [18] (Fig. 23.2). However, a commonly used entry

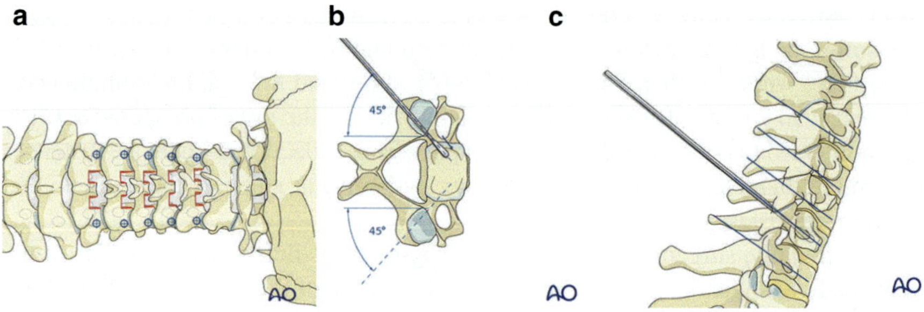

Fig. 23.1 Cervical pedicle screw placement. (**a**) Cervical spine pedicle screw entry points after laminotomy, just below the facet, midway between the medial and lateral margins of the lateral mass. (**b**) Medial-lateral inclination is roughly 45° depending on the level, but in general decreases while progressing cranial to caudal. (**c**) Cranial-caudal angulation should be perpendicular to the axis of the posterior elements. (**Reprinted with permission from AO Surgery Reference Online**. URL: https://surgeryreference.aofoundation.org/spine/trauma/subaxial-cervical/basic-technique/cervical-pedicle-screw-insertion#general-considerations)

Fig. 23.2 Thoracic pedicle screw placement. (**a**) In general, the entry point should be the center of a triangle formed by the pars interarticularis, the medial border of the transverse process, and the inferior border of the superior articular facet. (**b**) T1–T3 entry points are at the intersection of a horizontal line through the middle of the transverse process and a line slightly lateral to the center of the articular facet. (**c**) T1–T3 angulation is slightly medial and caudal. (**d**) T4–T6 entry points are similar to T1–T3 but more cranial and medial. (**e**) T4–T6 angulation is nearly vertical. (**f**) T7–T9 entry points are even more cranial and medial. (**g**) T7–T9 angulation is vertical. (**h**) T10–T12 entry points are at the intersection of the mamillary process and a vertical line. (**i**) T10–T12 angulation is vertical or slightly lateral. (**Reprinted with permission from AO Surgery Reference Online**. URL: https://surgeryreference.aofoundation.org/spine/deformities/scheuermann-kyphosis/further-reading/pedicle-screw-insertion?searchurl=%2fSearchResults)

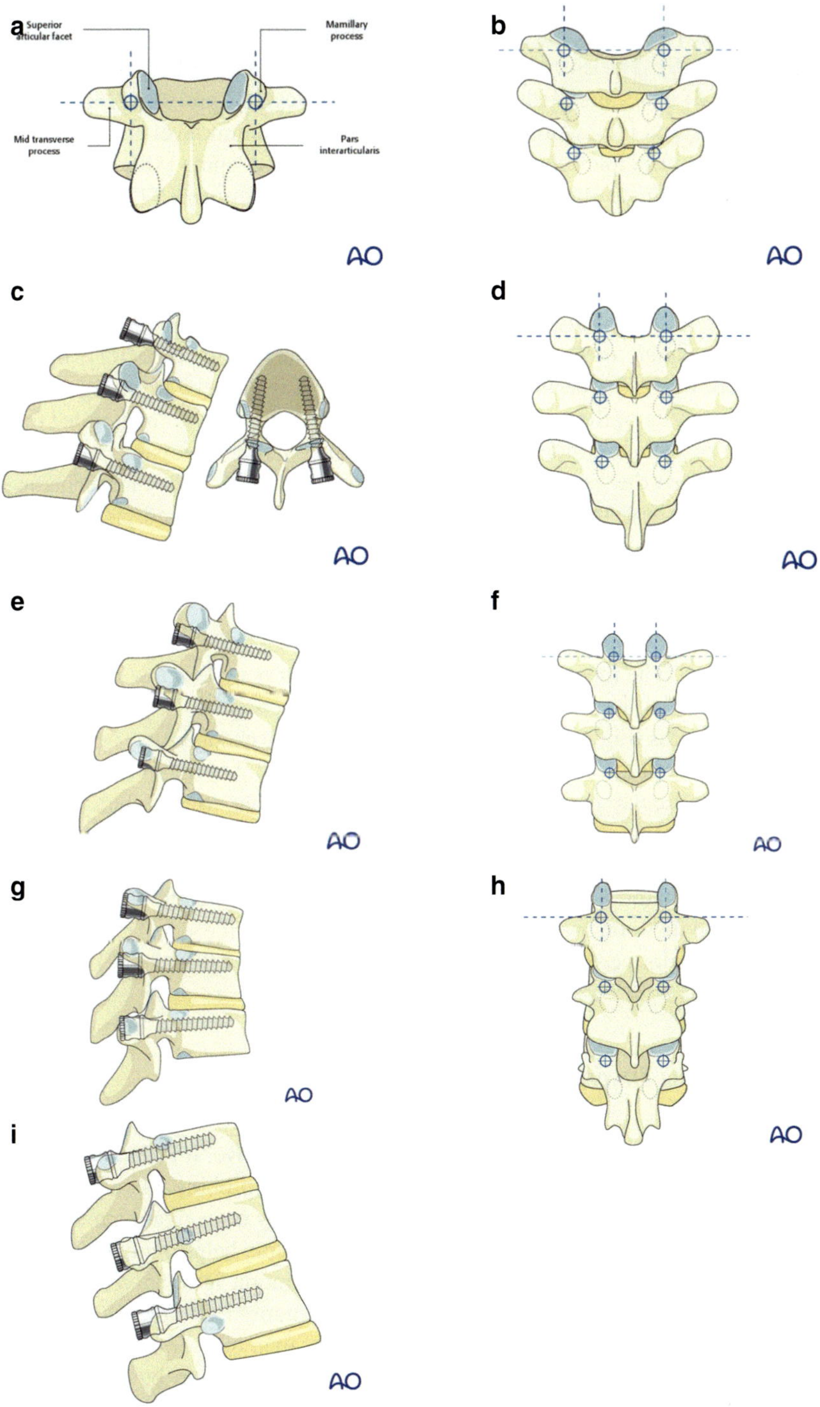
a
Superior articular facet
Mamillary process
Mid transverse process
Pars interarticularis
b
c
d
e
f
g
h
i

point is the center of a triangle formed by the pars interarticularis, the medial border of the transverse process, and the inferior border of the superior articular facet (Fig. 23.2a) [19]. The entry point is more lateral and caudal between T1 and T6 (Fig. 23.2b, d) and more medial and cephalad between T7 and T12 (Fig. 23.2f, h) [19]. Mediolateral inclination is dependent on the vertebral level and patient-specific anatomy, principles similar to those of the cervical spine [18]. Reported trajectories approximate 30° for T1 and T2 and 20° for T3 through T12 [20]. Another useful rule is that screw angulation is slightly medial and caudal for T1–T3 (Fig. 23.2c), almost vertical for T4–T6 (Fig. 23.2e), vertical for T7–T9 (Fig. 23.2g), and vertical/slightly lateral for T10–T12 (Fig. 23.2i). Cranial-caudal angulation can either be a "straightforward" trajectory, in which case the screw is parallel to the cranial endplate of the vertebral body, or an "anatomic" trajectory, in which case the screw follows the anatomic axis of the pedicle, thereby resulting in a more caudal positioning of the screw tip [18, 19]. Of special note, the "anatomic" trajectory does necessitate a more cephalad screw entry point. Compared to the "anatomic" trajectory, the "straightforward" trajectory is thought to be biomechanically superior [19]. These trajectories must be adapted to patient- and pathology-specific differences in pedicle size and angulations. Accordingly, the surgeon may find fluoroscopic, navigational, and robotic techniques to be helpful in fixation for complex pathologies.

Lumbar Spine The most widely used entry point for pedicle screw fixation in the lumbar spine is at the mamillary process, at the junction of the lateral facet and transverse process (Fig. 23.3a). Significant degenerative changes may necessitate an alternative entry point, in which case a more medial point at the inferior margin of the superior articular process may be used [21]. Similar to elsewhere along the spine, the angulation in the transverse plane is dependent on the vertebral level and patient-specific anatomy. The cranio-caudal angulation can follow either a "straightforward" or "anatomic" trajectory (Fig. 23.3b) [19]. Mediolateral inclination of screws should focus on avoiding superficial penetration of the spinal canal medially, and lateral/anterior perforation of the vertebral body cortex (Fig. 23.3c) [18].

Pedicle Screw Insertion Technique

In general, the entry site is confirmed anatomically as above. It is then decorticated with a high-speed drill or rongeur. During the process of probing, tapping, and placing pedicle screws, the use of intraoperative fluoroscopy or navigation may be used to ensure proper trajectory. On fluoroscopy, lateral films help to guide the sagittal angle through the pedicle as well as depth of penetration into the vertebral body, whereas AP films can aid with medial-lateral inclination. Of note, normal short-segment pedicle screws should not penetrate greater than 80% of the vertebral body length on lateral films, as there is risk of ventral penetration beyond this (it is

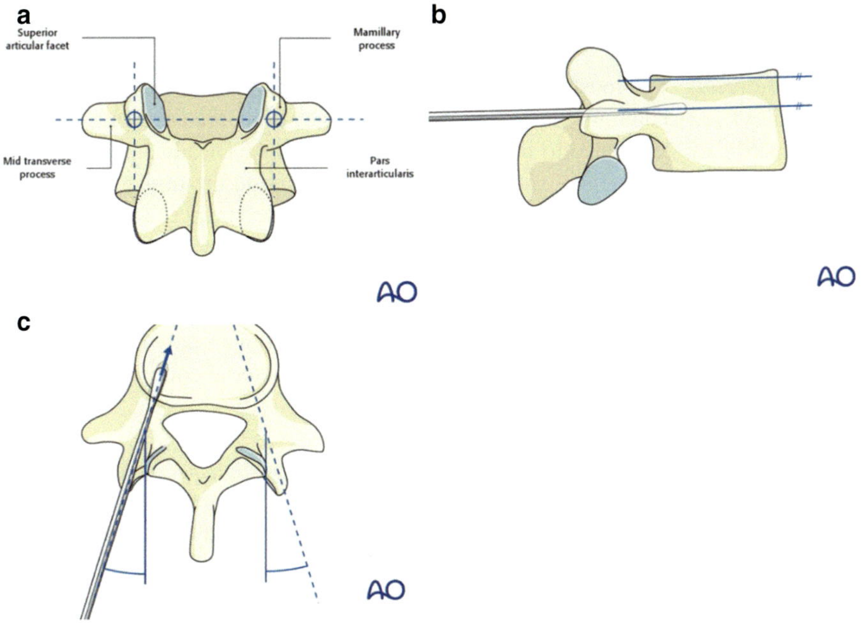

Fig. 23.3 Lumbar pedicle screw placement. (**a**) Pedicle screw entry points in the lumbar spine are at the mamillary process. (**b**) Cranio-caudal angulation is generally aimed parallel with the contralateral transverse process. (**c**) Mediolateral inclination should focus on avoiding superficial penetration of the spinal canal medially, and lateral/anterior perforation of the vertebral body cortex. (Reference: **Reprinted with permission from AO Surgery Reference Online**. URL: https://surgeryreference.aofoundation.org/spine/deformities/scheuermann-kyphosis/further-reading/pedicle-screw-insertion?searchurl=%2fSearchResults)

important to remember that the ventral surface of the vertebral body is convex and thus shorter on the sides than appears on lateral radiograph) [5].

After decortication, a curved or straight pedicle probe is used to create a path through the cancellous bone of the pedicle into the vertebral body. If a curved probe is used, it is initially pointed laterally while probing the pedicle down to roughly 30 mm in order to avoid the central canal, after which it is rotated 180° so that the curve now points medially toward the inner vertebral body. Next, a ball-tipped feeler is introduced into the pedicle to ensure there is no medial, lateral, cranial, caudal, or ventral breech through the floor of the hole. For screws that are not self-tapping, this is followed by tapping the hole with a tap that is smaller in diameter than the anticipated screw. The tap is introduced generally at the depth of the pedicle/vertebral junction. Tapping is then followed by screw placement, which again may be aided by the use of intraoperative fluoroscopy or navigation. After rod connection, the fusion bed is prepared by decorticating around the screw heads along the transverse processes, facet joints, pars, etc. Bone graft is then packed into the fusion bed and the incision is closed in typical fashion.

Technical Advances

Screw Materials The most widely utilized screw material is titanium and its associated alloys [22].Titanium confers several advantages to fixation systems, namely, biocompatibility, resistance to corrosion, and low density. Disadvantages include high elastic modulus, which causes stress shielding around the implant, and high radiodensity, which makes postoperative radiographic assessment of fusion difficult [23]. Recently, nonmetallic, carbon fiber-reinforced polyetheretherketone (CF-PEEK) pedicle screws have shown promise in reducing radiographic artifact while providing similar resistance to loosening as their titanium counterparts [22, 24]. CF-PEEK screw anchorage is substantially improved with polymethylmethacrylate cement augmentation [24], a remarkably strong material commonly used for implants in osteoporotic bone [25].

Fixation Systems Notable recent advances in fixation systems as a whole include wedge-shaped anterior lateral interbody fusion cages with "ratcheting" function to increase angulation in situ, utilization of CF-PEEK for interbody grafts and screws, nanometric roughening of titanium-coated surfaces to improve cellular adhesion and bone ingrowth, and utilization of silicon nitride implants to improve implant antimicrobial activity and biointegration [7]. The recent introduction of robotics to spine surgery has also fueled multiple early investigations into the application of this technology for bony decompression, transforaminal lumbar interbody fusion, facet decortication, and anterior approaches to the spine [26].

Navigation Intraoperative navigation confers the advantage of more accurate screw placement and reduced postoperative revision rates when compared to freehand technique [27]. Current intraoperative verification technologies include real-time, image-guided infrared navigation, O-arm-based navigation, and conventional fluoroscopy [28]. More recently, some headway has been made in the use of artificial/augmented reality for verification, though applications of this technology are varied and remain in early stages [29].

Percutaneous Screws Percutaneous pedicle screw placements have consistently demonstrated numerous advantages compared to open placements, including decreased operative time, blood loss, postoperative pain, infection rate, and length of hospital stay [26]. Although used in a myriad of pathologies, percutaneous pedicle screw placement in a degenerative setting typically requires the use of interbody grafting due to the limitation on posterolateral fusion options [7]. Recent developments of percutaneous screws with robotic assistance hold promise, demonstrating reduced length of hospital stays and radiation exposure compared to open fluoroscopy-guided screw placement [30].

Robotics There is not yet enough evidence to support the accuracy of robot-navigated pedicle screws over more traditional techniques. However, a recent meta-analysis did observe reduced postoperative revision rates with the use of a robot compared to freehand technique [27]. Although multiple robotics platforms have emerged over the past two decades, a steep learning curve exists for surgeons prior to achieving effective implementation of this technology into routine practice [26].

Special Considerations in the Elderly

Osteoporosis Probably the most important consideration in the elderly for pedicle screw placement is bone quality. The prevalence of osteoporosis in Americans >50 years old is as high as 10%, and osteopenia as high as 44% [31]. This becomes particularly important for spine surgeons as poor bone quality is associated with increased risk of kyphosis, fracture, instrument failure, pseudarthrosis, and adjacent level disc degeneration [32]. Furthermore, patients undergoing spinal surgery are more likely to have osteoporosis/osteopenia than aged-matched controls, increasing the likelihood of encountering one of these potential complications [33]. Pedicle screw failures in osteoporotic patients are often from screw pullout or loosening [34–36]. As such, there has been an increased focus on developing strategies to reduce these risks.

Increasing Points of Fixation One possible option to overcome the relatively low density of osteoporotic vertebrae is to increase the number of fixation points utilized. The addition of more fixation points can reduce the stress across any one point [37]. An optimal number of fixation points are three above and three below the apex of spinal deformity to be optimal, although this is not always possible [32].

Screw Selection Increasing the length or diameter of pedicle screws will naturally lead to larger forces required for pullout or screw loosening [9]. However, this also leads to an increased risk of fracture in already weakened bone [38, 39]. A pedicle screw that is tapered distally is believed to enhance fixation in the bone by compressing the surrounding bone structure. This idea appears to hold true in both preclinical models and postoperatively [38, 40–42]. Screw thread design and material makeup also play a role (see above section: *Screw Characteristics*). Taken together, the correct combination of screw length, diameter, thread design, tapering effect, and material makeup can substantially increase pullout strength and provide better rates of fusion and lower risk of instrumentation failure in the osteoporotic spine.

Screw Depth Increasing the depth of screw placement is an important factor for increasing pullout resistance. It appears that 80% pedicle screw insertion into the vertebral body is an appropriate balance to provide significantly increased pullout resistance (which significantly decreases with lesser penetration into the vertebral body) and avoid the risks associated with anterior perforation through vertebral body cortex [43]. Furthermore, it should be noted that the cancellous bone within the pedicle is responsible for affording the pullout resistance in the pedicle, not the pedicle's cortical bone [44]. In osteoporotic bone, bicortical penetration can further increase angular stiffness, although the theoretical risk of anterior cortex penetration is greater [45].

Screw Augmentations Osteoporotic effects on lumbar and thoracic vertebrae are almost exclusively found in trabecular bone [46]. Since the majority of thoracolumbar pedicle screws interface with trabecular bone, one option to improve screw pullout strength is to increase the density of trabecular bone. The use of bone cements or augmenting agents is one such technique. Cannulated or fenestrated screws allow for the injection of various substances that increase surrounding bone density and thus screw purchase. There have been several augmenting materials utilized that led to substantial improvements in pullout strength in both preclinical models and in patients. These include calcium phosphate, hydroxyapatite, and polymethylmethacrylate (PMMA) [47–49]. With regard to augmentation technique, pedicle screws augmented with kyphoplasty appear to have a stronger pullout strength than those with vertebroplasty or those augmented transpedicularly, although all techniques significantly improve pullout strength in osteoporotic bone [50, 51]. With regard to how much PMMA cement to use at each level, the data is inconclusive. Some studies cite significant increase in screw pullout strength with linear increase in amounts of cement from 0.5 to 4.5 cc, while other studies cite no change with these higher cement volumes [51]. In general, it would seem that cement volumes should be greater than 0.5 cc, but volumes greater than 5 cc are rarely indicated and theoretically increase the chance of neurological or cardiovascular adverse events.

Expandable Screws Preclinical studies of expandable pedicle screws have also demonstrated superior pullout strength in osteopenic or osteoporotic bone, although long-term clinical data is more scant [52, 53]. Such options may hold promise in the future with more clear evidence.

Screw Trajectory Another principle to reduce the risk of screw pullout is by altering the trajectory of the screw itself. If the screw threads can interface with more of the denser cortical bone, then pullout strength is theoretically increased [54, 55]. Toeing-in the screw by aiming it slightly more caudal in the sagittal plane will also aid in preventing screw/construct translocation from axial loading.

Challenges

Misplaced Screws The most common complication associated with pedicle screws is misplacement, although the actual rate is variable among different studies and is reasonably user and system dependent. It is important to note that any type of pedicle breech will result in decreased screw purchase and thus worsened pullout strength. Cranial breach of the pedicle screw will result in penetration of the intervertebral disc. Caudal misplacement can result in injury to the exiting nerve root or dura mater. Lateral misplacement can injure the surrounding viscera and segmental vessels. Medial misplacement risks injury to the spinal canal, including the thecal sac, spinal cord, or nerve roots depending on anatomical location.

Mechanisms of Failure Screw failure is usually designated by screw loosening, although the exact criteria for this are uncertain. Lack of good data on this metric in part stems from poorly defined clinical/radiographic standards for screw loosening. Nonetheless, it is generally accepted that screw loosening is associated with screw fracture, non-union, pseudoarthrosis, and progressive kyphosis [56]. In the majority of clinical cases, screw loosening is reported at <1% in non-osteoporotic patients [56]. This risk is increased in osteoporotic bone, reportedly 12.9% in the lumbar spine, although good meta-analyses are lacking [57].

Complication Rates and Safety Overall complication rates from pedicle screw fixation remain low, typically less than 3% [7]. These rates are higher in the setting of unstable injuries and in fixations at the cervical and mid-thoracic spines, where the pedicle morphology presents technical challenges [7]. Surgeons must be vigilant to avoid medial and lateral breaches during placement, which may result in neurovascular or visceral injury. Additionally, traditional open approaches to pedicle screw placement require extensive dissection and exposure of the posterior spinal elements; lengthy operative times, extended blood loss, and increased infection rates are not uncommon [5]. Rigid fixation also has the potential to accelerate adjacent segment degeneration, known as adjacent segment disease. These known risks of pedicle screw placement are generally justified due to the enhanced fusion rate and associated risks of pseudoarthrosis using other fixation techniques or where bone quality/comorbidities decrease fusion likelihood [7, 58].

Accuracy Pedicle screw placement has generally been shown to be more accurate in computer navigated versus freehand placement [59–61]. This increase in accuracy may carry over to robot-navigated screws as well, although current data is still inconclusive [7, 61]. Nonetheless, significantly reduced postoperative revision rates are observed in both robot-guided and robot-navigated placements compared to freehand placements, demonstrating the potential advantage of these technologies when used correctly [27].

Learning Curve A known modifier to accuracy rates is surgeon experience, which manifests as a learning curve. Multiple single-surgeon studies have demonstrated a positive correlation between number of freehand pedicle screw placements and accuracy rates, regardless of the anatomical region [16, 62]. Consequently, some surgeons advocate for the placement of a defined number of pedicle screws under the close supervision of an experienced surgeon prior to independent placements [63]. In the setting of deformative, degenerative, or rheumatic changes, however, this learning curve may, in fact, be steeper, requiring a greater number of repetitions prior to achieving acceptable accuracy rates [63].

Alternatives

Lateral Mass Screws Lateral mass screws are considered less technically challenging to place in the cervical spine than pedicle screws and demonstrate good fusion outcomes, explaining their long-standing popularity among surgeons [12, 64]. Multiple entry points and trajectories have been described in the literature, all of which carry varying risks of injury to neural, vascular, and articular components, but the goal of achieving bicortical screw purchase is shared among these techniques [64]. However, lateral mass screws have demonstrated biomechanical inferiority in comparison to pedicle screws, and the surgeon must weigh the individual risks and benefits on a case-by-case basis [12].

Cortical Screws Cortical pedicle screws are intended to maximize thread contact with hard cortical bone, thereby increasing screw pullout resistance [65]. They are inserted at the inferomedial aspect of the pedicle and follow an inferior-to-superior and medial-to-lateral trajectory (Fig. 23.4) [7].Compared to traditional pedicle screws, cortical pedicle screws have demonstrated similar clinical outcomes and fusion rates, along with decreased blood loss and length of hospital stay [7]. Definitive clinical data on superiority is still lacking.

Transfacet Screws Transfacet screws may be equivalent to pedicle screw fixation with respect to rigidity; however, pedicle screws demonstrate superiority in axial rotation and lateral bending, with no difference in flexion and extension [7]. They follow a trajectory through the facet joint and are typically employed unilaterally as adjuncts to interbody fusion. Transfacet screws are difficult to place at higher lumbar levels due to more vertical facet joint orientations, a challenge that contributes to greater entry point inaccuracies at these levels [7, 66].

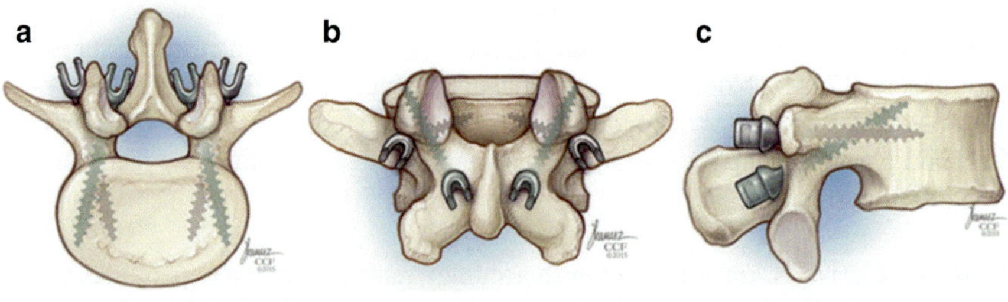

Fig. 23.4 Axial (**a**) and sagittal (**b**) schematics of pedicle screws versus axial (**c**) and sagittal (**d**) schematics of cortical screws and their respective trajectories. (Reference: From Chen Y, Deb S, Pham L, Singh H: Minimally Invasive Lumbar Pedicle Screw Fixation Using Cortical Bone Trajectory – A Prospective Cohort Study on Postoperative Pain Outcomes. *Cureus* 8(7): e714, 2016. **Reproduced with permission**)

Tanslaminar Fixation Similar to transfacet screws, translaminar screws are used as adjuncts to interbody fusion. In such constructs, they demonstrate either equivalent or inferior rigidity in comparison to pedicle screws [7].Translaminar screws are usually used in T1 or T2 alternately to pedicle screws [67]. They are inserted on the contralateral inferior spinous process and follow a trajectory through the ipsilateral lamina and facet joint (Fig. 23.5). The first screw entry point should be slightly cranial to the spinolaminar junction as to allow for placement of the contralateral screw below it (Fig. 23.5a) [67]. The anterior/posterior placement should be planned in the central plane of the contralateral lamina (Fig. 23.5b) [67]. As transmittal of screw forces relies on an intact pedicle, any damage to pedicles precludes use of this screw type [67].

Adjunctive Pelvic and Sacropelvic Fixation Adjunctive pelvic fixation is typically performed in lumbrosacral constructs that start above L3, in order to minimize stress on sacral fixation points which contributes to failure and development of pseudoarthrosis [7]. It is also performed in cases of high-grade spondylolisthesis and global sagittal and/or coronal imbalance [68]. The iliac wing represents the screw entry point and the trajectory is directed toward acetabular cortical bone (Fig. 23.6). Alternatively, S2-alar iliac screws that traverse the sacroiliac joint may also be used (Fig. 23.6). This option has the advantages of in-line screw head position with the remaining lumbrosacral pedicle screw construct, necessitating less dissection of the iliac wing. Furthermore, it may provide lower rates of screw fracture and reoperation compared to iliac wing fixation, and overall lower rates of complications [7, 69].

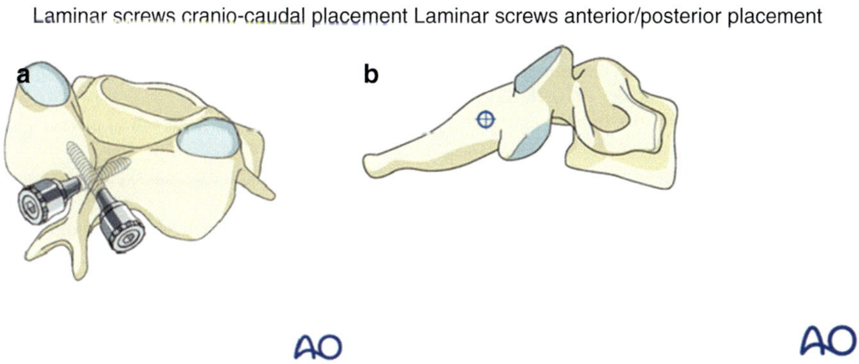

Fig. 23.5 Translaminar screws. (**a**) Laminar screw placement should allow positioning of one screw cranial to the other. (**b**) Anterior/posterior placement should begin slightly cranial at the spinolaminar junction for the first screw, in the central plane of the contralateral lamina. (Reference: **Reprinted with permission from AO Surgery Reference Online**. URL: https://surgeryreference.aofoundation.org/spine/trauma/subaxial-cervical/basic-technique/laminar-screws?searchurl=%2fSearchResults#screw-entry-point)

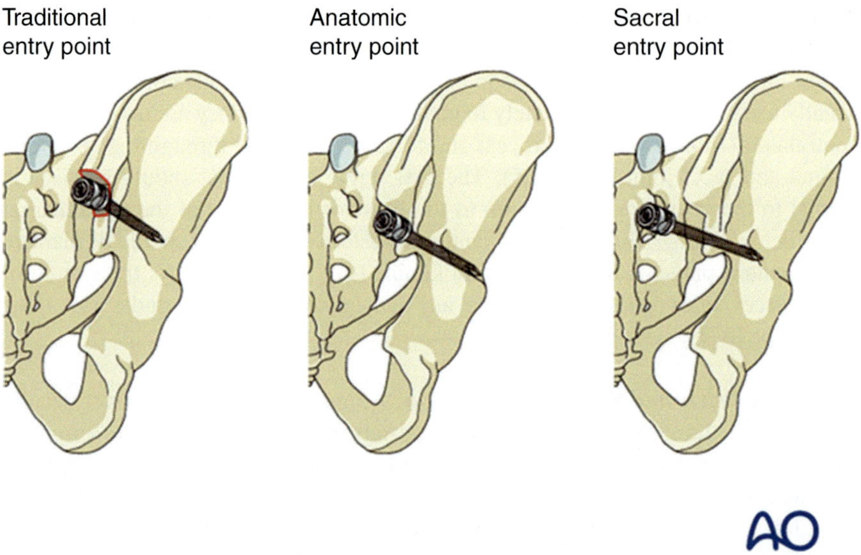

Fig. 23.6 Iliac screw entry points. The traditional entry point (**left**) is countersunk in the posterior iliac crest. The anatomic entry point (**middle**) is more caudal and medial to align better with the lumbar pedicles. The sacral entry point (**right**) is the inferolateral aspect of the S1 foramen. (Reference: **Reprinted with permission from AO Surgery Reference Online**. URL: https://surgeryreference.aofoundation.org/spine/deformities/spondylolisthesis/basic-technique/insertion-of-iliac-screw?searchurl=%2fSearchResults)

References

1. Roy-Camille R, Roy-Camille M, Demeulenaere C. [Osteosynthesis of dorsal, lumbar, and lumbosacral spine with metallic plates screwed into vertebral pedicles and articular apophyses]. La Presse medicale. 1970;78(32):1447–1448.
2. Louis R. Fusion of the lumbar and sacral spine by internal fixation with screw plates. Clin Orthop Relat Res. 1986;203:18–33.
3. Magerl FP. Stabilization of the lower thoracic and lumbar spine with external skeletal fixation. Clin Orthop Relat Res. 1984;189:125–41.
4. Steffee AD, Biscup RS, Sitkowski DJ. Segmental spine plates with pedicle screw fixation. A new internal fixation device for disorders of the lumbar and thoracolumbar spine. Clin Orthop Relat Res. 1986;203:45–53.
5. Benzel EC, Francis TB. Spine surgery: techniques, complication avoidance, and management. Philadelphia, PA: Elsevier/Saunders; 2012.
6. Vaccaro A, Garfin S. Pedicle-screw fixation in the lumbar spine. J Am Acad Orthop Surg. 1995;3:263–74.
7. Reid PC, Morr S, Kaiser MG. State of the union: a review of lumbar fusion indications and techniques for degenerative spine disease. J Neurosurg Spine. 2019;31(1):1–14. https://doi.org/10.3171/2019.4.Spine18915.
8. Krag MH, Weaver DL, Beynnon BD, Haugh LD. Morphometry of the thoracic and lumbar spine related to transpedicular screw placement for surgical spinal fixation. Spine. 1988;13(1):27–32. https://doi.org/10.1097/00007632-198801000-00007.

9. Benzel EC. Biomechanics of spine stabilization: principles and clinical practice. New York: McGraw-Hill; 1995.
10. Fogel GR, Reitman CA, Liu W, Esses SI. Physical characteristics of polyaxial-headed pedicle screws and biomechanical comparison of load with their failure. Spine. 2003;28(5):470–3. https://doi.org/10.1097/01.Brs.0000048652.45964.2e.
11. Bernard TN Jr, Seibert CE. Pedicle diameter determined by computed tomography. Its relevance to pedicle screw fixation in the lumbar spine. Spine. 1992;17(6 Suppl):S160–3. https://doi.org/10.1097/00007632-199206001-00017.
12. Ito Z, Higashino K, Kato S, Kim SS, Wong E, Yoshioka K, et al. Pedicle screws can be 4 times stronger than lateral mass screws for insertion in the midcervical spine: a biomechanical study on strength of fixation. J Spinal Disord Tech. 2014;27(2):80–5. https://doi.org/10.1097/BSD.0b013e31824e65f4.
13. Carlo Bellabarba M, Gruenberg CO. Cervical pedicle screw insertion. surgeryreference.aofoundation.org. Accessed Nov 2020.
14. Hojo Y, Ito M, Suda K, Oda I, Yoshimoto H, Abumi K. A multicenter study on accuracy and complications of freehand placement of cervical pedicle screws under lateral fluoroscopy in different pathological conditions: CT-based evaluation of more than 1,000 screws. Eur Spine J. 2014;23(10):2166–74. https://doi.org/10.1007/s00586-014-3470-0.
15. Abumi K. Cervical spondylotic myelopathy: posterior decompression and pedicle screw fixation. Eur Spine J. 2015;24(Suppl 2):186–96. https://doi.org/10.1007/s00586-015-3838-9.
16. Tan KA, Lin S, Chin BZ, Thadani VN, Hey HWD. Anatomic techniques for cervical pedicle screw placement. J Spine Surg. 2020;6(1):262–73. https://doi.org/10.21037/jss.2020.03.07.
17. Puvanesarajah V, Liauw JA, Lo SF, Lina IA, Witham TF. Techniques and accuracy of thoracolumbar pedicle screw placement. World J Orthop. 2014;5(2):112–23. https://doi.org/10.5312/wjo.v5.i2.112.
18. Vialle E. Pedicle screw insertion. https://surgeryreference.aofoundation.org/. Accessed Nov 2020.
19. Perna F, Borghi R, Pilla F, Stefanini N, Mazzotti A, Chehrassan M. Pedicle screw insertion techniques: an update and review of the literature. Musculoskelet Surg. 2016;100(3):165–9. https://doi.org/10.1007/s12306-016-0438-8.
20. Fennell VS, Palejwala S, Skoch J, Stidd DA, Baaj AA. Freehand thoracic pedicle screw technique using a uniform entry point and sagittal trajectory for all levels: preliminary clinical experience. J Neurosurg Spine. 2014;21(5):778–84. https://doi.org/10.3171/2014.7.Spine1489.
21. Parker SL, McGirt MJ, Farber SH, Amin AG, Rick AM, Suk I, et al. Accuracy of free-hand pedicle screws in the thoracic and lumbar spine: analysis of 6816 consecutive screws. Neurosurgery. 2011;68(1):170–8; discussion 8. https://doi.org/10.1227/NEU.0b013e3181fdfaf4.
22. Fleege C, Makowski M, Rauschmann M, Fraunhoffer KL, Fennema P, Arabmotlagh M, et al. Carbon fiber-reinforced pedicle screws reduce artifacts in magnetic resonance imaging of patients with lumbar spondylodesis. Sci Rep. 2020;10(1):16094. https://doi.org/10.1038/s41598-020-73386-5.
23. Rao PJ, Pelletier MH, Walsh WR, Mobbs RJ. Spine interbody implants: material selection and modification, functionalization and bioactivation of surfaces to improve osseointegration. Orthop Surg. 2014;6(2):81–9. https://doi.org/10.1111/os.12098.
24. Lindtner RA, Schmid R, Nydegger T, Konschake M, Schmoelz W. Pedicle screw anchorage of carbon fiber-reinforced PEEK screws under cyclic loading. Eur Spine J. 2018;27(8):1775–84. https://doi.org/10.1007/s00586-018-5538-8.
25. Liu D, Shi L, Lei W, Wei MQ, Qu B, Deng SL, et al. Biomechanical comparison of expansive pedicle screw and polymethylmethacrylate-augmented pedicle screw in osteoporotic synthetic bone in primary implantation: an experimental study. Clin Spine Surg. 2016;29(7):E351–7. https://doi.org/10.1097/BSD.0b013e31828bfc85.
26. Staub BN, Sadrameli SS. The use of robotics in minimally invasive spine surgery. J Spine Surg. 2019;5(Suppl 1):S31–s40. https://doi.org/10.21037/jss.2019.04.16.

27. Staartjes VE, Klukowska AM, Schröder ML. Pedicle screw revision in robot-guided, navigated, and freehand thoracolumbar instrumentation: a systematic review and meta-analysis. World Neurosurg. 2018;116:433–43.e8. https://doi.org/10.1016/j.wneu.2018.05.159.
28. Mao JZ, Agyei JO, Khan A, Hess RM, Jowdy PK, Mullin JP, et al. Technologic evolution of navigation and robotics in spine surgery: a historical perspective. World Neurosurg. 2020;145:159–67. https://doi.org/10.1016/j.wneu.2020.08.224.
29. Elmi-Terander A, Burström G, Nachabé R, Fagerlund M, Ståhl F, Charalampidis A, et al. Augmented reality navigation with intraoperative 3D imaging vs fluoroscopy-assisted freehand surgery for spine fixation surgery: a matched-control study comparing accuracy. Sci Rep. 2020;10(1):707. https://doi.org/10.1038/s41598-020-57693-5.
30. Hyun SJ, Kim KJ, Jahng TA, Kim HJ. Minimally invasive robotic versus open fluoroscopic-guided spinal instrumented fusions: a randomized controlled trial. Spine. 2017;42(6):353–8. https://doi.org/10.1097/brs.0000000000001778.
31. Wright NC, Looker AC, Saag KG, Curtis JR, Delzell ES, Randall S, et al. The recent prevalence of osteoporosis and low bone mass in the United States based on bone mineral density at the femoral neck or lumbar spine. J Bone Miner Res. 2014;29(11):2520–6. https://doi.org/10.1002/jbmr.2269.
32. DeWald CJ, Stanley T. Instrumentation-related complications of multilevel fusions for adult spinal deformity patients over age 65: surgical considerations and treatment options in patients with poor bone quality. Spine (Phila Pa 1976). 2006;31(19 Suppl):S144–51. https://doi.org/10.1097/01.brs.0000236893.65878.39.
33. Chin DK, Park JY, Yoon YS, Kuh SU, Jin BH, Kim KS, et al. Prevalence of osteoporosis in patients requiring spine surgery: incidence and significance of osteoporosis in spine disease. Osteoporos Int. 2007;18(9):1219–24. https://doi.org/10.1007/s00198-007-0370-8.
34. Coe JD, Warden KE, Herzig MA, McAfee PC. Influence of bone mineral density on the fixation of thoracolumbar implants. A comparative study of transpedicular screws, laminar hooks, and spinous process wires. Spine (Phila Pa 1976). 1990;15(9):902–7. https://doi.org/10.1097/00007632-199009000-00012.
35. Gilbert SG, Johns PC, Chow DC, Black RC. Relation of vertebral bone screw axial pull-out strength to quantitative computed tomographic trabecular bone mineral content. J Spinal Disord. 1993;6(6):513–21. https://doi.org/10.1097/00002517-199306060-00007.
36. Hitchon PW, Brenton MD, Coppes JK, From AM, Torner JC. Factors affecting the pullout strength of self-drilling and self-tapping anterior cervical screws. Spine (Phila Pa 1976). 2003;28(1):9–13. https://doi.org/10.1097/00007632-200301010-00004.
37. Hu SS. Internal fixation in the osteoporotic spine. Spine (Phila Pa 1976). 1997;22(24 Suppl):43S–8S. https://doi.org/10.1097/00007632-199712151-00008.
38. Hsu CC, Chao CK, Wang JL, Hou SM, Tsai YT, Lin J. Increase of pullout strength of spinal pedicle screws with conical core: biomechanical tests and finite element analyses. J Orthop Res. 2005;23(4):788–94. https://doi.org/10.1016/j.orthres.2004.11.002.
39. Patel PS, Shepherd DE, Hukins DW. The effect of screw insertion angle and thread type on the pullout strength of bone screws in normal and osteoporotic cancellous bone models. Med Eng Phys. 2010;32(8):822–8. https://doi.org/10.1016/j.medengphy.2010.05.005.
40. Krenn MH, Piotrowski WP, Penzkofer R, Augat P. Influence of thread design on pedicle screw fixation. Laboratory investigation. J Neurosurg Spine. 2008;9(1):90–5. https://doi.org/10.3171/SPI/2008/9/7/090.
41. Kim YY, Choi WS, Rhyu KW. Assessment of pedicle screw pullout strength based on various screw designs and bone densities-an ex vivo biomechanical study. Spine J. 2012;12(2):164–8. https://doi.org/10.1016/j.spinee.2012.01.014.
42. Chao CK, Hsu CC, Wang JL, Lin J. Increasing bending strength and pullout strength in conical pedicle screws: biomechanical tests and finite element analyses. J Spinal Disord Tech. 2008;21(2):130–8. https://doi.org/10.1097/BSD.0b013e318073cc4b.

43. Helton Defino FG, Wilke H-J. Lumbar spine online textbook. Section 11: surgery principles. Online: The International Society for the Study of the Lumbar Spine and Data Trace Internet Publishing; 2020.
44. Defino HL, Vendrame JR. Role of cortical and cancellous bone of the vertebral pedicle in implant fixation. Eur Spine J. 2001;10(4):325–33. https://doi.org/10.1007/s005860000232.
45. Karami KJ, Buckenmeyer LE, Kiapour AM, Kelkar PS, Goel VK, Demetropoulos CK, et al. Biomechanical evaluation of the pedicle screw insertion depth effect on screw stability under cyclic loading and subsequent pullout. J Spinal Disord Tech. 2015;28(3):E133–9. https://doi.org/10.1097/bsd.0000000000000178.
46. Chen LH, Tai CL, Lee DM, Lai PL, Lee YC, Niu CC, et al. Pullout strength of pedicle screws with cement augmentation in severe osteoporosis: a comparative study between cannulated screws with cement injection and solid screws with cement pre-filling. BMC Musculoskelet Disord. 2011;12:33. https://doi.org/10.1186/1471-2474-12-33.
47. Taniwaki Y, Takemasa R, Tani T, Mizobuchi H, Yamamoto H. Enhancement of pedicle screw stability using calcium phosphate cement in osteoporotic vertebrae: in vivo biomechanical study. J Orthop Sci. 2003;8(3):408–14. https://doi.org/10.1007/s10776-003-0639-6.
48. Hickerson LE, Owen JR, Wayne JS, Tuten HR. Calcium triglyceride versus polymethylmethacrylate augmentation: a biomechanical analysis of pullout strength. Spine Deform. 2013;1(1):10–5. https://doi.org/10.1016/j.jspd.2012.07.004.
49. Stadelmann VA, Bretton E, Terrier A, Procter P, Pioletti DP. Calcium phosphate cement augmentation of cancellous bone screws can compensate for the absence of cortical fixation. J Biomech. 2010;43(15):2869–74. https://doi.org/10.1016/j.jbiomech.2010.07.025.
50. Burval DJ, McLain RF, Milks R, Inceoglu S. Primary pedicle screw augmentation in osteoporotic lumbar vertebrae: biomechanical analysis of pedicle fixation strength. Spine. 2007;32(10):1077–83. https://doi.org/10.1097/01.brs.0000261566.38422.40.
51. Elder BD, Lo SF, Holmes C, Goodwin CR, Kosztowski TA, Lina IA, et al. The biomechanics of pedicle screw augmentation with cement. Spine J. 2015;15(6):1432–45. https://doi.org/10.1016/j.spinee.2015.03.016.
52. Vishnubhotla S, McGarry WB, Mahar AT, Gelb DE. A titanium expandable pedicle screw improves initial pullout strength as compared with standard pedicle screws. Spine J. 2011;11(8):777–81. https://doi.org/10.1016/j.spinee.2011.06.006.
53. Chen YL, Chen WC, Chou CW, Chen JW, Chang CM, Lai YS, et al. Biomechanical study of expandable pedicle screw fixation in severe osteoporotic bone comparing with conventional and cement-augmented pedicle screws. Med Eng Phys. 2014;36(11):1416–20. https://doi.org/10.1016/j.medengphy.2014.05.003.
54. Santoni BG, Hynes RA, McGilvray KC, Rodriguez-Canessa G, Lyons AS, Henson MA, et al. Cortical bone trajectory for lumbar pedicle screws. Spine J. 2009;9(5):366–73. https://doi.org/10.1016/j.spinee.2008.07.008.
55. Wray S, Mimran R, Vadapalli S, Shetye SS, McGilvray KC, Puttlitz CM. Pedicle screw placement in the lumbar spine: effect of trajectory and screw design on acute biomechanical purchase. J Neurosurg Spine. 2015;22(5):503–10. https://doi.org/10.3171/2014.10.SPINE14205.
56. Galbusera F, Volkheimer D, Reitmaier S, Berger-Roscher N, Kienle A, Wilke HJ. Pedicle screw loosening: a clinically relevant complication? Eur Spine J. 2015;24(5):1005–16. https://doi.org/10.1007/s00586-015-3768-6.
57. Wu ZX, Gong FT, Liu L, Ma ZS, Zhang Y, Zhao X, et al. A comparative study on screw loosening in osteoporotic lumbar spine fusion between expandable and conventional pedicle screws. Arch Orthop Trauma Surg. 2012;132(4):471–6. https://doi.org/10.1007/s00402-011-1439-6.
58. Groff MW, Dailey AT, Ghogawala Z, Resnick DK, Watters WC III, Mummaneni PV, et al. Guideline update for the performance of fusion procedures for degenerative disease of the lumbar spine. Part 12: pedicle screw fixation as an adjunct to posterolateral fusion. Journal of neurosurgery. Spine. 2014;21(1):75–8. https://doi.org/10.3171/2014.4.Spine14277.

59. Laine T, Lund T, Ylikoski M, Lohikoski J, Schlenzka D. Accuracy of pedicle screw insertion with and without computer assistance: a randomised controlled clinical study in 100 consecutive patients. Eur Spine J. 2000;9(3):235–40. https://doi.org/10.1007/s005860000146.
60. Rajasekaran S, Vidyadhara S, Ramesh P, Shetty A. Randomized clinical study to compare the accuracy of navigated and non-navigated thoracic pedicle screws in deformity correction surgeries. Spine. 2007;32:E56–64.
61. Perdomo-Pantoja A, Ishida W, Zygourakis C, Holmes C, Iyer RR, Cottrill E, et al. Accuracy of current techniques for placement of pedicle screws in the spine: a comprehensive systematic review and meta-analysis of 51,161 screws. World Neurosurg. 2019;126:664–78.e3. https://doi.org/10.1016/j.wneu.2019.02.217.
62. Samdani AF, Ranade A, Saldanha V, Yondorf MZ. Learning curve for placement of thoracic pedicle screws in the deformed spine. Neurosurgery. 2010;66(2):290–4.; discussion 4–5. https://doi.org/10.1227/01.Neu.0000363853.62897.94.
63. Gonzalvo A, Fitt G, Liew S, de la Harpe D, Turner P, Ton L, et al. The learning curve of pedicle screw placement: how many screws are enough? Spine. 2009;34(21):E761–5. https://doi.org/10.1097/BRS.0b013e3181b2f928.
64. Mikhail CM, Dowdell JE III, Hecht AC. Posterior fusion for the subaxial cervical spine: a review of the major techniques. HSS J. 2020;16(2):188–94. https://doi.org/10.1007/s11420-019-09722-x.
65. Hu JN, Yang XF, Li CM, Li XX, Ding YZ. Comparison of cortical bone trajectory versus pedicle screw techniques in lumbar fusion surgery: a meta-analysis. Medicine. 2019;98(33):e16751. https://doi.org/10.1097/md.0000000000016751.
66. Felbaum DR, Lajthia O, Syed HR, Voyadzis JM. Percutaneous lumbar transfacet screw fixation: a technique analysis of 176 screws in 83 patients with assessment of radiographic accuracy, hardware failure, and complications. Oper Neurosurg (Hagerstown). 2016;12(4):340–9. https://doi.org/10.1227/neu.0000000000001356.
67. Carlo Bellabarba M, Gruenberg CO. Laminar screws. surgeryreference.aofoundation.org. Accessed Nov 2020.
68. Lombardi JM, Shillingford JN, Lenke LG, Lehman RA. Sacropelvic fixation: when, why, how? Neurosurg Clin N Am. 2018;29(3):389–97. https://doi.org/10.1016/j.nec.2018.02.001.
69. Hasan MY, Liu G, Wong HK, Tan JH. Postoperative complications of S2AI versus iliac screw in spinopelvic fixation: a meta-analysis and recent trends review. Spine J. 2020;20(6):964–72. https://doi.org/10.1016/j.spinee.2019.11.014.

Chapter 24
Treatment of Spine Disease in the Elderly: Cutting-Edge Techniques and Technologies

Daniel B. C. Reid and Robert K. Eastlack

Introduction

The modern history of spine surgery is intimately intertwined with the development and application of advanced radiographic imaging modalities. Widely utilized radiographic techniques for diagnosis and treatment of spinal pathologies include plain radiographs, computed tomography (CT), myelography, magnetic resonance imaging (MRI), nuclear medicine, dual-energy X-ray absorptiometry (DEXA), and whole-body imaging modalities such as EOS. Further adding to the complex nature of imaging in the spine, a wide variability of techniques and protocols exists within each subcategory. Astute spine surgeons, neuroradiologists, and other clinicians managing spinal diseases must effectively manage the ever-expanding universe of anatomic and functional data in ways which are evidence-based, cost-effective, efficient, and patient-centered.

Plain Radiographs

Plain radiographs have been a mainstay in diagnosis and treatment of musculoskeletal and spinal pathologies since shortly after their discovery by Wilhelm Röntgen in 1895 [1]. Today, plain radiographs are available widely, even in most resource-poor areas. In comparison to other modalities, they remain inexpensive and efficient. While plain radiographs clearly lack the ability of CT and MRI to

D. B. C. Reid · R. K. Eastlack (✉)
San Diego Spine Foundation, San Diego, CA, USA
e-mail: Eastlack.Robert@scrippshealth.org

K.-M. G. Fu et al. (eds.), *Treatment of Spine Disease in the Elderly*,
https://doi.org/10.1007/978-3-031-12612-3_24

visualize bony structures in three dimensions or directly visualize soft tissues and neural structures, they nonetheless cheaply and efficiently provide critical information on alignment, instrumentation, and dynamic stability. Furthermore, X-rays are reasonable and cost-efficient modalities for routine postoperative follow-up care [2, 3].

Despite progress in advanced imaging, plain radiographs continue to drive spinal diagnosis, treatment, and research. They are particularly useful in determining stability and flexibility (Fig. 24.1). For example, in patients with degenerative spondylolisthesis and spinal stenosis, the determining factor between isolated decompressive procedures and instrumented fusion is often segmental motion on flexion-extension films or comparison of standing plain films to supine imaging modalities [4–6]. Similarly, in patients being considered for correction of spinal deformity, preoperative bending films may help surgeons determine the most appropriate surgical plan [7]. Finally, the various pelvic and spinal parameters which are widely used to assess global and focal spinal balance are most commonly measured on plain radiographs, both in the literature and in clinical practice [8–12].

Notably, various techniques for optimizing the results of long-alignment radiographs have been described. The supraclavicular placement of the hands by the patient during attainment of such imaging has been popularized as a method to reduce the artifact in alignment interpretation that may otherwise occur when leaning on objects or holding on to bars. Importantly, long-alignment and lumbar radiographs require the concomitant capture of both femoral heads in order to ascertain pelvic morphology parameters, such as pelvic incidence, as well as compensatory metrics like pelvic tilt. One of the challenges of standard radiography has been the inability to concurrently capture the position of the lower extremities. Given the importance of hip and knee flexion in altering spinopelvic parameters, most notably sagittal vertical axis, radiology technicians must be well-educated on the critical aspects of properly instructing patients during attainment of these radiographs. Newer technologies, such as EOS, which allow for full-body capture, allow for an improved awareness of these peripheral compensation or contributory alignment conditions.

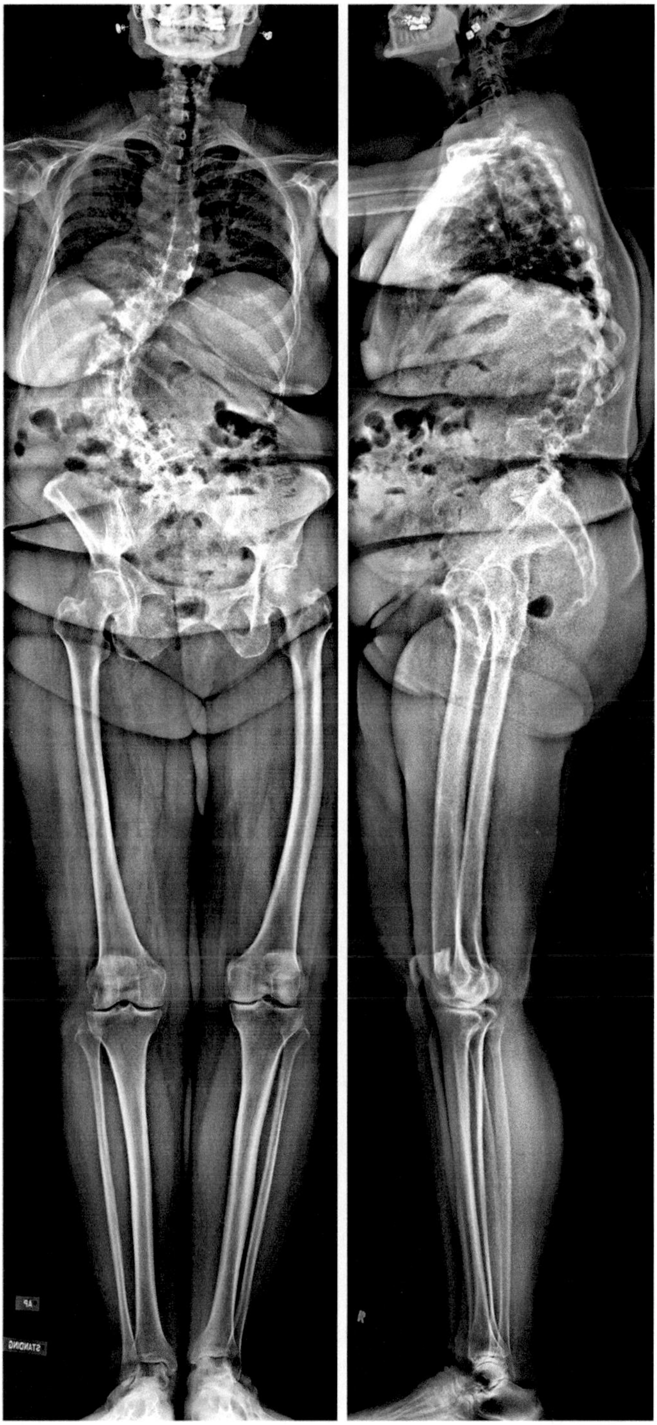

Fig. 24.1 Preoperative full-length standing anterior-posterior and lateral EOS films

Computed Tomography (CT)

The first CT was developed by Dr. Godfrey Hounsfield in the early 1970s [13]. In its most simple form, computed tomography utilizes a rotating X-ray source to capture radiographs at various angles to the body, and a computer to reconstruct the radiographs into cross-sectional images. This form of imaging has improved our ability to understand individualized bony anatomy from a three-dimensional perspective, enhanced the clarity over plain radiographs, increased the specificity and sensitivity for detecting fractures in trauma settings, and facilitated the intraoperative use navigation and robotics in spine surgery [14–19]. While CT does provide some enhanced ability to visualize structures which may compress on neural elements, particularly if such structures are bony or calcified [20, 21], the direct visualization of neural structures remains poor. CT myelography, in which contrast material is injected into the thecal sac prior to CT scanning, was developed to address this shortcoming. While still utilized for this purpose in patients unable to tolerate MRI, CT myelography is used less commonly today that in the past secondary to the widespread availability of MRI scanners (Fig. 24.2).

CT is often analyzed in conjunction with MRI to help differentiate between compressive pathologies which are bony/calcified and those which are soft tissue in nature [20, 21]. Recent use of CT scans to determine bone mineral density at the site of proposed surgery by measurement of Hounsfield units has been proposed for determining safe upper instrumented vertebrae in cases of adult spinal deformity to prevent screw pullout and proximal junctional kyphosis [22–24].

Preoperative CT findings may lead to an alteration in surgical approach, and may enable safer surgical techniques, with less chance for unexpected intraoperative findings. Additionally, the supine nature of the imaging capture can afford the perspective of a relaxed spine and thus provide a sense of dynamic flexibility within the imaged regions that may further inform the surgeon regarding corrective techniques required to realign the spine. Vacuum disk changes within individual motion segments provide helpful insight into motion capacity and typically suggest less rigorous requirement for inducing angular changes within those segments. Another important value of CT imaging is providing for better understanding of bony dysmorphology, such as coronal wedging of vertebra, or sacral promontory obliquity, which may also impact the choice of reconstructive methods. Finally, because of the high-resolution bone resolution rendering, CT can also be helpful in selecting fixation options that will be ideal and feasibly deployed during surgery. Although intraoperative CT is utilized in many centers for navigation while placing pedicle screws and other spinal instrumentation, its use remains controversial secondary to concerns regarding increased cost, radiation exposure, and operating time compared to traditional freehand or fluoroscopic techniques [25–27].

CT has improved significantly over the years in many facets; however, it is not without its disadvantages. These include substantial radiation exposure, increased cost, inability to perform dynamic or standing studies, and a frequent reliance on radiology technicians rather than surgeons to determine appropriate planes for multiplanar reconstructions.

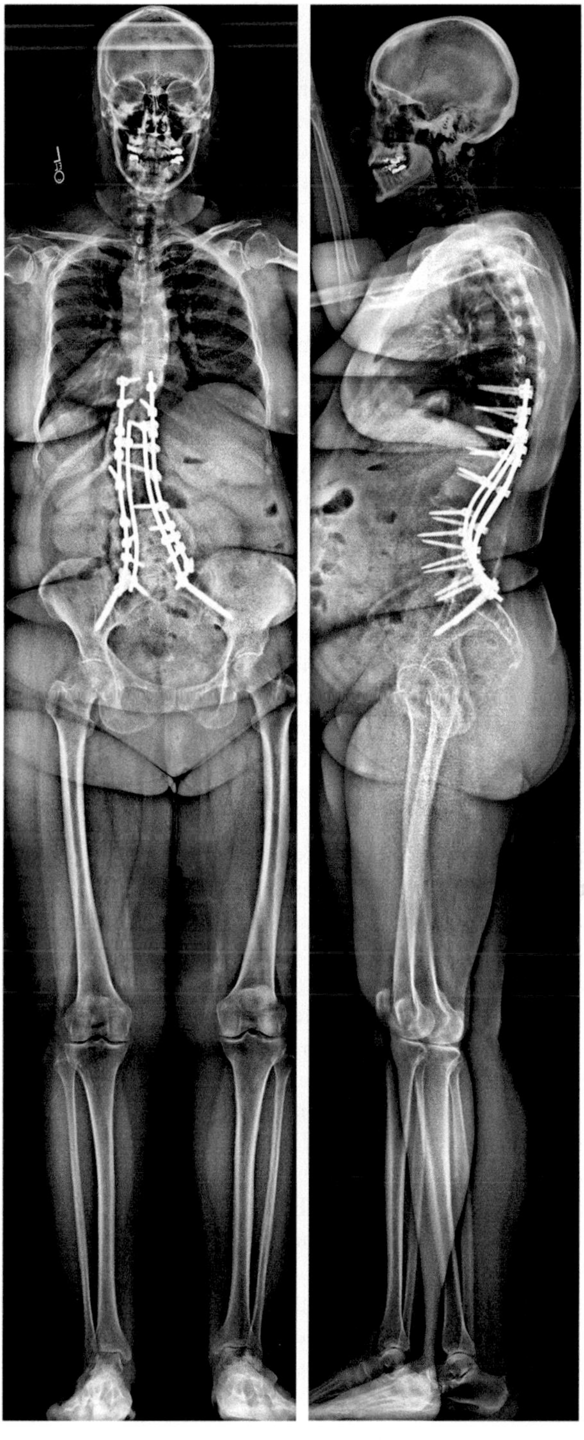

Fig. 24.2 One-year postoperative full-length standing anterior-posterior and lateral EOS films

Magnetic Resonance Imaging (MRI)

MRI utilizes strong magnetic fields to induce polarization in hydrogen molecules, which are localized in space by magnetic field gradients and used to generate anatomic imaging. While the MRI was first developed in the 1970s [28], it was not adapted for human use until the late 1980s and 1990s [29, 30]. MRI provides direct imaging of bone as well as soft tissue elements including disc spaces, cartilage, muscles, ligaments, and neural elements. As such, it has become the standard imaging modality for diagnosis of most spinal pathologies. In addition to localizing areas of neural compression, further progress in magnet strength and resolution of MRI imaging over the years has allowed for better characterization and classification of degenerative spinal changes associated with pain and disability [31–33].

While it is generally thought of as less useful than CT for evaluation of bony structures, MRI may be superior when evaluating bone marrow and determining acuity of injury in cases of fracture [34, 35]. For the majority of spinal imaging, MR pulse sequences include T1, T2, and short-tau inversion recovery (STIR). These sequences are frequently reconstructed in axial, sagittal, and coronal views for review. Unfortunately, as with CT, the specific cutlines (gantry) utilized to determine the axial cuts are most commonly determined by radiology technicians and may not be applicable for the needs of a reviewing surgeon. T1-weighted imaging may be obtained before and after administration of gadolinium in the setting of recent surgery or concern for infection/tumor in order to increase study sensitivity [36–38]. STIR sequence imaging is often utilized to determine injury acuity, integrity of the posterior osteo-ligamentous complex, and integrity of the anterior disco-ligamentous complex in the setting of suspected unstable spinal injury [34, 35, 39–42].

An important advantage of MRI is its ability to visualize surrounding anatomic soft tissue structures which may be germane to preoperative planning. For example, an adequate and individualized understanding of the great vessels, peritoneal contents, and iliopsoas anatomy is vital for safe anterior, oblique, and lateral approaches to the lumbar spine [43–46]. More advanced MRI modalities including dynamic MRI [47, 48], magnetic resonance myelography [49], magnetic resonance neurography [50], and MR spectroscopy [51] have been described and may be helpful for specific indications. Nonetheless, routine MRI continues to be among the mainstays for diagnosis for the large majority of spinal conditions secondary to its availability, lack of ionizing radiation, direct view of neural elements, and high sensitivity.

The primary disadvantage of MRI includes potential incompatibility with certain metallic implants and foreign bodies. MRI in the setting of such devices may result in implant movement, increased implant temperature, and patient harm. While recent evidence has called such strict contraindications to MRI into question [52], few centers routinely perform MRIs on patients with non-MRI-conditional implants. Furthermore, a rare but potentially damaging complication of gadolinium contrast used with MRI in some patients, nephrogenic systemic fibrosis, has been described [53]. From a logistical standpoint, MRI examination of the spine typically takes significantly longer to perform than plain films or CT, which may affect access and timely acquisition of imaging, especially in cases of trauma. Additionally, claustrophobia in MRI tubes is relatively common among patients and may affect the quality and/or availability of imaging for review [54, 55]. Other factors which may affect image quality for interpretation include magnet strength, operator experience, patient motion, and imaging artifact from implants. Stainless steel implants, in particular, are known to result in significant artifact; however, other materials may also result in varying levels of image degradation. Such artifact may severely compromise the utility of spinal MRIs in patients with a history of spinal instrumentation, particularly if the area of concern is in the vicinity of said implants. Finally, MRIs have been shown to be highly sensitive for picking up anatomic abnormalities of which the clinical relevance is questionable. Degenerative pathologies seen on MRI do not always correlate with patient symptoms, and MRI findings are commonly clinically insignificant [32, 56, 57]. As such, a careful and evidence-based synthesis of MRI findings, clinical history, and physical examination remains important for clinicians determining optimal treatment options.

Nuclear Medicine

The use of nuclear medicine in evaluation of the spine has historically been focused on evaluating spinal metastatic disease. Specifically, bone scintigraphy with technetium 99 and 18F-fluorodeoxyglucose positron emission tomography (PET) imaging are commonly utilized, with other radiotracers available for niche indications [58]. Indium-111-labeled white blood cell tracers are also available and have shown high specificity but low sensitivity for detection of spinal infection [59, 60]. Recent use of single-photon emission computed tomography (CT-SPECT) scanning for evaluation of discogenic and facet-mediated pain has been described, but its specificity and sensitivity for various degenerative spinal pathologies remain incompletely understood [61–63]. Recently, there have been reports of utilizing SPECT to provide guidance on selective fusions within the context of spinal deformity, which may lead to more cost-effective and less morbid applications of surgical intervention [64].

Dual-Energy X-Ray Absorptiometry (DEXA)

As opposed to the modalities discussed earlier in this chapter, DEXA scans do not provide especially relevant anatomic information. Rather, they are utilized to determine bone mineral density and diagnose osteopenia and osteoporosis, which is of critical importance when planning deformity surgery in the elderly. DEXA scores are typically reported in T-scores which refer the standard deviation of a patient's bone mineral density compared to a young adult at peak bone health of the same gender [65]. Generally, osteopenia is defined by a T-score of −1.0 to −2.5, whereas osteoporosis is defined by a T-score below −2.5 [65]. Such information is especially useful for those caring for patients sustaining fragility fractures as well as those planning for surgery requiring spinal instrumentation. Common targets for DEXA scanning include the lumbar spine, hip, and wrist. Importantly, clinicians should be aware of and account for the fact that the reported bone mineral density may be artificially elevated in areas of osteoarthritis. This is especially relevant to spine surgeons, as the lumbar spine DEXA score may be reported within normal limits, while the patient scores in the osteopenic or osteoporotic range in the hip or wrist. Furthermore, because concomitant lumbar spine and hip arthritis is common, DEXA scans of the wrist may provide the most accurate assessment of bone mineral density in many spine patients [66].

Patients being treated for fragility fractures, including spinal compression fractures, should undergo an assessment of their bone mineral density as part of routine preventative measures against further fragility fractures [67, 68]. DEXA scanning is also useful in preoperative planning prior to instrumented spinal fusion cases. Patients with osteoporosis may benefit from medical treatment, particularly with anabolic agents, prior to surgery [69, 70]. Even in patients who are not candidates for preoperative treatment of osteoporosis, such knowledge may result in alteration of surgical plans. Longer fusion constructs, vertebroplasty, ligament augmentation, hook fixation, and terminal rod contouring, for example, have all been proposed to prevent proximal junctional kyphosis in adult spinal deformity patients with poor bone quality [69, 71].

Full-Body Imaging and EOS

The importance of the use of full-length supine and standing spinal films for accurate evaluation of global sagittal and coronal alignment has been known for some time [72–74]. Furthermore, a recent expansion in evidence-based literature quantifying the important role of the hips and lower extremities in determining global spinal alignment, balance, and function has increased interest in evaluating the spine and lower extremities in unison [75–78]. However, until recently, the ability to obtain full-body imaging efficiently and effectively was largely unattainable at most institutions. The recent advent of the EOS imaging system (EOS Imaging, Paris, France) has shifted this paradigm. The EOS imaging system is a low-dose biplanar digital X-ray system. It consists of a booth in which the patient is positioned either standing, sitting, or both. Two biplanar X-ray sources move together with their associated detectors to scan the patient simultaneously. This allows for full-length 2D sagittal and coronal images of the whole body with significantly less distortion (e.g., parallax) than traditional radiographs [79]. Furthermore, because the booth is calibrated and the AP and lateral images are obtained simultaneously, stereoradiography can be utilized to create 3D reconstructions of the spine and lower limbs [79, 80]. The patient's radiation dose is thought to be 50–80% lower than with conventional radiographs [79], which may be clinically relevant in young patients and those requiring frequent X-rays. Software-based calculations of spinal parameters are also available and have been shown to be similar to manual measurements by surgeons [81–83]. The effect of gravity on global and focal spinal alignment as determined by comparison of supine to standing imaging has been described and is important for surgeons when evaluating dynamic spinal instability, flexibility of curves, and dynamic loss of disc height [84]. Such comparisons have been shown to alter management of multiple spinal pathologies [4, 84–88]. Because EOS imaging is typically obtained in an upright (standing or sitting) position, the imaging may be compared to supine imaging in order to understand the effect of gravity on spinal pathology. A recent study comparing standing EOS films to supine CT scans in adult spinal deformity patients found that standing position resulted in significantly greater mean cobb and rotational angles in the major curve, more loss of lumbar lordosis, and increased pelvic tilt [84].

Shortcomings of EOS include a lack of detail for focal segments secondary to decreased radiation dosage protocols. Thus, in cases in which detailed views of focal pathology are necessary, targeted radiographs are still often required.

Conclusion

The advancement in diagnosis and treatment of spinal disease has occurred in tandem with the development of novel imaging techniques. The complexity inherent to managing spinal conditions is accompanied by a complicated armamentarium of imaging options. Clinicians treating patients with spinal pathology must assess diagnostic accuracy, cost, efficiency, invasiveness, and availability of various imaging modalities to provide the best care to their patients. While this task is fundamentally challenging and requires lifelong learning to keep up with technologic and evidence-based advancement, it is undeniably crucial in the care of our patients.

References

1. Harada GK, Siyaji ZK, Younis S, et al. Imaging in spine surgery: current concepts and future directions. Spine Surg Relat Res. 2020;4:99–110.
2. Rhee JM, Chapman JR, Norvell DC, et al. Radiological determination of postoperative cervical fusion: a systematic review. Spine (Phila Pa 1976). 2015;40:974–91.
3. Venu V, Vertinsky AT, Malfair D, et al. Plain radiograph assessment of spinal hardware. Semin Musculoskelet Radiol. 2011;15:151–62.
4. Chan V, Marro A, Rempel J, et al. Determination of dynamic instability in lumbar spondylolisthesis using flexion and extension standing radiographs versus neutral standing radiograph and supine MRI. J Neurosurg Spine. 2019;31:229–35.
5. Wood KB, Popp CA, Transfeldt EE, et al. Radiographic evaluation of instability in spondylolisthesis. Spine (Phila Pa 1976). 1994;19:1697–703.

6. Burhan Janjua M, Tishelman JC, Vasquez-Montes D, et al. The value of sitting radiographs: analysis of spine flexibility and its utility in preoperative planning for adult spinal deformity surgery. J Neurosurg Spine. 2018;29:414–21.
7. Yao G, Cheung JPY, Shigematsu H, et al. Characterization and predictive value of segmental curve flexibility in adolescent idiopathic scoliosis patients. Spine (Phila Pa 1976). 2017;42:1622–8.
8. Schwab FJ, Blondel B, Bess S, et al. Radiographical spinopelvic parameters and disability in the setting of adult spinal deformity: a prospective multicenter analysis. Spine (Phila Pa 1976). 2005;38(13):E803–12. https://doi.org/10.1097/BRS.0b013e318292b7b9.
9. Rothenfluh DA, Mueller DA, Rothenfluh E, et al. Pelvic incidence-lumbar lordosis mismatch predisposes to adjacent segment disease after lumbar spinal fusion. Eur Spine J. 2015;24:1251–8.
10. Lafage R, Schwab F, Challier V, et al. Defining spino-pelvic alignment thresholds should operative goals in adult spinal deformity surgery account for age? Spine (Phila Pa 1976). 2016;41:62–8.
11. Protopsaltis TS, Lafage R, Smith JS, et al. The lumbar pelvic angle, the lumbar component of the T1 pelvic angle, correlates with HRQOL, PI-LL mismatch, and it predicts global alignment. Spine (Phila Pa 1976). 2018;43:681–7.
12. Koller H, Pfanz C, Meier O, et al. Factors influencing radiographic and clinical outcomes in adult scoliosis surgery: a study of 448 European patients. Eur Spine J. 2016;25:532–48.
13. Rubin GD. Computed tomography: revolutionizing the practice of medicine for 40 years. Radiology. 2014;273:S45–74.
14. McCulloch PT, France J, Jones DL, et al. Helical computed tomography alone compared with plain radiographs with adjunct computed tomography to evaluate the cervical spine after high-energy trauma. J Bone Joint Surg Ser A. 2005;87:2388–94.
15. Takami M, Nohda K, Sakanaka J, et al. Usefulness of full spine computed tomography in cases of high-energy trauma: a prospective study. Eur J Orthop Surg Traumatol. 24 Suppl 1:S167–71. https://doi.org/10.1007/s00590-013-1268-0.
16. Sartoris DJ, Resnick D. Computed tomography of the spine: an update and review. Crit Rev Diagn Imaging. 1987;27:271–96.
17. Shah LM, Ross JS. Imaging of spine trauma. Neurosurgery. 2016;79:626–42.
18. Mao JZ, Agyei JO, Khan A, et al. Technologic evolution of navigation and robotics in spine surgery: a historical perspective. World Neurosurg. 2021;145:159–67.
19. Adamczak SE, Bova FJ, Hoh DJ. Intraoperative 3D computed tomography: spine surgery. Neurosurg Clin N Am. 2017;28:585–94.
20. Hida K, Iwasaki Y, Koyanagi I, et al. Bone window computed tomography for detection of dural defect associated with cervical ossified posterior longitudinal ligament. Neurol Med Chir. 1997;37:173–6.
21. Chen Y, Guo Y, Chen D, et al. Diagnosis and surgery of ossification of posterior longitudinal ligament associated with dural ossification in the cervical spine. Eur Spine J. 2009;18:1541–7.
22. Wang Q, Wang C, Zhang X, et al. Correlation of vertebral trabecular attenuation in Hounsfield units and the upper instrumented vertebra with proximal junctional failure after surgical treatment of degenerative lumbar disease. J Neurosurg Spine. 2020;1–8.
23. Duan PG, Mummaneni PV, Rivera J, et al. The association between lower Hounsfield units of the upper instrumented vertebra and proximal junctional kyphosis in adult spinal deformity surgery with a minimum 2-year follow-up. Neurosurg Focus. 2020;49:1–7.
24. Zaidi Q, Danisa OA, Cheng W. Measurement techniques and utility of hounsfield unit values for assessment of bone quality prior to spinal instrumentation: a review of current literature. Spine. 2019;44:E239–44.
25. Verma SK, Singh PK, Agrawal D, et al. O-arm with navigation versus C-arm: a review of screw placement over 3 years at a major trauma center. Br J Neurosurg. 2016;30:658–61.
26. Pitteloud N, Gamulin A, Barea C, et al. Radiation exposure using the O-arm® surgical imaging system. Eur Spine J. 2017;26:651–7.

27. Laudato PA, Pierzchala K, Schizas C. Pedicle screw insertion accuracy using O-arm, robotic guidance, or freehand technique. Spine (Phila Pa 1976). 2018;43:E373–8.
28. Lauterbur PC. Image formation by induced local interactions: examples employing nuclear magnetic resonance. Nature. 1973;242:190–1.
29. Edelman RR, Shoukimas GM, Stark DD, et al. High-resolution surface-coil imaging of lumbar disk disease. Am J Roentgenol. 1985;144:1123–9.
30. Modic MT, Steinberg PM, Ross JS, et al. Degenerative disk disease: assessment of changes in vertebral body marrow with MR imaging. Radiology. 1988;166:193–9.
31. Mok FPS, Samartzis D, Karppinen J, et al. Modic changes of the lumbar spine: prevalence, risk factors, and association with disc degeneration and low back pain in a large-scale population-based cohort. Spine J. 2016;16:32–41.
32. Jensen RK, Kent P, Jensen TS, et al. The association between subgroups of MRI findings identified with latent class analysis and low back pain in 40-year-old Danes. BMC Musculoskelet Disord. 2018;19(1):62. https://doi.org/10.1186/s12891-018-1978-x.
33. Dudli S, Fields AJ, Samartzis D, et al. Pathobiology of Modic changes. Eur Spine J. 2016;25:3723–34.
34. Brinckman MA, Chau C, Ross JS. Marrow edema variability in acute spine fractures. Spine J. 2015;15:454–60.
35. Joshi A, Kulkarni S, Dedhia T, et al. Role of 3T MRI in evaluation of bone marrow changes in spine in various diseases. J Assoc Physicians India. 2019;67:46–51.
36. Donovan Post MJ, Sze G, Quencer RM, et al. Gadolinium-enhanced MR in spinal infection. J Comput Assist Tomogr. 1990;14:721–9.
37. Defroda SF, Depasse JM, Eltorai AEM, et al. Evaluation and management of spinal epidural abscess. J Hosp Med. 2016;11:130–5.
38. Numaguchi Y, Rigamonti D, Rothman MI, et al. Spinal epidural abscess: evaluation with gadolinium-enhanced MR imaging. Radiographics. 1992;13(3):545–59. https://doi.org/10.1148/radiographics.13.3.8316663.
39. Henninger B, Kaser V, Ostermann S, et al. Cervical disc and ligamentous injury in hyperextension trauma: MRI and intraoperative correlation. J Neuroimaging. 2020;30:104–9.
40. Crosby CG, Even JL, Song Y, et al. Diagnostic abilities of magnetic resonance imaging in traumatic injury to the posterior ligamentous complex: the effect of years in training. Spine J. 2011;11:747–53.
41. Vaccaro AR, Lee JY, Schweitzer KM, et al. Assessment of injury to the posterior ligamentous complex in thoracolumbar spine trauma. Spine J. 2006;6:524–8.
42. Arnold PM. Commentary: Validating the use of magnetic resonance imaging in making treatment decisions in patients with spine trauma. Spine J. 2011;11:754–5.
43. Nourian AA, Cunningham CM, Bagheri A, et al. Effect of anatomic variability and level of approach on perioperative vascular complications with anterior lumbar interbody fusion. Spine (Phila Pa 1976). 2016;41:E73–7.
44. Mai HT, Schneider AD, Alvarez AP, et al. Anatomic considerations in the lateral transpsoas interbody fusion: the impact of age, sex, BMI, and Scoliosis. Clin Spine Surg. 2019;32:215–21.
45. Louie PK, Narain AS, Hijji FY, et al. Radiographic analysis of psoas morphology and its association with neurovascular structures at L4–5 with reference to lateral approaches. Spine (Phila Pa 1976). 2017;42:E1386–92.
46. Kepler CK, Bogner EA, Herzog RJ, et al. Anatomy of the psoas muscle and lumbar plexus with respect to the surgical approach for lateral transpsoas interbody fusion. Eur Spine J. 2011;20:550–6.
47. Ali HI, Saleh A. Lumbar spine MRI axial loading in patients with degenerative spine pathologies: its impact on the radiological findings and treatment decision. Egypt J Radiol Nucl Med. 2015;46:1065–9.
48. Hiwatashi A, Danielson B, Moritani T, et al. Axial loading during MR imaging can influence treatment decision for symptomatic spinal stenosis. Am J Neuroradiol. 2004;25:170–4.

49. Algin O, Turkbey B. Intrathecal gadolinium-enhanced MR cisternography: a comprehensive review. Am J Neuroradiol. 2013;34:14–22.
50. Chhabra A, Andreisek G, Soldatos T, et al. MR neurography: past, present, and future. Am J Roentgenol. 2011;197:583–91.
51. Rhodes CJ. Magnetic resonance spectroscopy. Sci Prog. 2017;100:241–92.
52. Russo RJ, Costa HS, Silva PD, et al. Assessing the risks associated with MRI in patients with a pacemaker or defibrillator. N Engl J Med. 2017;376:755–64.
53. Beam AS, Moore KG, Gillis SN, et al. GBCAs and risk for nephrogenic systemic fibrosis: a literature review. Radiol Technol. 2017;88:583–9.
54. Nguyen XV, Tahir S, Bresnahan BW, et al. Prevalence and financial impact of claustrophobia, anxiety, patient motion, and other patient events in magnetic resonance imaging. Top Magn Reson Imaging. 2020;29:125–30.
55. Thorpe S, Salkovskis PM, Dittner A. Claustrophobia in MRI: the role of cognitions. Magn Reson Imaging. 2008;26:1081–8.
56. Berg L, Hellum C, Gjertsen Ø, et al. Do more MRI findings imply worse disability or more intense low back pain? A cross-sectional study of candidates for lumbar disc prosthesis. Skeletal Radiol. 2013;42:1593–602.
57. Suri P, Boyko EJ, Goldberg J, et al. Longitudinal associations between incident lumbar spine MRI findings and chronic low back pain or radicular symptoms: retrospective analysis of data from the longitudinal assessment of imaging and disability of the back (LAIDBACK). BMC Musculoskelet Disord. 2017;15:152. https://doi.org/10.1186/1471-2474-15-152.
58. Chang CY, Gill CM, Joseph Simeone F, et al. Comparison of the diagnostic accuracy of 99 m-Tc-MDP bone scintigraphy and 18F-FDG PET/CT for the detection of skeletal metastases. Acta Radiol. 2016;57:58–65.
59. Whalen JL, Brown ML, McLeod RI, et al. Limitations of indium leukocyte imaging for the diagnosis of spine infections. Spine (Phila Pa 1976). 1991;16:193–7.
60. Datz FL. Indium-111-labeled leukocytes for the detection of infection: current status. Semin Nucl Med. 1994;24:92–109.
61. Brusko GD, Perez-Roman RJ, Tapamo H, et al. Preoperative SPECT imaging as a tool for surgical planning in patients with axial neck and back pain. Neurosurg Focus. 2019;47(6):E19. https://doi.org/10.3171/2019.9.FOCUS19648.
62. Tender GC, Davidson C, Shields J, et al. Primary pain generator identification by CT-SPECT in patients with degenerative spinal disease. Neurosurg Focus. 2019;47:1–6.
63. Kato S, Demura S, Matsubara H, et al. Utility of bone SPECT/CT to identify the primary cause of pain in elderly patients with degenerative lumbar spine disease. J Orthop Surg Res. 2019;14(1):185. https://doi.org/10.1186/s13018-019-1236-4.
64. Ratnayake R, Mundis GM, Shahidi B, et al. 264. Assessment of impact of single photon emission computed tomography (SPECT) on management of degenerative cervical and lumbar disease: a multi-institution survey of spine surgeons. Spine J. 2020;20:S130–1.
65. WHO. Assessment of fracture risk and its application to screening for postmenopausal osteoporosis. Report of a WHO study group. World Health Organization—technical report series, vol. 843. Geneva: WHO; 1994. p. 1–129.
66. Gupta A, Upadhyaya S, Patel A, et al. DEXA sensitivity analysis in patients with adult spinal deformity. Spine J. 2020;20:174–80.
67. Francis RM, Baillie SP, Chuck AJ, et al. Acute and long-term management of patients with vertebral fractures. QJM. 2004;97:63–74.
68. Mears SC, Kates SL. A guide to improving the care of patients with fragility fractures, edition 2. Geriatr Orthop Surg Rehabil. 2015;6:58–120.
69. Karikari IO, Metz LN. Preventing pseudoarthrosis and proximal junctional kyphosis: how to deal with the osteoporotic spine. Neurosurg Clin N Am. 2018;29:365–74.
70. Seki S, Hirano N, Kawaguchi Y, et al. Teriparatide versus low-dose bisphosphonates before and after surgery for adult spinal deformity in female Japanese patients with osteoporosis. Eur Spine J. 2017;26:2121–7.

71. Safaee MM, Osorio JA, Verma K, et al. Proximal junctional kyphosis prevention strategies: a video technique guide. Oper Neurosurg. 2017;13:581–5.
72. Legaye J, Duval-Beaupère G, Hecquet J, et al. Pelvic incidence: a fundamental pelvic parameter for three-dimensional regulation of spinal sagittal curves. Eur Spine J. 1998;7:99–103.
73. Roussouly P, Gollogly S, Berthonnaud E, et al. Classification of the normal variation in the sagittal alignment of the human lumbar spine and pelvis in the standing position. Spine (Phila Pa 1976). 2005;30:346–53.
74. Jackson RP, McManus AC. Radiographic analysis of sagittal plane alignment and balance in standing volunteers and patients with low back pain matched for age5 sex, and size: a prospective controlled clinical study. Spine (Phila Pa 1976). 1994;19:1611–8.
75. Redmond JM, Gupta A, Nasser R, et al. The hip-spine connection: understanding its importance in the treatment of hip pathology. Orthopedics. 2015;38:49–55.
76. Buckland AJ, Vigdorchik J, Schwab FJ, et al. Acetabular anteversion changes due to spinal deformity correction: bridging the gap between hip and spine surgeons. J Bone Joint Surg Am. 2014;97:1913–20.
77. Buckland AJ, Steinmetz L, Zhou P, et al. Spinopelvic compensatory mechanisms for reduced hip motion (ROM) in the setting of hip osteoarthritis. Spine Deform. 2019;7:923–8.
78. Buckland AJ, Abotsi EJ, Vasquez-Montes D, et al. Lumbar spine degeneration and flatback deformity alter sitting-standing spinopelvic mechanics—implications for total hip arthroplasty. J Arthroplasty. 2020;35:1036–41.
79. Melhem E, Assi A, El Rachkidi R, et al. EOS® biplanar X-ray imaging: concept, developments, benefits, and limitations. J Child Orthop. 2016;10:1–14.
80. Chaibi Y, Cresson T, Aubert B, et al. Fast 3D reconstruction of the lower limb using a parametric model and statistical inferences and clinical measurements calculation from biplanar X-rays. Comput Methods Biomech Biomed Engin. 2012;15:457–66.
81. Kim SB, Heo YM, Hwang CM, et al. Reliability of the EOS imaging system for assessment of the spinal and pelvic alignment in the sagittal plane. Clin Orthop Surg. 2018;10:500–7.
82. Vidal C, Ilharreborde B, Azoulay R, et al. Reliability of cervical lordosis and global sagittal spinal balance measurements in adolescent idiopathic scoliosis. Eur Spine J. 2013;22:1362–7.
83. Michael N, Carry P, Erickson M, et al. Spine and thoracic height measurements have excellent interrater and intrarater reliability in patients with early onset scoliosis. Spine (Phila Pa 1976). 2018;43:270–4.
84. Hasegawa K, Okamoto M, Hatsushikano S, et al. Difference in whole spinal alignment between supine and standing positions in patients with adult spinal deformity using a new comparison method with slot-scanning three-dimensional X-ray imager and computed tomography through digital reconstructed radiography. BMC Musculoskelet Disord. 2018;19(1):437. https://doi.org/10.1186/s12891-018-2355-5.
85. Tarpada SP, Cho W, Chen F, et al. Utility of supine lateral radiographs for assessment of lumbar segmental instability in degenerative lumbar spondylolisthesis. Spine. 2018;43:1275–80.
86. Yasuda T, Hasegawa T, Yamato Y, et al. Effect of position on lumbar lordosis in patients with adult spinal deformity. J Neurosurg Spine. 2018;29:530–4.
87. Segebarth B, Kurd MF, Haug PH, et al. Routine upright imaging for evaluating degenerative lumbar stenosis: incidence of degenerative spondylolisthesis missed on supine MRI. J Spinal Disord Tech. 2015;28:394–7.
88. Finkenstaedt T, Del Grande F, Bolog N, et al. Correlation of listhesis on upright radiographs and central lumbar spinal canal stenosis on supine MRI: is it possible to predict lumbar spinal canal stenosis? Skeletal Radiol. 2018;47:1269–75.

Chapter 25
Robotics and Navigation

Robert M. Koffie, S. Harrison Farber, Jakub Godzik, and Juan S. Uribe

Abbreviations

CT Computed tomography
TLIF Transforaminal lumbar interbody fusion

Introduction

The complexity of spinal pathologies seen in elderly patients is increasing. Fortunately, various surgical and nonsurgical technologies to help treat these patients have also emerged. Some of the technologies build on what has been known for decades, making surgery more efficient and safer. Others, such as robotics, have been repurposed and adapted from other medical subspecialties into spine surgery to help patients. Elderly patients, who have a higher risk of complications from spine surgery than other patients, can benefit the most from technologies that improve the accuracy, precision, and safety of surgery. Here we review a subset of these technologies.

R. M. Koffie · S. H. Farber · J. Godzik
Department of Neurosurgery, Barrow Neurological Institute, St. Joseph's Hospital and Medical Center, Phoenix, AZ, USA

J. S. Uribe (✉)
Department of Neurosurgery, Barrow Neurological Institute, St. Joseph's Hospital and Medical Center, Phoenix, AZ, USA

Neuroscience Publications at Barrow Neurological Institute, St. Joseph's Hospital and Medical Center, Phoenix, AZ, USA
e-mail: Neuropub@barrowneuro.org

K.-M. G. Fu et al. (eds.), *Treatment of Spine Disease in the Elderly*,
https://doi.org/10.1007/978-3-031-12612-3_25

Minimally Invasive Spine Surgery

Elderly patients are typically not able to easily tolerate large open operations, which are often accompanied by high-volume blood loss and intraoperative complications. Tubular approaches to the spine have made simple but necessary surgical procedures that are often required by elderly patients, such as spinal decompressions and fusions, safer. Tubular decompressions, whether laminectomies or diskectomies, have become the preferred surgical approach in elderly patients with degenerative spinal stenosis. Tubular technology allows surgeons to localize directly on the target pathology and, with serial dilations and minimal tissue distraction, surgically address the pathology with minimal injury to surrounding tissues, which promotes rapid recovery. Tubular approaches to the spine have been demonstrated in cervical, thoracic, and lumbosacral pathology [1–4]. The tubular approach has also been extended to interbody fusions. The minimally invasive transforaminal lumbar interbody fusion (TLIF) technique allows direct and indirect decompression and fusion of the spine through a small incision. The minimally invasive TLIF technique is associated with shorter operating room time, less blood loss, and improved outcomes compared to the open TLIF operation [5].

Another innovative technique for treating elderly patients with lumbar pathology involves the lateral access operation using minimally invasive techniques. Lateral access to the spine traditionally has required large "shark bite" incisions, which are often associated with bowel and large-vessel injury as well as lumbar plexus injuries. With the development of innovative minimally invasive retractors and highly sensitive neuromonitoring paradigms, lateral access surgeries are associated with less morbidity and greater safety [6]. Lateral lumbar interbody fusion, which is effective at treating spondylolisthesis, adjacent level degeneration, and other spinal pathologies that are prevalent among elderly patients, has also become very safe and efficient when used to indirectly decompress nerve roots and fuse diseased segments [6].

Navigation and Image Guidance

Elderly patients typically present with symptoms associated with changes in the spine that are not easy to understand anatomically. Age-related degeneration is associated with osteophyte formation in unusual locations of the spine, which can pose a challenge when operating without image guidance. The development of navigation has therefore increased the safety of many spine operations in elderly patients, particularly patients with adult degenerative spinal deformity. Computed tomography (CT)-guided navigation allows the surgeon to quickly obtain intraoperative CT images and then use fiducial markers during surgery to guide and obtain direct anatomical information about the spinal pathology. Navigation provides a facile way to place pedicle screws with better accuracy, decompress the spine, and perform complex osteotomies with laser-focused accuracy. The ease of using intraoperative navigation in spine surgery has led to the birth of robotic spine surgery, which promises to be the future of spine surgery.

Robotic Spine Surgery

The use of robotic systems in surgical fields continues to evolve [7]. Robotics have been used for years in general surgery and in specialties such as urology and gynecology, where it has become a standard of care for procedures such as prostatectomies and hysterectomies [8–10]. The adoption of robotics technology in spine surgery was very slow until recently, when the use of navigation allowed robotic technology to add enormous value [11]. Among the multiple applications of robotics, the use of robotics for pedicle screw placement during simple and complex spine operations appears to be growing.

In elderly patients with degenerative processes such as lumbar spondylolisthesis, treatment entails instrumented fixation, which often requires the placement of pedicle screws. Techniques for pedicle screw placement were first described in the late 1950s and have evolved substantially over the years. Historically, placement of pedicle screws required a careful open technique with tissue dissection to allow anatomical visualization of critical spinal structures, such as the transverse process, pars interarticularis, and facet, for screw placement. Since then, the technique has undergone significant technical advances, including the description of open and percutaneous approaches using a variety of navigated techniques [12–17]. The evolution of minimally invasive spine techniques and navigation has now made percutaneous screw placement possible, opening the door for the use of robotics in spine surgery.

Pedicle screw malposition can lead to serious adverse complications, including nerve or cord injury, cerebrospinal fluid leak, vessel injury, the need for reoperations, and worsening patient outcomes. Although these issues can be addressed with relative ease in younger patients, elderly patients experience much worse outcomes when such complications occur because of screw malpositioning [18]. Accurate screw placement is therefore of utmost importance to reduce iatrogenic complications and to improve surgical outcomes in all patients, but this is critical in elderly patients.

Although open surgical techniques make it relatively easy to place pedicle screws, such techniques require a large incision, which is associated with greater blood loss and risk of intraoperative complications. Thus, elderly patients may benefit from less invasive approaches for spinal fixation, such as percutaneous pedicle screw placement. Accuracy of percutaneous pedicle screw placement depends largely on adequate imaging and intraoperative accuracy of localizing the screw trajectory, which makes the use of robotics very exciting.

To be adopted, any new technology for pedicle screw placement must have similar or better performance when compared to available techniques, such as open freehand, fluoroscopically assisted, or CT-assisted screw placement. Robotic systems offer the theoretical advantage of automating inherently repetitive tasks that are subject to human error, thereby increasing accuracy and precision during pedicle screw placement; however, robotics is not yet widely adopted, and a learning curve is required to perfect the robotic pedicle screw placement technique. Early reports of the use of robotic technologies in spine surgery have shown equivalent accuracy compared with other methods of screw placement [17]. Below we summarize the operative techniques and nuances, as described elsewhere [19].

Operative Technique

Robotic systems are most useful in thoracolumbar fusion, where anatomical variants make it challenging to navigate screw placement. As robotic systems are becoming more prevalent, they are also being used to place pedicle screws in routine and simple cases with accuracy. Robotics also can be incorporated into lumbar fusion procedures, including lateral lumbar interbody fusion [20] and TLIF [21]. Robotic techniques can be used for percutaneous pedicle screw fixation or as a complement to the open technique when it is difficult to identify critical anatomical structures, as required to place a screw safely with the freehand technique.

As we have described elsewhere [19], patient positioning and operating room setup are shown in Fig. 25.1. After the patient is prepped and draped in the usual sterile fashion, two bilateral subcentimeter incisions are made over the posterior

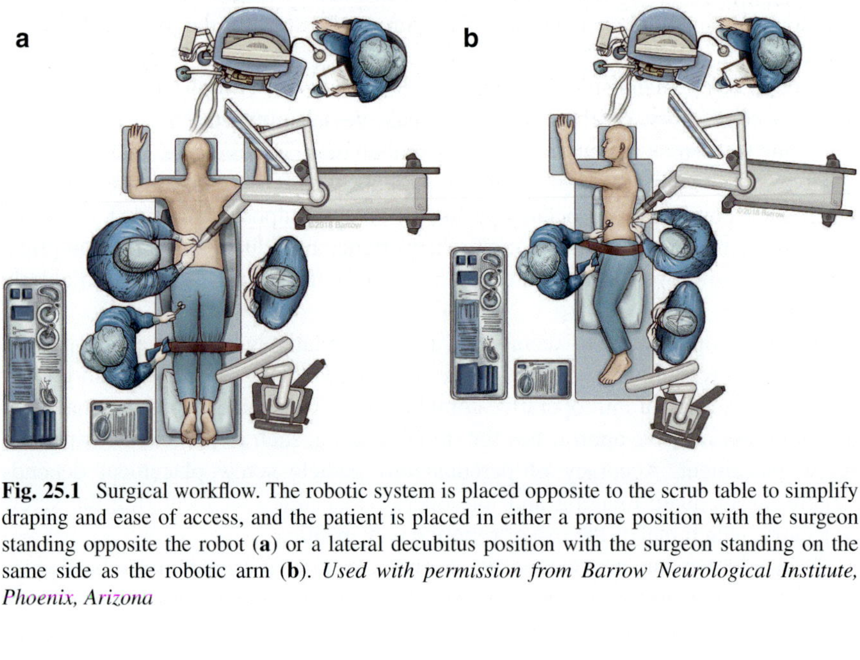

Fig. 25.1 Surgical workflow. The robotic system is placed opposite to the scrub table to simplify draping and ease of access, and the patient is placed in either a prone position with the surgeon standing opposite the robot (**a**) or a lateral decubitus position with the surgeon standing on the same side as the robotic arm (**b**). *Used with permission from Barrow Neurological Institute, Phoenix, Arizona*

superior iliac spine. The dynamic reference base array and the surveillance marker are then affixed to the posterior superior iliac spine bilaterally with a superolateral trajectory for navigation. Intraoperative CT registration is then attached to the dynamic reference array and an intraoperative CT is obtained using an O-arm (Medtronic; Dublin, Ireland). The patient's intraoperative images are then co-registered to the patient's preoperative imaging, which aids in creating a trajectory plan. Preoperative CT can also be used to plan the trajectory of the pedicle screws, which can then be confirmed using intraoperative images during surgery (Fig. 25.2). The robotic end effector arm moves into position to guide all movements along this planned trajectory with all subsequent steps performed through the end effector arm.

With regard to the step for actually placing the screw, a stab incision is made, and the Bovie electrocautery is used to dissect through the subcutaneous tissue and the fascia, making the fascial incision slightly medial to the skin incision. Using a high-speed drill with a bur, a small pilot hole is placed on the bone at the screw entry point, which prevents skiving of the drill off of the cortical bone and allows uninhibited entry into cancellous bone. Tapping, which is an optional step, can be performed using a navigated tap that matches the planned trajectory. The pedicle screw can then be placed through the tapped corridor using navigation. A force meter is also available to the surgeon to confirm that an appropriate amount of force is applied during the placement of the pedicle screw. The correct position of the pedicle screw is then confirmed by the robotic system and subsequently confirmed by intraoperative CT.

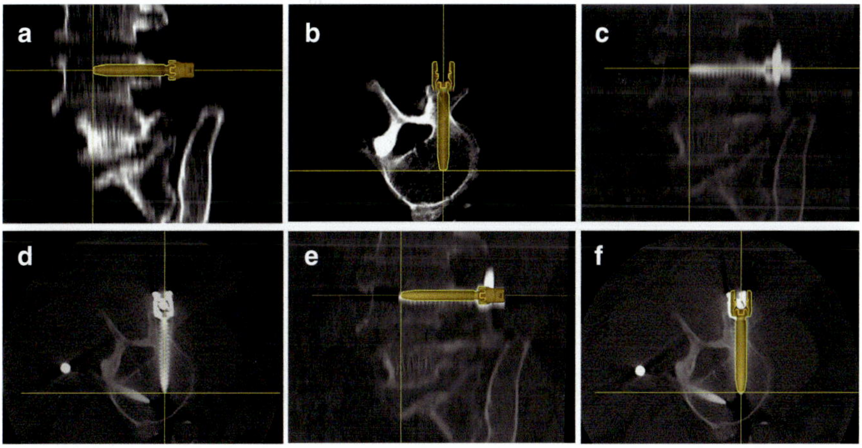

Fig. 25.2 Screw planning and accuracy assessment. Left L4 screw placement is planned using intraoperative software in sagittal (**a**) and axial (**b**) planes. The screw trajectory is lateral to medial to facilitate purchase along the medial pedicle wall. The crosshairs indicate the screw tip. Postoperative sagittal (**c**) and axial (**d**) CT scans demonstrate screw placement without a medial or lateral breach. Accuracy is assessed using image overlay analysis between preoperative planning and postoperative sagittal (**e**) and axial (**f**) CT scans, which show minimal error with a near-overlap of the planned trajectory and the resultant screw. *Used with permission from Barrow Neurological Institute, Phoenix, Arizona*

Pedicle Screw Placement Accuracy

Pedicle screw placement accuracy is very important in all patients, but even more so in elderly patients. Most elderly patients have degenerative changes and osteophytes that can affect the usual plans for traditional pedicle screw placement. Furthermore, because of the low bone density of elderly patients, screw accuracy is very important insofar as these patients do not tolerate reoperations well, least of all a reoperation for screw placement issues. Classification systems have been developed to determine the accuracy of screw placement after a robotic system has been used. The most commonly used classification system is the Gertzbein-Robbins classification [22]. Pedicle screw placement using robotic systems generally has very high accuracy, with literature reporting rates from 94% to 98% [23–28], which is superior to the accuracy achieved with a freehand technique. One randomized controlled trial compared pedicle screw placement using the robotic system versus a freehand technique and found that 93% of pedicle screws placed with the freehand technique were Gertzbein-Robbins A or B, compared with 85% for those placed with the robot [29]. A meta-analysis that included ten studies found that robotically assisted pedicle screw placement performed better than freehand screw placement in terms of "perfect accuracy" (odds ratio 95% confidence interval: 1.38–2.07; $P < 0.01$) as well as "clinically acceptable" (odds ratio 95% confidence interval: 1.17–2.08; $P < 0.01$) [30]. Two other meta-analyses reported similar results, showing increased accuracy of robotically assisted pedicle screw placement compared with freehand screw placement [17, 31]. A more recent meta-analysis that included nine randomized controlled trials with a total of 696 patients also found the accuracy of pedicle screw placement to be higher with use of robotic systems than with freehand techniques, although results varied on the basis of the different robotic systems used [32].

Operative Time

One disadvantage of using current robotic systems for pedicle screw placement is the longer operative time observed with the robotic systems. Several investigators have reported [33–35] that increased operative times were associated with robotic systems. Given the extra steps required to ensure accuracy, this finding is not surprising. However, as robotic systems continue to evolve with new updates, the amount of time needed to place pedicle screws is decreasing. Another factor that underlies the inherently longer time required to place pedicle screws using a robot is the steep learning curve associated with using this technology, which is expected to improve as the use of robotics for spine surgery becomes commonplace [36, 37].

Radiation Exposure

Although using robotic systems for pedicle screw placement is associated with longer operative time, the system decreases radiation exposure to surgeons, operating room staff, and patients. With robotic system use, the surgeon is not exposed to the initial (preoperative or intraoperative) CT, and only minimal intraoperative radiation is used during the fluoroscopic portion of the operation. When intraoperative CT is used, no additional fluoroscopy is required for registration. Studies have indeed validated that use of robotics decreases radiation exposure [38] both on a per-screw basis and with respect to overall radiation exposure [39, 40]. For example, in one randomized controlled trial, radiation exposure to the surgeon was found to be ten times lower during robotic procedures compared with fluoroscopy-guided screw placement, which adds enormous value when extrapolated across the career lifespan of a surgeon [33].

Conclusions

Robotic systems can increase the accuracy of pedicle screw placement, decrease the amount of radiation exposure to the surgeon, and decrease the need for reoperation for pedicle screw malpositioning. Given the steep learning curve required to perfect the robotic technique, using robotics in spine surgery is currently associated with a longer operative time. Nonetheless, as the robotic technology evolves, the systems will inevitably become more user-friendly and intuitive, hopefully decreasing the operative time required to use them. The use of robotics may also extend beyond pedicle screw placement to include techniques such as decompressions and osteotomies. These advances in robotics and minimally invasive spine surgery will complement the progress that has been made in treating elderly patients with spinal pathologies and will greatly improve how we care for our elderly spine patients.

Acknowledgments We thank the staff of Neuroscience Publications at Barrow Neurological Institute for assistance with manuscript preparation.

Disclosures No protected health information is disclosed in this chapter.

Financial Support Dr. Uribe is a consultant for, receives royalties from, and has direct stock ownership in NuVasive and is a consultant for Misonix and SI-BONE.

References

1. Paullus P, Wilson TA, Lee P, Gunasekaran A, Kazemi N. Minimally invasive approach to resection of paraspinal schwannoma. Neurosurg Focus. 2018;44(VideoSuppl1):V5. https://doi.org/10.3171/2018.1.FocusVid.17572.
2. Alvi MA, Kerezoudis P, Wahood W, Goyal A, Bydon M. Operative approaches for lumbar disc herniation: a systematic review and multiple treatment meta-analysis of conventional and minimally invasive surgeries. World Neurosurg. 2018;114:391–407.e2. https://doi.org/10.1016/j.wneu.2018.02.156.
3. Hussain I, Schmidt FA, Kirnaz S, Wipplinger C, Schwartz TH, Hartl R. MIS approaches in the cervical spine. J Spine Surg. 2019;5(Suppl 1):S74–83. https://doi.org/10.21037/jss.2019.04.21.
4. Fong S, DuPlessis SJ. Minimally invasive anterior approach to upper cervical spine: surgical technique. J Spinal Disord Tech. 2005;18(4):321–5. https://doi.org/10.1097/01.bsd.0000169062.77005.78.
5. Jin-Tao Q, Yu T, Mei W, Xu-Dong T, Tian-Jian Z, Guo-Hua S, et al. Comparison of MIS vs. open PLIF/TLIF with regard to clinical improvement, fusion rate, and incidence of major complication: a meta-analysis. Eur Spine J. 2015;24(5):1058–65. https://doi.org/10.1007/s00586-015-3890-5.
6. Xu DS, Walker CT, Godzik J, Turner JD, Smith W, Uribe JS. Minimally invasive anterior, lateral, and oblique lumbar interbody fusion: a literature review. Ann Transl Med. 2018;6(6):104. https://doi.org/10.21037/atm.2018.03.24.
7. Childers CP, Maggard-Gibbons M. Estimation of the acquisition and operating costs for robotic surgery. JAMA. 2018;320(8):835–6. https://doi.org/10.1001/jama.2018.9219.
8. Trastulli S, Farinella E, Cirocchi R, Cavaliere D, Avenia N, Sciannameo F, et al. Robotic resection compared with laparoscopic rectal resection for cancer: systematic review and meta-analysis of short-term outcome. Color Dis. 2012;14(4):e134–56. https://doi.org/10.1111/j.1463-1318.2011.02907.x.
9. Sammon J, Trinh QD, Menon M. Robotic radical prostatectomy: a critical analysis of surgical quality. Curr Opin Urol. 2011;21(3):195–9. https://doi.org/10.1097/MOU.0b013e328344e570.
10. Lowery WJ, Leath CA 3rd, Robinson RD. Robotic surgery applications in the management of gynecologic malignancies. J Surg Oncol. 2012;105(5):481–7. https://doi.org/10.1002/jso.22080.
11. Roser F, Tatagiba M, Maier G. Spinal robotics: current applications and future perspectives. Neurosurgery. 2013;72(Suppl 1):12–8. https://doi.org/10.1227/NEU.0b013e318270d02c.
12. Boucher HH. A method of spinal fusion. J Bone Joint Surg Br. 1959;41-B(2):248–59.
13. Roy-Camille R, Roy-Camille M, Demeulenaere C. Osteosynthesis of dorsal, lumbar, and lumbosacral spine with metallic plates screwed into vertebral pedicles and articular apophyses. Presse Med. 1970;78(32):1447–8.
14. Magerl FP. Stabilization of the lower thoracic and lumbar spine with external skeletal fixation. Clin Orthop Relat Res. 1984;189:125–41.
15. Foley KT, Gupta SK. Percutaneous pedicle screw fixation of the lumbar spine: preliminary clinical results. J Neurosurg. 2002;97(1 Suppl):7–12. https://doi.org/10.3171/spi.2002.97.1.0007.
16. Schwarzenbach O, Berlemann U, Jost B, Visarius H, Arm E, Langlotz F, et al. Accuracy of computer-assisted pedicle screw placement. An in vivo computed tomography analysis. Spine (Phila Pa 1976). 1997;22(4):452–8. https://doi.org/10.1097/00007632-199702150-00020.
17. Verma R, Krishan S, Haendlmayer K, Mohsen A. Functional outcome of computer-assisted spinal pedicle screw placement: a systematic review and meta-analysis of 23 studies including 5,992 pedicle screws. Eur Spine J. 2010;19(3):370–5. https://doi.org/10.1007/s00586-009-1258-4.
18. Cloyd JM, Acosta FL Jr, Ames CP. Complications and outcomes of lumbar spine surgery in elderly people: a review of the literature. J Am Geriatr Soc. 2008;56(7):1318–27. https://doi.org/10.1111/j.1532-5415.2008.01771.x.

19. Farber SH, Pacult MA, Godzik J, Walker CT, Turner JD, Porter RW, Uribe JS. Robotics in spine surgery: a technical overview and review of key concepts. Front Surg. 2021;8:578674.
20. Walker CT, Godzik J, Xu DS, Theodore N, Uribe JS, Chang SW. Minimally invasive single-position lateral interbody fusion with robotic bilateral percutaneous pedicle screw fixation: 2-dimensional operative video. Oper Neurosurg (Hagerstown). 2019;16(4):E121. https://doi.org/10.1093/ons/opy240.
21. Godzik J, Walker CT, Theodore N, Uribe JS, Chang SW, Snyder LA. Minimally invasive transforaminal interbody fusion with robotically assisted bilateral pedicle screw fixation: 2-dimensional operative video. Oper Neurosurg (Hagerstown). 2019;16(3):E86–E7. https://doi.org/10.1093/ons/opy288.
22. Gertzbein SD, Robbins SE. Accuracy of pedicular screw placement in vivo. Spine (Phila Pa 1976). 1990;15(1):11–4. https://doi.org/10.1097/00007632-199001000-00004.
23. Tsai TH, Wu DS, Su YF, Wu CH, Lin CL. A retrospective study to validate an intraoperative robotic classification system for assessing the accuracy of Kirschner wire (K-wire) placements with postoperative computed tomography classification system for assessing the accuracy of pedicle screw placements. Medicine (Baltimore). 2016;95(38):e4834. https://doi.org/10.1097/MD.0000000000004834.
24. Kuo KL, Su YF, Wu CH, Tsai CY, Chang CH, Lin CL, et al. Assessing the intraoperative accuracy of pedicle screw placement by using a bone-mounted miniature robot system through secondary registration. PLoS One. 2016;11(4):e0153235. https://doi.org/10.1371/journal.pone.0153235.
25. Keric N, Doenitz C, Haj A, Rachwal-Czyzewicz I, Renovanz M, Wesp DMA, et al. Evaluation of robot-guided minimally invasive implantation of 2067 pedicle screws. Neurosurg Focus. 2017;42(5):E11. https://doi.org/10.3171/2017.2.FOCUS16552.
26. van Dijk JD, van den Ende RP, Stramigioli S, Kochling M, Hoss N. Clinical pedicle screw accuracy and deviation from planning in robot-guided spine surgery: robot-guided pedicle screw accuracy. Spine (Phila Pa 1976). 2015;40(17):E986–91. https://doi.org/10.1097/BRS.0000000000000960.
27. Devito DP, Kaplan L, Dietl R, Pfeiffer M, Horne D, Silberstein B, et al. Clinical acceptance and accuracy assessment of spinal implants guided with SpineAssist surgical robot: retrospective study. Spine (Phila Pa 1976). 2010;35(24):2109–15. https://doi.org/10.1097/BRS.0b013e3181d323ab.
28. Kantelhardt SR, Martinez R, Baerwinkel S, Burger R, Giese A, Rohde V. Perioperative course and accuracy of screw positioning in conventional, open robotic-guided and percutaneous robotic-guided, pedicle screw placement. Eur Spine J. 2011;20(6):860–8. https://doi.org/10.1007/s00586-011-1729-2.
29. Ringel F, Stuer C, Reinke A, Preuss A, Behr M, Auer F, et al. Accuracy of robot-assisted placement of lumbar and sacral pedicle screws: a prospective randomized comparison to conventional freehand screw implantation. Spine (Phila Pa 1976). 2012;37(8):E496–501. https://doi.org/10.1097/BRS.0b013e31824b7767.
30. Fan Y, Du JP, Liu JJ, Zhang JN, Qiao HH, Liu SC, et al. Accuracy of pedicle screw placement comparing robot-assisted technology and the free-hand with fluoroscopy-guided method in spine surgery: an updated meta-analysis. Medicine (Baltimore). 2018;97(22):e10970. https://doi.org/10.1097/MD.0000000000010970.
31. Shin BJ, James AR, Njoku IU, Hartl R. Pedicle screw navigation: a systematic review and meta-analysis of perforation risk for computer-navigated versus freehand insertion. J Neurosurg Spine. 2012;17(2):113–22. https://doi.org/10.3171/2012.5.SPINE11399.
32. Li HM, Zhang RJ, Shen CL. Accuracy of pedicle screw placement and clinical outcomes of robot-assisted technique versus conventional freehand technique in spine surgery from nine randomized controlled trials: a meta-analysis. Spine (Phila Pa 1976). 2020;45(2):E111–E9. https://doi.org/10.1097/BRS.0000000000003193.
33. Villard J, Ryang YM, Demetriades AK, Reinke A, Behr M, Preuss A, et al. Radiation exposure to the surgeon and the patient during posterior lumbar spinal instrumentation: a prospective

randomized comparison of navigated versus non-navigated freehand techniques. Spine (Phila Pa 1976). 2014;39(13):1004–9. https://doi.org/10.1097/BRS.0000000000000351.

34. Siddiqui MI, Wallace DJ, Salazar LM, Vardiman AB. Robot-assisted pedicle screw placement: learning curve experience. World Neurosurg. 2019;130:e417–e22. https://doi.org/10.1016/j.wneu.2019.06.107.
35. Yu L, Chen X, Margalit A, Peng H, Qiu G, Qian W. Robot-assisted vs freehand pedicle screw fixation in spine surgery: a systematic review and a meta-analysis of comparative studies. Int J Med Robot. 2018;14(3):e1892. https://doi.org/10.1002/rcs.1892.
36. Hu X, Lieberman IH. What is the learning curve for robotic-assisted pedicle screw placement in spine surgery? Clin Orthop Relat Res. 2014;472(6):1839–44. https://doi.org/10.1007/s11999-013-3291-1.
37. Schatlo B, Martinez R, Alaid A, von Eckardstein K, Akhavan-Sigari R, Hahn A, et al. Unskilled unawareness and the learning curve in robotic spine surgery. Acta Neurochir. 2015;157(10):1819–23; discussion 23. https://doi.org/10.1007/s00701-015-2535-0.
38. Han X, Tian W, Liu Y, Liu B, He D, Sun Y, et al. Safety and accuracy of robot-assisted versus fluoroscopy-assisted pedicle screw insertion in thoracolumbar spinal surgery: a prospective randomized controlled trial. J Neurosurg Spine. 2019:1–8. https://doi.org/10.3171/2018.10.SPINE18487.
39. Fan Y, Du J, Zhang J, Liu S, Xue X, Huang Y, et al. Comparison of accuracy of pedicle screw insertion among 4 guided technologies in spine surgery. Med Sci Monit. 2017;23:5960–8. https://doi.org/10.12659/msm.905713.
40. Hyun SJ, Kim KJ, Jahng TA, Kim HJ. Minimally invasive robotic versus open fluoroscopic-guided spinal instrumented fusions: a randomized controlled trial. Spine (Phila Pa 1976). 2017;42(6):353–8. https://doi.org/10.1097/BRS.0000000000001778.

Chapter 26
Awake Spine Surgery in the Elderly

Clayton L. Haldeman and Michael Y. Wang

Introduction

The first awake, minimally invasive spine (MIS) procedure was, arguably, reported in 1958 by Ralph Cloward in his early description of anterior cervical discectomy and fusion [1]. He describes a muscle-sparing approach which he first performed awake on a "stoic" individual. Since that time, indications and techniques for MIS surgery have greatly expanded, and improvements in tools and technology have made awake surgery safer and more comfortable for patients [2]. More recently, awake spinal surgery has been incorporated into an entire suite of care known as Enhanced Recovery After Surgery (ERAS), a multimodal system designed to reduce the impact of surgery on patients resulting in earlier mobilization and decreased length of stay [3]. These techniques have the potential to ease the burden of surgery in all patient populations; however, they have the potential to be especially powerful in the elderly, who are disproportionately impacted by general anesthetics.

Supplementary Information The online version contains supplementary material available at [https://doi.org/10.1007/978-3-031-12612-3_26].

C. L. Haldeman (✉)
University of Miami Miller School of Medicine, Miami, FL, USA

M. Y. Wang
Departments of Neurosurgery and Rehabilitation Medicine, University of MiamiMiller School of Medicine, Miami, FL, USA
e-mail: MWang2@med.miami.edu

K.-M. G. Fu et al. (eds.), *Treatment of Spine Disease in the Elderly*,
https://doi.org/10.1007/978-3-031-12612-3_26

History and Impetus

Concerns over the harmful effects of general anesthesia have been growing during the last decade, particularly in two patient populations—the young and the old [4, 5]. Multiple studies have raised the specter of long-term cognitive impairment in children as a result of exposure to general anesthetics [6–8]. These concerns culminated in 2016 when the FDA issued a public warning urging healthcare providers to "balance the benefits of appropriate anesthesia in young children and pregnant women against the potential risks, especially for procedures that may last longer than 3 h or if multiple procedures are required in children under 3 years" [9].

As the structure and reserve capacity of all organs diminish over time, the adverse effects of general anesthesia in geriatric population can be multiple. In a study of 367 patients who underwent general anesthesia over the age of 80, 25% developed adverse postoperative outcomes, and the mortality rate was 4.6% [10]. Postoperative delirium is one of the most common concerns for elderly undergoing general anesthetic, and the incidence is estimated to be at around 30% [11]. Initially thought to be transient, evidence is mounting that delirium can have long-term morbidity in this population and can result in an inability to return to independent living [12]. For elderly patients with preexisting coronary artery disease or a history of heart failure, adverse cardiac outcomes and in-hospital and out-of-hospital 90-day mortality are increased. Pulmonary complications are also disproportionately increased in the elderly population and range from 5 to 10%. Postoperative pneumonias are the most common event; however, pulmonary embolism, acute respiratory distress syndrome (ARDS), and need for reintubation following surgery also occur.

Among the elderly population, spine surgery is one of the top five procedures performed [13]. Despite growing concern from the harmful effects of general anesthesia mentioned above, the majority of elective spine surgery is performed under general anesthetic. This likely has to do with multiple factors, including custom and the desire to secure the airway for procedures planned in the prone position, anesthesiologist's comfort or familiarity with the technique, surgeon's perception of compromised surgical technique or concerns for surgical time length, limitation on neuromonitoring, or patient preference [14]. However, awake spinal surgery is not a new concept. The use of spinal anesthesia for lumbar spine surgery was first described in 1959 by Ditzler et al. in a review of 20 years of experience operating on 766 patients who received either laminectomy, discectomy, or fusion [15]. They concluded that "spinal anesthesia in these operations neither complicates nor adversely effects the postoperative results." While general anesthetic techniques and safety have improved vastly since 1939, there remain multiple potential benefits to this approach. Without general anesthetics, the patient maintains spontaneous respirations, thus avoiding the need to instrument the airway. The decreased thoracic pressure from spontaneous ventilation (compared to mechanical) has the potential to reduce blood loss as well [16]. Additionally, the use of spinal anesthesia for lumbar spine surgery is associated with a lower incidence of intraoperative hypertension and tachycardia, reduced opioid and other analgesic requirements in the PACU, less postoperative nausea and vomiting (PONV) at 24 h, and a shorter hospital length of stay compared with general anesthesia [17]. While waking from general anesthesia, patients may have mental confusion and temporary alterations of sensory and motor function [18]. Blood pressure changes, electrolyte disturbances, and resulting cardiac dysrhythmias can also occur during emergence from general anesthesia. As such, general anesthesia may be contraindicated in certain patients, particularly in the elderly or those with multiple comorbidities.

Enhanced Recovery After Surgery

ERAS, initially developed in Denmark, gained momentum in the 1990s with the goal of integrating multidisciplinary, perioperative care programs. The ultimate aim of this effort was to reduce the length of hospitalization after elective abdominal surgery through integrated approaches to maintain cardiovascular, pulmonary, neurological, gastrointestinal, and endocrine homeostatic functions [19, 20]. See Chap. 6 for a full discussion and history of ERAS. Below, we will review its implementation at University of Miami, specifically for minimally invasive transforaminal lumbar interbody fusion (MIS TLIF). This operation was chosen due to the widespread application of this technique, its versatility for treating diverse lumbar spine pathologies, and its existing development as an MIS approach. There are six core components (Table 26.1).

Table 26.1 Adverse events associated with use of general anesthesia in the elderly [10]

Organ system	Adverse events
CNS	Stroke, delirium
Cardiovascular	Myocardial infarction, arrhythmia, heart failure, intraoperative hypotension/hypertension
Pulmonary	Pulmonary embolism, ARDS, pneumonia, reintubation
Renal	Acute kidney injury

Anesthetic Technique

Conscious sedation for awake spinal surgery consists of a continuous infusion of propofol and ketamine. Supplemental oxygen is delivered via nasal cannula. Medications are titrated to achieve a moderate sedation level. The optimal level of sedation is one where patients are kept comfortable but maintain spontaneous ventilation and respond purposefully to verbal or noxious stimuli. Gabapentin 600 mg is given orally prior to surgery and 1 g IV Tylenol is given immediately postoperatively with the goal of decreasing the need for narcotics after surgery (Table 26.2). Ondansetron, glycopyrrolate, and oxymetazoline nasal spray are all given preoperatively to prevent intraoperative emesis and epistaxis that would force conversion to general anesthesia. For lumbar fusions, a thoracolumbar interfascial plane (TLIP) block is performed with liposomal bupivacaine prior to the creation of any soft tissue tract [21]. Injecting prior to any muscle trauma maintains a pressure gradient and allows for more efficient diffusion and delivery of the drug. No opioid medication or additional spinal, epidural, or general analgesic is used (Table 26.3). As the

Table 26.2 Six components of awake MIS TLIF

Component	Advantages	Disadvantages	FDA clearance
Working channel endoscope	8 mm incision, allows for a formal discectomy and clear visualization	Limited decompression capability, capital equipment cost, learning curve	On-label
Awake surgery	Patient neuromonitoring, limited anesthetic side effects, minimal disturbance of homeostasis	Limited working time, airway not secured, learning curve for anesthetist	On-label
Expandable cage	Implantable through 8 mm tract, increased foraminal height, spinal alignment correction	Cage resorption and subsidence, risk of bone allograft, not available in all countries	Off-label
BMP	Robust osteogenesis, no need for autograft	Heterotopic bone formation, cost, question of teratogenesis	Off-label
Small caliber percutaneous screws	Premium implant cost	Learning curve	On-label
Liposomal bupivacaine	72 h of local anesthesia, reduced narcotic and NSAID use	Cost, risk of intrathecal injection	Off-label

Table 26.3 Medications

Pre-op	Intra-op	Post-op
Gabapentin 600 mg Ondansetron Glycopyrrolate Oxymetazoline nasal spray	TLIP block with liposomal bupivacaine prior to any incision Propofol infusion Ketamine infusion	Tylenol IV 1 g immediate post-op Gabapentin, tramadol, Tylenol Avoidance of narcotics

patient is positioned prone without an advanced airway, the experience and comfort level of the anesthesia team are critical to this technique. Continuous patient monitoring and communication between surgeon and anesthesiologist allow for the safety and success of the procedure. In addition to avoiding the complications of general anesthesia, awake surgery has the advantage of immediate feedback via painful stimuli if there is any irritation of nerve or dorsal root ganglion, thus providing real-time nerve monitoring without the need of a neurophysiologist.

Surgical Technique (See Video 26.1)

The patient is awake and therefore able to position himself on the Jackson table in a comfortable position, minimizing the possibilities of peripheral nerve injury or pressure ulcers (Fig. 26.1). Kambin's triangle is accessed on the symptomatic side [22] (Fig. 26.2). A series of successive dilators is used to dilate the tract up to 8 mm, which is the size of the working cannula of the endoscope (joimax). The disc space is entered and unpacked with a pituitary rongeur (Fig. 26.3). Fluoroscopic shots are taken intermittently to confirm the depth and location of instruments as needed. A series of manual drills, automatic steel brushes, and cutting instruments are used to perform an efficient discectomy (Fig. 26.4). An inflatable balloon is placed into the

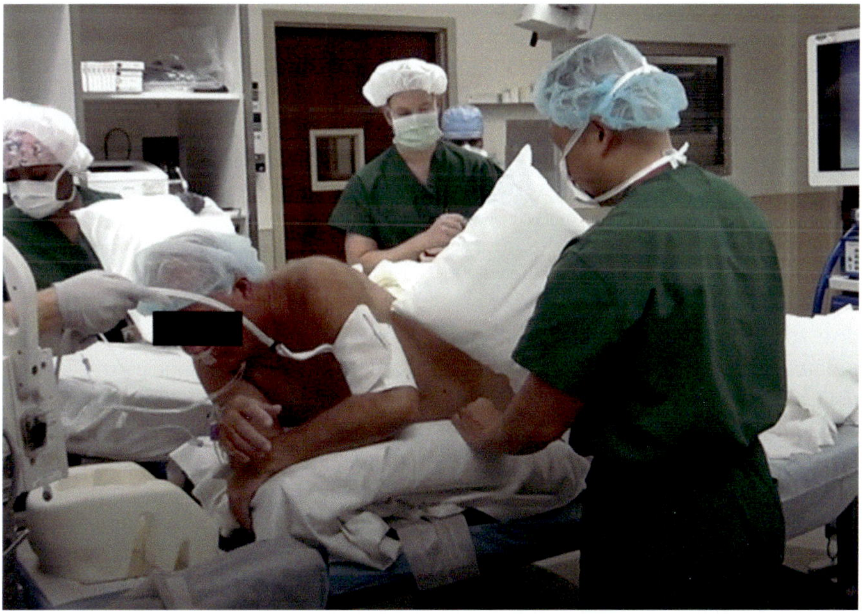

Fig. 26.1 The patient is awake and therefore able to position himself on the Jackson table in a comfortable position, minimizing the possibilities of peripheral nerve injury or pressure ulcers

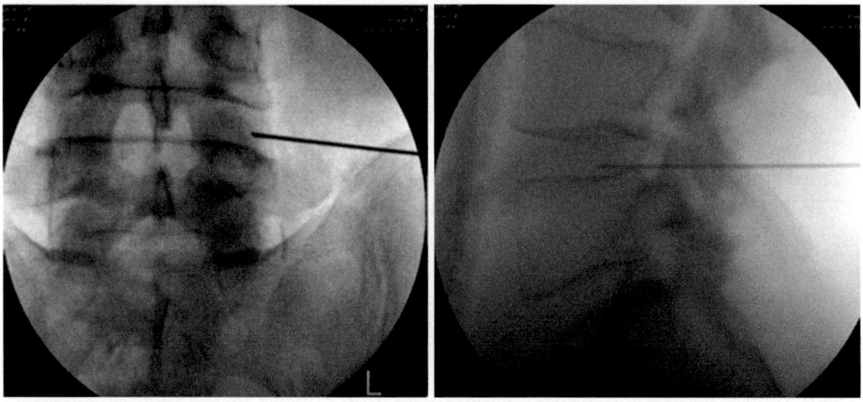

Fig. 26.2 AP and lateral fluoroscopy showing percutaneous access to the disc space via Kambin's triangle

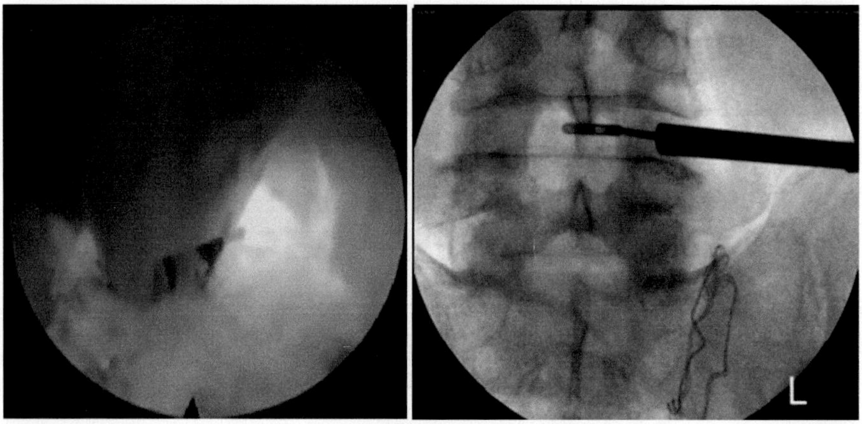

Fig. 26.3 Initial endoscopic view of the discectomy and AP fluoroscopic view of the pituitary rongeur crossing midline during the discectomy

disc space and subsequently expanded using radiopaque contrast material. Once inflated, an anteroposterior radiograph is obtained, and, if there appears to be residual cartilaginous endplate, additional endplate preparation is performed (Fig. 26.5). The endoscope is reinserted, and the endplates are surveyed to ensure they are well prepared and there are no cartilaginous fragments left (Fig. 26.6). These additional steps help ensure adequate endplate preparation and help prevent early cage migration [23].

Following disc removal, 2.1 mg of rhBMP-2 (recombinant human bone morphogenetic protein-2, InFuse, Medtronic SofamorDanek) is placed into the anterior disc space as far away from any neural structures as possible. This is followed by placement of an OptiMesh (Spineology) cage. The mesh expandable cage is filled

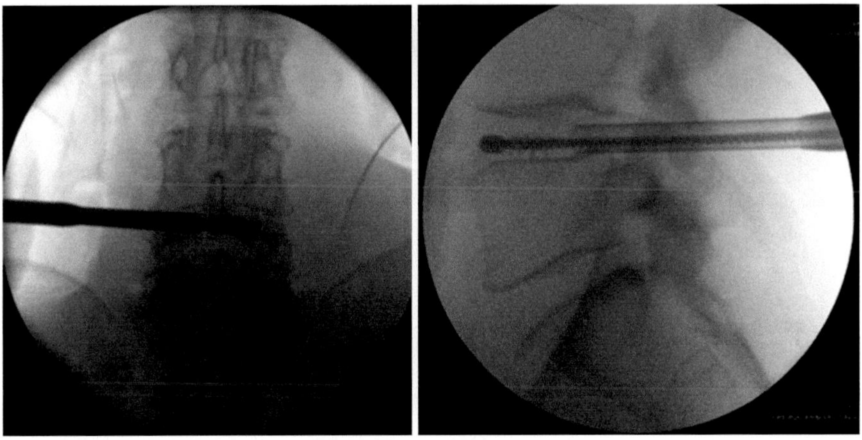

Fig. 26.4 AP view of manual drill and lateral view of automated steel brush used for efficient discectomy

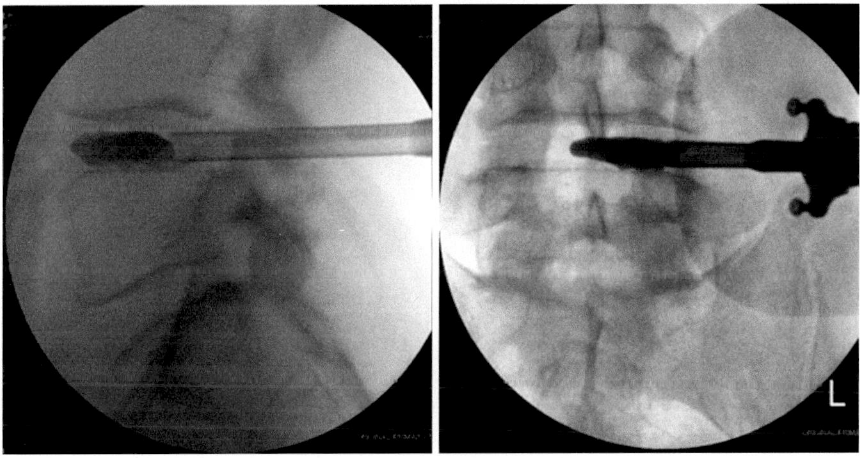

Fig. 26.5 AP and lateral fluoroscopy of radiopaque balloon inflated in the disc space. The balloon is to the front of the canal on the lateral image. The AP image shows some remaining disc fragments left to be cleared, so further discectomy is needed

internally with premachined allograft matrix to increase interbody height (Fig. 26.7). Appropriate placement and expansion allow for re-establishment of disc space height, additional indirect neural element decompression, and correction of any concomitant spondylolisthesis. Pedicle screws are subsequently placed percutaneously using anteroposterior fluoroscopic guidance; bilateral connecting rods are inserted subfascially; and set screws are placed to secure the construct (Fig. 26.8). A total of five incisions are then closed with subcuticular sutures.

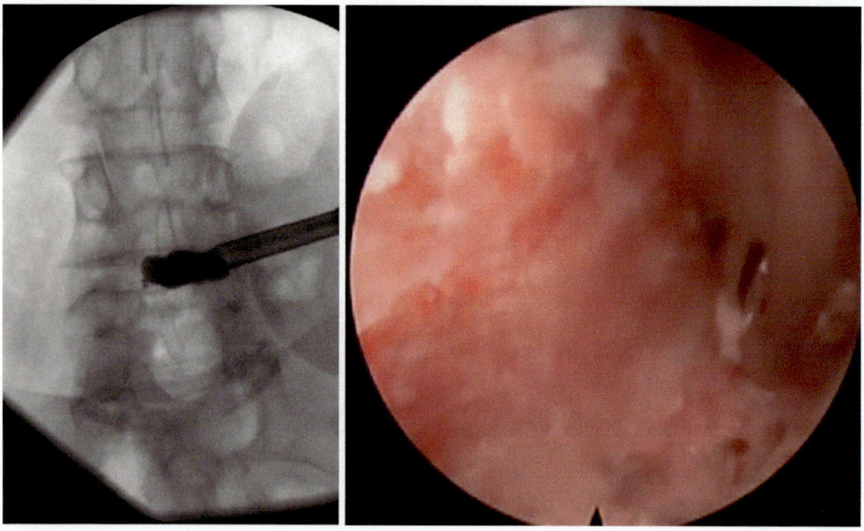

Fig. 26.6 AP fluoroscopy showing good apposition of the endplate by the inflatable balloon indicating adequate endplate preparation (left) and an endoscopic view of the final endplate preparation (right)

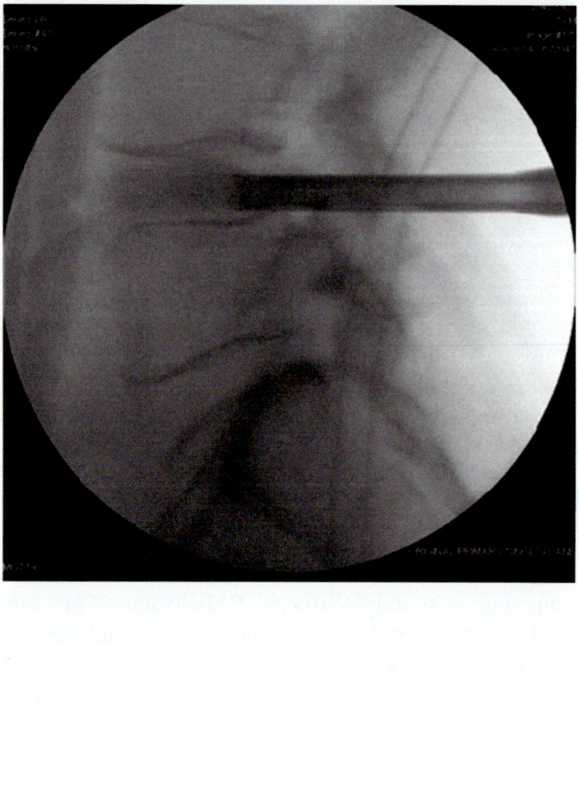

Fig. 26.7 Lateral view of OptiMesh cage being deployed in the disc space

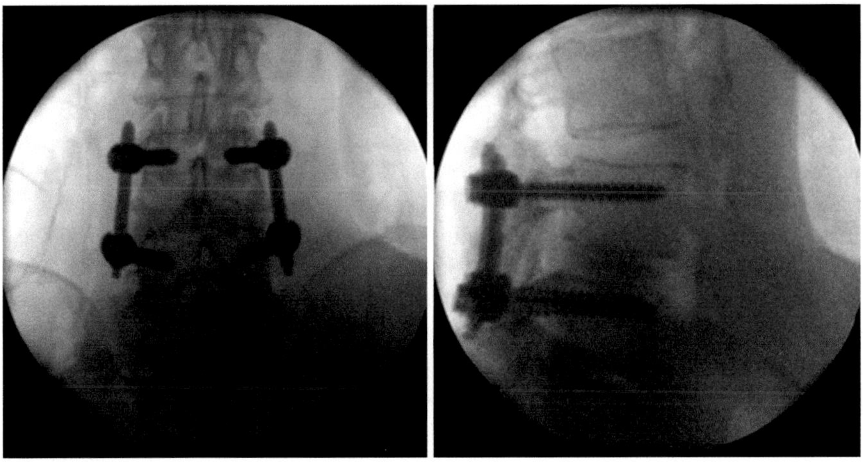

Fig. 26.8 AP and lateral view of the final construct showing bilateral pedicle screws and interbody graft

Postoperative Care

The goal of minimal disturbance of physiological homeostasis continues in the postoperative period. Surgical drains and Foley catheters are not placed during surgery so there is nothing to remove postoperatively resulting in minimal impediments to mobilizing the patient. Gabapentin and Tylenol are given post-op. No IV narcotics are given, and oral narcotic use is minimized. Each patient receives a daily postoperative visit from a member our ERAS care team consisting of medical students working closely with the neurosurgical resident staffing the floor. The goal of these visits is to ensure that patients have adequate pain management and receive early mobilization from the physical therapy and occupational therapy teams. Additionally, the ERAS care team can aid in discharge planning and help facilitate patient discharge plans, ensuring appropriate medical devices such as braces and walkers are delivered on time.

Outcomes

Initial outcomes of MIS TLIF using ERAS principles have been encouraging. Analysis of the first 100 procedures performed by a single surgeon (MYW) demonstrate overall positive results with regard to clinical outcome, complication rate, and overall reduction in perioperative morbidity [23]. Of these 100 cases, single-level fusion was performed in 84 patients and two-level fusion in 16 patients. L4–5 was the most common level, representing 77% of all fused levels. The mean (± standard deviation) operative time was 84.5 ± 21.7 min for one-level fusions and

128.1 ± 48.6 min for two-level procedures. The mean intraoperative blood loss was 65.4 ± 76.6 ml for one-level fusions and 74.7 ± 33.6 ml for two-level fusions. And the mean length of hospital stay was 1.4 ± 1.0 days. Four patients died from causes unrelated to surgery or spinal pathology prior to 1-year follow-up. Four patients required conversion to general anesthesia intraoperatively and the surgery was completed on the same day. The reasons for conversion were two patients had emesis, one had epistaxis, and one experienced extreme anxiety. These four cases resulted in changes to the ERAS protocol (addition of oxymetazoline nasal spray and ondansetron pre-op). Surgical complications included two cases of early cage migration, one case of osteomyelitis, and one endplate fracture. There were no cases of delayed non-union or hardware breakage.

In a further review of all 1- to 3-level lumbar fusions done using the ERAS protocol (57 patients) at University of Miami, patients had a significantly shorter length of stay (2.9 days vs 3.8 days), consumed significantly less oxycodone-acetaminophen, had lower pain scores recorded by the PT/OT teams and nursing, consumed less meperidine and ondansetron, and ambulated farther on postoperative day 1 compared to a similar group of patients who underwent the same procedures 6 months prior to implementation [24].

Mummaneni et al., in an attempt to address limitations of endoscopic surgery, have reported successful awake MIS TLIF using tubular retractors to achieve direct decompression [25]. They achieve analgesia using spinal anesthetic in addition to liposomal bupivacaine. The potential advantage of this approach is the ability to allow for longer operative times (>2 h), avoid the steep learning curve required for endoscopic procedures, and provide direct as well as indirect decompression. The drawbacks include the increased invasiveness of the approach (compared to endoscopy) and the potential complications of spinal anesthesia.

Conclusions

Elderly patients are disproportionally impacted by the harmful effects of general anesthesia. As population pyramids in most developed countries continue to invert, novel surgical solutions will be required to safely take care of the world's aging population. Awake surgery and ERAS concepts have the potential to become a powerful tool to expand surgical care to those who might otherwise not be optimal candidates for intervention. These techniques also allow for shorter length of hospital stay. In some instances, surgeries that previously required admission are converted into outpatient procedures. This results in cost savings and reduced burden on strained medical resources. Finally, initial data has shown these procedures to be efficacious, with significant reductions in ODI, resulting in meaningful quality of life improvement for patients [23].

References

1. Cloward RB. The anterior approach for the removal of ruptured cervical discs. J Neurosurg. 1958;15(6):602–17.
2. Oppenheimer JH, DeCastro I, McDonnell DE. Minimally invasive spine technology and minimally invasive spine surgery: a historical review. Neurosurg Focus. 2009;27(3):E9.
3. Wang MY, Grossman J. Development of an enhanced recovery after surgery (ERAS) approach for lumbar spinal fusion. J Neurosurg Spine. 2017;26(4):411–8.
4. Inouye SK, Westendorp RGJ, Saczynski JS. Delirium in elderly people. Lancet. 2014;383(9920):911–22.
5. Lee JR, Loepke AW. Does pediatric anesthesia cause brain damage?—addressing parental and provider concerns in light of compelling animal studies and seemingly ambivalent human data. Korean J Anesthesiol. 2018;71(4):255–73.
6. Jevtovic-Todorovic V, Olney JW. PRO: anesthesia-induced developmental neuroapoptosis: status of the evidence. Anesth Analg. 2008;106(6):1659–63.
7. Loepke AW, McGowan FX Jr, Soriano SG. CON: the toxic effects of anesthetics in the developing brain: the clinical perspective. Anesth Analg. 2008;106(6):1664–9.
8. Vutskits L. Anesthetic-related neurotoxicity and the developing brain: shall we change practice? Paediatr Drugs. 2012;14(1):13–21.
9. US Food and Drug Administration. FDA drug safety communication: FDA review results in new warnings about using general anesthetics and sedation drugs in young children and pregnant women. White Oak, MD: US Food and Drug Administration; 2017.
10. Liu LL, Leung JM. Predicting adverse postoperative outcomes in patients aged 80 years or older. J Am Geriatr Soc. 2000;48(4):405–12.
11. Brown CH 4th, et al. Delirium after spine surgery in older adults: incidence, risk factors, and outcomes. J Am Geriatr Soc. 2016;64(10).2101–8.
12. Lipowski ZJ. Delirium in the elderly patient. N Engl J Med. 1989;320(9):578–82.
13. Deiner S, Westlake B, Dutton RP. Patterns of surgical care and complications in elderly adults. J Am Geriatr Soc. 2014;62(5):829–35.
14. Tetzlaff JE, et al. Spinal anesthesia for elective lumbar spine surgery. J Clin Anesth. 1998;10(8):666–9.
15. Ditzler JW, et al. Should spinal anesthesia be used in surgery for herniated intervertebral disk? Anesth Analg. 1959;38(2):118–24.
16. Jellish WS, et al. A prospective randomized study comparing short- and intermediate-term perioperative outcome variables after spinal or general anesthesia for lumbar disk and laminectomy surgery. Anesth Analg. 1996;83(3):559–64.
17. Walcott BP, et al. Cost analysis of spinal and general anesthesia for the surgical treatment of lumbar spondylosis. J Clin Neurosci. 2015;22(3):539–43.
18. Wang H, et al. Cervical plexus anesthesia versus general anesthesia for anterior cervical discectomy and fusion surgery: a randomized clinical trial. Medicine (Baltimore). 2017;96(7):e6119.
19. Kehlet H. Multimodal approach to control postoperative pathophysiology and rehabilitation. Br J Anaesth. 1997;78(5):606–17.
20. Kehlet H, Wilmore DW. Multimodal strategies to improve surgical outcome. Am J Surg. 2002;183(6):630–41.
21. Hand WR, et al. Thoracolumbar interfascial plane (TLIP) block: a pilot study in volunteers. Can J Anesth. 2015;62(11):1196–200.
22. Fanous AA, Tumialán LM, Wang MY. Kambin's triangle: definition and new classification schema. J Neurosurg. 2020;32(3):390.
23. Kolcun JPG, et al. Endoscopic transforaminal lumbar interbody fusion without general anesthesia: operative and clinical outcomes in 100 consecutive patients with a minimum 1-year follow-up. Neurosurg Focus. 2019;46(4):E14.

24. Brusko GD, et al. Reductions in length of stay, narcotics use, and pain following implementation of an enhanced recovery after surgery program for 1- to 3-level lumbar fusion surgery. Neurosurg Focus. 2019;46(4):E4.
25. Kai-Hong Chan A, et al. A novel technique for awake, minimally invasive transforaminal lumbar interbody fusion: technical note. Neurosurg Focus. 2019;46(4):E16.

Chapter 27
Endoscopic Spine Surgery in the Geriatric Population

Jacob L. Goldberg and Eric Elowitz

Introduction

The most common indication for spinal surgery in the elderly population is lumbar spine stenosis (LSS) [1]. Lumbar stenosis is most commonly diagnosed in adults 65 years and older, a cohort of the population which is expected to dramatically increase in the coming years [1]. Over the past few decades, the most rapidly increasing type of lumbar spine surgery was for stenosis [2]. In appropriately selected patients, surgery for decompression is superior to nonoperative management [3–6]. Despite the clear benefits of surgery, the older population is at increased risk of perioperative complications due to increased rate of medical comorbidities, immobility, and overall poor nutritional status [7]. In fact, patients older than 65 years who undergo surgery for LSS face increased risks of complications and/or rehospitalizations [8] which can negatively impact quality of life. Further, among adults older than 80 years, this increased risk is directly correlated with the number of medical comorbidities, surgical invasiveness, and operative time [9].

Endoscopic spine surgery in the elderly population is an attractive alternative to conventional spine surgery as it offers a therapeutic treatment with less tissue trauma and hopefully quicker recovery. As a result of the small diameter of the endoscope, less soft tissue, muscle, and ligamentous dissection is required which translates into less blood loss and reduced length of hospital stay [10]. In fact, many endoscopic procedures can be performed in the outpatient surgical center setting. These

J. L. Goldberg
Department of Neurosurgery, New York Presbyterian Hospital, New York, NY, USA
e-mail: jag9177@nyp.org

E. Elowitz (✉)
Department of Neurosurgery, New York Presbyterian Hospital, New York, NY, USA

Department of Neurological Surgery, Weill Cornell Medicine, New York, NY, USA
e-mail: ere2006@med.cornell.edu

K.-M. G. Fu et al. (eds.), *Treatment of Spine Disease in the Elderly*,
https://doi.org/10.1007/978-3-031-12612-3_27

qualities alone mitigate a significant amount of risk in the elderly as their tolerance of blood loss is lower and their propensity to develop delirium in the inpatient hospital setting has been well documented [11–16]. The evidence base for endoscopy in the geriatric population is growing, with current results consistently indicating comparable outcomes, similar complication profile, and significantly shorter lengths of stay [17, 18].

The two most common endoscopic approaches used to treat degenerative lumbar pathology are the interlaminar and transforaminal approaches. The interlaminar approach is similar to the more conventional tubular laminectomy or discectomy approach and allows for good central decompression and access to paracentral disc herniations. The transforaminal approach is more lateral, uses Kambin's triangle as a safe working corridor, and provides access to foraminal pathology as well as central and paracentral disc herniations. If a patient has both central stenosis and a foraminal disc herniation, a procedure using both approaches may be employed (Fig. 27.1).

Here we discuss the two most common endoscopic approaches used to address the lumbar degenerative pathology commonly encountered in the elderly. We review their advantages and disadvantages, preoperative considerations and preparation, and key surgical steps. Finally, we detail the decision-making, considerations, and techniques involved in an illustrative example case.

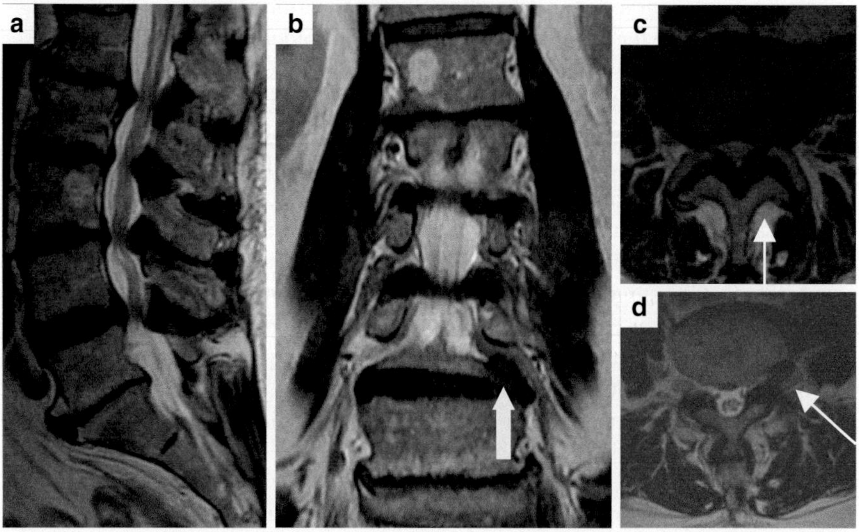

Fig. 27.1 (**a**) Sagittal T2 MRI lumbar spine demonstrating degenerative changes throughout most notably loss of lumbar lordosis, degenerative disc disease at all visualized levels, and severe stenosis at L3–4 and L4–5. (**b**) Coronal T2 MRI lumbar spine with foraminal disc herniation on left side at L4–5 (arrow) compressing the exiting L4 nerve root. (**c**) Axial T2 MRI with severe central stenosis at L3–4. The white arrow indicates the trajectory for the interlaminar approach. (**d**) Axial T2 MRI with a foraminal disc herniation at L4–5. The white arrow indicates the trajectory for a transforaminal approach

Advantages and Disadvantages of Endoscopic Discectomy and Decompression

Conventional open and tubular spine surgical techniques are important as not all pathology can be treated endoscopically. However, when the anatomy and pathology are amenable, endoscopic technique offers several unique advantages. First, visualization of anatomy is superb owing to powerful light sources, high-resolution camera and display, and the ability to position the endoscope in very close working distance to the pathology (Fig. 27.2). In addition to the obvious benefits to the surgeon, the easy visibility of the procedure on the monitor facilitates resident and medical student training and allows a more seamless integration with regard to the surgical assistant and/or scrub technician participation in the case. Second, after the initial learning curve is overcome, this procedure is cost-effective as a result of lower operating room costs and postoperative costs associated with length of stay. Importantly, fully endoscopic is less invasive compared with traditional microscope-assisted approaches resulting in less injury to surrounding tissues and stabilizing ligaments. This facilitates easier revision surgery if required. It also leaves less dead space for fluid to collect and become infected. The lack of dead space is also helpful in containing small CSF leaks as there is less space for fluid to collect. Lastly, there is significant and growing interest among patients in pursuing increasingly MIS procedures with patients indicating they would travel significant distances in pursuit of an MIS procedure [19].

Several disadvantages to endoscopic approaches are worth noting. First, endoscopy offers a limited number of techniques/maneuvers to deal with significant intraoperative complications. A significant complication such as uncontrolled bleeding may necessitate a more invasive approach to address the problem. As a result, patients should be counseled preoperatively regarding the possibility of conversion

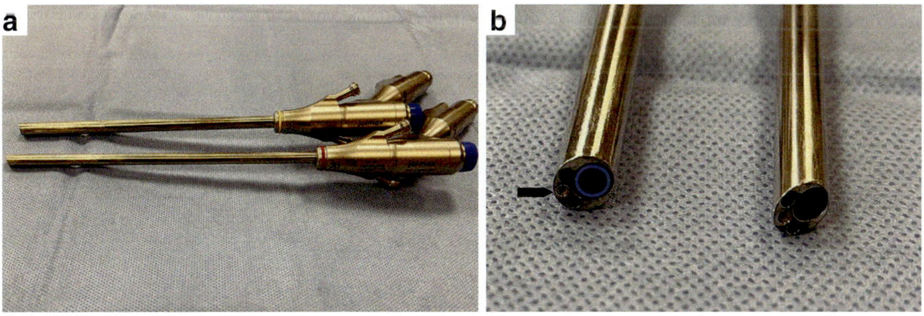

Fig. 27.2 (**a**) Endoscopes with 15° (top) and 30° (bottom) viewing angles ideal for interlaminar and transforaminal procedures, respectively. (**b**) Head on view of the 15° (left) and 30° (right) endoscopes. On the 15° endoscope, one of the two paired light sources is highlighted in yellow, one of the paired irrigation channels is highlighted in green, the working channel is outlined in blue, and a black arrow indicates the single camera. These same components are found on the 30° endoscope

to open surgery. Similarly, options for dealing with large dural lacerations are limited as it is not currently possible to effectively suture dura endoscopically. While economic barriers to endoscopic surgery are low relative to other new technologies (such as intraoperative navigation), there is a notably steep but surmountable learning curve. Though there is a lower cost to entry, additional resources are required for the safe performance of endoscopic surgery. For example, in the transforaminal approach, intraoperative monitoring can be useful if the patient is under anesthesia. In the event of an awake transforaminal surgery, special skill is needed on the part of the anesthesia team to manage the patient's conscious sedation in order to strike the correct balance of maintaining the patient in a lucid state to report pain but with enough sedation to remain still during the operation. Lastly, it is worth noting that many of the complications associated with traditional microdiscectomy need to be considered during endoscopy including re-herniation, dural tear, nerve root injury, hematoma, and poor wound healing or infection [20]. However, some of these risks, specifically hematoma in the surgical bed and issues related to wound healing, are mitigated by the lack of dead space and small stab incision associated with endoscopic surgery.

Preoperative Considerations

Imaging

As is the case with all surgery aimed at addressing lumbar pathology, imaging must be tailored to the patients presenting symptoms, clinical concerns, and neurological exam. MRI with axial, sagittal, and coronal imaging remains the gold standard for identifying lumbar spinal pathology. In the case of patients with comorbid conditions precluding MRI, CT myelogram with full reconstructions can be obtained. In cases amenable to the transforaminal approach, particularly above L4/5, it is imperative to ensure that no abdominal contents obstruct the ideal path. If this is unclear, additional imaging should be obtained.

Anesthesia

While many centers perform endoscopic spinal procedures under local anesthesia with conscious sedation, the authors use general anesthesia for their surgeries. Local anesthesia with conscious sedation presents unique anesthetic challenges as patients must be "light" enough to be able to communicate neurologic symptoms encountered but "deep" enough to be able to remain still during the procedure. This is only possible with careful patient selection and high familiarity with the procedure and anesthetic needs on the part of the anesthesiologist. Additionally, elderly patients may become confused with sedation leading to an uncooperative patient unable to safely remain still.

Endoscopic Approach

A widely accepted algorithm to determine the optimal endoscopic approach is not yet available. However, there are several factors to consider when selecting an approach. A key consideration is the site of the pathology. In general, foraminal or extraforaminal stenosis due to disc material or joint cysts is more amenable to a transforaminal approach. If the pathology extends toward the canal, it can be safely accessed if it is located between the lower aspect of the cranial pedicle (beneath the nerve root) and superior aspect of the caudal pedicle. Another somewhat obvious consideration is the presence of obstructing structures. For endoscopy performed at the rostral or caudal extremes of the lumbar spine, the transforaminal approach may be obstructed by the ribs or iliac crests, respectively. Additionally, abdominal contents may obstruct the transforaminal approach and need to be considered especially in very thin patients. The interlaminar approach is useful in addressing pathology causing central stenosis without a foraminal or extraforaminal component. Lastly, it should be noted that the interlaminar space increases in area when moving in a rostral to caudal direction. As a result, the space is readily accessible at L5–S1 often without additional bone resection when performed at this level.

Operative Considerations

For both interlaminar and transforaminal approaches, the patient is secured prone on an X-ray compatible table with careful padding of the hips, chest, knees, elbows, and wrists. The transforaminal approach can be performed in the lateral position depending on surgeon preference. Care is taken not to hyperextend the shoulder greater than 90°. Sequential compression boots are applied unless contraindicated. Of note, slight kyphosis should be either induced in the lumbar spine by choice of table or created by the placement of a hip roll to aid in opening the interlaminar or foraminal window.

For the interlaminar approach, a slightly paramedian stab incision is made at the level of the interlaminar space. This is determined using AP and lateral fluoroscopy. The authors aim to minimize the skin incision to reduce the egress of irrigation solution in order to maintain a constant pressure. Conversely, a larger fascial incision is performed to allow for mobility of the endoscope. As the patient's lumbar spine is in slight kyphosis due to positioning, the rostral spinous process should project over the disc space of interest and roughly approximate the border of the interlaminar space. Ensuring the optimal approach to the lateral recess decreases the need for bony resection. The rostro-caudal starting point will be determined by patient-specific pathology. Once determined and confirmed by palpation (if body habitus allows), a stab incision is made down through the fascial layer and serial dilators advanced to the inferomedial edge of the lamina. The working channel is placed with the bevel optimizing the medial view. Next bipolar cautery and pituitary rongeurs are used to clear connective tissue. Next, the high-speed drill with diamond burr attachment is used for medial facetectomy. For microdiscectomy, a micro-punch is used to enter the ligamentum flavum with care taken to avoid durotomy. At this time, coagulation of epidural veins is performed as needed. The remainder of the operation depends on patient-specific pathology. However, there are several foundational maneuvers to note. Retraction of nerve roots can be accomplished by rotating the beveled outer sleeve 180° compared with its orientation on insertion. Most minor bleeding quickly tamponades with the hydrostatic pressure applied by the irrigation but coagulation can also be used. While starting from the optimal point will minimize need for bony resection, if the size of the interlaminar window is not large enough to allow removal of a large disc fragment, additional drilling may be necessary, or the fragment may be removed piecemeal. In the case of spinal stenosis, "over the top" decompression by undercutting the spinous process (unilateral approach for bilateral decompression) can be performed as has been described for open and tubular microscope-assisted discectomy.

As compared to the interlaminar approach, trajectory planning for the transforaminal approach has a steeper learning curve as it differs significantly by both spinal level and site of pathology. Especially during the transforaminal approach, the proper trajectory is essential to ensure safely avoiding exiting nerve root injury or injury to abdominal contents. With a combination of AP and lateral fluoroscopy, a beveled spinal needle (facing ventrally) is advanced to the superior articular process (SAP), rotated 180°, and advanced into Kambin's triangle. Dilation is performed after a guidewire is inserted through the needle. Manual bone reamers can be used to remove the inferior aspect of the SAP. The outer sleeve and endoscope can now be inserted, and the remainder of the procedure is performed as dictated by patient-specific pathology.

Interlaminar Endoscopic Discectomy: Illustrative Case

Brief Clinical History

A 67-year-old male with no past medical history presented with 1 month of severe and worsening debilitating radicular pain which failed to improve with conservative management. MRI revealed a large L5–S1 left paracentral disc herniation with resultant lateral recess stenosis without significant foraminal involvement (Fig. 27.3).

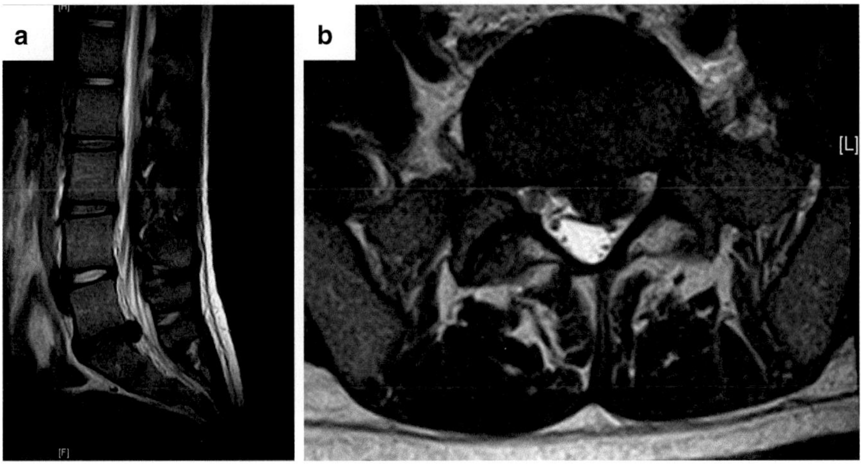

Fig. 27.3 (**a**) Sagittal T2 MRI lumbar spine demonstrating large disc herniation at L5–S1. (**b**) Axial T2 MRI demonstrating L5–S1 disc herniation causing lateral recess stenosis causing mass effect on the traversing nerve root without a significant foraminal or extraforaminal component

Indication for Surgery

As is the case for most surgeries for microdiscectomy, the patient has severe radicular pain with failure to improve with conservative management; MRI scans generally indicate a large herniated disc causing significant compression of the cauda equina nerve roots. While the literature indicates sciatica referable to a lumbar herniated disc will improve with time, it also suggests quicker resolution of symptoms with surgery. Further, a large herniation of this size is unlikely to resorb in an expedient fashion without surgical intervention. Though it is compressing the cauda equina nerve roots, the patient does not endorse symptoms of cauda equina syndrome; therefore, surgery can be offered on an elective basis.

Surgical Approach

This pathology is amenable to open, tubular, or endoscopic treatment depending on surgeon comfort, skill, and equipment availability. Considering endoscopic approaches, this pathology is amenable to an interlaminar approach for several important reasons. First, this patient's iliac crest (Fig. 27.4b) limits the transforaminal approach to L5–S1. Even if that were not the case and the disc space was easily accessible transforaminally, the authors generally prefer the interlaminar approach at L5–S1 due to the large interlaminar window for strictly paracentral herniated discs. Similarly, the slight caudal migration is a factor that may make

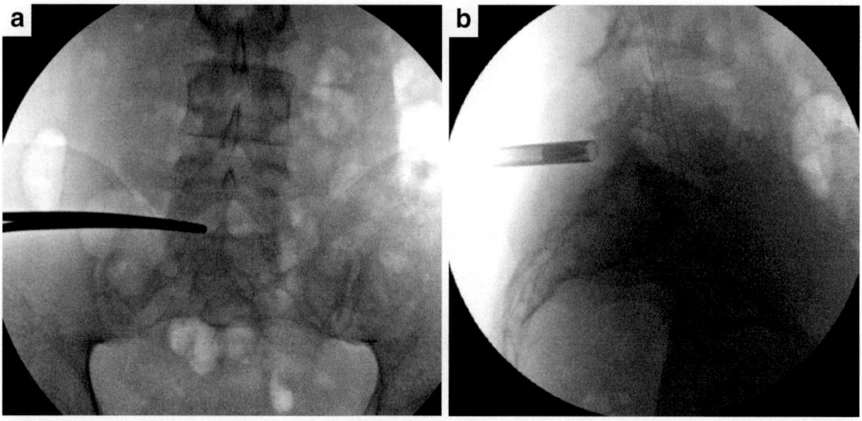

Fig. 27.4 (**a**) AP fluoroscopy with a clamp used to localized the surgical level. The dashed yellow line is placed along the inferior border of the L5 lamina, immediately cranial to the interlaminar space (green dot). (**b**) Lateral fluoroscopy demonstrating the dilator within the outer sleeve directed at the L5–S1 disc space. Note the iliac crest (dashed red line) obstructing lateral access to the L5–S1 disc space

the transforaminal approach more challenging in this case. The large interlaminar space at L5–S1 increases the ease of performance of interlaminar endoscopic discectomy as no bone resection is usually required for optimal access (Fig. 27.4a). The caudal migration of the fragment may pose a challenge to the transforaminal approach.

Operative Procedure

Following the induction of general anesthesia, the patient was placed in prone position. The L5–S1 interlaminar space was confirmed via AP and lateral intraoperative X-ray (Fig. 27.4). A sub-centimeter incision, carried through the skin and fascia, was made slightly left of midline which was the side of the sequestered disc fragment. After serial dilations, the outer sleeve was inserted, and the level and trajectory were confirmed via lateral view X-ray. The endoscope, directed toward the interlaminar space, revealed an intact ligamentum flavum which was cleared of connective tissue with bipolar cautery (Fig. 27.5a, b). All of the subsequent instruments used are modified to function in the endoscope's working channel. A forceps and Kerrison are used to create a window in the ligamentum flavum approximately at the level of the traversing nerve root (Fig. 27.5c). The traversing nerve root is inspected and bluntly mobilized with a ball tip probe (Fig. 27.5d). The tip of the endoscope, beveled to function as a nerve root retractor, is used to medialize and protect the traversing nerve root. Next, the

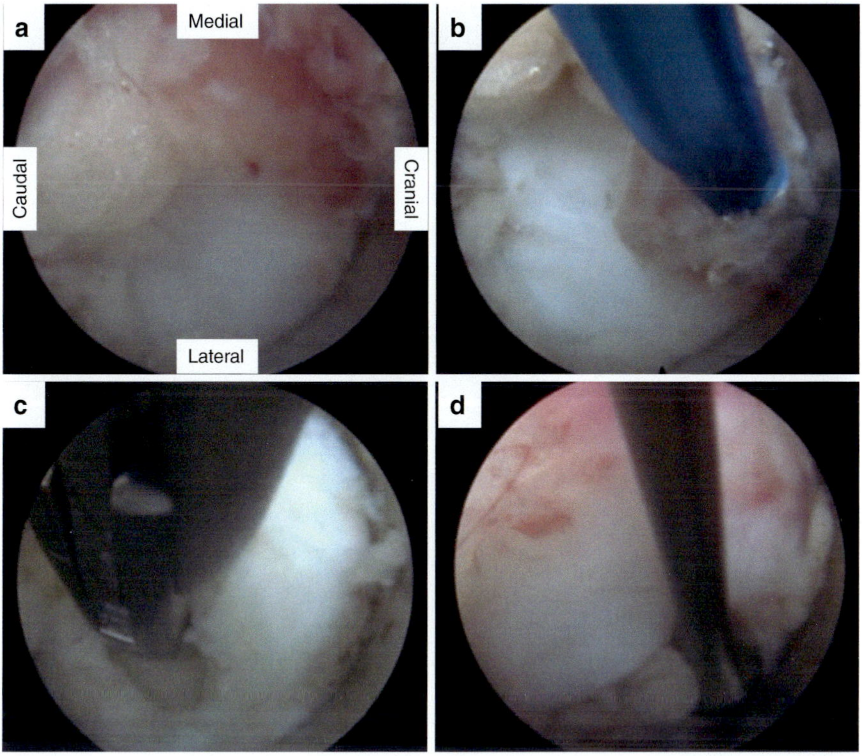

Fig. 27.5 (**a**) Intact ligament with connective tissue/fat overlying medially. (**b**) Bipolar cautery used to clear connective tissue from ligament. (**c**) Ligament entered with blunt forceps. (**d**) Blunt ball dissector used to mobilize traversing nerve root

sequestered disc fragment can be removed through the endoscope's working channel (Fig. 27.6). After adequate decompression has been achieved, careful inspection for hemostasis is performed. Bleeding is addressed with the application of hydrostatic pressure supplied by the constant saline irrigation through the endoscope in combination with bipolar cautery. After hemostasis was obtained, the endoscope was removed, and the incision was closed with a deep fascial suture followed by a running subcuticular suture.

Postoperative Care

After surgery, the patient awoke with immediate relief of symptoms and neurologically intact. After uneventful recovery, the patient was discharged home on the day of surgery and experienced no postoperative complications.

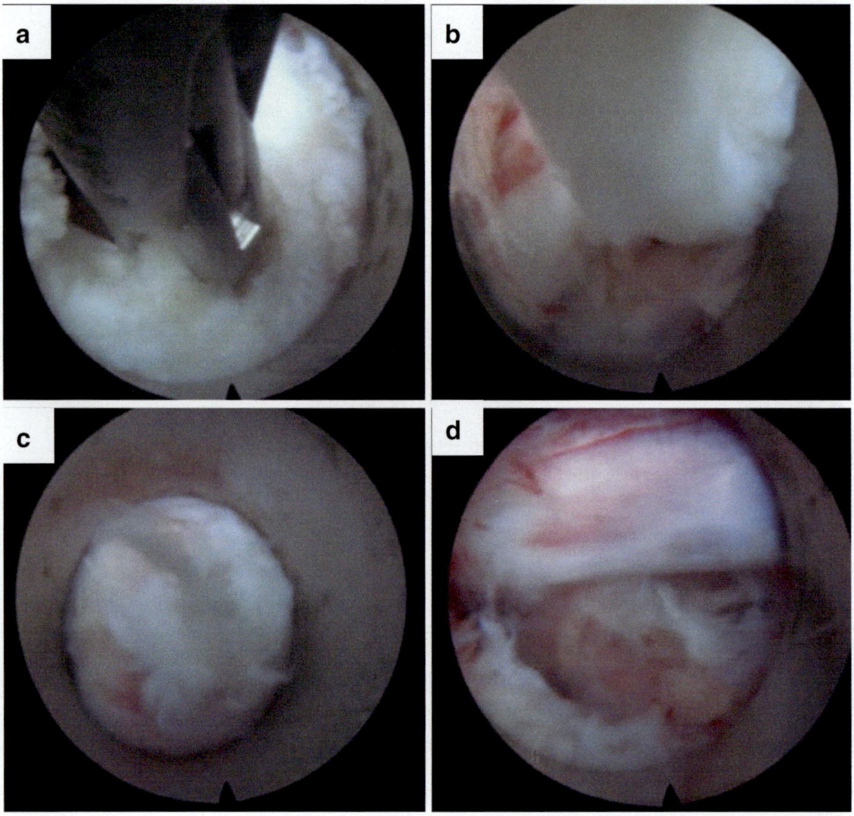

Fig. 27.6 (**a**) Blunt forceps used to grasp disc fragment. (**b**) Disc fragment being pulled into working channel. (**c**) Disc fragment filling working channel. (**d**) Decompressed traversing nerve root after disc removed

References

1. Deyo RA. Treatment of lumbar spinal stenosis: a balancing act. Spine J. 2010;10(7):625–7.
2. Taylor VM, Deyo RA, Cherkin DC, Kreuter W. Low back pain hospitalization. Recent United States trends and regional variations. Spine. 1994;19(11):1207–12. discussion 13
3. Atlas SJ, Keller RB, Wu YA, Deyo RA, Singer DE. Long-term outcomes of surgical and nonsurgical management of lumbar spinal stenosis: 8 to 10 year results from the maine lumbar spine study. Spine. 2005;30(8):936–43.
4. Atlas SJ, Keller RB, Robson D, Deyo RA, Singer DE. Surgical and nonsurgical management of lumbar spinal stenosis. Spine. 2000;25(5):556–62.
5. Weinstein JN, Tosteson TD, Lurie JD, Tosteson ANA, Blood E, Hanscom B, et al. Surgical versus nonsurgical therapy for lumbar spinal stenosis. N Engl J Med. 2008;358(8):794–810.
6. Malmivaara A, Slätis P, Heliövaara M, Sainio P, Kinnunen H, Kankare J, et al. Surgical or nonoperative treatment for lumbar spinal stenosis? A randomized controlled trial. Spine. 2007;32(1):1–8.

7. Smith ZA, Fessler RG. Paradigm changes in spine surgery: evolution of minimally invasive techniques. Nat Rev Neurol. 2012;8(8):443–50.
8. Deyo RA, Mirza SK, Martin BI, Kreuter W, Goodman DC, Jarvik JG. Trends, major medical complications, and charges associated with surgery for lumbar spinal stenosis in older adults. JAMA. 2010;303(13):1259–65.
9. Kobayashi K, Imagama S, Ando K, Ishiguro N, Yamashita M, Eguchi Y, et al. Complications associated with spine surgery in patients aged 80 years or older: Japan Association of Spine Surgeons with ambition (JASA) multicenter study. Global Spine J. 2017;7(7):636–41.
10. Choi G, Pophale CS, Patel B, Uniyal P. Endoscopic spine surgery. J Korean Neurosurg Soc. 2017;60(5):485–97.
11. Wu W-C, Schifftner TL, Henderson WG, Eaton CB, Poses RM, Uttley G, et al. Preoperative hematocrit levels and postoperative outcomes in older patients undergoing noncardiac surgery. JAMA. 2007;297(22):2481–8.
12. Foss NB, Kristensen MT, Kehlet H. Anaemia impedes functional mobility after hip fracture surgery. Age Ageing. 2008;37(2):173–8.
13. Hagino T, Ochiai S, Sato E, Maekawa S, Wako M, Haro H. The relationship between anemia at admission and outcome in patients older than 60 years with hip fracture. J Orthop Traumatol. 2009;10(3):119–22.
14. Dunne JR, Malone D, Tracy JK, Gannon C, Napolitano LM. Perioperative anemia: an independent risk factor for infection, mortality, and resource utilization in surgery. J Surg Res. 2002;102(2):237–44.
15. Collier R. Hospital-induced delirium hits hard. Can Med Assoc J. 2012;184(1):23–4.
16. Vijayakumar B, Elango P, Ganessan R. Post-operative delirium in elderly patients. Indian J Anaesth. 2014;58(3):251–6.
17. Yang F, Chen R, Gu D, Ye Q, Liu W, Qi J, et al. Clinical comparison of full-endoscopic and microscopic unilateral laminotomy for bilateral decompression in the treatment of elderly lumbar spinal stenosis: a retrospective study with 12-month follow-up. J Pain Res. 2020;13:1377–84.
18. Kim JH, Kim HS, Kapoor A, Adsul N, Kim KJ, Choi SH, et al. Feasibility of full endoscopic spine surgery in patients over the age of 70 years with degenerative lumbar spine disease. Neurospine. 2018;15(2):131–7.
19. Narain AS, Hijji FY, Duhancioglu G, Haws BE, Khechen B, Manning BT, et al. Patient perceptions of minimally invasive versus open spine surgery. Clin Spine Surg. 2018;31(3):E184–92.
20. Shriver MF, Xie JJ, Tye EY, Rosenbaum BP, Kshettry VR, Benzel EC, et al. Lumbar microdiscectomy complication rates: a systematic review and meta-analysis. Neurosurg Focus. 2015;39(4):E6.

Part V
Advances in Pain Management Treatments for Elderly Patients

Chapter 28
CT-Guided Radiofrequency Ablation

Michelle Roytman and J. Levi Chazen

Introduction to Ablation

Ablation therapy is a minimally invasive technique commonly used in the treatment of benign and malignant tumors, with emerging use in the realm of pain management. A number of ablative modalities exist, generally comprising a generator and needlelike device delivering energy directly to targeted tissue to cause acute cellular necrosis [1]. Radiofrequency (RF), microwave, laser, and high-intensity focused ultrasound (HIFU) systems apply energy to heat tissue to cytotoxic temperatures (e.g., at least 60 °C for maximal efficacy of protein denaturation and immediate coagulative necrosis), while cryoablation systems cool tissues to less than −40 °C to cause tissue necrosis via ice crystal formation and osmotic shock [2]. Irreversible electroporation (IRE) is an additional nonthermal technique that induces cell apoptosis through the formation of permanent nanopores within the cell membrane utilizing a high-voltage electrical current. These ablative techniques can be performed percutaneously, endoscopically, laparoscopically, or via a celiotomy incision, with the exception of HIFU which is performed extracorporeally utilizing a specialized ultrasound probe [1]. Though similar in purpose, each technique has its own specific and optimal indications. This chapter will review CT-guided RF ablation, including a discussion of RF ablative principles and frequently performed procedures, focusing on its use as a cutting-edge technique for the treatment of spine disease in the elderly.

M. Roytman
Department of Radiology, Weill Cornell Medicine, New York, NY, USA
e-mail: mir9146@med.cornell.edu

J. L. Chazen (✉)
Department of Radiology, Weill Cornell Medicine, New York, NY, USA

Department of Radiology, Hospital for Special Surgery, New York, NY, USA
e-mail: chazenjl@hss.edu

K.-M. G. Fu et al. (eds.), *Treatment of Spine Disease in the Elderly*,
https://doi.org/10.1007/978-3-031-12612-3_28

Principles of RF Ablation

RF ablation relies on a complete electrical circuit created through the body to conduct RF current [2]. An RF generator is used to deliver high-frequency, alternating current (375–600 kHz) through an RF probe, with current passing through the uninsulated active tip of the probe and resulting in oscillation of charged tissue molecules (ions) within the ablative zone [3]. RF current is able to pass through tissue due to the abundance of ionic fluid present; however, tissues are poor conductors of electricity, leading to ionic agitation and resistive heating (the Joule heating effect). Areas closest to the electrode (within several millimeters) experience the highest current and greatest rise in temperature via direct RF heating, while tissues farther away in the final ablation zone are primarily heated via thermal conduction [1, 2, 4].

RF current can be applied using "monopolar" or "bipolar" systems [2]. In the monopolar system, a single interstitial electrode is used to deliver current at the target site, and the circuit is completed using surface electrodes (ground pads) applied onto the patient's skin. In the bipolar system, current flows between two interstitial electrodes, either within the same applicator or between two separate applicators, thereby increasing the invasive nature of the procedure. Bipolar mode has advantages by heating the area between the electrodes, reduced dependence on background conductivity, and reduced likelihood of skin burns by eliminating the use of a grounding pad [1, 2]. However, bipolar systems do not heat well outside of this array and often require saline infusion to improve results. Benefits of the monopolar system include its wide clinical availability, broader zone of ablation around each electrode, and decreased invasiveness given its use of a single electrode [1, 2]. Currently available RF systems typically utilize monopolar electrodes in three general varieties: straight needlelike, multitined, or multitined expandable. Expandable multitined and non-deployable multitined electrodes increase the electrode-tissue contact surface area, dispersing the current over a greater volume which can increase the ablation zone size [1].

While RF ablation has been shown to be clinically effective in the treatment of small tumors (<2 cm), principles of electrical and thermal conductivity may hinder its success [1, 2, 4]. RF ablation relies on the flow of current through tissue for adequate heating and cell death. Tissues with high water and ion contents (e.g., liver) are able to more effectively transmit current than those with lower water and ion contents (e.g., lung, fat, and bone) which demonstrate a higher electrical impendence. As tissues become heated and char (carbonization), water vapor is generated and tissue becomes dehydrated, resulting in a rapid increase in electrical impedance limiting flow of electrical current. Therefore, RF ablation can be a self-limiting process [1, 2]. Cooling the electrode with circulating water has been shown to decrease temperatures at the electrode-tissue interface, reducing char and improving current over time [5].

Char can be further minimized by modifying the RF generator output [1, 2]. Impedance-controlled systems, or "pulsed RF ablation," utilize a power pulsing algorithm to achieve a goal maximum impedance while allowing tissue to cool and rehydrate as needed, generating greater energy deposition with decreased average impedance. Power is initially set to a relatively low level (20–50 W) with temporary suspension of power output as impedance rapidly rises. This power pulsing technique can be sequentially performed with multiple electrodes to create multiple independent ablations or one large ablation, increasing procedural efficiency. Temperature-controlled systems, or "thermal RF ablation," alternatively aim to achieve a preset target temperature at the tip(s) of the electrode(s). Power is gradually increased until the target temperature is obtained, which can be modulated to maintain target temperature for the duration of ablation [1, 2, 6].

A critical consideration for spinal RF ablation is the potential for spinal cord injury [7]. RF heating has been shown to be cytotoxic to the spinal cord and peripheral nerves at around 45 °C [8], and a lesion-to-spinal cord distance of less than 10 mm has previously been reported as an exclusion criteria for RF ablation in some series [9]. A number of neuroprotective maneuvers have been explored, such as instillation of epidural/periradicular carbon dioxide or cooled 5% dextrose in water during ablation and/or use of thermocouples for continuous temperature monitoring as an extra margin of safety [10–12]. However, a retrospective review of 17 patients treated for spinal osteoid osteoma demonstrated RF ablation to be a safe procedure, even with lesions located within 10 mm of neural structures, without differences in outcome or complication with use of epidural air as a neuroprotective agent [7]. In fact, the authors reported instances of thecal sac and cord displacement toward the lesion by instilled air, contrary to the desired effect, potentially raising temperatures reaching the neural elements. When neurological injury does occur, literature reports it to be typically transient in nature, noting at least one case report of permanent lower extremity paralysis due to RF ablation-induced thermal injury [13].

Use of moderate or general anesthesia has also been suggested to further mitigate possible risk of neural injury due to patient movement related to procedural pain at the time of ablation [3, 14], noting sedation may be associated with its own risks. Limiting RF ablation time, for example, under 2 min in one series [14], has been reported as an additional neuroprotective measure. Presence of intact cortical bone between target lesion and neural structures provides an additional margin of safety [8]. However, osteolysis with cortical destruction, frequently encountered in the setting of osseous metastases, compromises this protective boundary from undesired RF energy propagation [3, 15, 16].

The high impedance of bone is an additional limiting factor of spinal RF ablation, with resultant poor thermal conduction and diminished ablative margins [1, 2]. However, procedural modifications and maneuvers have been implemented to improve intraprocedural conductivity. Infusion of normal saline (0.9%) has been shown to successfully enlarge the area of necrosis during RF ablation, serving as a liquid electrode with conductivity 3–5 times greater than that of blood and 12–15 times greater than that of soft tissues [17]. Use of hypertonic saline (6–36%), in combination with the bipolar technique, has demonstrated faster and more extensive ablation with less heat loss as compared to the monopolar technique in an animal liver model. Use of hypertonic saline has also been shown to reduce volume of saline required for desired decrease in impedance [17]. Simultaneous use of multiple applicators has been shown to result in thermal synergy as the cumulative effect of overlapping ablation zones leads to increased temperatures [6].

Efficacy of tissue heating can further be affected by adjacent vasculature, such as large blood vessels which may dissipate thermal energy [1]. In fact, tumors adjacent to large vessels have been shown to demonstrate increased local recurrence rates, demonstrating the significant impact of these thermal energy sinks [18]. The thermal energy sink phenomenon is relevant in spine interventions, given the presence of epidural venous plexus and movement of cerebral spinal fluid within the spinal canal [8]. However, some authors hypothesize this heat sink effect of spinal fluid and venous plexus is protective and allows for the ability to safely perform RF ablation in lesions as close as 2 mm away from nerve roots [19].

Safety and efficacy of spinal RF ablation has been further improved by the development of novel navigational bipolar electrode systems designed specifically for ablation of osseous spinal lesions [12, 20]. One such system (STAR ablation device, DFINE, Inc., San Jose, CA, comprised of SpineSTAR electrode and MetaSTAR generator) contains a pair of built-in active thermocouples positioned along the length of the electrode at either 5 and 10 mm (smaller version) or 10 and 15 mm (larger version) from the center of the ablation zone, allowing for real-time monitoring of sufficiently high temperature and ablative volume while minimizing risk of thermal injury. The navigating tip of the probe can be articulated in different orientations through the same entry site with the ability to cross midline, allowing for electrode placement in challenging locations that may be otherwise difficult to access. Another novel ablation system utilizes cooled RF needles (OsteoCool, Medtronic, Inc., San Jose, CA). While not flexible, the system comes in different lengths to control the ablation zone and can be used in a unipedicular approach, though bipedicular access is desired to achieve a larger zone of ablation. A separate thermocouple is attached to the system and can be introduced into the epidural space for real-time monitoring [21]. These novel RF ablation devices ultimately provide smaller and more predictable ablation zones, thereby improving feasibility and success of spinal RF ablation.

An additional safety consideration when performing RF ablation, particularly in the elderly, is the presence of cardiac implantable electrical devices (CIEDs). While the potential for electromagnetic interference affecting CIED function is known with RF ablation procedures, available guidelines do not specifically address management of RF ablation for certain procedures, such as zygapophyseal (facet) joint pain. In a web-based survey sent to interventionalists from varying subspecialties who perform this procedure (e.g., radiology, pain anesthesia, and physiatry), practice patterns regarding CIED management in ambulatory spine RF ablation procedures were found to vary [22]. While the presence of CIED is not a contraindication for spine RF ablation, it does increase the complexity of the procedure and necessitates added precautions.

Image guidance with computed tomography (CT) is a key component of CT-guided RF ablation. Pre-procedural planning utilizing CT allows for determination of osseous lesion density (e.g., osteoblastic, osteolytic, or mixed) as well as the identification of cortical discontinuities from tumor erosion and pathologic fracture clefts [3]. Use of CT guidance during the procedure further allows visualization of needle positioning. However, post-procedural RF ablative margins can be poorly visualized with CT and use of CT guidance may result in increased radiation exposure [23].

With this foundation of the principles of RF ablation, we will now review its role as a cutting-edge technique for the treatment of spine disease in the elderly.

Spinal Metastases

Spinal metastases are the most commonly encountered tumor of the spine, typically occurring in the elderly and affecting up to 40% of patients with cancer [24]. Patients with spinal metastases may experience severe and often debilitating tumor-associated pain, pathologic vertebral fractures, and neurologic deficits related to nerve root or spinal cord compression with resultant significant reduction in quality of life [24–26]. Goals of treatment in patients with spinal metastases include pain palliation, local tumor control, mechanical stability, and improvement or maintenance of function. Current standard of care involves a variety of treatment strategies, including a combination of analgesics, bisphosphonates, radiation therapy (RT), and/or surgical intervention, which may be extensive [24]. Palliative RT is reported to have response rates of 50–90% [24]; however, RT has critical limitations. Therapeutic effect of RT may be delayed 10–14 days with recurrence of pain in up to 57% of patients [24]. Specific tumor histologies demonstrate a poor response to RT, notably melanoma, sarcoma, non-small cell lung cancer, and renal cell carcinoma [27]. Additionally, RT to the spine is limited by cumulative tolerance of the spinal cord with potential for radiation-induced myelopathy.

Multiple series have been published in recent years demonstrating the role of minimally invasive, percutaneous, image-guided procedures, such as RF ablation and vertebral augmentation. These techniques have demonstrated progressive success in pain reduction and improved function with high technical success and low complication rates [25, 28]. RF ablation with concurrent vertebral augmentation has been advocated as a combined treatment given the advantageous antitumoral effect of heat and mechanical stabilization by cement injection (Fig. 28.1). RF ablation and vertebroplasty have demonstrated independent efficacy in pain palliation [28, 29], with some studies suggesting synergy in degree of pain palliation when performed concurrently. Furthermore, these procedures can be conveniently performed in tandem in an outpatient setting. Comparative trials have not yet been performed to date to establish superiority of this combined therapy [24]. RF ablation as an adjuvant to palliative RT has also been reported to improve patient pain scores with more rapid palliation as compared with local RT alone [13].

It is evident that RF ablation of spinal metastases has a clear therapeutic role, particularly for nonsurgical candidates and/or for those who failed chemoradiation. In addition to the percutaneous approach, RF ablation has been reported as an adjunct treatment intraoperatively at the time of surgical decompression and

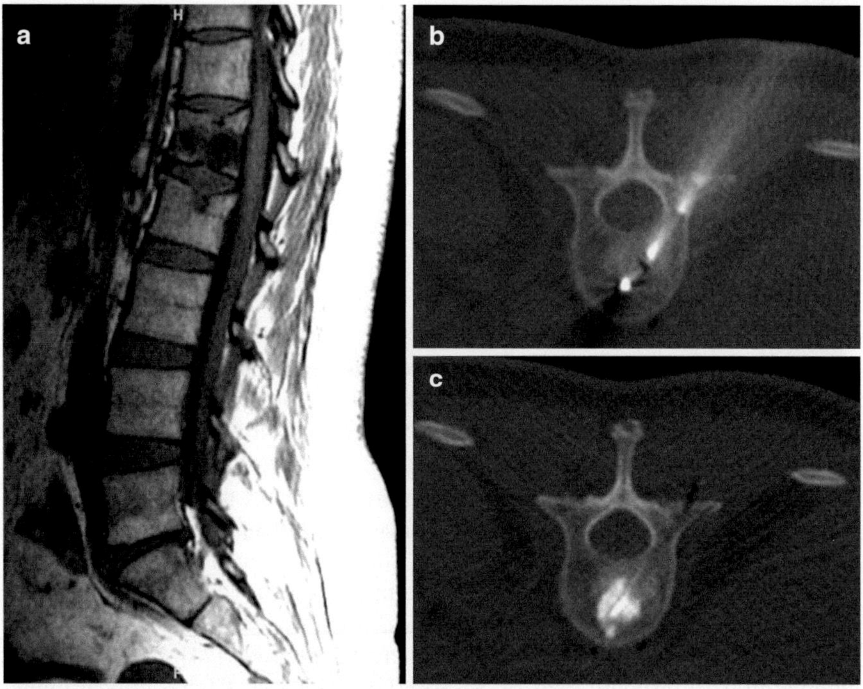

Fig. 28.1 Sagittal T1 (**a**) demonstrating a T1 hypointense metastasis in the L1 vertebral body. Axial procedural CT images (**b** and **c**) show the DFINE STAR ablation device entering the vertebral body via a transpedicular approach with deployment of the curved RF cannula (**b**). Following the ablation, cement augmentation is administered (**c**)

stabilization [30] as well as via a transoral approach for treatment of a lesion involving the lateral mass of the C1 vertebral body [31].

It is important to note that osteoblastic/sclerotic lesions exhibit higher intrinsic impedance than do osteolytic/lucent lesions, rendering them more challenging to treat as the RF circuit is unable to generate sufficiently high temperatures to ensure cell death [32]. Many series list osteoblastic metastases as an exclusion criteria for RF ablation, suggesting cryoablation or microwave ablation as the preferred thermal ablative modality for their treatment [3].

Malignant Primary Osseous Lesions

Chordoma

Chordomas are the most common primary malignant spinal tumor, representing 1–4% of primary bone tumors and more than half of primary sacral tumors [33]. Chordomas originate from notochordal remnants and arise within the axial skeleton, most frequently in the sacrococcygeal region (50–66%) and skull base (35%), with a metastatic rate of 5–43% [34]. Age at detection ranges from 30 to 70 years, more often found in males (2–3:1; M/F) [33]. Chordomas are locally aggressive and resistant to RT with high recurrence rates, low disease-free survival, and high rates of morbidity from conventional treatments.

A number of case reports and small case series suggest RF ablation as an effective therapeutic option for painful or rapidly growing chordomas, with evidence of radiographic success, reduction of tumor pain, decrease in tumor burden, and arrest in tumor growth [33, 35, 36]. RF ablation has also been shown to help achieve tumor-free exposed margins for gross-total excision, particularly critical for chordomas given their high recurrence rate and associated morbidity [35]. It is hypothesized that the high-water content of this tumor (e.g., classically very T2 hyperintense lesion) and lack of vascularity contribute to its favorable dielectric properties with a treatment volume larger than expected [33]. Additional larger prospective studies will be needed to validate efficacy of these initial observations.

Plasmacytoma and Myeloma

Plasmacytoma and myeloma are hematologic malignancies resulting in skeletal destruction with osteolytic lesions and/or pathologic fractures, involving the vertebra in 60% of cases at time of diagnosis [37]. Two-thirds of patients with myeloma report bone pain, frequently in the back or pelvis [38]. While RT is the current gold standard treatment for cancer patients with localized bone pain, 20–30% do not experience relief with this approach [39]. RT can further result in early bone loss due to inflammation and possible RT-related pathological fractures. Similar to pain associated with spinal metastases, additional conventional treatment options such as surgical excision, systemic chemotherapy, bisphosphonates, and analgesics are often unsuccessful in providing complete pain relief. Therefore, minimally invasive percutaneous techniques such as RF ablation and vertebroplasty have been explored as additional therapeutic options.

RF ablation is a favorable modality in the treatment of multiple myeloma as the lesions are osteolytic with associated low intrinsic impedance; therefore, myeloma is a frequently included diagnosis in case series of RF ablation with or without concurrent vertebroplasty [3, 5, 9, 28, 40–43]. Vertebroplasty alone has been demonstrated to provide improved pain relief in patients with myeloma, hypothesized to occur due to its increased internal trabecular stabilization. In a prospective series of 36 patients receiving concurrent RF ablation with vertebroplasty versus vertebroplasty alone, use of percutaneous vertebroplasty alone appeared to be effective for the pain management of patients with vertebral involvement of multiple myeloma [37]. The authors suggested the additional use of RF ablation for treatment of myelomatous lesions included cost and time without clear added benefit. Further larger prospective studies are needed to validate these initial observations. To our knowledge, there is no published literature describing use of RF ablation for treatment of plasmacytoma; however, RF ablation could theoretically serve as an additional therapeutic option in the appropriate clinical setting.

Aggressive Intraosseous Venous Malformations (Vertebral Hemangioma)

Intraosseous venous malformations, formerly known as vertebral hemangiomas, are benign angiomatous lesions involving the spine. They have an estimated incidence of 10–12%, commonly occurring in young adults with slight female predilection [44]. The vast majority of lesions are asymptomatic and detected as an incidental finding during imaging examinations. However, approximately 1% of cases can be aggressive, defined as symptomatic with extraosseous extension or significant osseous expansion owing to pathological fracture, osseous expansion, and/or extraosseous extension resulting in mass effect upon adjacent neural structures [44]. Use of RF ablation of a sacral S1–S2 aggressive hemangioma has been reported via robotic-assisted placement of a 10-mm bipolar probe providing an ablation zone of 17 × 13 mm, covering nearly the entire hemangioma [44]. Additional larger prospective studies will be needed to validate the efficacy of this initial case report.

Benign Primary Osseous Lesions

Benign tumors comprise 4–13% of spinal lesions and are treated with curative intent [3, 45]. Pain secondary to benign spine lesions is commonly managed with nonsteroidal anti-inflammatory drug (NSAID) therapy and opioids titrated to achieve relief while minimizing side effects [46]. When pharmacologic therapy is inadequate or contraindicated, minimally invasive, percutaneous, image-guided interventions, such as RF ablation, are indicated [3]. Though many of the following entities infrequently affect the elderly, they are briefly mentioned to comprehensively review the many potential uses of CT-guided RF ablation in the spine.

Osteoid Osteoma and Osteoblastoma

Osteoid osteoma (OO) is a benign bone-forming tumor composed of a central nidus generally less than 15 mm in diameter surrounded by reactive bone [14]. OOs represent 3% of all primary bone tumors with 10% arising in the spine, most commonly in the posterior elements [12]. OOs classically occur in young adult males (2–4:1; M/F) under the age of 30 presenting with constant or episodic bone pain, typically worsening at night or with physical activity and alleviated with NDSAIDs. Initially reported in 1992 [47], RF ablation of OOs is a frequently performed procedure with numerous papers advocating its efficacy and safety [7, 10–12, 14, 16, 19, 48–50]. RF ablation is now considered standard of care for most osteoid osteomas, with success rates equaling or surpassing those of surgery as well as decreased morbidity and shorter hospitalizations [15].

Osteoblastoma (OB) is a rare benign tumor strikingly similar in histology to OO but biologically more aggressive [3, 51]. OBs most commonly occur in the second or third decades of life with a slight male predilection (2:1; M/F). OBs are typically larger (>1.5 cm) and more expansile as compared to OOs and may be associated with aneurysmal bone cysts. The entire osteolytic and soft tissue components, when present, must be ablated for definitive cure. Due to its larger size, a more radical ablative approach is required including at least two ablations with straight unipolar probes covering the entire lesion at a recommended temperature of 90 °C for 6 min [3]. Use of the previously described novel navigational bipolar RF ablation probe with articulation of probe tip in different orientations through a single-entry site has been reported for successful RF ablation of OBs. A prospective series of 11 patients with OBs undergoing RF ablation demonstrated complete success in terms of pain relief with RF ablation alone [51].

Aneurysmal Bone Cyst and Giant Cell Tumor

Aneurysmal bone cyst (ABC) is a benign expansile vascular tumor of bone which can be locally aggressive, typically occurring in patients younger than 20 years of age [3]. ABCs involve the spinal column in 20–30% of cases, typically affecting posterior elements. ABCs can be challenging lesions to manage due to their large size and close proximity to neurovascular structures. While limited literature exists on use of RF ablation for its treatment, a case series of 20 patients with ABCs receiving RF ablation with or without concomitant vertebroplasty demonstrated RF ablation to be clinically successful and curative with reduction in mean visual analog scale pain score in all treated cases [52]. No post-procedural complications or recurrence was reported within this cohort. Additional larger prospective studies will be needed to validate these initial findings.

Giant cell tumor (GCT) is a primary skeletal neoplasm representing 5% of all primary bone tumors [23]. Most commonly occurring in the long bones near articulations, it comprises fewer than 5% of primary bone tumors in the spine, predominantly occurring in the sacrum [53]. These uncommon osteolytic lesions occur primarily in females in their twenties and thirties, often presenting with complaints of back pain. GCT can be associated with high recurrence rates (30–50%), with preoperative RF ablation suggested to ensure adequate tumor removal and reduction in local recurrence [23]. Preoperative RF ablation was reported to enable easier curettage of necrotic tumor with decreased potential blood loss, minimal surgical trauma, and preservation of osseous continuity allowing for rapid functional recovery and reduction of morbidity [23]. Further studies are required to better define the role of RF ablation in the treatment of GCT.

Intraosseous Spinal Glomus Tumors

Glomus tumors, also known as angioglomoid tumors, are benign vascular neoplasms arising from smooth muscle cells of the neuromyoarterial glomus [54]. Glomus tumors are most frequently located in the subcutaneous tissues of the extremities, especially the palmar, plantar, and subungual regions. However, glomus tumors have been reported in an intraosseous location, though uncommon and possibly related to secondary involvement of a soft tissue lesion. While treatment of choice is complete surgical resection by curettage or en bloc resection, Becce et al. report a case of biopsy-proven intraosseous spinal glomus tumor successfully treated with RF ablation with improved pain and without evidence of residual or recurrent disease at 6-month follow-up [54]. Additional larger prospective studies will be needed to validate this case report.

Chronic Back Pain and Degenerative Spine Disease

Chronic low back pain affects more than 30 million people, approximately 10–13% of the adult US population [55, 56]. There is a substantial body of evidence supporting vertebral body endplates and nociceptors arborizing from the basivertebral nerve (BVN) to be a significant source of low back pain [56–58]. Therefore, disruption of the BVN signaling pathway via RF ablation has been hypothesized as a therapeutic option for chronic low back pain. Industry-sponsored studies [56, 57] have been performed to investigate this theory, including the INTRACEPT trial: a prospective, parallel, randomized, controlled, open-label, multicenter clinical trial of 140 patients with suspected vertebrogenic chronic low back pain as well as Modic Type 1 or 2 changes from L3 to S1 randomized to either RF ablation of the BVN or continuation of standard care [56]. An interim analysis at 3 months posttreatment identified a clear statistical superiority for all primary and secondary patient-reported outcome measures in the RF ablation arm compared with standard care, thereby halting enrollment and allowing early crossover from the control arm. Analysis of control subjects who elected to crossover to treatment as well as subsequent follow-up of treatment arm patients at 5 years will be performed, which will provide additional long-term data on this promising novel treatment.

Additional RF ablations performed for the treatment of degenerative spine disease include RF ablation of the medial branch of the dorsal ramus, which provides sensory innervation to the zygapophyseal (facet) joint [59–61]. Medial branch RF ablation has been performed in patients with centralized pain (e.g., fibromyalgia-like phenotype), demonstrating less improvement in overall pain but equal improvement in site-specific pain levels within this cohort after localized interventions [62].

Targeted intraspinal RF ablation for lumbar spinal stenosis has been reported as an effective percutaneous alternative for treatment of spinal stenosis by reducing intraspinal soft tissue and creating relatively more epidural space [63]. Similarly, CT-guided RF nucleoplasty has been performed for the treatment of lumbar disc herniation, demonstrating relative efficacy and safety for treatment of leg pain caused by radicular encroachment [64]. These minimally invasive nonsurgical treatment options are especially useful in high-risk surgical candidates, often including elderly patients.

Coccydynia and Pudendal Neuralgia

Coccydynia, pain within the coccyx area, has a multitude of different causes and can affect a wide range of ages [65, 66]. Primary treatment is conservative therapy, including rest, decreased time in the sitting position, physical therapy, usage of seat cushions, and NSAIDs. Several interventional therapies, including local injection of local anesthetics and steroids, neurolysis of sacral nerve roots, caudal epidural block, and RF ablation, have been suggested for patients who do not respond to initial conservative therapy. In a retrospective review of 12 patients who underwent pulsed or thermal RF ablation for coccydynia, average pain relief experienced was 55.5% with positive outcomes more likely in patients who received prognostic blocks, suggesting sacrococcygeal nerve RF ablation may be a useful treatment option for patients with coccydynia who have failed more conservative measures [66]. Within this cohort, two cases of transient neuritis were reported. Additional larger prospective studies will be needed to validate these initial findings.

Pudendal neuralgia (PN), or “Alcock’s canal syndrome,” results from pudendal nerve entrapment or injury. Common areas of nerve compression include the interspace between the sacrotuberous and sacrospinous ligaments as well as within the pudendal canal of Alcock [67]. A variety of etiologies are attributable to PN, including mechanical injury, prolonged compression, trauma during childbirth, and

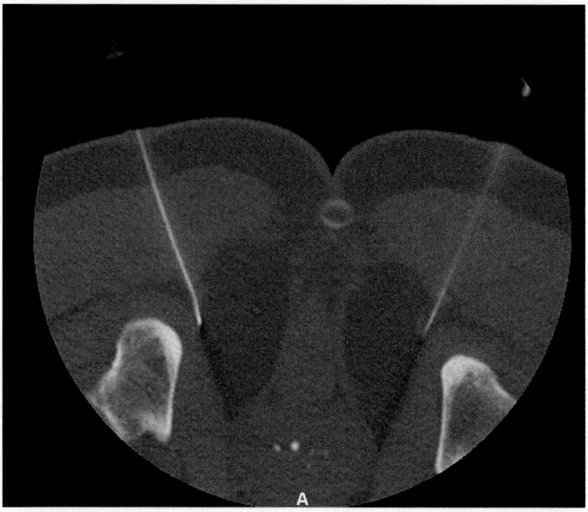

Fig. 28.2 Radiofrequency ablation cannulas are placed bilaterally at the proximal aspect of Alcock's canal for pulsed radiofrequency ablation of the pudendal nerves

iatrogenic during surgical procedures. PN can result in chronic pain that may be debilitating, often affecting the elderly. Initial management is usually conservative, including a combination of lifestyle modifications and pharmacologic options. If conservative measures do not provide adequate pain relief, invasive treatment such as local steroid injections and surgical decompression are typically performed. Pulsed RF ablation has been shown to be safe and efficacious in the treatment of chronic recalcitrant pelvic pain [67, 68] (Fig. 28.2).

Cervicogenic Headache

Cervicogenic headache is a secondary headache syndrome attributable to upper cervical spine pathology, with an estimated prevalence of up to 4% of the general population and 20% of patients with chronic headache [69]. Due to the convergence of upper cervical segment nociceptive afferents with the trigeminal complex, pain from the upper cervical nerves may be referred to the occipital, orbital, frontal, and/or parietal regions [70]. Potential culprit nerves include the greater occipital nerve, lesser occipital nerve, and third occipital nerves, with the greater and lesser occipital nerves both receiving contributions from the C2 dorsal root ganglion [71]. While cervicogenic headaches may occur from a variety of pathologies (e.g., tumors, fractures, infections, and arthritides), osteoarthritis of the lateral atlantoaxial joint with resultant C2 dorsal root ganglion irritation is an important, and potentially treatable, cause of cervicogenic headaches [72].

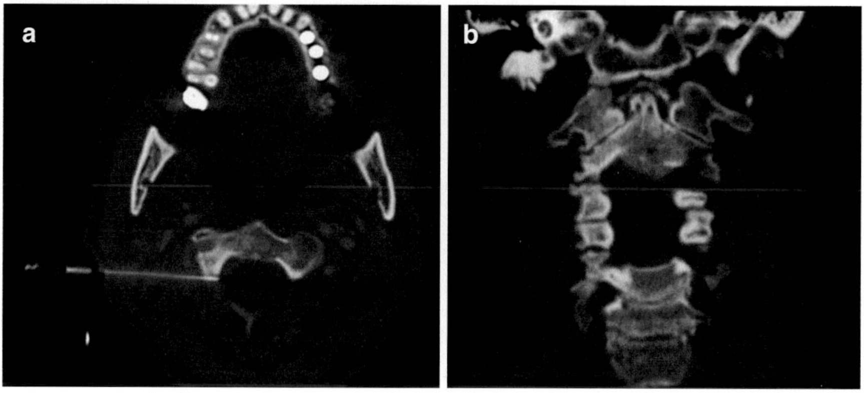

Fig. 28.3 Axial CT image (**a**) showing appropriate placement of a radiofrequency cannula for thermal ablation of the right C2 dorsal root ganglia for cervicogenic headache. Coronal CT reformation (**b**) shows severe asymmetric osteoarthrosis of the right C1–C2 articulation

CT-guided RF ablation of the C2 dorsal root ganglion for treatment of cervicogenic headache has been described [72]; however, to date, there is no high-quality randomized control trial and/or strong non-randomized control trial supporting use of these techniques [73, 74] (Fig. 28.3).

Trigeminal Neuropathic Pain

Trigeminal neuropathic pain is a syndrome of unilateral, paroxysmal, stabbing facial pain, originating from the trigeminal nerve [75]. Most cases are caused by vascular compression of the trigeminal root entry zone and most patients respond well to pharmacotherapy. However, in the setting of refractory trigeminal neuropathic pain, surgical options or neurostimulation may be explored. Neurostimulation directed to the trigeminal nerve itself intracranially or to its peripheral branches subcutaneously has been reported to be efficacious. Additionally, RF ablation of the spinal trigeminal tract/nucleus, by way of percutaneous CT-guided trigeminal nucleotractotomy of the spinal trigeminal tract, has been described as an additional treatment option for refractory cases [76], which may be a useful treatment option for elderly patients experiencing debilitating pain.

The sphenopalatine ganglion can be targeted in a similar fashion with promising efficacy in the treatment of cluster headaches and a variety of pain syndromes [77] (Fig. 28.4).

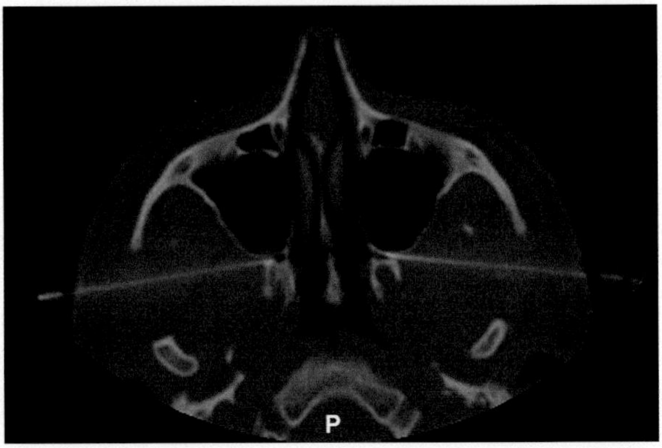

Fig. 28.4 Axial CT image showing placement of bilateral radiofrequency cannula within the sphenopalatine ganglion via the pterygomaxillary fissure

Conclusion

CT-guided RF ablation is an emerging cutting-edge technique and therapeutic option for a variety of benign and malignant entities affecting the elderly. The above-described literature strongly supports its use as a safe, resource-saving, and highly effective therapeutic option that should be considered in the appropriate clinical setting. It is important to note that while RF ablation is often performed for treatment of painful osseous lesions, RF ablation in itself can induce significant peri-procedural and immediate post-procedural pain [3]. This is in part due to a significant inflammatory reaction that occurs post-ablation, though short-term corticosteroid therapy immediately after treatment has been reported to be effective for pain management and allows for prompt hospital discharge [51].

Ultimately, healthcare utilization has been shown to significantly decrease post-RF ablation, including complete elimination of opioid use in some patients due to alleviation of pain with a corresponding improvement in quality of life [78]. For these reasons, RF ablation should be highly considered in the management of spine disease in the elderly.

References

1. Knavel EM, Brace CL. Tumor ablation: common modalities and general practices. Tech Vasc Interv Radiol. 2013;16(4):192–200.
2. Brace CL. Radiofrequency and microwave ablation of the liver, lung, kidney, and bone: what are the differences? Curr Probl Diagn Radiol. 2009;38(3):135–43.
3. Tomasian A, Wallace A, Jennings J. Benign spine lesions: advances in techniques for minimally invasive percutaneous treatment. Am J Neuroradiol. 2017;38(5):852–61.
4. Eckmann M, Martinez M, Lindauer S, et al. Radiofrequency ablation near the bone-muscle interface alters soft tissue lesion dimensions. Reg Anesth Pain Med. 2015;40(3):270–5.

5. David E, Kaduri S, Yee A, et al. Initial single center experience: radiofrequency ablation assisted vertebroplasty and osteoplasty using a bipolar device in the palliation of bone metastases. Ann Palliat Med. 2017;6(2):118–24.
6. Brace CL, Sampson LA, Hinshaw JL, et al. Radiofrequency ablation: simultaneous application of multiple electrodes via switching create larger, more confluent ablations than sequential application in a large animal model. J Vasc Interv Radiol. 2009;20(1):118–24.
7. Vidoni A, Grainer M, James S. Experience of neuroprotective air injection during radiofrequency ablation (RFA) of spinal osteoid osteoma. Eur Radiol. 2018;28(10):4146–50.
8. Dupuy DE, Hong R, Oliver B, Goldberg SN. Radiofrequency ablation of spinal tumors: temperature distribution in the spinal canal. Am J Roentgenol. 2000;175(5):1263–6.
9. Gronemeyer DHW, Schirp S, Gevargez A. Image-guided radiofrequency ablation of spinal tumors: preliminary experience with an expandable array electrode. Cancer J. 2002;8(1):33–9.
10. Rybak LD, Gangi A, Buy X, et al. Thermal ablation of spinal osteoid osteomas close to neural elements: technical considerations. Am J Roentgenol. 2010;195(4):W293–8.
11. Klass D, Marshall T, Toms A. CT-guided radiofrequency ablation of spinal osteoid osteomas with concomitant perineural and epidural irrigation for neuroprotection. Eur Radiol. 2009;19(9):2238–43.
12. Pipola V, Tedesco G, Spinnato P, et al. Surgery versus radiofrequency ablation in the management of spinal osteoid surgery versus radiofrequency ablation in the management of spinal osteoid osteomas: a spine oncology referral center comparison analysis of 138 cases. World Neurosurg. 2020;145:E1–7.
13. Huntoon K, Eltobgy M, Mohyeldin A, Elder JB. Lower extremity paralysis after radiofrequency ablation of vertebral metastases. World Neurosurg. 2019;133:178–84.
14. Cuesta HE, Villagran JM, Horcajadas AB, et al. Percutaneous radiofrequency ablation in osteoid osteoma: tips and tricks in special scenarios. Eur J Radiol. 2018;102:169–75.
15. Rybak LD. Fire and ice: thermal ablation of musculoskeletal tumors. Radiol Clin N Am. 2009;47(3):455–69.
16. Wallace AN, Tomasian A, Chang RO, Jennings JW. Treatment of osteoid osteomas using a navigational bipolar radiofrequency ablation system. Cardiovasc Intervent Radiol. 2016;39(5):768–72.
17. Buy X, Basile A, Bierry G, et al. Saline-infused bipolar radiofrequency ablation of high-risk spinal and paraspinal neoplasms. Am J Roentgenol. 2006;186:S322–6.
18. Lu DSK, Raman SS, Limanond P, et al. Influence of large peritumoral vessels on outcome of radiofrequency ablation of liver tumors. J Vasc Interv Radiol. 2003;14(10):1267–74.
19. Vanderschueren GM, Obermann WR, Dijkstra SPD, et al. Radiofrequency ablation of spinal osteoid osteoma: clinical outcome. Spine (Phila Pa 1976). 2009;34(9):901–3.
20. Anchala PR, Irving WD, Hillen TJ, et al. Treatment of metastatic spinal lesions with a navigational bipolar radiofrequency ablation device: a multicenter retrospective study. Pain Physician. 2014;17(4):317–27.
21. Georgy BA, Marini S, Piras E. RF for treatments of malignant lesions. In: Marcia S, Saba L, editors. Radiofrequency treatments on the spine. Cham: Springer; 2017. p. 95–105.
22. Friedrich J, Itano EM, Lynn RR, Friedrich J. Management of cardiac implantable electrical devices in patients undergoing radiofrequency ablation for spine pain: physician survey and review of guidelines. Pain Physician. 2020;23(4):E335–42.
23. Zhao Q, Wang L, Chen F, Jiang T. Percutaneous radiofrequency ablation for treatment of giant cell tumor of bone guided by real-time US fused with CT. J Med Ultrason. 2014;41(2):223–7.
24. Kam NM, Maingard J, Kok HK, et al. Combined vertebral augmentation and radiofrequency ablation in the management of spinal metastases: an update. Curr Treat Options in Oncol. 2017;18(12):74.
25. Bagla S, Sayed D, Smirniotopoulos J, et al. Multicenter prospective clinical series evaluating radiofrequency ablation in the treatment of painful spine metastases. Cardiovasc Intervent Radiol. 2016;39(9):1289–97.

26. Gazis AN, Beuing O, Franke J, et al. Bipolar radiofrequency ablation of spinal tumors: predictability, safety and outcome. Spine J. 2014;14(4):604–8.
27. Gerszten PC, Mendel E, Yamada Y. Radiotherapy and radiosurgery for metastatic spine disease: what are the options, indications, and outcomes? Spine (Phila Pa 1976). 2009;34(22S):S78–92.
28. Burgard CA, Dinkel J, Strobl F, et al. CT fluoroscopy-guided percutaneous osteoplasty with or without radiofrequency ablation in the treatment of painful extraspinal and spinal bone metastases: technical outcome and complications in 29 patients. Diagn Interv Radiol. 2018;24(3):158–65.
29. Callstrom MR, Charboneau JW, Goetz MP, et al. Painful metastases involving bone: feasibility of percutaneous CT- and US-guided radiofrequency ablation. Radiology. 2002;224(1):87–97.
30. Ha K-Y, Kim Y-H, Yoo T-W. Intraoperative radiofrequency ablation for metastatic spine disease: report of 4 cases and review. Eur J Orthop Surg Traumatol. 2013;23(Suppl 2):S129–34.
31. Bundy JJ, Griauzde J, Srinivasa RN, et al. Transoral radiofrequency ablation and cementoplasty for lateral mass of the C1 vertebral body. J Vasc Interv Radiol. 2018;29(9):1246–7.
32. Singh S, Saha S. Electrical properties of bone. Clin Orthop Relat Res. 1984;186:249–71.
33. Neeman Z, Patti JW, Wood BJ. Percutaneous radiofrequency ablation of chordoma. Am J Roentgenol. 2002;179(5):1330–2.
34. Hug EB, Slater JD. Proton radiation therapy for chordomas and chondrosarcomas. Neurosurg Clin N Am. 2000;11(4):627–38.
35. Zhou H, Yang X, Jiang L, et al. Radiofrequency ablation in gross total excision of cervical chordoma: ideas and technique. Eur Spine J. 2018;27(12):3113–7.
36. Anis N, Chawki N, Antoine K. Use of radio-frequency ablation for the palliative treatment of sacral chordoma. Am J Neuroradiol. 2004;25:1589–91.
37. Orgera G, Krokidis M, Matteoli M, et al. Percutaneous vertebroplasty for pain management in patients with multiple myeloma: is radiofrequency ablation necessary? Cardiovasc Intervent Radiol. 2014;37:203–10.
38. Santiago FR, del Garcia MMC, Montes JLM, et al. Treatment of bone tumours by radiofrequency thermal ablation. Curr Rev Musculosket Med. 2009;2(1):43–50.
39. Callstrom MR, Charboneau JW, Goetz MP, et al. Image-guided ablation of painful metastatic bone tumors: a new and effective approach to a difficult problem. Skelet Radiol. 2006;35(1):1–15.
40. Gevargez A, Groenemeyer DHW. Image-guided radiofrequency ablation (RFA) of spinal tumors. Eur J Neurol. 2008;65(2):246–52.
41. Wallace AN, Tomasian A, Vaswani D, et al. Radiographic local control of spinal metastases with percutaneous radiofrequency ablation and vertebral augmentation. Am J Neuroradiol. 2016;37(4):759–65.
42. Tomasian A, Hillen TJ, Chang RO, Jennings JW. Simultaneous bipedicular radiofrequency ablation combined with vertebral augmentation for local tumor control of spinal metastases. Am J Neuroradiol. 2018;39(9):1768–73.
43. Sayed D, Jacobs D, Sowder T, et al. Spinal radiofrequency ablation combined with cement augmentation for painful spinal vertebral metastasis: a single-center prospective study. Pain Physician. 2019;22(5):E441–9.
44. Kaoudi A, Capel C, Chenin L, et al. Robot-assisted radiofrequency ablation of a sacral S1-S2 aggressive gemangioma. World Neurosurg. 2018;116:226–9.
45. Kelley SP, Ashford RU, Rao AS, Dickson RA. Primary bone tumours of the spine: a 42-year survey from the Leeds regional bone tumour registry. Eur Spine J. 2007;16(3):405–9.
46. Hara S. Opioids for metastatic bone pain. Oncology. 2008;74(Suppl 1):52–4.
47. Rosenthal DI, Alexander A, Rosenberg AE, Springfield D. Ablation of osteoid osteoma with a percutaneously placed electrode: a new procedure. Musculoskelet Radiol. 1992;183(1):29–33.
48. Martel J, Bueno A, Nieto-Morales L, Ortiz EJ. Osteoid osteoma of the spine: CT-guided monopolar radiofrequency ablation. Eur J Radiol. 2009;71(3):564–9.
49. Yu X, Wang B, Yang S, et al. Percutaneous radiofrequency ablation versus open surgical resection for spinal osteoid osteoma. Spine J. 2019;19(3):509–15.

50. Wang B, Han SB, Jiang L, et al. Percutaneous radiofrequency ablation for spinal osteoid osteoma and osteoblastoma. Eur Spine J. 2017;26(7):1884–92.
51. Arrigoni F, Barile A, Zugaro L, et al. CT-guided radiofrequency ablation of spinal osteoblastoma: treatment and long-term follow-up. Int J Hyperth. 2018;34(3):321–7.
52. Zarzour OA, Santiago FR, Serrano NO, et al. CT-guided radiofrequency ablation in patients with aneurysmal bone cysts. Eur J Radiol. 2018;100:116–23.
53. Luther N, Bilsky MH, Hartl R. Giant cell tumor of the spine. Neurosurg Clin N Am. 2008;19(1):49–55.
54. Becce F, Richarme D, Letovanec I, et al. Percutaneous radiofrequency ablation of primary intraosseous spinal glomus tumor. Skelet Radiol. 2012;41(4):467–72.
55. Freburger JK, Holmes GM, Agans RP, et al. The rising prevalence of chronic low back pain. Arch Intern Med. 2009;169(3):251–8.
56. Khalil JG, Smuck M, Koreckij T, et al. A prospective, randomized, multicenter study of intraosseous basivertebral nerve ablation for the treatment of chronic low back pain. Spine J. 2019;19(10):1620–32.
57. Becker S, Hadjipavlou A, Heggeness MH. Ablation of the basivertebral nerve for treatment of back pain: a clinical study. Spine J. 2017;17(2):218–23.
58. De Vivo AE, D'Agostino G, D'Anna G, et al. Intra-osseous basivertebral nerve radiofrequency ablation (BVA) for the treatment of vertebrogenic chronic low back pain. Neuroradiology. 2021;63(5):809–15.
59. Stolzenberg D, Ahn JJ, Kurd M. Lumbar radiofrequency ablation: procedural technique. Clin Spine Surg. 2020;33(1):20–3.
60. Cohen SP, Raja SN. Pathogenesis, diagnosis, and treatment of lumbar zygapophysial (facet) joint pain. Anesthesiology. 2007;106(3):591–614.
61. Nguyen T, Chan K, Chryssidis S, Selby M. CT guided radiofrequency ablation of the cervical medial branch using a lateral approach in the supine patient. J Spine Surg. 2017;3(3):463–7.
62. Morffi D, Larach DB, Moser SE, et al. Medial branch radiofrequency ablation outcomes in patients with centralized pain. Reg Anesth Pain Med. 2019;44:730–5.
63. Jacobson RE, Granville M, Hatgis J. Targeted intraspinal radiofrequency ablation for lumbar spinal stenosis. Cureus. 2017;9(3):e1090.
64. Wu S, Li X, Lin C, et al. CT-guided nucleoplasty with radiofrequency energy for the treatment of lumbar disk herniation. J Spinal Disord Tech. 2015;28(1):9–16.
65. Elkhashab Y, Ng A. A review of current treatment options for coccygodynia. Curr Pain Headache Rep. 2018;22(4):1–8.
66. Chen Y, Huang-lionnet JHY, Cohen SP. Radiofrequency ablation in coccydynia: a case series and comprehensive, evidence based review. Pain Med. 2017;18(6):1111–30.
67. Petrov-Kondratov V, Chhabra A, Jones S. Pulsed radiofrequency ablation of pudendal nerve for treatment of a case of refractory pelvic pain. Pain Physician. 2017;20(3):E451–4.
68. Collard MD, Xi Y, Patel AA, et al. Initial experience of CT-guided pulsed radiofrequency ablation of the pudendal nerve for chronic recalcitrant pelvic pain. Clin Radiol. 2019;74(11):897e19–23.
69. Haldeman S, Dagenais S. Cervicogenic headaches: a critical review. Spine J. 2001;1(1):31–46.
70. Barmherzig R, Kingston W. Occipital neuralgia and cervicogenic headache: diagnosis and management. Curr Neurol Neurosci Rep. 2019;19(5):20.
71. Blumenfeld A, Siavoshi S. The challenges of cervicogenic headache. Curr Pain Headache Rep. 2018;22(7):1–5.
72. Chazen JL, Ebani EJ, Virk M, et al. CT-guided block and radiofrequency ablation of the C2 dorsal root ganglion for cervicogenic headache. Am J Neuroradiol. 2019;40(8):1433–6.
73. Grandhi RK, Kaye AD, Abd-elsayed A. Systematic review of radiofrequency ablation and pulsed radiofrequency for management of cervicogenic headaches. Curr Pain Headache Rep. 2018;22(3):18.

74. Nagar VR, Birthi P, Grider JS, Asopa A. Systematic review of radiofrequency ablation and pulsed radiofrequency for management of cervicogenic headache. Pain Physician. 2015;18(2):109–30.
75. Al-quliti KW. Update on neuropathic pain treatment for trigeminal neuralgia. Neurosciences. 2015;20(2):107–14.
76. Larkin MB, North RY. Radiofrequency ablation of spinal trigeminal tract and nucleus caudalis for refractory trigeminal neuropathic pain: 2-dimensional operative video. Oper Neurosurg. 2020;19(5):2019–20.
77. Tolba R, Weiss AL, Denis DJ. Sphenopalatine ganglion block and radiofrequency ablation: technical notes and efficacy. Ochsner J. 2019;19(1):32–7.
78. Loh E, Reid JN, Alibrahim F, Welk B. Retrospective cohort study of healthcare utilization and opioid use following radiofrequency ablation for chronic axial spine pain in Ontario, Canada. Reg Anesth Pain Med. 2019;44:398–405.

Chapter 29
Dorsal Root Ganglion and Peripheral Nerve Stimulation in the Treatment of Low Back and Leg Pain

Neel D. Mehta and Rohit Aiyer

Introduction

Spinal cord stimulation (SCS) has been commonly used in the treatment of low back pain for many years in patients suffering from post-laminectomy syndrome (see Chap. 30). These devices utilize placement of electrode leads in the epidural space of the spinal cord to stimulate near the dorsal column. Historically, while leg pain could be adequately treated using this therapy, low back pain relief had mixed results. Newer and emerging technologies have improved treatment effect and durability and have been utilized in patients previously not operated on as a surgical alternative in elderly patients. These treatments can be less invasive and often completed under sedation anesthesia with minimal blood loss.

Recently, two therapies have been utilized in the treatment of spine pain utilizing neuromodulation techniques with differing targets and purpose. While the overall treatment leads to improved quality of life and functional improvement, one therapy (DRGS) reduces pain, while the other is focused on restorative treatment of chronic mechanical low back pain (CMLBP). These two concepts will be discussed in detail in the below sections.

Over the past several years, there has been an abundance of research on the causes for chronic low back pain. There are several potential causes for chronic low back pain, which include mechanical stress; damage to joints, ligaments, muscles, and fascia; compression of nerve roots in the spinal canal; and neuropathic pain [1].

N. D. Mehta (✉)
Pain Management, Weill Cornell Medicine, NewYork-Presbyterian Hospital, New York, NY, USA
e-mail: nem9015@med.cornell.edu

R. Aiyer
Pain Medicine, Henry Ford Health System, Detroit, MI, USA

K.-M. G. Fu et al. (eds.), *Treatment of Spine Disease in the Elderly*,
https://doi.org/10.1007/978-3-031-12612-3_29

It should be noted that pain that is worsened on certain movements is generally nociceptive in character and therefore is known as mechanical low back pain. One area that has been extensively investigated is the lumbar multifidus (LM) muscle group. The muscle is divided into three layers: superficial, intermediate, and deep fibers [2]. The intermediate and superficial fibers span three to five vertebral levels and function phasically, while the deep fibers span over two vertebral levels and function tonically [2]. The LM is the most medial and largest muscle in the back, as it is spread over the lumbosacral junction. There has been good evidence to show that this muscle group is inhibited in patients with acute low back pain [3]. Other research has also shown that a change in neuromuscular recruitment of the LM can contribute to injury and instability of the lumbar spine and may be worse in elderly patients [1]. There is literature that suggests a patient's inability to properly recruit the affected LM can lead to accelerated muscle fatigue, maladaptive recruitment patterns, and muscle atrophy and is known as motor control impairment [4]. As a result, spine stability and loading is negatively impacted, and furthermore, this leads to a cyclical process of chronic low back pain as patients also have an increased risk of reinjury while having this pain, often leading to chronic disability in the elderly [1].

Neurophysiology of Low Back Pain

Neurophysiological research suggests that cerebral processing of the motor control system is altered which can lead to a loss of discrete cortical organization of inputs to the lumbar paraspinal muscles. There is also a phenomenon known as reflex inhibition, which has been studied and demonstrates that during injury to spine structures, there can be a reduction in electrical activity (which is confirmed with electromyography studies) [4]. As a result, to allow for a person to recover from their chronic low back pain, motor control impairment has to be suppressed [1].

Dorsal Root Ganglion Stimulation

The treatment of chronic pain using DRGS has primarily focused on conditions involving severe neuropathic pain including complex regional pain syndrome [5, 6]. However, emerging evidence has focused this therapy in the treatment of spine pain, especially difficult to treat low back pain [7, 8]. The dorsal root ganglion (DRG) focuses on the primary sensory neurons transmitting afferent nociception, and could better treat beyond strictly neuropathic pain, including nociceptive or mixed nociceptive/neuropathic pain conditions involved in chronic low back pain (CLBP) [9].

Dorsal root ganglion stimulation involves similar technology as SCS, including electrodes and a pulse generator. However, leads are often smaller, with shorter spacing between electrodes, and more flexibility in steering toward the DRG. Techniques can involve placement from outside of the foramen entering inward, or from medial to lateral via the interlaminar space. Leads are secured either through redundant loops or anchoring to fascia.

Target DRG can be identified based on the dermatome pattern (S1 typically for lower radicular pain); however, back pain targets have been debated between T12 and L2. Dermatome maps show the low back area innervation by L1–L5 dermatome levels [10]. A case series of 17 consecutive patients with primary targets at T12 with CLBP and additional leads at either L1 or S1 as needed were trialed and subsequently implanted for DRG-S. Subthreshold stimulation was utilized with no perceived paresthesias. Last follow-up times averaged 8.3 months. More than half of the patients experienced pain relief ≥80%, with an average low back pain relief of 78%, with improvements in physical and mental functioning, disability, and quality of life [11]. A 12-patient case series of targets for low back pain at L2 or L3 was less effective with 46% patients reporting 50% pain relief [8]. Focal discogenic back pain following micro discectomy surgery treated with DRG-S was studied in a 13-patient case series showing 85% of patients showing 50% relief of pain when targeting L2 [12]. The same authors studied low back pain treatment using DRG-S in non-operated discogenic back pain patients by once again targeting L2 in a case series of 20 patients, in which 63% experienced significant back pain relief [13].

Of the case series listed above, T12 appears to be the most likely target for success in low back pain relief using DRG-S. The authors of the T12 case series further hypothesized a mechanism of action. Branches of individual spinal nerve roots innervate facet joints and other posterior spinal structures, yet painful discs and anterior vertebral bodies travel via L2 and converge at the T8–9 spinal cord dorsal horn. The T12 nerve root contains cutaneous afferents from the low back and enters the DH of the spinal cord at T10. Low back Aδ and C-fibers travel via Lissauer's tract (LT) to T8-T9, converging with other low back afferents. DRG-S at T12, then, results in inhibition of the converged low back fibers via endorphin-mediated and GABAergic frequency-dependent mechanisms. Therefore, T12 lead placement may be the optimal location for DRG-S to treat LBP [14].

Peripheral Nerve Stimulation

A new method that has been recently analyzed is the utilization of an implant device to stimulate the medial branch of the dorsal ramus nerve which overrides the reflex inhibition [1]. Anatomically, it is thought that the clinically most effective target for stimulation in chronic low back pain is the deep fibers in the LM [1]. As a result, peripheral nerve stimulation (PNS) has evolved over the past few years, a method to treat chronic low back pain. This intervention is beneficial as it is minimally invasive and stimulates nerve fibers to modulate central sensitization [15]. The PNS system activates signals in the medial branch nerves which innervate the multifidus muscles. The PNS leads can be inserted to target the medial branches as it travels over the lamina, medial, and inferior part of the facet joint, which then activates the medial branch nerves [15]. Anatomic landmarks for this procedure include the spinous process and lamina, and imaging is either ultrasound or fluoroscopy [15]. It is thought that stimulating afferent sensory fibers initiate the gate mechanism, which in return decreases pain signals. Concurrently, efferent nerve fibers activate the multifidus muscles which indirectly produces physiological and proprioceptive afferent signals [10]. Consequently, this neuromodulation technique is unique in that it stimulates both motor and sensory fibers [15]. The additive effect of stimulating both fibers is thought to modulate synaptic transmission via gate control and therefore helps return membrane excitability of neurons and circuits in nociceptive pathways in the central nervous system to baseline [15].

As of present, there are several case series and case reports, as well as few randomized controlled trials that have evaluated the use of PNS for chronic pain, and not limited to just low back pain. One large international multicenter prospective clinical trial that studied 54 patients with an implanted neurostimulator for low back pain showed good results, with over 61% relief at 6 months and 57% relief at 1 year [16]. The clinicians and researchers utilized an implanted pulse generator (IPG) and two leads, which contained four electrodes and was placed near the medial branch of the L2 dorsal ramus nerve as it crosses the L3 transverse process. More specifically, the distal end of each lead was fixated in the intertransversarii muscles that are located between the transverse processes, and therefore away from the dorsal root ganglion and neural foramen [17].

Another study investigated the use of peripheral nerve stimulation as alternative to patients with chronic low back pain that failed radiofrequency ablation [16]. As opposed to having another ablation, these patients underwent implantation of PNS percutaneous leads that targeted the medial branch nerves within the multifidus muscles. The stimulation therapy then activated the multifidus muscles for 6–12 h daily for 60 days. After 2 months, the leads were withdrawn. The results showed that among the 15 patients, 10 had over 50% reduction in average pain intensity and 13 showed improvement in disability, while 12 patients had improvement in pain interference [16].

As with any procedure in neuromodulation, clinicians should be aware of potential risks, with the common ones being lead fracture, migration, and infection. These adverse events can be mitigated, such as treating an infection with antibiotics or having a lead replaced if the patient experiences lead migration.

Conclusion

PNS and neuromodulation of the multifidus muscle for chronic low back pain appears to be a promising new treatment that is relatively low risk for elderly patients, especially as a potential less invasive surgical option. While the intervention is relatively new for alleviation of chronic low back pain, further research over the next few years should help further establish the effectiveness of this treatment. Similarly, DRG-S targeting of the T12 or L2 DRG is promising for low back pain treatment and further studies are underway.

References

1. Deckers K, De Smedt K, Van Buyten JP, et al. Chronic low back pain: restoration of dynamic stability. Neuromodulation. 2015;18:476–86.
2. Macdonald DA, Hodges PW, Moseley GL. The lumbar multifidus: does the evidence support clinical beliefs? Man Ther. 2006;11:254–6.
3. Rosatelli AL, Ravichandiran K, Agur AM. Three-dimensional study of that musculotendinous architecture of lumbar multifidus and its functional implications. Clin Anat. 2008;21:539–46.
4. O'Sullivan PB. Diagnosis and classification of chronic low back pain disorders: maladaptive movement and motor control impairments as underlying mechanism. Man Ther. 2005;10:242–55.
5. Deer TR, Grigsby E, Weiner RL, Wilcosky B, Kramer JM. A prospective study of dorsal root ganglion stimulation for the relief of chronic pain. Neuromodulation. 2013;16:67–72.
6. Liem L, Russo M, Huygen FJPM, et al. A multicenter, prospective trial to assess the safety and performance of the spinal modulation dorsal root ganglia neurostimulator system in the treatment of chronic pain. Neuromodulation. 2013;16:471–82.
7. Weiner RL, Yeung A, Montes Garcia C, Tyler Perryman L, Speck B. Treatment of FBSS low back pain with a novel percutaneous DRG wireless stimulator: pilot and feasibility study. Pain Med. 2016;17:1911–6.
8. Huygen F, Liem L, Cusack W, Kramer J. Stimulation of the L2-L3 dorsal root ganglia induces effective pain relief in the low back. Pain Pract. 2018;18:205–2013.
9. Kent AR, Min X, Hogan QH, Kramer JM. Mechanisms of dorsal root ganglion stimulation in pain suppression: a computational modeling analysis. Neuromodulation. 2018;21:234–46.
10. Keegan JJ, Garrett FD. The segmental distribution of the cutaneous nerves in the limbs of man. Anat Rec. 1948;102:409–37.
11. Chapman KB, Groenen PS, Patel KV, Vissers KC, van Helmond N. T12 dorsal root ganglion stimulation to treat chronic low back pain: a case series. Neuromodulation. 2020;23:203–12.
12. Kallewaard JW, Nijhuis H, Huygen F, et al. Prospective cohort analysis of DRG stimulation for failed back surgery syndrome pain following lumbar discectomy. Pain Pract. 2019;19:204–10.
13. Kallewaard JW, Edelbroek C, Terheggen M, Raza A, Geurts JW. A prospective study of dorsal root ganglion stimulation for non-operated discogenic low back pain. Neuromodulation. 2020;23:196–202.
14. Chapman KB, Groenen PS, Vissers KC, van Helmond N, Stanton-Hicks MD. The pathways and processes underlying spinal transmission of low back pain: observations from dorsal root ganglion stimulation treatment. Neuromodulation. 2021;24(4):610–21. https://doi.org/10.1111/ner.13150.
15. Deer TR, Gilmore CA, Desai MJ, et al. Percutaneous peripheral nerve stimulation of the medial branch nerves for the treatment of chronic axial back pain in patients after radiofrequency ablation. Pain Med. 2021;22(3):548–60.
16. Gilmore CA, Patel J, Esebua LG, Burchell M. A review of peripheral nerve stimulation techniques targeting the medial branches of the lumbar dorsal rami in the treatment of chronic low back pain. Pain Med. 2020;21(1):S41–6.
17. Deckers K, De Smedt K, Mitchell B, et al. New therapy for refractory chronic mechanical low back pain—restorative neurostimulation to activate the lumbar multifidus: one year results of a prospective multicenter clinical trial. Neuromodulation. 2018;21(1):48–55.

Chapter 30
SI Joint in the Elderly

Kenneth J. Holton and David W. Polly Jr

The sacroiliac (SI) joint is the largest joint by surface area in the body. It transfers significant loads from axial spine to the lower extremities. In the situation of positive sagittal imbalance or flatback syndrome, the forces are increased as the erector spinae muscles are constantly firing generating increased cantilever loads to maintain erect posture. In men typically S1–S3 have articulations between the sacrum and the ilium (Fig. 30.1a), but in women it is often only S1–S2 (Fig. 30.1b). The surface has various undulations or grooves and is not simply a smooth surface.

The SI joint is stabilized by a combination of form and force closure [1]. The form closure is the keystone shape of the sacrum within the pelvis. The force closure is the surrounding musculature and fascia exerting a compressive force across the joint. Ligamentous contributions to stability include the anterior joint capsule and the posterior interosseous ligament. These are supplemented by the sacrotuberous and sacrospinous ligaments, all of which help to stabilize the entire pelvis. With aging or degeneration, there is probably an alteration in the function of the ligaments [2].

The SI joint has a small range of motion. It has been studied using radiostereometric analysis, external fixator differential movement, and electrogoniometer and by CT scans [3–6]. It is 1.1° to 2.2° in flexion extension (nutation/counternutation), 0.5° to 8.0° in lateral bending, and 0.8° to 4.0° in axial rotation. This is in normal individuals. Mikula has reported changes in pelvic incidence of 7.1° supine versus upright in patients with bilateral vacuum signs on CT scans [7]. This may be a good indication of instability.

The SI joint is innervated by ventral and dorsal structures. Ventral innervation comes from direct branches off of the lumbosacral trunk to the anterior capsule and

K. J. Holton (✉) · D. W. Polly Jr
Department of Orthopaedic Surgery, University of Minnesota, Minneapolis, MN, USA
e-mail: pollydw@umn.edu

K.-M. G. Fu et al. (eds.), *Treatment of Spine Disease in the Elderly*,
https://doi.org/10.1007/978-3-031-12612-3_30

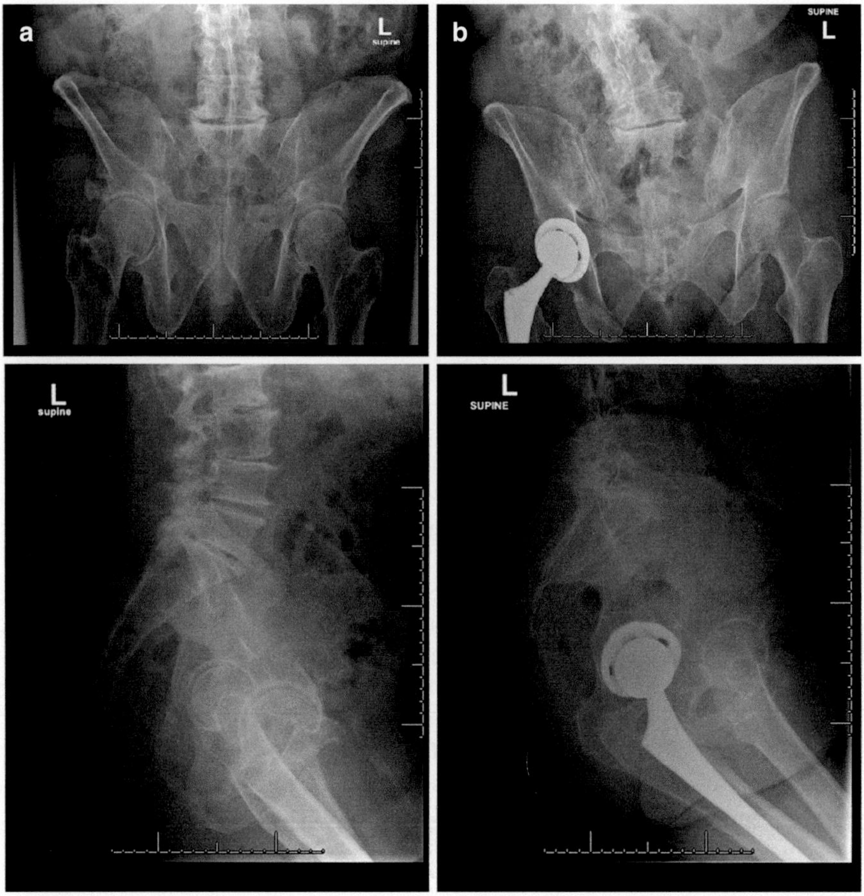

Fig. 30.1 (**a**) Ferguson or inlet view of 76-year-old male. This demonstrates S1–S3 articulation with the ilium. Incidentally seen is avulsion of the anterior inferior iliac spine on the right (Corresponding lateral view). (**b**) Ferguson view of 81-year-old female. Clear articulation of S1–2 with ilium but only partial S3 articulation (Corresponding lateral image)

to the articular cartilage [8]. Dorsal rami from S1 to S4 (and possibly L5) provide dorsal innervation. The joint has mechanoreceptors and nocioceptors [9–11].

Radiographic degeneration is prevalent with aging and not necessarily associated with pain [12]. Pain can be present radiographically in normal joints and no imaging study modality is definitive for painful versus non-painful SI joints. Computed tomography (CT) imaging is challenging (Fig. 30.2). It has been reported to have a sensitivity of 57.5% and specificity of 69% in patients with SI joint-mediated pain. The value of radionuclide imaging is debated [13, 14]. Perhaps vacuum sign may be prognostic. Recently, it has been shown to be associated with change in PI supine vs upright perhaps representing instability [7]. There is profound regional bone mineral density variation within the sacrum [15] (Fig. 30.3).

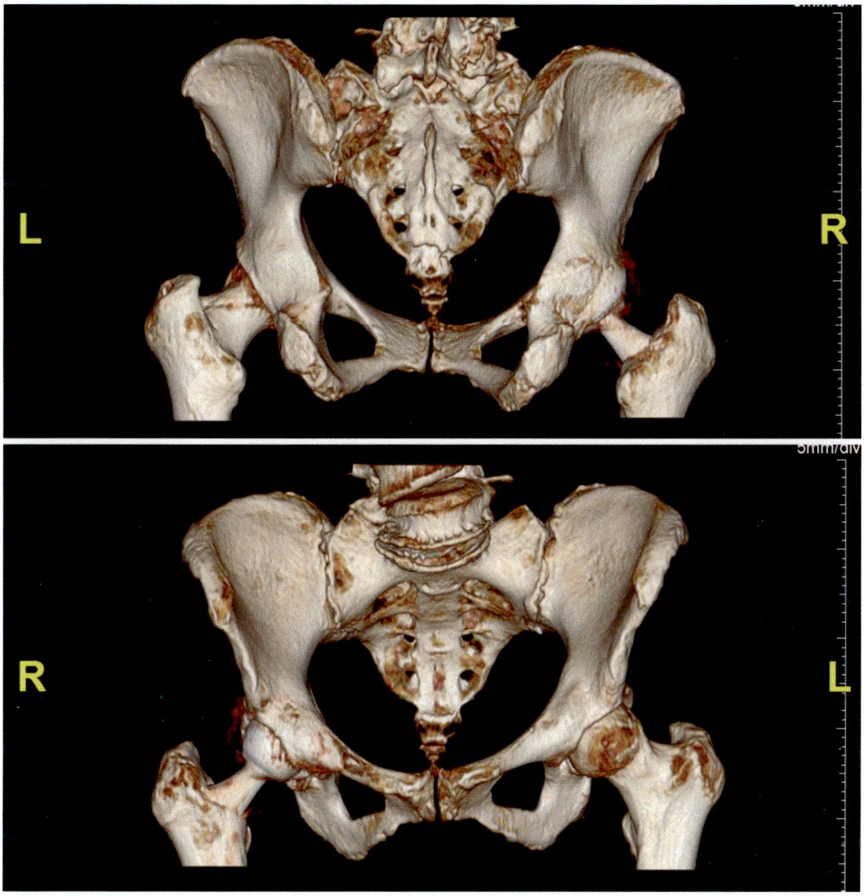

Fig. 30.2 3D CT images from 81-year-old female patient

Confirmatory SI joint image-guided injection is the current reference standard [16]. The injection needs to be done under image guidance to confirm location within the joint (Fig. 30.4). Typically, a confirmatory arthrogram is done. If there is significant extravasation of the contrast outside of the joint, then it is unclear where the local anesthetic is going and should not be considered an adequate study. If there is any doubt or there is technical difficulty in accessing the joint, using CT guidance for the injection can be quite helpful. There is some debate about what amount of pain relief constitutes a positive response. This was studied in patients participating in two randomized controlled trials and used patient-reported outcomes as the reference standard and then looked at level of block response (50–75% vs 75–100%) [17]. No difference was seen between these groups suggesting that a 50% response is the appropriate threshold.

Physical exam can reliably diagnose the SI joint as the pain generator [18]. It begins with asking the patient to point to the one spot that hurts the most. This is the

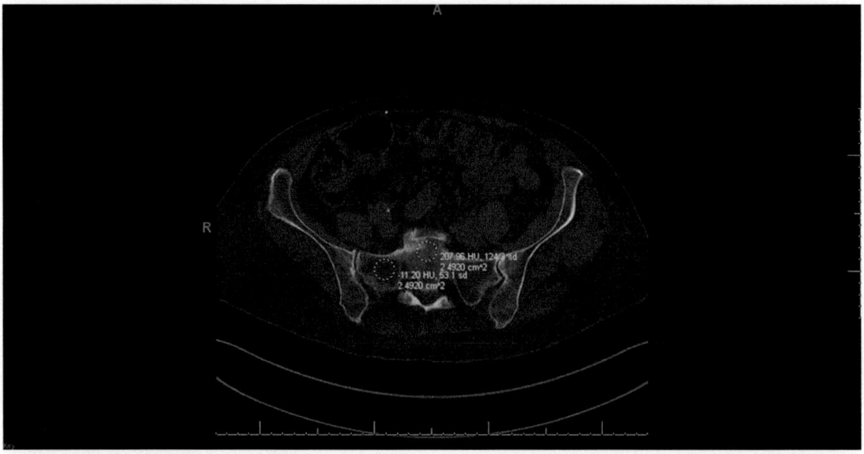

Fig. 30.3 Opportunistic bone mineral density comparing the sacral ala (−11.20 Hounsfield units) to the S1 body (207.96 Hounsfield units)

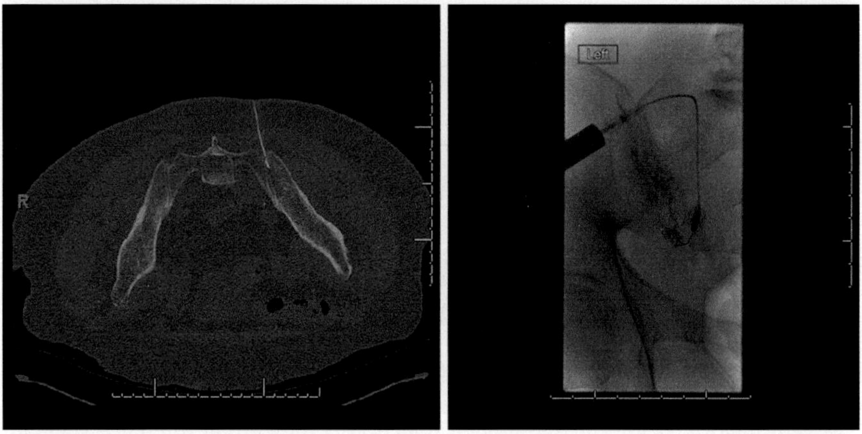

Fig. 30.4 (Left) CT-guided diagnostic injection. (Right) Fluoroscopically guided SI injection with arthrogram outlining the joint

so-called Fortin finger sign when they point directly to the posterior superior iliac spine. No single physical exam maneuver is sensitive and specific, but if five tests are used as a multitest survey, the reliability and specificity are high (85% positive predictive value of a positive response to injection). These tests include thigh thrust, flexion abduction external rotation (FABER), pelvic gapping, pelvic compression, and Gaenslen's test (Fig. 30.5). Some studies have also added sacral thrust as a sixth test. In Europe, the active straight leg raise test is frequently used. Care must be exercised to rule out hip and spine pathology. The hip scour test examines for pain with hip range of motion (differentiating the posterior hip capsule vs the posterior

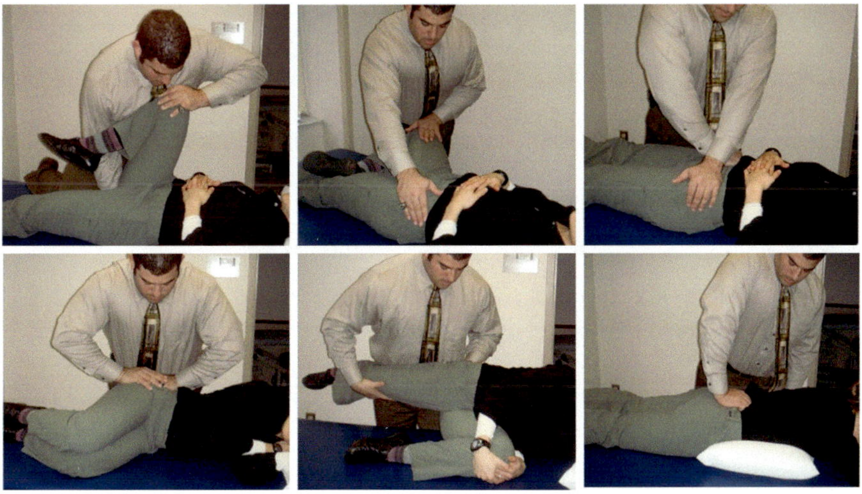

Fig. 30.5 Physical exam maneuvers including thigh thrust, FABER, pelvic gapping, pelvic compression, Gaenslen's maneuver, and sacral thrust

superior iliac spine). Similarly, exam of the spine is specifically looking at facet loading, radiculopathy (which can be present from SI joint pathology as well) [19], and spine range of motion. Specifically looking for quadratus lumborum tenderness/spasm is a common finding in these patients due to altered gait pattern. Appropriate spine and hip imaging is necessary depending on the physical exam findings.

The differential diagnosis of buttock pain is complex. In addition to SI joint pain, other common entities include piriformis syndrome, femoroacetabular impingement, labral tears within the hip, ischial tuberosity bursitis, hip osteoarthritis, referred spine pain, and sacralgia.

In patients with primary SI pain, fusion has been shown to have a high rate of success. There have been two randomized controlled trials compared to nonoperative treatment, and one prospective cohort study looking at fusion with triangular titanium rods and 2-year results [20–22]. These studies were aggregated into a pooled analysis [23] (Fig. 30.6). Approximately 85% of patients saw a 50% reduction in visual analog pain scales and in Oswestry Disability Index scores. Both of these were clinically significant differences being greater than the minimally clinically important differences. These results have been durable through 5 years [24].

Patients with spine fusions increase load across the SI joint. Ivanov, using a finite element model, showed that fusing the L5–S1 increases the stress on the SI joint by 52% and fusing L4–S1 increases it by 168% [25]. Conversely, fusing the SI joint increases the stress on the spine by 2–4% [26] and on the hip by 5% [27]. Ha [28] showed that in patients undergoing floating fusions, the CT-based radiographic degeneration rate was 38%, whereas fusion to the sacrum resulted in a 75% rate of degeneration.

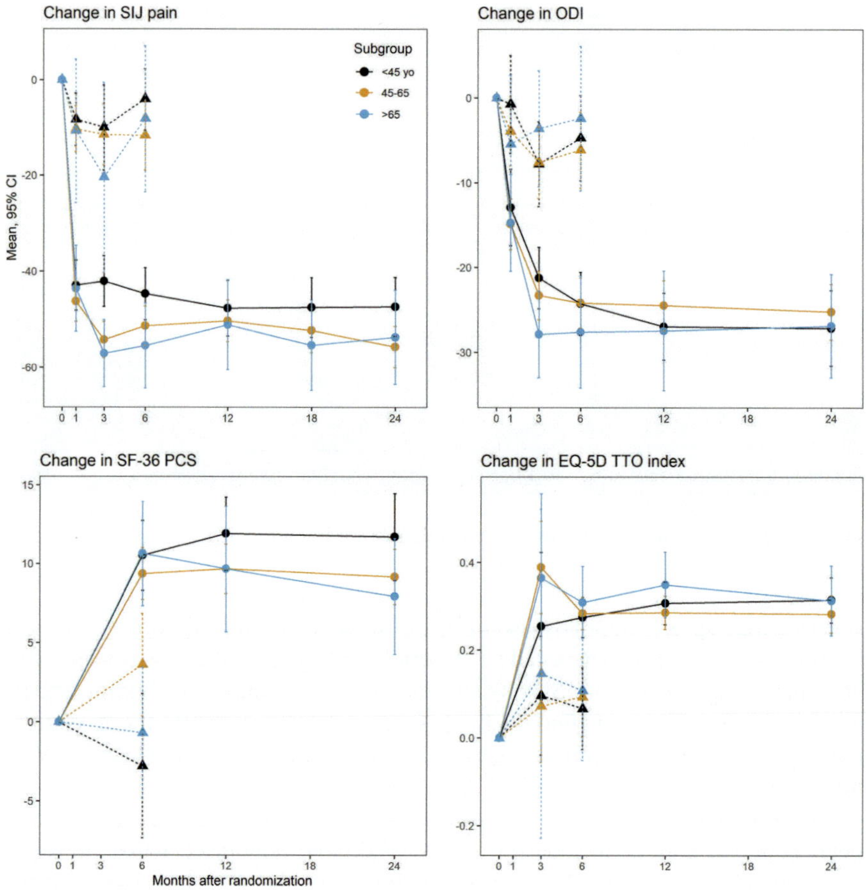

Fig. 30.6 Results of data pooled from two randomized controlled trials, INSITE and iMIA, and one prospective cohort study, SIFI, of minimally invasive SI joint fusion using triangular titanium rods. Data is broken down by age of <45, 45–65, and >65 [23]

Long fusions to the sacrum have a historically high rate of pseudarthrosis. Lee showed that four level fusions or greater had a 30% or greater rate of pseudarthrosis [29]. This high rate of pseudarthrosis has led to the search for strategies to improve spinopelvic fixation (Fig. 30.7). This began with the Galveston technique of bending rods so that they could be directly inserted into the sacrum [30]. This then morphed into the initial use of iliac bolts, followed by iliac screws. McChord [31] showed that iliac fixation was significantly superior to other forms of sacral fixation and established the concept of the pivot point located at the posterior portion of the L5–S1 disc. Fixation extending anterior to the pivot point is far more robust and experiences cantilever loading rather than just in line pullout.

Iliac fixation spans an unfused SI joint. As such, there is still motion present. This motion leads to halo formation around iliac fixation. In addition, there is

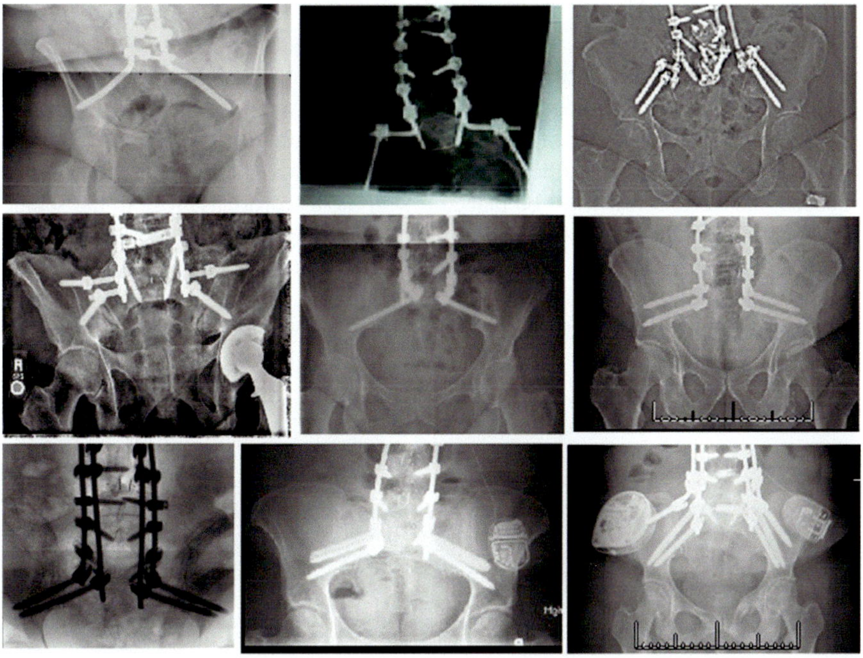

Fig. 30.7 Evolution of pelvic fixation (top—left to right), classic Galveston, iliac screws, stacked iliac and screws; (middle—left to right), divergent stacked iliac screws, S2AI screws, and stacked S2AI screws; (bottom—left to right), stacked S2AI screws with quad rods, S2AI screws with triangular titanium rods, and stacked S2AI and iliac screws

typically prominence of iliac fixation. There can be a high revision and/or failure rate of iliac fixation. These rates can be as high as 30–35% (personal experience Polly unpublished data and podium#23 presented at the Scoliosis Research Society 2020 annual meeting by Eastlack et al.).

The next development in pelvic fixation by Sponseller and Kebaish has been the use of the S2 alar iliac (S2AI) screw [32]. This screw requires less lateral dissection and crosses the sacrum, through the SI joint, and into the ilium. The biomechanics are at least as good as conventional iliac screws [33]. Systematic review has shown a lower revision and failure rate of S2AI screws compared to conventional iliac screws [34]. But S2AI screws have problems as well. A recent study demonstrated a failure rate due to set plug extrusion, screw breakage below the tulip head, and fracture where the screw crosses the SI joint [35]. These are all locations where finite element modeling has demonstrated increased stress.

Unoki showed longer fusions' higher rate of new onset SI pain with 1 level being 6%, 2 levels 10%, 3 levels 20%, and >4 levels 23% [36]. Finger showed 32% of persisting or new SI pain in 32% [37]. This has led to strategies such as stacked ipsilateral iliac or S2AI screws with the hope of eliminating this pain. There is no compelling data yet on the effectiveness of such a strategy.

Given this rate of pelvic fixation and loosening, there is increased interest in concomitant SI joint fusion. Biomechanically, this has been shown in a finite element model to decrease strain on the S1 screws and the rods at the lumbosacral junction [38]. Similar findings on a cadaveric model were also found (Fig. 30.8). Our group at the University of Minnesota has been doing this technique for more than a year. We utilize intraoperative navigation to place the implants. In order to succeed, the S2AI screw must be placed low in the teardrop, as close to the sciatic notch as possible. This allows for placement of a triangular titanium rod above the S2AI screw and just below the iliopectineal line. As the triangular titanium rod crosses the SI joint, there is a tendency for it to want to skive anteriorly, and this must be carefully controlled. Our group had 3/38 of our initial triangular titanium

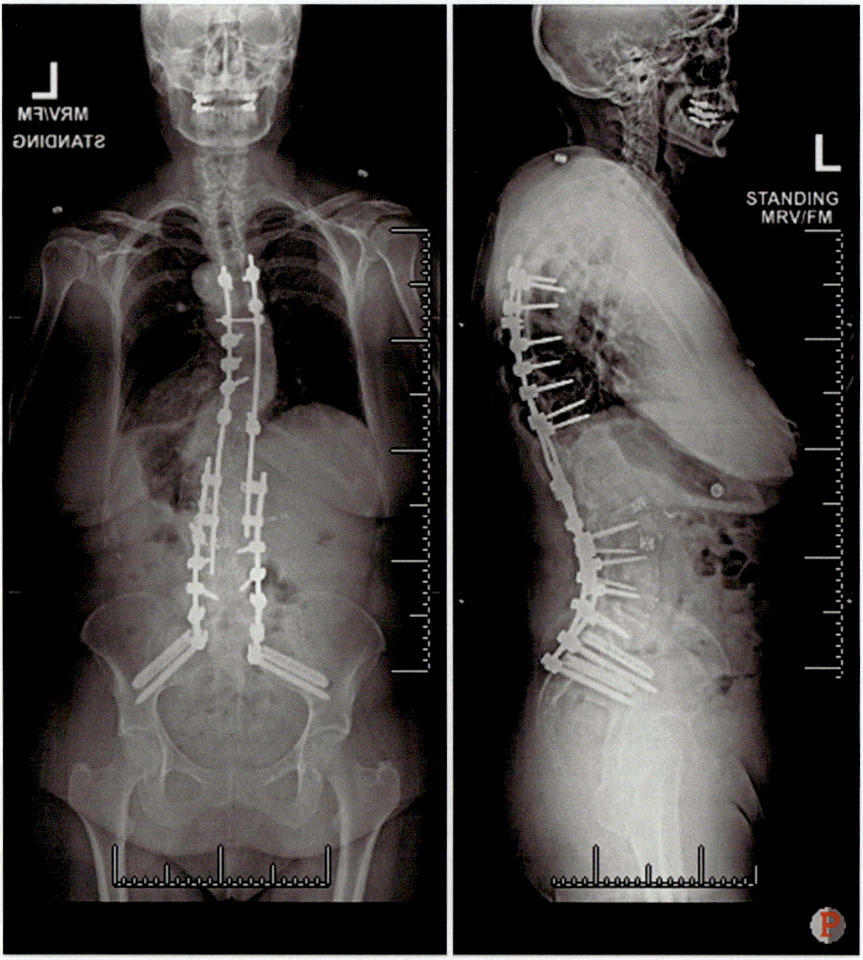

Fig. 30.8 Post revision imaging showing revision instrumentation and pelvic fixation with S2alar iliac screws and triangular titanium rods for concomitant SI joint fusion

rods malpositioned. This was determined intraoperatively and all were able to be successfully repositioned. We have not had that issue recur in subsequent cases. Clinical results are not yet available to demonstrate whether or not this technique lessens screw loosening or the rate of SI joint pain. A randomized, multicenter clinical trial is currently underway.

In summary, the SI joint can be a source of pain. This can be determined by physical exam and confirmed with a diagnostic injection. SI joint fusion has clinical data demonstrating meaningful clinical benefit. Spinal fusion places significantly more stress on the joint. Pelvic fixation has a significant rate of loosening and a need for revision. Strategies to lessen this rate include stacked screws or screws and concomitant SI joint fusion. There is biomechanical data to support this strategy. Clinical efficacy remains to be determined.

References

1. Vleeming A. The sacroiliac joint: a clinical anatomical biomechanical and radiological study. Thesis. Rotterdam: Erasmus University Rotterdam; 1990.
2. Hammer N, Ondruschka B, Fuchs V. Sacroiliac joint ligaments and sacroiliac pain: a case-control study on micro- and ultrastructural findings on morphologic alterations. Pain Physician. 2019;22(6):E615–25.
3. Sturesson B, Udén A, Onsten I. Can an external frame fixation reduce the movements in the sacroiliac joint? A radiostereometric analysis of 10 patients. Acta Orthop Scand. 1999;70:42–6.
4. Jacob H, Kissling R. The mobility of the sacroiliac joints in healthy volunteers between 20 and 50 years of age. Clin Biomech. 1995;10:352–61.
5. Wilke HJ, Fischer K, Jeanneret B, Claes L, Magerl F. In vivo measurement of 3-dimensional movement of the iliosacral joint. Z Orthop Ihre Grenzgeb. 1997;135:550–6.
6. Smidt GL, Wei SH, McQuade K, Barakatt E, Sun T, Stanford W. Sacroiliac motion for extreme hip positions: a fresh cadaver study. Spine. 1997;22:2073–82.
7. Mikula AL, Fogelson JL, Oushy S, Pinter ZW, Peters PA, Abode-Iyamah K, Sebastian AS, Freedman B, Currier BL, Polly DW, Elder BD. Change in pelvic incidence between the supine and standing positions in patients with bilateral sacroiliac joint vacuum signs. J Neurosurg Spine. 2021;34(4):617–22. https://doi.org/10.3171/2020.8.SPINE20742. PMID: 33450735.
8. Szadek KM. Sacroiliac joint pain: anatomy, diagnosis and treatment. PhD thesis. 2016.
9. Vilensky JA, O'Connor BL, Fortin JD, et al. Histologic analysis of neural elements in the human sacroiliac joint. Spine (Phila Pa 1976). 2002;27(11):1202–7.
10. Szadek KM, Hoogland PV, Zuurmond WW, de Lange JJ, Perez RS. Nociceptive nerve fibers in the sacroiliac joint in humans. Reg Anesth Pain Med. 2008;33(1):36–43.
11. Szadek KM, Hoogland PV, Zuurmond WW, De Lange JJ, Perez RS. Possible nociceptive structures in the sacroiliac joint cartilage: an immunohistochemical study. Clin Anat. 2010;23(2):192–8. https://doi.org/10.1002/ca.20908.
12. Cohen AS, et al. The "normal" sacroiliac joint analysis of 88 sacroiliac roentgenograms. Am J Roentgenol Radium Ther. 1967;100(3):559–63.
13. Maigne JY, Boulahdour H, Chatellier G. Value of quantitative radionuclide bone scanning in the diagnosis of sacroiliac joint syndrome in 32 patients with low back pain. Eur Spine J. 1998;7(4):328–31.
14. Puhakka K, Jurik A, Schiøttz-Christensen B, et al. MRI abnormalities of sacroiliac joints in early spondyloarthropathy: a 1-year follow-up study. Scand J Rheumatol. 2004;33(5):332–8.

15. Hoel RJ, Ledonio CG, Takahashi T, Polly DW Jr. Sacral bone mineral density (BMD) assessment using opportunistic CT scans. J Orthop Res. 2017;35(1):160–6. https://doi.org/10.1002/jor.23362. Epub 2016 Aug 26.
16. Jung MW, Schellhas K, Johnson B. Use of diagnostic injections to evaluate sacroiliac joint pain. Int J Spine Surg. 2020;14(Suppl 1):30–4. https://doi.org/10.14444/6081. PMID: 32123655; PMCID: PMC7041665.
17. Polly D, Cher D, Whang PG, Frank C, Sembrano J, INSITE Study Group. Does level of response to SI joint block predict response to SI joint fusion? Int J Spine Surg. 2016;10:4. https://doi.org/10.14444/3004. PMID: 26913224; PMCID: PMC4752015.
18. Petersen T, Laslett M, Juhl C. Clinical classification in low back pain: best-evidence diagnostic rules based on systematic reviews. BMC Musculoskelet Disord. 2017;18(1):188. https://doi.org/10.1186/s12891-017-1549-6. PMID: 28499364; PMCID: PMC5429540.
19. Dengler J, Sturesson B, Kools D, Prestamburgo D, Cher D, van Eeckhoven E, Erk E, Pflugmacher R, Vajkoczy P, the iMIA study group. Referred leg pain originating from the sacroiliac joint: 6-month outcomes from the prospective randomized controlled iMIA trial. Acta Neurochir. 2016;158(11):2219–24. https://doi.org/10.1007/s00701-016-2953-7. Epub 2016 Sep 15
20. Polly DW, Swofford J, Whang PG, Frank CJ, Glaser JA, Limoni RP, Cher DJ, Wine KD, Sembrano JN, INSITE study group. Two-year outcomes from a randomized controlled trial of minimally invasive sacroiliac joint fusion vs. non-surgical management for sacroiliac joint dysfunction. Int J Spine Surg. 2016;10:28.
21. Dengler J, Kools D, Pflugmacher R, Gasbarrini A, Prestamburgo D, Gaetani P, Cher D, Van Eeckhoven E, Annertz M, Sturesson B. Randomized trial of sacroiliac joint arthrodesis compared with conservative management for chronic low back pain attributed to the sacroiliac joint. J Bone Joint Surg Am. 2019;101(5):400–11. https://doi.org/10.2106/JBJS.18.00022. PMID: 30845034; PMCID: PMC6467578.
22. Duhon BS, Bitan F, Lockstadt H, Kovalsky D, Cher D, Hillen T, SIFI Study Group. Triangular titanium implants for minimally invasive sacroiliac joint fusion: 2-year follow-up from a prospective multicenter trial. Int J Spine Surg. 2016;10:13. https://doi.org/10.14444/3013. PMID: 27162715; PMCID: PMC4852595.
23. Dengler J, Duhon B, Whang P, Frank C, Glaser J, Sturesson B, Garfin S, Cher D, Rendahl A, Polly D, INSITE, iMIA, SIFI Study Groups. Predictors of outcome in conservative and minimally invasive surgical management of pain originating from the sacroiliac joint: a pooled analysis. Spine (Phila Pa 1976). 2017;42(21):1664–73. https://doi.org/10.1097/BRS.0000000000002169.
24. Whang PG, Darr E, Meyer SC, Kovalsky D, Frank C, Lockstadt H, Limoni R, Redmond AJ, Ploska P, Oh M, Chowdhary A, Cher D, Hillen T. Long-term prospective clinical and radiographic outcomes after minimally invasive lateral transiliac sacroiliac joint fusion using triangular titanium implants. Med Devices (Auckl). 2019;12:411–22. https://doi.org/10.2147/MDER.S219862. PMID: 31576181; PMCID: PMC6769032.
25. Ivanov AA, Kiapour A, Ebraheim NA, Goel V. Lumbar fusion leads to increases in angular motion and stress across sacroiliac joint: a finite element study. Spine (Phila Pa 1976). 2009;34(5):E162–9. https://doi.org/10.1097/BRS.0b013e3181978ea3.
26. Lindsey DP, Kiapour A, Yerby SA, Goel VK. Sacroiliac joint fusion minimally affects adjacent lumbar segment motion: a finite element study. Int J Spine Surg. 2015;9:64. https://doi.org/10.14444/2064. PMID: 26767156; PMCID: PMC4710165.
27. Joukar A, Chande RD, Carpenter RD, Lindsey DP, Erbulut DU, Yerby SA, Duhon B, Goel VK. Effects on hip stress following sacroiliac joint fixation: a finite element study. JOR Spine. 2019;2(4):e1067. https://doi.org/10.1002/jsp2.1067.
28. Ha KY, Lee JS, Kim KW. Degeneration of sacroiliac joint after instrumented lumbar or lumbosacral fusion: a prospective cohort study over five-year follow-up. Spine (Phila Pa 1976). 2008;33(11):1192–8. https://doi.org/10.1097/BRS.0b013e318170fd35.

29. Lee CS, Chung SS, Choi SW, Yu JW, Sohn MS. Critical length of fusion requiring additional fixation to prevent nonunion of the lumbosacral junction. Spine (Phila Pa 1976). 2010;35(6):E206–11. https://doi.org/10.1097/BRS.0b013e3181bfa518.
30. Allen BL Jr, Ferguson RL. The Galveston technique of pelvic fixation with L-rod instrumentation of the spine. Spine (Phila Pa 1976). 1984;9(4):388–94. https://doi.org/10.1097/00007632-198405000-00011.
31. McCord DH, Cunningham BW, Shono Y, Myers JJ, McAfee PC. Biomechanical analysis of lumbosacral fixation. Spine (Phila Pa 1976). 1992;17(8 Suppl):S235–43. https://doi.org/10.1097/00007632-199208001-00004.
32. Chang TL, Sponseller PD, Kebaish KM, Fishman EK. Low profile pelvic fixation: anatomic parameters for sacral alar-iliac fixation versus traditional iliac fixation. Spine (Phila Pa 1976). 2009;34(5):436–40. https://doi.org/10.1097/BRS.0b013e318194128c.
33. JR OB, Yu W, Kaufman BE, Bucklen B, Salloum K, Khalil S, Gudipally M. Biomechanical evaluation of S2 alar-iliac screws: effect of length and quad-cortical purchase as compared with iliac fixation. Spine (Phila Pa 1976). 2013;38(20):E1250–5.
34. Keorochana G, Arirachakaran A, Setrkraising K, Kongtharvonskul J. Comparison of complications and revisions after sacral 2 alar iliac screw and iliac screw fixation for sacropelvic fixation in pediatric and adult populations: systematic review and meta-analysis. World Neurosurg. 2019;132:408–420.e1.
35. Hyun SJ, Jung JM, Kim KJ, Jahng TA. Durability and failure types of S2-alar-iliac screws: an analysis of 312 consecutive screws. Oper Neurosurg (Hagerstown). 2020;20(1):91–7. https://doi.org/10.1093/ons/opaa251. Epub ahead of print
36. Unoki E, Abe E, Murai H, Kobayashi T, Abe T. Fusion of multiple segments can increase the incidence of sacroiliac joint pain after lumbar or lumbosacral fusion. Spine (Phila Pa 1976). 2016;41(12):999–1005. https://doi.org/10.1097/BRS.0000000000001409.
37. Finger T, Bayerl S, Bertog M, Czabanka M, Woitzik J, Vajkoczy P. Impact of sacropelvic fixation on the development of postoperative sacroiliac joint pain following multilevel stabilization for degenerative spine disease. Clin Neurol Neurosurg. 2016;150:18–22.
38. Casaroli G, Galbusera F, Chande R, Lindsey D, Mesiwala A, Yerby S, Brayda-Bruno M. Evaluation of iliac screw, S2 alar-iliac screw and laterally placed triangular titanium implants for sacropelvic fixation in combination with posterior lumbar instrumentation: a finite element study. Eur Spine J. 2019;28(7):1724–32. https://doi.org/10.1007/s00586-019-06006-0. Epub 2019 May 15.

Index

K.-M. G. Fu et al. (eds.), *Treatment of Spine Disease in the Elderly*, https://doi.org/10.1007/978-3-031-12612-3

D

T